P. A. T. H.
Wellness Manual

Second Edition

Compiled and Written by:

Eric R. Braverman, M.D., Director

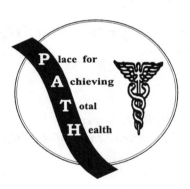

Patient Care Centers
New York, NY
Penndel, PA (metro-Philadelphia)
Naples, FL

For information call (888) 231-PATH
Visit our website at http://www.pathmed.com

Table of Contents

Approbations . . . . *xvi*

The PATH Concept in Health Care . . . . *xvii*

Note to Patients . . . . *xix*

P. A. T. H. Services . . . . *xix*

Materials Available from Path . . . . *xxi*

Directions to PATH Medical Center . . . . *xxii*

Map of Location of the PATH Medical Center . . . . *xxiii*

Acknowledgments . . . . *xxiv*

Introduction to the PATH Wellness Manual . . . . *xxv*

1. Allergic Disorders *1*

How to Discover a Food Allergy or Food Addiction 1
Allergy Tests 1
Allergies and Treatment 2
Allergy: Low Histamine Diet 2
Asthma 3
Dust Precautions for Allergy 5
Methods for Treating Cat Allergy 5
How to Avoid a Mold Allergy 5
Food Allergy: Concomitant and Synergistic Foods 6
Classification of Allergic Reactions and Spectrum of Antihistamines 7

2. Brain Diseases -- Drug Abuse and Others *11*

Alcoholism 11
The Amino Acid Blood Test 11
Brain Fatigue 11
DHEA -- Adrenopause -- Protecting Your Brain 11
Benzodiazepine Addiction 12
Adrenalin and the Brain 12
Brain Mapping: A Short Guide to Interpretation, Philosophy and Future 13
Brain Electrical Activity Mapping (BEAM) 22
BEAM EEG (Electroencephalography) 23
BEAM Topography EEG Spectral Analysis 24
References for BEAM and Nutrition: How the Brain Waves are Corrected 24
An Analysis of Consciousness 25
Imaging the Brain 25

P300 Test 26
Variables That Affect Individual Subject P300 Measurements 26
P300 Diagnosis Based on Voltage and Time 27
Nutrients and Drugs that Can Change P300 27
Behavioral Disorders 28
Addiction: Gambling 28
Chronic Lead Poisoning as a Cause of Bulimia: Hair Test and Brain Electrical Activity Mapping
    as a Diagnostic Aid 29
Chronic Fatigue Syndrome 31
Chocolate Addiction 32
Marijuana and Cocaine 32
The Significance of Having the A1 Allele of the D2 Dopamine Receptor Gene 32
Can Brain Biochemical Imbalance
    be a Causal/Contributory Factor in Homosexuality? 33
Sleep Apnea Syndrome 34
A Cause of National Drug Abuse 34
The Path to Live Again: Nutritional Detoxification from Drugs 34
Classification of Common Tremors 35
Factors Increasing Physiological Tremor 35
Minor and Severe Head Injuries 36
References for BEAM and Head Injury 36
Head Trauma and Heart Trauma 37
Whiplash and Head Trauma 37
Emotional Trauma Damages the Immune System 37
Attention Deficit Disorder (ADD) in Adults 38
Attention Deficit Disorder Resources 39
Temporal Lobe Abnormalities 40
Head Trauma BEAM Bibliography 41

3. *Brain -- General, and Eye Health* **43**

Alpha Waves 43
Alzheimer's Disease and Change in Mental Status 43
Psychiatry and the Doctor-Patient Relationship 46
Biological Psychiatry: Ideal Testing to Uncover Medical Basis in the Brain of Mood Problems 46
Healing Your Abnormal Brain Maps 46
Biological Rhythms 48
Brain Stimulants 48
Eldepryl: An Anti-Aging Compound 48
Feel Good Response (FGR) 49
Brain Waves and States of Consciousness 49
Neurotransmitter-Associated Symptoms and Signs 50
Neurotransmitters: Sources and Major Metabolites 51
Neurotransmitters: Regulating Cofactor and Enzymes 51
Core Laboratory Studies for Clinical Management of Mood Disorders Such as the Schizophrenias 52
Handicapping Effects of Brain Injury and Psychological Disorders Resulting from Traumatic Experiences . . . 53
Neuropsychological Evaluation 54
Neuropsychological Screening 55
Neurological and Psychometric Techniques 55
Advanced Cognitive Remediation System 56
Brain Biofeedback Exercises and Training: How to Heal, Rebuild, and Maximize Brain Potential 57

The Brain Beats on the Path 57
Eye Health 57
Hemorrhage of the Eye 57
Nutrition: Glaucoma And Other Eye Diseases 57

4. Cancer and Oncology -- Hematology **59**

Cancer: Diagnosing Gastrointestinal Malignancies 59
Idiopathic Thrombocytopenic Purpura (ITP) 59
Polycythemia 60
Anti-Cancer Diet & Nutrients 60
Potential Cancer Fighters in Foods 61
Anti-Cancer Polyamine Diet 62
Cancer: New Treatments and Notes on Nutritional Deficiencies 62
Natural Cancer Therapies 63
Tamoxifen and Megace: Hormonal Manipulation for Treatment of Cancer 64
Cancer Treatments -- Shark Cartilage 64
Screening for Testicular Cancer 64
Reversal of Preleukemia with Antioxidants: A Case Report 65
New Era in Cancer Diagnosis and Prevention 66
Prostate Cancer 67
Cancer Information 67
Cancer Referrals: Where to Check the Promises 68
Whole Body PET Scan 68

5. Childhood Disorders **69**

Hyperactivity 69
Attention Deficit Disorder With Hyperactivity Symptoms 69
Children and Childhood Diseases and Nutrition: Notes on Autism, Attention Deficit, and Depression 70

6. Dentistry **71**

Periodontal Disease (Gum Health) and Dental Care 71
Temporal-Mandibular Joint Dysfunction (TMJ) 71

7. Dermatology and Skin Disease **73**

Acne 73
Acne Treatments 73
Risk Factors for Acne 74
Acne Rosacea 74
Atopic Dermatitis 75
Contact Dermatitis 75
Dermatology and Nutrition 75
Dermatology and Diet Update 76
New Studies in Dermatology 76
Retin-A: Instruction Information 76
Moles 77
Hair 77
Eczema 77
Psoriasis 78

8. *Diabetes and Hypoglycemia* **79**

Diabetes 79
Glycemic Index of Foods 80
Glucose Tolerance Test 82
Guar Gum - The Most Valuable Fiber 82
Sugar Content in Certain Manufactured Foods 83
Foods and Insulin Control 83
The Use of Nutrient Supplements for Diabetes 84

9. *Dieting, Weight Loss, and Eating Disorders* **87**

Anorexia 87
Anti-Hyperactivity Diet 87
Obesity 87
The Fast Path to Weight Loss 88
Appetite Suppressants that May Alter Brain Chemistry 88
Avoiding Fungus 88
The Yeast Connection 89
Basic Health and Diet Rules 89
Breaking Your Bad Addictive Habits 90
Other Techniques for Breaking a Bad Dietary Habit 91
Addiction: The Most Critical Dimension of Nutrition and Preventative Medicine ... 91
Carbohydratism and Alcoholism 92
Fiber 93
Fiber for a Healthier You 94
Trimming the Fat 95
Dietary Information for Meats, Fish, and Poultry 96
Dietary Information for Salad Dressings 97
Body Composition Analysis 98
Dietary Fats 99
Nutritional Facts and Fancies 99
Sugar Cravings 100
Mastering Desserts 100
Some New Ideas on Weight Loss 100
Feingold Anti-Hyperactivity Diet 101
Oxy-Cholesterol in Food 101
Oxy-Cholesterol Foods 101
Bone Spurs 102
PATH High Protein (Protein Sparing), Low Carbohydrate, High Fiber Diet ... 102
Sample Menus for General High Protein Diet 104
Additional Menu Ideas 109
Health Spa 110
The Fast PATH to Dieting 111
Depression Diet: The Mood Foods 111
An Explanation of The Low Carbohydrate Diet: With Individualized Portions for Hypertension,
   Obesity, Anxiety, Depression, and Hypoglycemia 112
The Low Carbohydrate and High Blood Pressure Diet 112
Program for Hypertension 114
Hypertension Diet 114
Herpes Diet 115

Low Tyramine Diet (Low Headache Diet) 115
Low Monamine Diet 116
Foods with Monamine Oxidase Inhibitors to be Avoided 116
The Princeton Plan Diet 117
Moderate Protein, Moderate Complex Carbohydrate, High Fiber Diet 118
The Benefits of Fasting 120
Therapeutic Fasting 120
Food Diaries: Keeping a Food Diary Helps Dietary Compliance 121
Supplemental Food Diary 122
Eating Out Tips 123
The Problem of Vegetarianism 124
B-6 and Zinc Deficiency and Vegetarianism 124
Reducing Allergy to Protein 125
The Healthiest Choice 125
Problems With Vegetarianism 125
Cardiac Patients and a Vegetarian Diet 126
Dr. Fuhrman's Strict Vegetarian Diet 126
The Much Maligned Egg: The Best Amino Acid Food 127
Lactobacillus for Antibiotic Side Effects and for Indigestion 128
The Diet Almanac: Finding the Diet for Life, Health, and Combating Disease: There is a
    Diet for All Occasions 129
Recipes 151
PATH to Healthier Food Choices 158
Brand New High Protein Breakfast 159
Healthy Choice Shopping List 160

10. Electromedicine **161**

What Most Doctors Won't Tell You: The New PATH -- Our PATH -- in Medicine and Science 161
Electromedicine at PATH 161
Electromagnetic Pollution: Is There an Electromagnetic Antidote? 162
Cranial Electrical Therapy Stimulation (CES): A Brief Summary 167
Cranial Electrical Stimulation 168
Pulsing Brain Hormones by CES? 169
Cranial Electrotherapy Stimulation 170
CES Placement Important to Health 177
Use of 3M Corporation CES/TENS Device 178
TENS Settings 178
Electrical Parameters of CES Devices 179
Electromedicine: Some Frequencies of Reported Benefits 180
Transcutaneous Electrical Nerve Stimulation (TENS) For the Treatment of Primary Dysmenorrhea (Menstrual
Cramps) 182
Electrolytes and Nutrients 182
Adrenalin System and the CES Device 182

11. Endocrinology **183**

Aging Reversal Services 183
Adrenal Gland Stress Tests 183
New Testing for Blood Sugar Tolerance 183
Natural Steroid Therapy 184
What is Aging? -- The Signs of Aging 184

Breaking the Aging Barrier 185
Eldepryl and Brain Aging 185
Tofranil Protocol 185
DHEA Deficiency is also a Factor in Control of Blood Pressure and Heart Disease 186
Male Menopause (Andropause) 186
Male Menopause 186
Adrenopause 187
DHEA -- Adrenopause: Protecting Your Brain 187
DHEA and Adrenopause: A New Sign of Aging and a New Treatment 187
DHEA -- Treatment for Obesity and Adrenopause 189
Update on DHEA 189
DHEA Supplements 189
DHEA and Other Hormones: Availability 190
DHEA References 192
Melatonin: A Modified Amino Acid 194
Melatonin Deficiency 195
Biological Rhythms 195
Hypothyroidism: Notes on Iodine and Thyroid 196
Thyroid Hormones and Iodine 197
The Thyroid Stress Test or TRH Screen 197
Psychiatric Diagnostic Lab of America 198
Hydroxycortisone: For Allergies, Depression, and Chronic Fatigue Disorder 198
Nutrition and Endocrinology 199
Estrogen: Natural Hormones for Lowering Blood Pressure and Stabilizing Heart Disease 200
Rosacea 200
Pharmaceutical Purchases 200

12. *Environment and Toxins* **201**

Air Pollutants 201
Toxic Metals 201
Chelation: Heavy Metal Toxicity 201
Chelation: Side Effect 201
Mercury Toxicity 202
Cigarette Smoking 202
Environmental Sensitivities 203
Radiation 203
Household Appliances 204
Chlorine 204
Indoor Air Pollutants and Sources 205

13. *Food* **207**

Biologic Classification of Foods: Establishing a Food Rotation Diet 207
Plants 208
Foods with Monamine Oxidase Inhibitors to be Avoided 210
Corn 210
Food Groups: Guide to Labels 210
Yeast: A Brief Description of Common Sources of Contacts 211
Tips for Cooking 212
Microwave Radiation 213

14. Gastroenterology -- Stomach, Colon, and Intestine ... 215

Constipation: Some Causes ... 215
Cystic Fibrosis and Nutrition ... 215
Dry Mouth ... 216
Flatulence or Gas ... 216
Heartburn ... 216
Gastrointestinal Dysbiosis ... 216
Lactose Intolerance ... 217
Inflammatory Bowel Disease ... 217
Nutrition and Gastrointestinal Diseases ... 218
Gallstones ... 220
Motion Sickness ... 220
Ulcers ... 221
Conventional Treatment of Ulcers ... 221
Heidelberg Test ... 221
Flexible Sigmoidoscopy: Patient Preparation Instructions ... 222
Guaiac Card or Hemoccult: Stool Blood Test ... 223

15. Heart Disease, Cardiovascular and Peripheral Vascular Health ... 225

Cardiac Disease Reversal Program ... 225
Doppler Test ... 225
Doppler Testing -- Vascular Screening ... 226
Indications for Non-Invasive Vascular Testing ... 227
Vascular Patient History ... 228
Vascular and Venous Blood Testing ... 228
Chelation Therapy ... 234
Chelation Therapy Facts ... 235
Chelation: Side Effect ... 237
Stroke ... 237
Blood Clots ... 239
EKG and Echocardiogram (Echo) ... 241
Exercise ... 241
Exercise: A Summary ... 242
Leg Cramps ... 242
Diet and Anticoagulants ... 243
High Triglycerides and High Cholesterol ... 243
Causes Of High Cholesterol Levels ... 244
Causes of Low Cholesterol Levels ... 244
Cholesterol ... 244
Cholesterol Update ... 244
Pregnancy/Cholesterol ... 245
Angina ... 245
Heart Disease Prevention ... 245
The Physical Link Between Stress and Heart Attacks ... 246
Sudden Death ... 246
Fish Oil and Sudden Death ... 246
Nutrients to Prevent Heart Attacks ... 247
Thrombosis ... 247
PET Scanning at PATH ... 247

Whole Body PET Scan 248
Pre-PET Scan Instructions 248
Body Composition Analysis 249
Body Composition -- Addendum 250
Pretest Instructions for Body Composition Analysis 251
Twenty-Four Hour Blood Pressure Monitor 251
Holter Monitors 252

16. *Infectious Disease and the Immune System* *253*

Immunology 253
Autoimmune Disorders 254
EMS (Eosinophilia Myalgia Syndrome) 254
Middle Ear Infections 254
Infection: Modification by Food, Nutrients, and Behavior 255
AIDS 255
Lyme Disease 256
Chronic Fatigue Syndrome 257
Important Information About Pneumococcal Disease and Pneumococcal Polysaccharide Vaccine 258
Lupus 259
Sporonox 259
Rare Diseases Information 260
The Immune System as Regulator of Homeostasis: Implications for Nutritional Therapy 261
Immunoglobulins and Disease 262
Building and Maintaining an Effective Immune System 264
Immunoglobulins 265
T-Cell or Immune System Ratios and Health 267
Thymus Hormone and T-cell Life 267
Vaccines 268
Ways to Improve the Immune System When You're Sick 270
Balancing Your Immune System 270
Ratios of T-Helper to T-Suppressor Ratios in Various Diseases 271
The Immune System -- Imbalance of Autoimmune Disorders 272
Serum IgE Levels in Disease 272
T-Cell Ratios: Modulation by Nutrition: Case Report 273

17. *Kidney Disease* *277*

Kidneys and Kidney Stones 277
Kidney Stones: Questions and Answers 277
Creatinine Clearance (For Kidney Function) 278
Monitoring Renal Function for Chelation Therapy Infusion 279
Calcium Oxalate Kidney Stones and the Breast 279
Cystitis 279
Dialysis and Transplantation 280
Chronic Renal Failure 280

18. *Neurology and Brain Disorders* *281*

Depression, Addiction, and Anticonvulsants 281
Temporal Lobe Abnormalities 281

Felbamate: A New Antidepressant 282
The Neuropsychological Examination 282
The One-Hour Test 283
Psychoneuroimmunology 285
Lithium 287
Tegretol Protocol 288
Tegretol Protocol -- Revised: For the Individual Who is Extra-Sensitive to Medication 288
Magnetic Resonance Imaging (MRI) 289
Chiropractic 289
Tourette's Syndrome 290
Neurological Obesity 290
Multiple Sclerosis 291
Parkinson's Disease 292
Epilepsy 293
Kinds of Seizures 295
Seizures - Nutritional Control 295
Dyslexia 295
Tinnitus 296
Sleeping Better 296

19. Nutrients and Drugs **297**

The Nutrient Beatitudes 297
Elements of Good Nutrition and Malnutrition 298
Marginal Nutrition/Malnutrition: Basic Causes -- Past and Present 298
Essential Amino Acids: The Protein You Need to Live 300
The Amino Acid Blood Test 301
Acute and Chronic Supplementation of Amino Acids 302
Branched Chain Amino Acid (BCAA), Anabolic Properties, and Future First Thought for I. V. Feeding 307
Cysteine - Glutathione: The Body's Strongest Antioxidant 308
5-Hydroxytryptophan 308
Histidine: Vasodilator and Antirheumatism 309
L-Carnitine: An Oxidizer of Fat 309
Deanol 310
Methionine: for Arthritis, Parkinson's and Depression 310
Pain and Nutritional Supplements 311
Phenylalanine: Fatigue and Pain Relief 311
Taurine: for High Blood Pressure, Seizures, and Depression 312
Tryptophan: A Sleep and Anti-Aggression Nutrient 313
Tyrosine: Anti-Fatigue Adrenalin Builder 314
Proline 315
Threonine 315
Arginine 315
N-Acetylcysteine 315
Amino Acids Build Neurotransmitters That Initiate Behavioral Response(s) 316
Stress Causes Imbalances of Neurotransmitters Therapy Impairing Brain Functions 317
Uses of Fish Oil 318
Products for Achieving Total Health (PATH): Supplements and Their Possible Benefits 319
Formula Contents 322
Mineral Analysis 325
More Mineral Analysis 326

Hair Testing 326
Some Guidelines for Selecting a Specimen 327
Magnesium 328
Magnesium Found To Aid Bypass Patients 328
Manganese 329
Zinc 329
Selenium 330
Your Trace Element Study 330
Vitamins Boost the Immune System 331
Taking Your Vitamins 331
Niacin Therapy 331
The Wonders of Niacin 332
Vitamin Testing 332
Benefits of Nutritional Testing for Vitamins 332
Urinary Methylmalonic Acid: To Detect B-12 333
Nutrition: Glaucoma And Other Eye Diseases 333
Light as a Nutrient 334
Light Levels in Our Environment 335
Prescribing Nutrients and Drugs 335
Your Pharmacist and This Office 335
Drugs for Many Purposes 336
Symptoms and Side Effects of Medications 336
Beta Carotene 337
Choline 337
Quercetin 337
Dandruff 338
Nicotine 338
Diet Pills and Obesity 338

20. Obstetrics, Gynecology and Women's Health 339

Estrogen and Testosterone Therapy at the Menopause 339
Effects of Estrogen 340
New Age in Natural Estrogen Hormone Therapy 340
The Hormone Diet: Influencing Foods and Herbs 341
Treating Menopause with Hormone Replacement Therapy -- Continuous, Daily,
    Oral, Micronized Estradiol and Progesterone 342
Natural Hormone Preparations 343
Most Asked Questions About Natural Oral Progesterone 343
The Use of Progesterone for Post-Partum (Postnatal) Depression 344
Why Oral Progesterone? 345
Progesterone Administration 345
Natural Progesterone: New Ideas 345
Progesterone Dosage 346
Side Effects of Progesterone Therapy 347
Overdose of Progesterone 347
Synthetic Progestogens 347
Progesterone Differs from Progestogens 347
Conception on Progesterone 348
Update on Progesterone and Miscarriages 348
The Physiological Effects of Estrogen and Progesterone 348

Premenstrual and Perimenstrual Tension 349
PMS and BEAM 349
PMS -- Current Research into Its Physical and Psychological Aspects 349
Endometriosis 350
Hair Loss in Women 350
Using Natural Progesterone For Premenstrual Syndrome 351
Daily Symptom Record 352
Pregnancy 353
Utilization by Pregnancy Trimester Markers for Gestational Health and Disease 354
Nutrition and Pregnancy 355
Sex as a Mood Healer 355
Substance Abuse and Pregnancy 355
Protocol for Fibroids 357
The Benefits of Iron Therapy 357
Understanding Pap Smears 358
Mammography 359
Women and Heart Disease 359

21. Osteoporosis and Bone Diseases 361

Bone Health 361
Osteoporosis 361
Causes of Osteoporosis 362
Osteoporosis and Nutrients 362
Osteoporosis and Diet 363

22. Psychological Therapy, Problems and Factors in Disease 365

Anxiety 365
Hypochondriasis: Depression and Anxiety 365
Physical Causes of Anxiety-Like Symptoms 366
Depression and Manic Depression 366
MHPG Urine Test for Depression: Method and Explanation 367
Portrait of Aggressiveness 367
Forms of Aggressiveness 367
Medical Syndromes of Aggression 368
Dissociation 368
Organic Etiology of Psychotic Symptoms 369
Seasonal Affective Disorder 370
Be Your Own Doctor? 370
Baseline Coping Repertoire 370
Cognitive Remediation: Brain Rehabilitation 371
Design and Content of the Remediation Program 371
The Neuropsychological Examination 372
A New Science of Personality 372
Psychometric Testing 372
Psychotherapy 372
The Psychodiagnostic Examination 373
Information About the Myers-Briggs Type Indicator (MBTI) 373
How the Myers-Briggs is Used for Evaluating Patient Compliance 374
Five Symptoms of Psychiatric Disorders 376
The Millon Test and Heart Disease 376

Computerized Psychological Tests 376
Clozaril Dose Schedule 377
Diary for Neurological/Somatization Disorders 378
Link Support Group Listing 379
Personality Disorders 380
Multiple Personality Disorder 384
References Regarding Personality Disorders 384
Neuropsycho-Spiritual Development 385
For Further Reading 387

23. Pulmonary Disorders **389**

Spirometry or PFT 389
The Benefits of Spirometry 389
Asthma and Anxiety 391
Asthma and Exercise 391

24. Rheumatological Disorders and Arthritis **393**

Gout and Elevated Uric Acid 393
Nutrition and Osteoarthritis 393
Rheumatoid Arthritis 394
Fibromyalgia Syndrome (FMS) 394
Capsaicin 395

25. Sex **397**

Sexual Brain Health and Increasing The Sex Drive 397
Sex, Infertility and Impotence 397
Prostate Problems 398
Basic Rules of Sex Drive 398
Family Planning and Safe Sex 399
Birth Control Pills 400

26. Surgery **401**

Nutrition and Wound Healing 401

27. Sports and Exercise **413**

Sports and Exercise: Nutritional Augmentation and Health Benefits 413

28. Spirituality **423**

Psychoneuroimmunology 423
Abridged Spiritual Behavior Inventory 423
Spiritual Distress Diagnosis 425
Proverbs and Healthy Emotions 425
The Biological, Psychological, and Spiritual Bases of Death 426
Breaking Addictions: 12 Steps on the Path to Wellness 427
Controlling Appetite with the Word of the Lord 428
Nutritional Ten Commandments 428

Verses of Peace and Healing 429
The Application of Intelligence to the Development of
    Character: Breaking the Cycle of Anxiety and Anger 429
The Three Paths to Healing Model 430
Holy Medicine 430
Treatment of Disease by Jesus 430
Character and Communication 430
Conventional Medicine and Foolishness 431
Faith in Medicine 432
Family Matters 432
Vaccines, Medicines, and Religion 432
Religious Addiction 433
Some Signs of Inner Peace 433
Dedication of the P.A.T.H. Wellness Manual 433
Scriptures on Abortion 434
Relationships Between Biofeedback and Religious Terminology 435
The Brain Controls the Body as the Mind and Spirit Control Health 436
Medicine 436
Biofeedback 436
PATH'S Guide to Biofeedback 437
Biblical or PATH Therapy Versus Conventional or Freudian Psychotherapy: Their Differences and
    Similarities, Their Strengths and Weaknesses 441
The Electrical Basis of the Holy Spirit: Rauch Ha Kodesh 445

Appendices *447*

Appendix 1: Eric R. Braverman, M. D. 449
Appendix 2: The Place for Achieving Total Health: Multimedia Projects 459

Subject Index *461*

Dear friends on the PATH to Wellness:

It is with great pleasure we bring you this second edition of the PATH Wellness Manual, which I believe is the most comprehensive wellness medical book available today. We believe that you will find more information from this one source related to your total wellbeing than anywhere else.

Sincerely,

[signature]

Eric R. Braverman, M.D.

Dept of Family Practice
Helene Fuld Hosp/Robt. Wood Johnson Medical School

Dept of Psychiatry, NYU Medical School

Fellow -- American College of Nutrition

Diplomat -- American Board of Chelation

Approbations

I like the format and the emphasis on upon "Healing comes from the Most High." It is mysterious that for disease there is healing by faith and physical means. We have, and are, the means of responding to God and our various environments. Well done!

Rev. Ernest Gordon, Ph.D, Princeton NJ.

It combines three essential elements of your professional and intellectual world: sophisticated modern medicine, creative utilization of alternative medical options including traditional remedies, et al., and spiritual fusion of mind and body. It is an impressive and elegant book and I hope it has great success both in the number of people who use it and in delivering to each of them a better physical, emotional, and spiritual life.

David J. Steinberg, President, Long Island University

. . . a terrific manual for anyone's home medical library. Here we discover the holistic way to health seldom followed by the majority of health practitioners today. Beginning with "Allergies," their symptoms and preventative measures the manual goes through the alphabet discussing treatments for a majority of the ailments that cause modern man to weaken and become victims of ill health. The section on "Dieting and Eating Disorders" is a most useful help to anyone on the search for new energy and vitality. Your family will certainly benefit from this book affirming the transitional period through which medicine is traveling and championing the combination of high technology and the naturalistic manner of healing.

Total Health, June 1994.

We welcome a new book of practical information from the author of the outstanding *The Healing Nutrients Within*. The author uses advanced neuroelectronic diagnostic techniques that we didn't think existed outside of university research laboratories.

Durk Pearson, author of *Life Extension*.

The PATH Concept in Health Care

The Place for Achieving Total Health – PATH Medical – is a family center for complete health care devoted to body and mind wellness. We offer complete primary care, and treat neurological, psychiatric, cardiovascular, gastroenterological, nutritional, pediatric infectious, pulmonary, gynecological, oncological, and hematological disorders.

PATH Medical offers a unique approach to both the treatment of existing illness and the prevention of degenerative disease. PATH combines the best of both orthodox and alternative medicine. Hence, our acronym P.A.T.H. -- the true path to wellness must incorporate the best that all fields of medicine has to offer.

The PATH philosophy is to address the body and mind as an integrated system, not as two isolated entities. We rely on both conventional and alternative medical approaches, including nutritional and life-style counseling, and state-of-the-art technology to evaluate and treat patients.

We prevent and treat illness aggressively. All of our patients are evaluated for the nutritional content of their diet, corrections and fine tuning are suggested accordingly. We offer vitamin, mineral, and amino acid supplementation to ensure that all methods of optimal nutrition are met in both the prevention and treatment of illness. We seek to correct biochemical or metabolic malfunctioning that may be contributing to the disease process. PATH Medical has pioneered the use of natural estrogen and natural testosterone for female and male menopause as well as DHEA for adrenopause.

We, at PATH, use medications when necessary, while striving to use the smallest dosages possible for the shortest practical periods of time. Medication can provide quick relief for the individual suffering from emotional symptoms or drastic reduction in blood pressure in the dangerously hypertensive individual. Thanks to the interludes of relief provided by the prudent use of medicine, we are able to achieve prompt symptomatic relief while attacking the cause of disease on other levels.

"We believe that wellness is best achieved through preventive and diagnostic medicine, discovering and treating the underlying basis of illness," explains Eric R. Braverman, M.D., medical director of PATH. "Too often a medicine is prescribed as a quick, short-term solution to symptoms. Instead, we seek long-term answers through identifying and eliminating, if possible, the cause of the illness."

General Medical Services

PATH is a general medical and nutritional practice, offering comprehensive diagnostic and therapeutic services for children and adults.

"We begin by giving each patient a complete physical examination so we are familiar with his or her overall health," explains Dr. Braverman. "We often recommend that patients undergo a psychological screening -- many patients have psychological and emotional needs which their physicians should be aware of before evaluating medical symptoms."

Diagnostic Services

Comprehensive understanding of a patient's condition is fundamental to well being. PATH offers an extensive array of diagnostic and treatment services, from spirometry and nutritional blood analysis to innovative techniques such as 24-hour blood pressure monitoring, neuropsychological testing, and Brain Electrical Activity Mapping (BEAM). PATH has now expanded its services to include Positron Emission Tomography (PET) scanning of the heart and whole body cancer screening, stress testing, biofeedback, and computerized personality profiles (Millon), etc.

The center also has comprehensive (live again) substance abuse prevention, treatment, and counseling programs.

"Because we have a wide variety of diagnostic techniques available, we can better identify the underlying cause of a patient's illness," states Dr. Braverman.

Our most innovative work lies in the area of Brain Electrical Activity Mapping. BEAM testing provides us with the most sophisticated look at brain functioning available today. This completely non invasive procedure, developed at Harvard Medical School, allows us to see what areas of the brain may be contributing to or causing an individual's difficulties. It can be likened in a way to computerized electroenceptolography, and as such, probably makes current EEG testing obsolete.

One of the interesting new therapies that we employ, based on BEAM results, is Cranial Electrical Stimulation. Know as CES, this treatment involves the introduction of a gentle, healing electrical current that stimulates the brain into a more normalized and ultimately more optimized functioning. This treatment is not to be confused with electroconvulsive therapy, known as ECT. ECT is probably damaging to the brain while CES is healing. The current is delivered via two electrodes. One is placed on the forehead just above the bridge of the nose centered between the eyebrows. The second electrode is placed on the left wrist over the radial artery. This is the area one locates to take his/her pulse. This placement of electrodes is an improvement over the original electrode position which dictated that the electrodes be placed on the mastoid areas behind the ears. CES is a self applied prescription treatment F.D.A. approved for anxiety, depression, and insomnia. That is, patients take the units home with them and apply the therapy for one hour each evening. This may be continued for a period from three to nine months and then applied at intervals of perhaps two to three times weekly to maintain the achieved improvements. We at PATH know that virtually any stress related illness is likely to respond favorably to CES (anxiety relief). Another exciting application lies in the area of substance abuse. CES has a normalizing effect on the brain's addiction areas and may offer the key to unlocking the mystery of craving and addiction to food and drugs.

PET Scan is another great innovation at PATH Medical. Positron Emission Tomography can show the amazing break through in cardiovascular reversal. We are able to provide for PET Scanning which we believe replaces cardiac catheterization and stress thallium testing virtually completely. We have been able to achieve cardiovascular reversal using this non-invasive, nontoxic technique. The PET scanner is capable of diagnosing cancer malignancies and may obviate the need for much of today's cancer biopsy and staging techniques.

Another PATH innovation is Doppler non-invasive intravascular ultrasound screening of blood vessels. Stroke is all to common in our society, especially in people in their sixth and seventh decade. Risk factors for a stroke include: diabetes, being overweight, having high cholesterol, high blood pressure, being inactive or bed ridden, and having a family history of heart attack and perioral vascular disease. Deposits build up in the walls of our arteries and veins decreasing blood flow to our toes, fingers, and brain. Vascular blockage can be diagnosed early in the course of the disease. It probably occurs in at least one of four Americans and can be reversed with the PATH program of exercise, chelation, diet, special vascular stockings, medications, nutrients, and methods of ceasing smoking. It is very simple to test for both peripheral and carotid vascular disease with the new Doppler equipment. Get your circulatory "pipes" checked at PATH Medical and prevent the disease that once acquired is often irreversible, except at PATH.

PATH Medical has extensive neurological and psychometric computerized techniques which provides state of the art diagnosis and may help to reveal the biochemical basis of the disease process. New attention deficit testing called the TOVA (test of variables of attention), is a test that detects variations in attention. Neuro-psych evaluation tests for learning educational evaluation and prediction of dimension with memory testing. Testing includes cognitive rehabilitation, personality testing (Myers-Briggs), career testing, and behavior testing. Today PATH Medical can tell you more about your long term behavior than ever before and how that interrelates to your total health and physical well being. Take care of your mental, emotional, and neurological health and you are taking care of your total health and your life.

Nutritional Services

A well-balanced diet is a primary factor in maintaining a healthy body and mind. Our team of dieticians and nutritionists work with a computerized analytical system to interpret each patient's diet and target nutritional deficits. Often a controlled, individualized diet is prescribed to address a specific medical problem, but diets are also available for those who want to lose weight and increase vitality.

"We can design a diet for every disease and every need," states Dr. Braverman.

PATH offers specialized testing to detect nutritional imbalances, allergens, amino acids, vitamins, fatty acids, trace metals, pesticides, and other pollutants.

Educational and Research Services

An extensive medical library and more than 100 informational handouts are available to our patients. To stay at the forefront of medical sciences PATH professionals are involved in ongoing research (the PATH Foundation is nonprofit) studying natural electrical therapy -- exploring the role of brain chemistry in overall wellness -- and maintain staff privileges at an area hospital.

Clearly, PATH Medical offers the cutting edge approach to both the prevention and treatment of the diseases which are eliminating our families and loved ones. We resolve to continue our endeavors in these areas and invite inquiries from both the lay and professional communities. Our commitment to health and the public is alive and growing.

Note to Patients

We recommend to our patients that each time you come to the office, you bring your *PATH Wellness Manual* with you so that Dr. Braverman or his colleagues may point out other articles pertinent to your health education and understanding. Dr. Braverman has written extensively on the subjects dealt with in this manual. Anyone wanting more scientific description and treatment of these matters, rather than the simple lay style employed in the manual, will find such articles listed in Appendix 1 of his Curriculum Vitae.

P. A. T. H. Services

Audiometry: Basic screening for hearing loss.

Biofeedback: Alpha-theta relaxation training and attention deficit recovery training. This is a good technique for achieving reduction of drugs for many conditions.

Body Fat Composition: Analyzed percentage of body fat and muscle. Analyzes conditioning and shows redistribution of body fat with weight loss.

Brain Electrical Activity Mapping (BEAM): BEAM® is a technique to visualize the brain and how it functions. It is useful in all psychiatric and neurological conditions, particularly to determine which medication or treatment to utilize. It is helpful in following the state of recovery of the brain's health or a patient's level of anxiety.

Chelation: A controversial technique thought to help remove toxic metals like lead, clean out plaques in the blood, open clogged vessels, and possibly prevent Alzheimer's disease.

Computerized Nutritional Evaluation: Computerized program analyzing your diet over the past month to show strengths and weaknesses in your dietary nutrient selection.

Cranial Electrical Stimulation (CES): A technique which is FDA-approved for anxiety, depression, and insomnia. It provides mild, gentle electrical stimulation that is also helpful in reducing drug use.

® **Nicolet Instrument Corp.**

Doppler: Safe ultrasound studies of circulation of the blood vessels of the neck (carotids), legs, hands, feet, and male genitals.

EKG: Electrocardiogram -- an ultrasound study of the ejection function of the heart, its valve function and its chamber size.

Fasting: Supervised distilled water fasting.

Holter Monitoring: Used to analyze a person's cardiac arrhythmia over the course of an entire day or a 24/12-hour period. It is the test of choice for evaluating heart palpitations, etc.

Medifast, High Protein Diet: These techniques are used for weight loss, and can be combined with other techniques such as medications and Fast Path.

Neuropsychological Evaluation: Comprehensive examination of neurobehavioral/neurocognitive functions and overall assessment of brain integrity.

Nutritional Blood Analysis: Comprehensive testing for nutrients, vitamins, amino acids, trace metals, toxins, etc.

Physical Examination: A complete physical exam is an essential part of PATH services because it rules out basic diseases and identifies the early signs of medical disease.

Positron Emission Tomography (PET): PET scanning is available at a site in New York City and is the best breakthrough in stress testing ever devised. It is probably more accurate than cardiac catheterization for evaluating the heart, and has no significant side effects.

Proctosigmoidoscopies: Done by flexible sigmoidoscopes which are useful for identifying colon cancer, monitoring individuals at high risk for colon cancer, and monitoring internal hemorrhoids, polyps, inflammatory bowel disease, etc.

Psychodiagnostic Evaluation: A comprehensive analysis of current cognitive and psychological functioning which provides information regarding contribution of psychological and physiological factors in a patient's presenting problems.

Psychological Screening: Clinical assessment using personality inventories and clinical interview.

Psychotherapy: A range of treatment services are provided, including individual, marital, family, and group therapy.

Spirometry: Spirometry, or pulmonary function test, is used to identify early lung disease, damage from smoking, problems related to allergies, asthma, etc. (It may be a predictor of longevity.)

24-Hour Blood Pressure Monitor: The tool of choice for accurately analyzing a person's blood pressure. It is a computerized instrument which provides up to 40 blood pressure readings in one day.

Ultrasound Testing: Used for evaluating heart murmurs and other organs of the body.

Materials Available from Path

1. Video Tapes on PATH and Special Topics; Brain Electrical Activity Mapping (BEAM®) and Cranial Electrical Stimulation (CES)

- ■ "Late Night with David Letterman" -- BEAM

- ■ "Prime Time" -- BEAM/CES for Drug Addiction

- ■ "BEAM" -- by Nicolet

- ■ "Houston TV News" Crack/Cocaine Conference, Houston -- BEAM/CES

- ■ "CNBC" -- BEAM/CES

- ■ "Good Morning" -- BEAM/CES

2. Cassette tapes of the Total Health Show from WTTM and WMCA

3. All articles listed in Appendix 1: Curriculum Vitae

4. Nutrients

5. Books:

> *A Remarkable Medicine Has Been Overlooked* by Jack Dreyfus
>
> *Alcohol and the Addictive Brain* by Kenneth Blum, Ph.D.
>
> *Cancer and Nutrition* by Charles Simone, M.D.
>
> *Healing Nutrients Within: Facts, Findings and New Research on Amino Acids* by Eric Braverman, M.D.
>
> *How to Lower Your Blood Pressure and Reverse Heart Disease Naturally*, by Eric R. Braverman, M.D.
>
> *New Hope for Binge Eaters* by Harrison B. Pope, Jr., M.D., and James I. Hudson, M.D.
>
> *The Broad Range of Clinical Use of Phenytoin* by Barry Smith, M.D., Ph.D., and Jack Dreyfus
>
> *The Princeton Plan* by Edwin Heleniak, M.D.
>
> *What Your Doctor Won't Tell You* by Jane Heimlich
>
> *Nutritional Influences on Disease* by Melvyn Werback, M.D.

® Nicolet Instrument Corp.

Directions to PATH Patient Care Centers

Driving Directions

For the most up-to-date directions please call the office which you will visit.
You may also check the PATH Medical website at http://www.pathmed.com to obtain a map (courtesy of Yahoo!®).

New York City Office

274 Madison Avenue, Suite 402
New York, NY 10016
tel: (212) 213-6155

The New York City office is located between the New York Public Library and Grand Central Terminal
Parking garages are plentiful in the vicinity.

Metro-Philadelphia
Penndel, Pennsylvania Office

142 Bellevue Avenue
Penndel, PA 19047
tel: (215) 702-1344

The Penndel office is located approximately 20 miles north from downtown Philadelphia.
It is easily accessed from Interstate I-95.

Gulf Coast Florida
Naples, Florida Office

219 South Airport Road
Naples, FL 34102
tel: (941) 513-1661

Consultations at the Naples office are by appointment only. Please call in advance to make arrangements.

Notes

Acknowledgments

The *P.A.T.H Wellness Manual* would not have been possible without the inspiration, assistance, and brilliant ideas of my mentor Carl C. Pfeiffer, Ph.D., M.D. I am indebted also to:

- APA (American Psychiatric Association) for permission to print DSM-III-R criteria;
- Kenneth Blum, Ph.D., for amino acid references and permission to use the SAVE formula;
- Allison Braverman, M.A., for her contribution to the article entitled, "Biblical or PATH Therapy Verus Conventional or Freudian Psychotherapy: Their Differences and Similarities, Their Strengths and Weaknesses"; and for her input to the biofeedback articles, "Biofeedback from the Living God" and "Biofeedback Imagery for Christians";
- Fred Elbrecht for showing the amplitude and frequency of CES units;
- Kathleen Esposito, M.S., for recipes and for dietary information for meats and salad dressings;
- Joel Fuhrman, M.D., for helping us design a strict vegetarian diet;
- Frances Goulart for her assistance in preparing some recipes in this manual;
- Randy Gunsel for help in organizing the teaching material and for irreplaceable help;
- Martin Haydon, Ph.D., for his contribution to the article entitled, "The Neuropsychological Examination";
- Marty Hayt, for proofreading;
- Susan Laird, M.A., for organizational help;
- Janet Lupa, R.N., for her article on chelation, and for recipes and general assistance;
- Madison Pharmacy for the Daily Activity Planner;
- Robert Moss, C.A.D.C., M.A., for general wisdom and substance abuse related materials;
- Nicolet Instrument Corp for permission to use various BEAM maps. BEAM is a registered trademark of the Nicolet Instrument Corp.;
- Annie Schade, certified EEG technician, for help with the doppler and BEAM material;
- Richard Smayda for his contribution to the article entitled "Chronic Lead Poisoning as a Cause of Bulimia: Hair Test and Brain Electrical Activity Mapping as a Diagnostic Aid";
- Enid Sterling, Esq., for editing and proofreading this book;
- Karen Swansboro for help with the doppler and biofeedback material;
- Kristin Swartz for her contribution to the article, "Cranial Electrotherapy Stimulation";
- Matthew Taub, M.D., for editing this second edition;
- The entire staff at PATH for their help and support in the creation of this work.

Introduction to the PATH Wellness Manual

MEDICINE IN RELATIONSHIP WITH THIS OFFICE

The dosing of medication is very individual. One patient should start at one pill while another needs four pills. This will require constant communication with the office. Do not hesitate to call with any reactions, fears, and concerns. Sometimes medicine has to be started slowly and reactions will disappear and the medication can be gradually increased. Other times it just isn't the right medication despite the best of testing. Don't let this disappoint you.

COST OF TESTING

We were first able to do blood levels of calcium and phosphorus in the 1920's and 1930's, protein bound iodine and thyroid testing in the 1950's, and EKG's about 1915. Tests that were too expensive and not available for everybody, eventually became available. So we do our best to offer these tests as well as those that are currently available. What PATH testing includes and seeks to do today will be utilized by the rest of medicine in the future.

THE BEST WAYS TO GET HELP FROM YOUR DOCTOR

- Be as familiar as possible with your own medical history.

- Try to keep a list of your medications in your purse or wallet to review at each visit with your doctor.

- Jot down specific questions you have for the doctor to bring to each visit.

- If you have a new health concern, be as specific as possible. Bring in related articles you have found, write down your symptoms and the dates and times of each problem.

- Be certain you understand any new medical prescriptions. Ask for information and get prescription summaries from your pharmacist if possible. Remember that doctors prescribe most medications for reasons other than the typical indication of the drug.

- Find out what other resources are available to help you understand your condition. Ask your doctor about other associations where you can get information.

- Get copies of your test results, speak to the nurses, make sure you understand the results of your tests.

- Adopt a schedule for routine preventive health care. Follow your doctor's advice on routine preventive care.

- Get suggested second opinions from the doctor.

- Try to build a long-term relationship with the doctor so he can continue to benefit you.

1. *Allergic Disorders*

How to Discover a Food Allergy or Food Addiction

Many people are unaware that they have a food allergy or what may be termed a food addiction. A person may be eating a certain food several times a day not realizing that he is "addicted" to the food. It gives an increase in energy or a sense of well-being; and when the energy dwindles, he once again reaches for the food to boost his energy level.

Or, one may be presently experiencing ill health due to intolerance to certain foods. If one eliminates this particular food from the diet for several hours he would begin to experience withdrawal symptoms such as fatigue, irritability, anxiety, headache, upset stomach, muscle cramps, or almost any other ill feeling. These symptoms can be more acute after a shock to the system such as surgery, illness, pregnancy, accident, or some other form of stress.

A person may experience relief of symptoms when food is eliminated.

The problem is to discover what food (if any) is causing symptoms of ill health. The foods that usually cause the most problems are: 1) wheat, 2) dairy products, 3) corn, 4) sugar, 5) caffeine (coffee, tea, and cola drinks),

and 6) proteins (meat, fish, eggs, etc.); also citrus fruits, yeast, or any food in a daily diet. In order to determine if any of the above foods are causing problems you must go on an elimination diet. This means taking one food at a time, for example, wheat, out of your diet completely for four full days. (When omitting a particular food, be sure to omit all forms of that food.) On the fifth day starting with the noon meal, eat all you can eat of the particular food you have previously eliminated from your diet for the preceding four days. Eat the food by itself in its whole, natural form (organic if possible -- free from preservatives). Observe for any symptoms (untoward reaction). If no symptoms occur after one hour, eat more of the same food -- this time, one-half of the previous amount. If still no ill effects occur after a one-half hour period, eat a third feeding. If still no symptoms, wait until evening to eat the next normal meal. If one is allergic to a food, symptoms can occur anywhere from the moment the food is swallowed and up to 12 hours thereafter (although a rare possibility). The degree of reaction may vary from a mild discomfort or irritation to a severe discomfort. Keep a written record of what symptoms you experience on the day of testing.

Allergy Tests

Some allergy tests are: IgE, a general screen for inhalants and, to some degree, foods; IgE-RAST testing, which deals with immediate reactions to inhalants and foods, by which specific things are tested and identified; IgE-chicken or IgE-wheat. IGG, in general, deals with immune deficiencies, but also identifies food-delayed reactions if certain foods are chosen, such as chicken or wheat. Other allergy tests include IGA Gliadin of IGG, which relate to celiac disease, sprue, and wheat sensitivity. Allergy testing is thought to be approximately 60 to 70 percent accurate. PATH has new IgE food and allergy testing which may be more accurate.

Allergies and Treatment

Most people suffer from some allergies throughout the year due to mold, cat dander, rag weed, pollen, and house dust. Some ways to avoid allergies are to cover mattresses and box springs with dust proof covers, avoid upholstered head boards and feather pillows, avoid woolen blankets and down comforters, replace heavy draperies and slatted blinds, use mothproof paint, dust books, knick-knacks, and toys frequently, close forced air heating and air conditioning outlets covering them with double density air filters, keep bedroom doors shut to prevent dust and pets from entering, keep windows closed to prevent dust and pollen from entering, replace shower curtains and liners frequently to avoid mold growth.

If allergies are seasonal they are called Seasonal Allergic Rhinitis. Eight out of ten individuals have hay fever and itchy, scratchy eyes. For many with Allergic Rhinitis, indoor irritants are feathers, mold spores, animal dander, and minute insects that thrive on dust. Treatment is typically with natural antihistamines, e.g., vitamin C, methionine and quercetin. Using antihistamines to treat patients with high blood pressure can be very dangerous.

In patients with heart disease, they can cause worsening of angina, and in patients who have diabetes or thyroid problems, antihistamines may interfere to some degree with medication or give false signs suggesting the need for different medication dosages.

Light, wind-born pollens from trees, grasses, and weeds are the main causes of allergies. Colorful, scented flowers, like the goldenrod, have too heavy a pollen to be carried by the wind. Ragweed pollen may cause the most allergies, followed by various grass and tree pollens. Trees pollinate in the spring, grass in the summer, and ragweed from August to October. Pollen counts are highest on warm sunny days, and lowest on cool cloudy days or after a rainfall. Most radio stations warn of high pollen count days. Pollen counts are highest in the morning and gradually decrease throughout the day. Frost kills outdoor pollen-producing plants but allergies continue to be triggered by indoor allergens such as molds, animal dander, and dust. See Allergy or Low Histamine Diet, p. 132.

Allergy: Low Histamine Diet

Diet for elimination of additives and foods high in histamines which may provoke flushing and allergies

Permitted

Cereals: Fresh-baked breads and cereals (not packaged).

Fats: Butter, olive oil.

Fruits: Any in moderate quantities (many contain natural salicylates).

Meats: Fresh meat, eggs, and fish only, in small quantities (no luncheon meats).

Vegetables: Any in fresh state except cabbage (including sauerkraut), beans, and spinach. Tomatoes permitted in moderation.

Condiments: Salt, pepper; other condiments to be taken only as dried leaves; vinegar only if label indicates no additives.

Sweets: Homemade only, without additives.

Beverages: Fresh milk, tea, homemade fruit juice, mineral water.

Avoid

Food items: Colored beverages, wines and other alcoholic beverages, artificial sweeteners, ice cream, sweets, and ready-made, commercially available desserts.

Other items: Colored toothpaste, colored cosmetics.

Asthma

There are increasing numbers of asthma cases documented in the United States because of indoor and environmental pollution, outdoor pollution, molds, cat danders, house dust, mites, and multiple other factors. If it can make you allergic, you can get asthma from it.

Asthma is associated with sinusitis, hypertension, emphysema, heart failure, eczema, and respiratory failure. Asthma can occur in patients with pneumonia, fractured ribs, tuberculosis, and arthritis. All these conditions can interplay with asthma.

Asthmatic patients are frequently allergic to cockroaches, house dust, ragweed, rats, mice, etc.

Asthma is well known to be a brain disorder. If you deplete certain neurotransmitters in the brain, tyrosine, phenylalanine, dopamine, and noracymethadol, you can have a dramatic increase in asthma.

Asthma occurs during periods of stress and can be successfully treated by antidepressants. Medications like Dilantin and anticonvulsants can be dramatically helpful.

Yogurt has been shown to be helpful for bronchial asthma, as well as any relaxation technique, biofeedback, CES, prayer, etc.

Brain norepinephrine has been shown to be depleted in asthmatics, again pointing out the benefits of various asthmatic treatments. Antiasthmatic effects have been shown with onion extracts, as well as mustard oils. Acupuncture has been recommended for asthma. Vitamin C has been shown to reduce some of the lung hyper-responsiveness of asthmatics. Intravenous magnesium has been shown to be useful in asthmatics. Diets high in sodium are dangerous for asthmatics. Inhalants are used by doctors, but certain inhalants will actually result in rebound wheezing, palpitations, and serious side effects due to the drugs.

Avoidance of allergic foods can dramatically help asthmatics. As many as 93 percent are dramatically helped who have bronchial asthma. This can be tested through IGG testing.

Snow crab processing workers have a high rate of asthma. We recommend shell fishing be avoided by asthmatics. (Shell fish are essentially rodents.) Occupational hazard asthma occurs with exposure to nickel and other irritants.

White wine can sometimes help asthmatics and sometimes may harm asthmatics. Sulfites have been linked to worsening asthma. Sulfites are found in fruit juices, soft drinks, wines, beers, cider vinegar, potato chips, dried fruits, and various vegetables. There is no doubt that one of the few benefits of coffee is that it can help asthma.

Vitamin B-6 has been thought to be helpful for asthma. Low selenium levels have been linked to asthma. Bronchitis has been a cause of asthma and has been treated with N-acetylcystine. Asthma frequently goes undiagnosed and has been associated with depression. It is sometimes related to sleep disorder.

Allergic rhinitis can be relieved by aspirin and Motrin. It is important to treat asthma since you can have more permanent loss of pulmonary function.

There has been one study which has shown that fish oil can help relieve asthma. Calcium channel blockers have been used in asthma. Their action is like magnesium. Theophylline is still used in asthma, but it may be obsolete. Beta agonist drugs can sometimes worsen your overall mortality and risk from asthma. The reason is that inhaled beta agonists have been linked to deaths (fenoterol and albuterol). This is why we don't use albuterol. We will use a little bit of Proventil and asthma Cort.

Smoking has been linked to childhood asthma. Quinoline antibiotics, norfloxacin may be helpful in acute exacerbation of asthma. The CES device (see section 10) is an important dimension in asthma. Methotrexate has been used with severe pediatric asthma when it is being treated like an autoimmune disease. Low glutathione has been associated with asthma. Antioxidants have been shown to be imbalanced in asthmatics.

Seventy-four percent of asthmatics that were elite swimmers were diagnosed after swimming and chlorine was associated with the asthma. There is also evidence of exercise-induced asthma. Asthma has been shown to be relieved by aspirin in some cases. Physical exercise training can be very important in asthmatics.

Bacteria has been associated with the cause of asthma. Food sensitivities must be carefully evaluated. All antioxidants such as Vitamin E can be beneficial in asthmatics. Lithium has been used effectively to treat asthma.

The causes of occupational asthma are quite extensive. Sensitizing agents have been rats, mice, rabbits, guinea pigs, pigeons, chickens, grain, mites, moths, butterflies, crabs, prawns, wheat flour, rye flour, coffee beans, tea leaves, tobacco leaves, wood dust, biological enzyme, isothiocyanates which are in automobile spray paint, epoxy resins, plastics, metals, tanners, platinum refiners, metal platers, aluminum solderers, pharmaceutical workers, refrigeration workers, hairdressers, plastics and rubber workers, insulators and multiple chemicals of all types have been associated with asthma.

Asthma, of course can be very much linked to biological rhythms and therefore Melatonin which helps sleep can be useful in asthma.

Asthma is caused by spasm and narrowing of the airway in the lungs due to allergy. This spasm makes it hard to move air through the air passages out of the lungs.

Causes - cold, dust, pollen, chlorine, exercise, etc.
Symptoms - coughing, dry throat, trouble breathing.

Treatment includes:

1 - Shots (hyposensitization)
2 - Antihistamines
3 - Bronchodilators
4 - Avoiding the cause of the allergy.
5 - Fluids (medications do not work well during an attack complicated by dehydration) - and/or nasal douching with saline alkalor.
6 - Prophylaxis with the nutrients magnesium, vitamin C, bioflavonoids, and antioxidants.
7 - Trials of atypical medicine, e.g., Dilantin, Wellbutrin, and Prozac.

References:

1. Dolovich J, Evans S, Nieboer A, Occupational asthma from nickel sensitivity: I Human serum albumin in the antigenic determinant, *British Journal of Industrial Medicine* 41:51-55, 1984.

2. Cartier A, et al., Occupational asthma in snow crab processing workers, *J. Allergy Clin. Immunol.* September 1981.

3. Scanlon R, Chang S, Brain norepinephrine: a possible role in bronchial asthma, *Annals of Allergy* 60:333-338, 1988.

4. Kang B, Jones J, Johnson J, Kang I, Analysis of indoor environment and atopic allergy in urban populations with bronchial asthma, *Annals of Allergy* 62:30-34, 1989.

5. Barnes P, The role of neurotransmitters in bronchial asthma, *Lung* 57-65, 1990.

6. Nagarathna R, Nagendra H, Yoga for bronchial asthma: a controlled study. *British Medical Journal* 391:1077-1079, 1985.

7. Dorsch W, et al., Antiasthmatic effects of onion extracts -- detection of benzyl and other isothiocyanates (mustard oils) as antiasthmatic compounds of plant, *European Journal of Pharmacology* 107:17-24, 1985.

8. Tandon M, et al., Acupuncture for bronchial asthma? *Medical Journal of Australia* 154:409-412, 1991.

9. Al-Frayh A, IgE-Mediated skin reaction among asthmatic children in Riyadh, *Annals of Saudi Medicine* 11:448, 1991.

10. Mohsenin V, Effect of Vitamin C on No 2-induced airway hyperresponsiveness in normal subjects, *Am Rev Respir Dis.* 136:1408-1411, 1987.

11. Newman A, *Johns Hopkins Magazine* 4:43-8, 1987.

12. Burney P, A diet rich in sodium may potentiate asthma, *Chest.* 91:64, 1987.

13. Peliken M, Bronchial asthma due to food allergy, *XII International Congress of Allergy and Clinical Immunology*, 1985. Washington, D.C.

14. Burr M, et al., Food-allergic asthma in general practice, *Human Nutrition*, 39:349, 1985.

Dust Precautions for Allergy

1. Vacuum sleeping quarters daily.
2. Zippered plastic mattress and box spring covers.
3. Dacron, fluff-filled pillow, dry cleaned every 3 months.
4. Bedspread, removed from bed at night.
5. Washable mattress cover, washed monthly.
6. Washable curtains or drapes, washed monthly.
7. Bare floors or washable area rug.
8. Walls and wall hangings, books and bookcases, vacuum-dusted weekly.
9. Cold-steam vaporizer at night.
10. Electrostatic precipitator or filters.

Methods for Treating Cat Allergy

There is hope for teary-eyed cat lovers. If you are allergic to your cat, do not despair. A monthly rinse in distilled water may help rid your cat of the substance that causes allergic reactions. The cats bathed in one liter of distilled water once a month for 10 minutes demonstrated a substantial reduction in the amount of milliunits of cat allergen. Nine rinses of a cat resulted in the reduction of 3,000 milliunits of cat allergen to 400 milliunits. In addition, if the house is kept clean, this may result in a significant toleration of the cat.

How to Avoid a Mold Allergy

To avoid a mold allergy, first obtain a gauge to measure relative humidity. Keep humidity low, 35 percent, if possible. In addition, use dehumidifiers and empty the water regularly. Air conditioners can be sprayed at the air intake with mold killing spray if they develop a musty odor. Use a humidifier in winter, avoid over-humidification, and wash the humidifier and change the water frequently to prevent mold growth.

A very tightly insulated house will prevent the escape of moisture, thus encouraging mold growth. Allow adequate ventilation. In the kitchen, use an exhaust fan to remove water vapor when cooking. Mold grows in refrigerators and around door gaskets and garbage containers; these should be kept clean.

Use exhaust fans in the bathrooms, wash or replace shower curtains, and clean bathroom tiles and shower stalls. Repair any damage to caulking or grout. Do not carpet bathrooms.

In the laundry room, vent the clothes dryer to the outdoors. Dry clothing immediately after washing. In the basement, use a dehumidifier. Correct seepage or flooding problems. Keep the basement free of dust. Remove moldy stored items. Avoid storage of any unnecessary items in the house. Allergic individuals should avoid living in basement apartments or dormitories. Avoid window condensation. Mold grows well in closets, which are damp and dark. Dry shoes and boots thoroughly before storing. A low watt light bulb or chemical moisture remover can prevent mold growth in closets.

Indoor plants are not a major source of mold spores, but it is prudent to limit the number of house plants. Spores can be airborne when plants are watered. Molds are present in wood used in fireplaces. Good quality HEPA air cleaners can remove mold spores in the air. Inexpensive table top air cleaners are not effective.

Outdoors, avoid cutting grass and raking leaves, and correct drainage problems near the house. Pool water increases mold formation. When camping or walking in the woods, exposure to mold spores is increased. They are also increased on dry and windy days. Greenhouses are loaded with mold, as are summer cottages. Hotel rooms are sources of increased mold. Automobile air conditioners harbor mold. Gardeners, bakers, brewers, carpenters, mill workers, upholsterers, and paperhangers are all exposed to molds.

Products that kill mold: household bleach and water; commercially available products such as Exportine contain a similar solution combined with cleaning agents and a spray dispenser; Mildew Stop spray is also available.

Food Allergy:
Concomitant and Synergistic Foods

It has been suggested that there are some concomitant and synergistic foods that cause allergy, as listed in the following two tables. It will take some time to discover whether this is true or not.

CONCOMITANT FOODS

Pork, black pepper	Rhus allergy (poison ivy, oak, sumac)
Egg	Ragweed, short
Wheat	Ragweed, giant
Potato, tomato, tobacco (Chewing or snuff)	Iva Ciliata
Pork, black pepper	Sage
Legumes: beans, peas, soybean, cottonseed (cooking fats)	Pigweed
Beef, yeasts (baker's, brewer's, malt)	Cedar
Milk, mint	Elm
Lettuce	Cottonwood
Egg, apple	Oak
Corn, banana	Pecan
Cane sugar, orange	Mesquite
Oysters (seafood)	Dust
Cheese mushrooms, truffles	Molds

SYNERGISTIC FOODS

Banana	Corn
Baker's yeast, brewer's yeast	Beef
Orange	Cane sugar
Mint	Milk
Apple	Egg
Black Pepper	Pork

Reference:

King, W. P., Food Hypersensitivity in Otolaryngology, Manifestations, Diagnosis, and Treatment, *Otolaryngic Allergy* 25(1):163-179, 1992.

Classification of Allergic Reactions and Spectrum of Antihistamines

Studies now show that food allergy is common and can occur by either IgG or IgE response. Most food allergy is not type 1 but actually type 4, delayed hypersensitivity (see Table 1). Food allergy has been implicated in numerous diseases: dermatitis, herpetiformis, celiac disease, arthritis, short stature. Asthma in particular has been thought to be an IgE-related problem. Sixty percent of the population has known food intolerance. A surprising allergy is fruit juice intolerance. It has been shown that the elevated serum IgE levels in chronic alcoholics have been associated with food allergies. Mild allergies can be provoked even by nondairy foods that are parv (dairy free). Hot dogs, bologna, tuna, tofu, and rice-based ice cream substitutes all seem to have some mild proteins and can worsen milk allergy. Atopic, urticaria, and allergic rhinitis have all been linked to food allergy.

Pollens and apples can cross-react. Breast feeding may prevent food allergy from developing as frequently. Soy protein allergy is also common. IgE and IgG responses can identify even unusual allergies like watermelon, shellfish, etc. Tricyclic antidepressants, vitamin C, and calcium can help treat food allergies. Sodium cromolyn is also valuable. Allergies to fish can occur, and cow's milk and egg are the most common. Urticaria vasculitis can occur from food allergy. Antihistamines are common treatment. Phenothiazines (Prolixin, Mellaril, etc.) are available as antihistamines. Methdilazine, promethazine, and trimeprazine tartrate are phenothiazines (see Table 2). It is notable that ethanolamines are most related to choline, phenothiazines are antipsychotics, and alkylamines are probably more related to antidepressants.

TABLE 1: GELL AND COOMBS CLASSIFICATION OF ALLERGIC REACTIONS [1]

Reaction	Pathological Response
Type I: Anaphylactic	allergic rhinitis and conjunctivitis wheal and flare skin reactions anaphylaxis
Type II: Cytotoxic	blood transfusion reactions hemolytic disease of the newborn Coombs' positive hemolytic anemias drug-induced cytopenias
Type III: Immune complexes -- mediated	serum sickness hypersensitivity angitis hypersensitivity pneumonitis glomerulonephritis
Type IV: Delayed hypersensitivity	tuberculin-type hypersensitivity tissue transplantation rejection drug-induced reactions

1. Table 1 is from "Allergy Testing: From In Vivo to In Vitro," by Majid Ali, M.D., et al. Reprinted from *Diagnostic Medicine*, May/June 1982.

TABLE 2: SPECTRUM OF ANTIHISTAMINES [1]

Class	Generic name
Ethylenediamines	Methapyrilene Pyrilamine Tripelennamine citrate
Ethanolamines	Bromodiphenhydramine Hcl Carbinoxamine maleate Clemastine fumarate Diphenhydramine Hcl Doxylamine succinate
Alkylamines	Brompheniramine maleate Chlorpheniramine maleate Dexchlorpheniramine maleate Triprolidine Hcl
Piperazines	Hydroxyzine Hcl pamoate
Phenothiazines	Methdilazine Promethazine Hcl Trimeprazine tartrate
Piperidines	Azatadine maleate Cyproheptadine

Allergy References

1. Ali M, Nalebuff DJ, Fadal RG, Ramanarayanan MR. Allergy testing: From in vivo to in vitro. *Diagnostic Medicine*, 1982.

2. Nalebuff DJ. Keep allergic rhinitis in your practice. *Diagnosis* 1987.

3. Kniker WT. IgE-medicated allergy: *Diagnostic Tools and Strategies*, pp. 52-69.

4. Bachert C, et. al. Decreased reactivity in allergic rhinitis after intravenous application of calcium. A study on the alteration of local airway resistance after nasal allergen provocation. *Arzneimittelforsch*, 40:984-987, 1990.

5. Stenhammar L, et al. Celiac disease in children of short stature without gastrointestinal symptoms. *Eur J Pediatr*, 145:185-6, 1986.

6. Sampson HA, Cooke SK. Food allergy and the potential allergenicity-antigenicity of microparticulated egg and cow's mild proteins. *J of Amer Col of Nutrition*, 9(4):410-417, 1990.

7. Bock SA, Atkins FM. The natural history of peanut allergy. *J Allergy Clin Immunol.*, 83(5):900-904, 1989.

8. Burrows B, et al. Association of asthma with serum IgE levels and skin-test reactivity to allergens. *NE J of Medicine*, 320:271-277, 1989.

9. Magaziner A. *Food Allergies Linked to Common Medical Problems.*

10. Fruit juice intolerance. *Healthwise*. Indianapolis, IN: Alexander Grant, M.D. and Associates, Inc., 1988.

11. Metcalfe DD. Diseases of food hypersensitivity. *NE J of Medicine*, 321(4):255-257, 1989.

12. Kinoshita K, et al. Participation of food antigens in increased polyclonal antibody production induced by alcohol. *J Clin Lab Immunol*, 29:105-108, 1989.

13. Friend T. Mild allergies provoked by nondairy foods. *USA Today.*

14. Plebani A, Albertini A, Scotta S, Ugazio AG. IgE antibodies to dydrolysates of cow milk proteins in children with cow milk allergy. *Annals of Allergy*, 64:279-280, 1990.

---

1. Table 2 is from "Keep Allergic Rhinitis in Your Practice," by Donald J. Nalebuff, M.D. Reprinted from *Diagnosis*, March 1987.

15. Andre C, Heremans JF, Vaermann JP, Cambiaso CL. A mechanism for the induction of immunological tolerance by antigen feeding: Antigen-antibody complexes. *J of Experimental Medicine*, 142:1509-1519, 1975.

16. Atherton DJ. The role of foods in atopic eczema. *Clin and Exper Derm*, 8:227-232, 1983.

17. Atherton DJ, Sewell M, Soothill JF, Wells RS, Chilvers CE. A double-blind crossover trial of an antigen-avoidance diet in atopic eczema. *Lancet*, pp. 401-403, 1978.

18. Pagnelli R, Levinsky RJ, Brostoff J, Wraith DG. Immune complexes containing food proteins in normal and atopic subjects after oral challenge and the effect of sodium cromoglycate on antigen absorption. *Lancet*, p. 321, 1979.

19. Brostoff J, Carini C, Wraith DG, et al. Immune complexes in atopy. In: Pepys J, Edwards AM, eds. *Mast Cell*. London: Pitman, p. 380, 1979.

20. Ogle KA, Bullock JD. Children with allergic rhinitis and/or bronchial asthma treated with elimination diet, a five year follow-up. *Annals of Allergy*, 44:273-278, 1980.

21. Rowe AH. Bronchial asthma because of food and inhalant allergy and less frequent drug and chemical allergy. In: Rowe AH, ed., *Food Allergy*. Springfield: Charles C. Thomas, pp. 169-210, 1972.

22. Egger J, Carter CM, Wilson J, et al. Is migraine food allergy? A double-blind trial of oligoantigenic diet treatment. *Lancet*, pp. 865-868, 1983.

23. Rowe AH, Rowe A. Bronchial asthma in patients over age of 55 years: Diagnosis and treatment. *Annals of Allergy* 5:509-518, 1947.

24. Businco L, Marchetti F, Pellegrini G, et al. Prevention of atopic disease in "at risk newborns" by prolonged breast feeding. *Annals of Allergy*, 51:296, 1983.

25. Chandra RK. Prospective studies of the effect of breast feeding on incidence of infection and allergy. *Acta Paediatr Scandanavia*, 68:691, 1979.

26. Anderson LB, Dreyfus EM, Logan J, Johnston DE, Glaser. Melon and banana sensitivity coincident with ragweed pollinosis. *J Allergy Clin Immunol*, 45:310, 1970.

27. Lahti A, Bjorksten F, Hannuksela M. Allergy to birch pollen and apple, and cross-reactivity of the allergens studied with the RAST. *Allergy* 35:297, 1980.

28. Bahna SL. The diagnostic dilemma of milk allergy. *Annals of Allergy*, 63:475-476, 1989.

29. Richards DG, et al. Cow's mild protein/soy protein allergy: gastrointestinal imaging. *Radiology*, 167(3):721-723, 1988.

30. Enberg RN, McCullough J, Ownby DR. Antibody responses in watermelon sensitivity. *J Allergy Clin Immunol*, 82(5):795-800, 1988.

31. Geller-Bernstein C, et al. IgA, IgG, IgM, and IgE levels in normal, healthy, non-atopic Israeli children. *Annals of Allergy*, 61:296-299, 1988.

32. Pelikan Z. Nasal response to food ingestion challenge. *Arch Otolaryngol Head Neck Surg*, 114:525-530, 1988.

33. Rao KS, et al. Duration of the suppressive effect of tricyclic antidepressants on histamine-induced wheal-and-flare reactions in human skin. *J Allergy Clin Immunol*, 82(5):752-757, 1988.

34. Bjorksten B, Kjellman N-I M. Does breast-feeding prevent food allergy? *Allergy Proc*, 12(4):233-237, 1991.

35. Walker M. IgG bloodprint determination of adverse responses to foods. *Townsend Letter for Doctors*, pp. 566-568, July 1991.

36. Plebani A, et al. IgE antibodies to hydrolysates of cow milk proteins in children with cow milk allergy. *Annals of Allergy*, 64(3):279-280, 1990.

37. Bucca C, et al. Effect of vitamin C on histamine bronchial responsiveness of patients with allergic rhinitis. *Annals of Allergy*, 65:311-314, 1990.

38. Businco L, Cantani A. Food allergy in children: Diagnosis and treatment with sodium cromoglycate. *Allergol Et Immunopathol*, 18(6):339-348, 1990.

39. Bernhisel-Broadbent J, Strause D, Sampson HA. Fish hypersensitivity. II: Clinical relevance of altered fish allergenicity caused by various preparation methods. *J Allergy Clin Immunol*, 90(4):622-629, 1992.

40. Oranje AP, et al. Immediate contact reactions to cow's milk and egg in atopic children. *Acta Derm Venereol*, 71:263-266, 1991.

41. Epstein MM, Watsky KL, Lanzi RA. The role of diet in the treatment of a patient with urticaria and urticarial vasculitis. *J Allergy Clin Immunol*, 90(3):414-415, 1992.

42. Nalebuff DJ. In vitro tests and immunotherapy. *Ear, Nose, Throat J*, 67:33-40, 1988.

43. Bell IR, et al. Polysymptomatic syndromes and autonomic reactivity to nonfood stressors in individuals with self-reported adverse food reactions. *J Amer Coll Nutr*, 12(3):227-238, 1993.

44. Agata H, et al. Effect of elimination diets on food-specific IgE antibodies and lymphocyte proliferative responses to food antigens in atopic dermatitis patients exhibiting sensitivity to food allergens. *J Allergy Clin Immunol*, 91(2):668-679, 1993

45. Katsunuma T, et al. Wheat-dependent exercise-induced anaphylasix: Inhibition by sodium bicarbonate. *Annals of Allergy*, 68:184-188, 1992.

46. King HC. Skin endpoint titration and immunotherapy: An overview. *Ear, Nose Throat J*, 67:24-30, 1988.

47. Osguthorpe JD. Otolaryngic Allergy. *Ear, Nose, Throat J*, 67:7-8, 1988.

48. Trevino RJ. Food allergies and hypersensitivities. *Ear, Nose, Throat J*, 67:42-48, 1988.

49. Becker GD, Radford ER. An otolaryngic approach to the allergic patient. *Ear, Nose, Throat J*, 67:10-22, 1988.

2. *Brain Diseases -- Drug Abuse and Others*

Alcoholism

Alcoholism is a drug addiction to a substance that is metabolized like sugar and has the antianxiety effect of Valium. Alcohol is also a mild depressant. Hence, alcoholics usually have hypoglycemia (low blood sugar) and brain biochemical imbalances. Addicts to Valium, Xanax, or Librium are often called "dry drunks."

Nutritionally, alcoholics are depleted in virtually all nutrients, especially magnesium, B-vitamins, zinc, and selenium. Decreases in thiamine are related to memory loss and increasing tolerance to alcohol. Alcoholics usually need antianxiety or anticonvulsant medication (e.g., Klonopin), antidepressants or lithium in order to taper off alcohol. Taurine, GABA, inositol, tryptophan, and niacin (possible antianxiety nutrients) may supplement medication. Tegretol is particularly effective for reducing cravings for alcohol in individuals with mood swings.

Several researchers have also suggested that primrose oil or borage oil and/or niacin can help to reduce cravings for alcohol. Disulfiram (Antabuse), a sulfur compound, seems to decrease appetite for alcohol, yet its side effects, especially when combined with alcohol, can be deadly. Vitamin B-6 prevents the side effect of raising the cholesterol. To discover an alcoholic, an alcoholic screening test has been used.

Alcoholics become addicted for biochemical, psychological, and spiritual reasons. We can now treat the biochemical causes. Spiritually, Alcoholics Anonymous teaches the knowledge of a higher power. Twelve-step programs have been used for effective treatment of alcoholics. Psychologically, alcoholics need training in coping mechanisms.

The Amino Acid Blood Test

For a discussion of testing for the blood levels of amino acids, the building blocks of brain neurotransmitters necessary to brain health, see Section 19, p. 301.

Brain Fatigue

Emphasis on the brain in total functioning has been documented in a recent study on chronic fatigue syndrome. Dr. J. Goldstein of Southern California identified damage to the brain in puberty. Dr. Goldstein identified up to 4,000 patients with damage to the limbic system, which is an area that governs energy, motions, memory, and sleep. The limbic system is in the temporal region of the brain, deep within the temporal lobes. He was able to pick out scans that show abnormalities to the temporal lobe.

We have been showing this for years in the brain electrical activity map and are thankful to our patients who continue to alert us that the brain controls the body's energy level.

DHEA -- Adrenopause -- Protecting Your Brain

At the American Psychiatric Association, Biological Psychiatry Division, a new study was presented showing that low levels of DHEA correlate the cognitive deficit semantic and memory processes can be inhibited. Low levels of DHEA are associated with memory loss.

Low DHEA, like low thyroid, is a marker of aging and dying.

Benzodiazepine Addiction

In our society, in which addiction to alcohol, cocaine, heroin, marijuana, cigarettes, and caffeine has increasingly been held in low esteem, other ways of healing have been and will continue to be sought for abnormalities in brain chemistry. Therefore, other legal and medically appropriate addictions are occurring in our society.

Some people are getting addicted to 900 numbers and gambling; a great majority, particularly women who suffer from anxiety, are becoming addicted to Xanax, Librium, Valium, Halcion, Dalmane, etc. Fortunately, there is one benzodiazepine that is relatively nonaddictive -- namely, clonazepam. But the majority of these women need, instead, to treat their brain chemistry with an antidepressant, anticonvulsant, or Cranial Electrical Stimulation device, and, in some cases, even an antipsychotic would be preferable, because an abnormal brain chemistry leads to a craving for temporary healing through addiction.

Unfortunately, the addiction leads to increasing deterioration of health functions. Frequently, individuals who are addicted to benzodiazepines lose interest in sex, become carbohydrate addicts, gain a lot of weight, have slow mentation, frequently visit doctors, and have all the symptoms of anxiety and depression, even during periods when they are not using a drug to a great degree, and even when using the drug ceases to satisfy. We have consistently been able to remove benzodiazepines with a program of brain rehabilitation. The first step is to understand brain health through brain mapping and to get the individual who is afflicted to make a positive step and recognize that the drug has one hooked. CES with the amino acid GABA (all benzodiazepines work through the brain's natural GABA receptors) or hydroxytryptophan is probably the best natural route to follow, although diet, e.g., no caffeine, no liquor, etc., is also important.

Adrenalin and the Brain

The brain's neurotransmitter system produces two extremely important neurotransmitters, Adrenalin (epinephrine) and serotonin. Accumulation or depletion of either of these substances are thought to play a major role in virtually every psychological illness, including major depression and schizophrenia. Accumulation of neurotransmitters can be caused by amino acids, and drugs like antidepressants and anticonvulsants. Depletion of neurotransmitters can occur from stressful situations, med-ications, and organic disorders. Their depletion is associated with the increased use of Valium, Benzodiazepin and alcohol.

Repletion of these neurotransmitters occurs at an increased rate when the body is provided with a diet high in amino acids, the substates, or fuel, of the brain's neurotransmitter system.

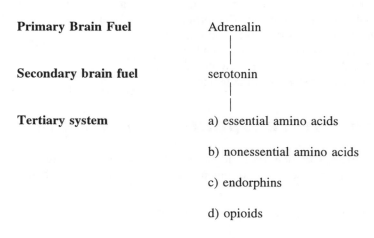

Primary Brain Fuel	Adrenalin
Secondary brain fuel	serotonin
Tertiary system	a) essential amino acids
	b) nonessential amino acids
	c) endorphins
	d) opioids

Brain Mapping: A Short Guide to Interpretation, Philosophy, and Future [1]

INTRODUCTION

Quantitative studies of EEG and evoked response, including spectral analysis and topographic mapping, are becoming increasingly popular in clinical practice. Recent studies have shown these techniques to be useful in cerebrovascular disease, [1][2] epilepsy, [3][4] headaches, [5] mass lesions, [6] and head injuries. [7] Perhaps the most important application has been in documenting organicity in patients with psychiatric syndromes or learning disabilities. [8][9]

Brain electrical activity mapping (BEAM), including computerized EEG and cortical evoked potentials, has demonstrated subtle neurological abnormalities in patients with schizophrenia, [10][11][12][13][14] depression, Parkinson's, Alzheimer's, [15] toxic exposures, [16][17] and more. Brain mapping is also useful in analyzing and assessing the function of drugs given to patients. [18] In many situations, the quantitative/topographical approach may be more sensitive than conventional test modalities, such as standard EEG, CT scanning, MRI, and neuropsychiatric testing. [19][20][21] Moreover, brain mapping may also be useful in monitoring patients having undergone neurosurgery or cardiovascular surgery. [22]

Brain mapping is a great medical breakthrough which "medicalizes" psychiatry. [24]

COMPONENTS

The ideal brain map is a full spectrum BEAM, which can be obtained by applying the principles from the Spectrum invented by E. Roy Johns, Ph.D., at NYU, and the BEAM invented by Frank Dully, M.D., at Harvard University. We utilize the BEAM with the full spectral components (Table 1) which were first developed as part of the SPECTRUM. Brain mapping consists of a computerized EEG (electroencephalograph), spectral computerized analysis of frequency bands, an auditory evoked potential (AER), and a visual evoked potential (VER), along with numerous spectral and accessory tests or components.

The P300 is part of the auditory evoked potential, and at 300 milliseconds there is a peak. There are many other periods of time (latencies) which may be measured in terms of an evoked potential response. Hence, there are a variety of brain stress tests (reaction of the brain when exposed to light, sound, or cognitive stresses) that can be done on the full spectrum BEAM. For example, EEG with hyperventilation and strobed or different colored lights may reveal things about the brain's ability to process information. Measuring brain waves after such stressors can be helpful just as heart stress tests reveal aspects of the heart. We hope to continue to improve upon the techniques used for measuring neurobiochemical imbalances.

IDENTIFICATION OF DISEASES

On the quantified EEG much can be learned about both diagnosis and potential treatments. For example, it is well known obsessive compulsive disorder individuals may have increased alpha waves. Drug abusers often have decreased alpha waves. There may be increased delta and theta waves in schizophrenics, although this is disputed, and deceased beta waves in Alzheimer's disease. Some researchers believe they can diagnose based on BEAM, but, more likely, each diagnosis is just a symptom of a heterogenous group of BEAM abnormalities. The effects of diseases on the spectral analysis is outlined in Table 9.

COMMENTARY ON MEDICATIONS, DRUGS, AND ELECTRICAL THERAPIES

There has been a tremendous amount of research done on the interactions of medications and EEG's. It is to be noted that individual drugs can have very different effects on different individuals' brain waves, although there are some general patterns. For example, barbiturates produce slowing of EEG background activity. Barbiturate overdose, ischemia, cortical irritability, and attention deficit disorder can be marked by the appearance of widespread beta dominance. Barbiturates increase beta activity over the anterior head region. Drugs like Dilantin overdosage enhance slow waves, such as delta and theta. Tegretol can cause a diffuse slowing. In general, anticonvulsants stabilize brain waves by decreasing beta. The dominant effect of neuroleptics is to increase delta

---

1. Reprinted by permission from *The Journal of Orthomolecular Medicine*, 5:4, 1990.

and theta, while decreasing beta and alpha activity. The dominant effect of antidepressants is to increase alpha activity and possibly all brain waves. The dominant effect of benzodiazepines is to decrease the slow waves such as slow alpha, delta, and theta, and increase the beta and alpha. The dominant effect of amphetamines, methylphenidate, and PCP is to tremendously decrease delta and theta.

Some other common drug effects include temporary increase in alpha which occurs with many addictive drugs, including morphine, heroin, and marijuana. There can be delta bursts with PCP (phencyclidine), and it should be noted that THC (Tetrahydrocannabinol), the active ingredient in marijuana, will actually decrease beta frequency. Overall, drugs can significantly affect quantified EEG's [25] (Tables 3-6).

Estrogen may increase seizures. Tyrosine may increase estrogen and therefore promote seizures, while progesterone decreases seizures. Steroids increase both tryptophan and tyrosine and raise blood sugar and help encephalopathy. Testosterone levels decrease thyroid, and estrogen increases thyroid. To identify the meaning of abnormalities on brain mapping it is important to know approximately what each region of the brain does.

PHYSIOLOGICAL ABNORMALITIES ASSOCIATED WITH ANATOMICAL REGIONS OF BRAIN IN CORRELATION WITH BEHAVIOR ON BEAM

Brain mapping can give clues in terms of treatment as well as to diagnosis of brain illnesses. Anyone with any type of serious behavioral disorder or deficit should have a brain map. In fact, brain mapping should probably be done on everyone as part of a total health check up. The brain is the most important part of the body and affects all diseases. A healthy brain is the first priority on the PATH to wellness.

Generally speaking, left hemisphere dysfunctions will largely impact language processing areas. These findings are generally suggested by increased delta and theta activity on spectral analysis, as well as excessive reactivity during auditory and visual stimulation components of the BEAM. Mid-temporal and posterior temporal are more likely to impact specific language and language processing functions and may also be seen in individuals with central auditory processing disorders, which are further and more clearly defined with speech and language assessments. More anterior left hemisphere dysfunction will likely impact language production (i.e., Broca's area involvement and aphasic disorders), as well as difficulty in learning and

executing a sequence task.

Right hemisphere disturbances may be frequently associated with emotional modulation difficulty and impulse control disorders. Most characteristic is episodic dyscontrol which may have a high correlation with physiologic disturbances in right anterior regions, specifically right anterior temporal and right frontal areas. These findings typically include increased theta activity on the spectral analysis and excessive reactivity in both auditory and visual stimulation components. Typically, the excessive reactivity occurs between a 150 and 350 milliseconds time frame and takes the form of excessive amplitude or aberrant wave forms in these regions. Right posterior physiologic dysfunctions may clinically be associated with visual-spatial analysis difficulties and the appreciation of social cues such as subtleties of individual facial expressions. Visual evoked responses showing excessive reactivity in these areas may therefore be correlated with these clinical findings.

EEG findings carry unusual implication of seizure disorders, but EEG's are frequently normal in the face of abnormal physiologic changes identified by spectral analysis and evoked potentials and are corroborated with neuropsychological and speech and language data.

Brain mapping reveals various effects of disease and drugs on brain mapping (Table 7). Tables 8-10 review regions of brain function which give clues to pathology.

PRESCRIPTION ELECTRICITY

The most exciting development in the field of BEAM research is that amino acids and electrical methods can more naturally change brain waves. Amino acids (phenylalanine, tyrosine, and tryptophane) affect alpha waves in particular. Other research is needed to help tailor nutrients to brain wave abnormalities. Also exciting is the concept of changing brain waves by cranial electrical stimulation (CES). The FDA has permitted the CES device for use in treating insomnia, anxiety, and depression. Our preliminary results have shown that, based on which device is used, we can demonstrate the ability to correct imbalances in delta, beta, anti-alpha waves. Furthermore, the electrical imbalances of substance abuse can be corrected. The age of prescription electricity for the brain seems to be dawning. [26] [27]

BRAIN REJUVENATION

Brain rejuvenation may sound like a faddish term, but in some ways it is a truism of advanced medical science. As the human brain ages or becomes diseased, it has reductions in neurotransmitters and functional neurons. Through neurotransmitter manipulation, amino acids, and nutrients, we are able to rejuvenate the memory in various individuals and improve their mental functioning. Virtually all aging is associated with some memory loss and neurological deterioration. Alzheimer's (senile dementia) has been increasing in our society, and we expect even more organic brain diseases to become prevalent due to the prevalence of toxins such as lead, mercury, pesticides, organics, etc., as well as drug abuse. Brain rejuvenation techniques may be augmented by bioelectrical devices, amino acid supplementation, and neurotransmitter augmenting medications. The neurotransmitter systems can be built up and rejuvenated by nutrients in a number of ways. Nutrients rejuvenate the brain and increase the levels that age, stress, and drug abuse have depleted, as well as balance an individual's neurotransmitters that have been deficient since birth. [28] Rejuvenation of the brain after drug abuse is another prime and critical example of the technique of reversing brain disease. [29] Tables 11 and 12 describe the relationship between drugs, nutrients, and brain chemistry, i.e., neurotransmitters.

PHILOSOPHY OF BRAIN MAPPING: AN ANALYSIS OF CONSCIOUSNESS

One can speculate that brain electrical mapping device or BEAM is a measurement of consciousness. Normally, beta and alpha waves are indicative of conscious processes, and theta and delta waves are indicative of unconscious processes. Abnormalities in brain waves are indicative of problems of consciousness. Consciousness raising in some ways is the proper balance of all levels of consciousness so that it can be raised mutually and jointly. We now know that in certain conditions medications that relieve anxiety or depression can raise beta waves, while antipsychotics decrease them. A person who has an excess of beta waves might be said to have a lack of tranquility. Unreality, irritability, hyperactivity, anesthesia, and ischemia produce increases in beta waves. We also know that an absence of alpha waves (alpha waves can be increased by certain techniques that relax the brain) can symbolize a lack of creativity, imagination, etc. An excess of alpha waves can occur in an overly-compulsive person and that overly-compulsive activity may likely be antidoted by anxiety reduction techniques. Individuals with spikes in their consciousness or irregular overconcentrated consciousness might be thought to need to defocus their attention or antidote this with an anticonvulsant. Antianxiety medicines also widen out consciousness by decreasing delta and theta and increasing

alpha and beta. Deficiencies in theta and delta waves may also indicate a lack of tranquility as an excess of those waves can symbolize a lack of arousal. Both antipsychotic and antidepressants increase delta and theta waves. Excess delta and theta waves without a drug source might symbolize a person who has too much involvement with his or her unconscious. Brain waves symbolize various dimensions of our consciousness, and with knowledge and treatment of these we may get closer to our own balanced brain waves or happiness. Prescription electrical devices, with amino acids, may be the best natural way to "raise consciousness" or "heal consciousness" by changing brain waves.

SUMMARY

Brain mapping is a new technique which measures the electrical waves of the brain. It is able to diagnose and predict future prognosis of brain biochemical imbalances and provide clues to treatment of learning disabilities, Alzheimer's, schizophrenia, epilepsy, drug abuse, depression, anxiety, Parkinson's, multiple sclerosis, etc. All brain diseases are both chemical and electrophysiological in their makeup. The brain's chemistry and electrophysiology affect the immune system, appetite control, and virtually every illness interacts in the chemistry and biology of the brain. The brain is the chief organ of the body: chief endocrine gland, cardiovascular regulator, and immunodefense. Therefore, the most important part of the health of every individual is the brain's balance. Brain imbalances are a factor in virtually all diseases.

A full spectrum BEAM is the best path to brain analysis because it sheds light on brain function and helps reveal the tendency for drug abuse and many other important aspects of brain health. Brain electrical wave abnormalities are identified and this information is combined with blood testing for biochemical abnormalities to provide a complete understanding of the brain's function. A dynamic integrative treatment can then be implemented, using a nutritional, electrical, and/or drug approach. If the patient is not interested in the bioelectrical or nutritional approach, one can use a heavier biochemical treatment which can overcome the biochemical and even some of the electrical imbalances. We try to stay away from the current electrical treatments in psychiatry such as electroconvulsive shock therapy. Sledge hammer approaches with drugs (i.e., polypharmacy, overmedicating) or shock therapy can often be replaced by more subtle treatments. The ideal treatment of all brain disease is both electrical and biochemical (bioelectrical) because the brain is electrical and biochemical. Eventually we hope to develop a collection site which will go into the various physicians' offices where individuals will be able to have brief brain wave checks as a measure of their brain health.

ADDENDUM ON BEAM TEST AND MEDICATIONS

All brain mapping patients, unless they are completely broken down, should stop all medications 24 hours before the Beam test. If the patient is unstable in any way, they should call Randy Gunsel or speak with Dr. Braverman directly.

REFERENCES

1. Ahn SS, Jordan SE, Nuwer MR, Computerized EEG topographic brain mapping. Moore W., (ed.). *Surgery for Cerebrovascular Disease.* New York: Churchill Livingstone, 1987, 275-280.
2. Nuwer MR, Jordan SE, Ahn SS, Evaluation of stroke using EEG frequency analysis and topographic mapping. *Neurology,* 37:1153-1159, 1987.
3. Kowell AP, Reveler MJ, Nuwer MR, Topographic mapping of EEG and evoked potentials in epileptic patients. *J Clin Neurophysiol,* 4:233-234, 1987.
4. Nuwer MR, Frequency analysis and topographic mapping of EEG and evoked potentials in epilepsy. *Electroenceph Clin Neurophysiol,* 69:118-126, 1988.
5. Braverman ER, Remission of forty years of headaches with divalproex sodium. *Brain Dysfunct,* 2:55, 1989.
6. Nagata K, Gross C, Kindt G, Geier J, Adey G, Topographic electroencephalographic study with power ratio index mapping in patients with malignant brain tumors. *Neurosurg,* 17:613-619, 1985.
7. Houshmand W, Director K, Becknet E, Radfar F, Topographic brain mapping in head injuries. *J Clin Neurophysiol,* 4:228-229, 1987.
8. Duffy FH, The BEAM method for neurophysiological diagnosis. *Ann NY Acad Sci,* 457:19-34, 1985.
9. Duffy FH, *Brain Electrical Activity Mapping: Issues and Answers.* Topographic Mapping of Brain Electrical Activity, Duffy, FH (ed.), Boston: Butterworth, 401-418, 1986.
10. Daniels EK, et al., Patterns of thought disorder associated with right cortical damage, schizophrenia, and mania. *Amer Journal of Psychiatry,* 145:944-918, 1988.
11. Stoudemire A, et al., Interictal schizophrenia-like psychoses in temporal lobe epilepsy. *Psychosoma,* 24:331-338, 1983.
12. Braverman ER, Brain electrical activity mapping in treatment resistant schizophrenics. *J Orthom Med,* 5(1):46-48, 1990.
13. Morstyn R, et al., Altered P300 topography in schizophrenia. *Arch Gen Psychiatry,* 40:729-734, 1983.
14. Karson CN, et al., Computed electroencephalographic activity mapping in schizophrenia. *Arch Gen Psychiatry,* 14:514-517, 1987.
15. Duffy FH, et al., Brain electrical activity in patients with presenile and senile dementia of the Alzheimer type. *Annals of Neurology,* 16:439-448, 1984.
16. Bernad PG, Review: EEG and pesticides, *Clin Electroenceph* 20: ix-x, 1989.
17. Knoll O, et al., EEG indicates aluminum load in long term hemodialysis patients, *Trace Elements in Med.* 1:54-58,1984.
18. Saletu B, et al., Topographic brain mapping EEG in neuropsychopharmacology - Part II, Clinical applications (Pharmaco EEG imaging), *Meth and Find Expt Clin Pharm* 9:385-408, 1987.
19. Lombroso CT, Duffy FH, Brain electrical activity mapping as an adjunct to CT scanning, Advances in Epileptology, XIth Epilepsy International Symposium, Cangor R, Angeheri F, Pentry JK (eds.), New York: Raven Press, 83-88, 1982
20. Fisch BJ, Pedley TA, Keller DL, A topographic background symmetry display for comparison wilt routine EEG, *Electroenceph Clin Neurophysiology,* 69:491-494, 1988.
21. Nuwer MR, Frequency analysis and topographic mapping of EEG and evoked potentials in epilepsy. *Electroenceph Clin Neurophysiol,* 69:118-126, 1988.
22. John ER, et al., Monitoring brain function during cardiovascular surgery: Hypoperfusion vs Microembolism as the major cause of neurological damage during cardiopulmonary bypass, *Heart & Brain,* 405-421, 1989.
23. John ER, et al., Real-time intraoperative monitoring during neurosurgical and neuroradiological procedures, *J Clin Neurophysio,* 125-158, 1989.
24. Garber HJ, Weilburg JB, Duffy FH, Clinical use of topographic brain electrical activity mapping in psychiatry, *J Clin Psychiatry,* 50:205-211, 1989.
25. Herman WM, Itil TM, *Biological Psychiatry Today,* Obiols, et al., (ed.), Elselvier, North Holland: Medical Press, 1317-1327, 1979.
26. Braverman ER, Blum K, Smayda RJ, A commentary on brain mapping in sixty substance abusers: Can the potential for drug abuse be predicted and prevented by treatment? *Curr Ther Res,* October 1990.

27. Braverman ER, Smith RB, Smayda RJ, Blum K, Modifications of P300 amplitude and other electrophysiological parameter of drug abuse by cranial electrical stimulation (CES), *Curr Ther Res*, October 1990.
28. Braverman ER, Pfeiffer CC, *The Healing Nutrients Within*, New Cannan: Keats Publishing, 1987.
29. Blum K, A commentary on neurotransmitter restoration as a common mode of treatment for alcohol, cocaine and opiate abuse, *Integr Psychiatry* 6:199-204, 1989.

Table 1

BEAM Components

EEG	P300 (Oddball Paradigm)
Spectral Analysis	Statistical Tests
AER	(comparing one BEAM to another)
VER	

Full Spectral Components

Total Frequency, Power and Percent Power
Coefficient of Variation and % Coefficient of Variation
Asymmetry and % Asymmetry
Coherence and Phase Coherence

Supplemental Components

Hyperventilation	Brain Stem Evoked Potentials
Coloured Lights	P200, N100, N450, etc.

Table 2
Clinical Diseases and QEEG

	Alzheimer's	Hyperactivity	Parkinson's	Drug Abuse	Schizophrenia	Depression	Hepatic Coma
Beta	▼	▲				▼	▼
Alpha	▼		▼	▼		▼	▼
Theta	▼▲				▲	▼	▲
Delta	▼▲				▲	▼	▲

Table 3
The Effects of Drugs on QEEG

	30 mg. Chlorprothixene	75 mg. Imipramine	10 mg. Diazepam	250 mg. Caffeine	600 mg. Pyritinol
Beta1	▼		▲		
Beta2	▼	▲	▲	▼	▲
Beta3	▼	▲	▲	▲	▲
Alpha-Fast	▼				▲
Alpha-Slow		▲		▼	▲
Theta	▲	▲	▼		▲
Delta	▲	▲	▼		▲

Table 4
The Effects of Drugs on QEEG

	L-Dopa	L-Phenylalanine	Anticonvulsants	Estrogen	Progesterone
Beta					
Alpha-Fast	▲	▲	▼	▲	▼
Alpha-Slow			▲	▼	▲
Theta					
Delta					

Table 5
The Effects of Drugs on QEEG

	Inderal	Aspirin	Chlortrimeton	Oxiractam	Prednisone
Beta1					▲
Beta2					
Beta3		▼			
Alpha-Fast	▲			▲	
Alpha-Slow		▼		▲	
Theta		▲	▲	▼	
Delta	▼		▲	▼ .	

Table 6
The Effects of Drugs on QEEG

	Elavil	Antimotion Scopolamine	Lithium	Prozac	Cocaine	Amphetamines
Beta	▲		▼		▲	▲
Alpha	▼	▼▼	▼		▲	▲
Theta	▲	?▼	▲?			
Delta	▲	?▼	▲			

Table 7
The Effects of Disease on Brain Regions

	Depression	Schizophrenia	Cocaine	Marijuana	Alcohol	Lead	Dyslexia
Frontal		X		X	XX		
Temporal	X	X	X		X	X	X
Parietal	X	X	X		X		
Occipital	X		X				

Table 8
Frontal Lobe — Behavioural Effects

Aphasia
Auditory Hallucination and
    Illusion
Psychotic Behaviour

Aggression
Rage Reaction
Apathy
Placidity

Table 9
Temporal Lobe — Behavioural Effects

Difficulties in Adapting
Loss of Initiative
Lack of Tact
Bland Affect

Labile Mood
Rigidity of Thinking
Lack of Ability to Sit Still
Lack of Problem Solving Ability

Table 10
Parietal Lobe — Behavioural Effects

Disorders of Language
Memory Loss
Emotional Ability

Loss of Logic
Loss of Emotional Well-Being

Table 11

Neurotransmitter/ central action	Drug of abuse that affects neurotransmitter action	Central location
Gamma Aminobutyric acid (GABA) General inhibition of other neurotransmitters	Alcohol Barbiturates Benzodiazepines Chloral hydrate Ethchlorvynol Meprobamate Methaqualone (?) Phencyclidine	Throughout brain
Acetylcholine Counterbalances dopamine Maintains memory Initiates short-term memory	Phencyclidine	Caudate nucleus Lentiform nucleus Cerebral cortex Nucleus basalis of Meynert Nigrostriatal tract Reticular activating substance
Norepinephrine Modulates mood Maintains sleeping state	Amphetamines Cocaine Opiates Phencyclidine	Nucleus locus ceruleus Pontine and medullary cell groups
Dopamine Counterbalances acetylcholine Stimulates pleasure center Modulates mood Affects intellectual processes Inhibits prolactin release	Amphetamines Cocaine Phencyclidine	Caudate nucleus Lentiform nucleus Nucleus accumbens Basal Ganglia Tuberoinfundibular pathway Nigrostriatal tract
Serotonin Modulates mood Initiates sleep Involved in REM sleep	Psychedelic agents Phencyclidine Alcohol	Pontine raphe nuclei
Beta-Endorphin Modulates mood Modulates pain perception Inhibits norepinephrine release	Opiates Phencyclidine Nucleus locus ceruleus	Thalamus Arcuate and premamillary nuclei Hippocampus Nucleus solitarius Substantia gelatinosa

Table 12

Neurotransmitter/ central action	Nutrients that affect that action	Drugs that affect that action
Gamma Aminobutyric acid (GABA) General inhibition of other neurotransmitters	Taurine, manganese, B6, gamma-amino butyric acid, glutamine, glutamic acid	Anticonvulsants, bensodiazepines, Lioresal, Valium
Acetylcholine Counterbalances dopamine Maintains memory Initiates short-term memory	Choline, manganese, B6, lysine, threonine, niacin	Prostigmin, tetrahydroacridine Neostigmin
Norepinephrine Modulates mood Maintains sleeping state	L-dopa, tyrosine, phenylalanine, folic acid, thiamine, copper	Desipramine, Pamelor
Dopamine Counterbalances acetylcholine Stimulates pleasure center Modulates mood Affects intellectual processes Inhibits prolactin release	L-dopa, tyrosine, phenylalanine, folic acid, thiamine, copper	Desipramine, Pamelor, Parlodel, Parsidol, Symmetrel, Sinemet, Artane
Serotonin Modulates mood Initiates sleep Involved in REM sleep	Tryptophan, Zinc, B6, Niacin	Prozac, Fenfluramine, Desyrel, Alcohol
Beta-Endorphin Modulates mood Initiates sleep Involved in REM sleep	d, l-phenylalanine, branched-chain amino acids, enkephalins	Trexan heroin, alcohol
Histamine Modulates mood, appetite, sleep, immune system, cognition	Histidine, methionine, niacin, calcium, magnesium, zinc, copper, vitamin C	Periactin, Benedryl, Haldol, Elevil, ephedrine, adrenalin, terfenadine, astemizole

Reprinted from *The Journal of Orthomolecular Medicine*, 5:4, 1990.

Brain Electrical Activity Mapping (BEAM)

Brain Electrical Activity Mapping is a technique to evaluate the electrophysiological function of the brain. Computerized evaluation of the brain electrical activity is performed in the eyes open and eyes closed state (Spectral Analysis). The brain is stimulated with flashes of light (visual evoked response or VER) and clicks (auditory evoked response or AER) and the processing of this information by the brain is tracked by computer. The data is compared with normalized age and sex controls, and the statistical probability mapping of the abnormalities is demonstrated on color maps of the brain. The technique is particularly effective even in the presence of a completely normal EEG. Brain function is evaluated, unlike imaging, such as MRI, which shows anatomy but not function. While many causes of brain dysfunction, such as tumor, infection, stroke, degenerative disease, and trauma can be detected, the greatest use of the technique is to detect brain dysfunction, that is not able to be detected by other means. Changes can be followed sequentially over time.

Head trauma is sometimes associated with brain dysfunction and accompanied by normal neurological, MRI and other tests. Brain Electrical Activity Mapping will often show areas of malfunction giving objective evidence of brain dysfunction.

Disorders for which BEAM testing can give useful information:

- Any so-called treatment-resistant psychiatric condition
- Head trauma
- Change in behavior
- Alzheimer's disease
- Parkinson's disease
- Dyslexia
- Schizophrenia
- Surgical or anesthesia injury
- Any psychotic condition
- Abnormal EEG
- Temporal lobe disorder
- Mood swings
- Whiplash
- Personality disorder
- Depression
- Anxiety
- Cerebral allergies

In PATH's laboratory, Brain Electrical Activity Mapping includes the following:

(1) BEAM EEG. This is a detailed EEG and differs from the "routine" in the following ways:

    (a) Recorded for 3-4 times as long.
    (b) Many more electrodes are used to sample the data.
    (c) Many artifact channels are used simultaneously to assist in the interpretation of electrical events recorded from the scalp.

(2) BEAM Spectral Analysis (computerized EEG). The EEG data is processed by the computer, artifact is removed and the data is displayed in the form of a map of the electrical activity of the brain. In this way electrical activity is shown which the human eye is often not able to appreciate. This leads to more accurate diagnosis and less human interpreter error.

(3) BEAM Visual Evoked Responses (VER)

(4) BEAM Auditory Evoked Responses (AER)

These latter two tests probe the brain by stimulating with light or sound respectively and provide information about the way in which the brain processes information; this information cannot be obtained in any other way. This testing differs from conventional VER and AER (or BAER) in the following ways:

    (a) The hemispheres of the brain, where most of the processing of information occurs, are tested.
    (b) Numerous channels (electrodes) sample this activity allowing an easily viewed image of the electrical function of the brain to be demonstrated.
    (c) The processing of the stimulus by the brain can be followed as if it were a "movie" or "cartoon" enabling the sequence of events to be easily understood. The function of the brain can thus be studied, not only in terms of the voltage generated, but also the exact timing and the location can be determined as the stimulus passes through the brain.

These four tests, plus the P300 and CES challenge, together provide a very comprehensive testing of the electrical function of the brain and help us to understand brain processing of information, diagnose dysfunction of the brain and its causes in some instances, locate the problem, and also provide a quantitative measure to follow progress of disease or treatment.

BEAM EEG (Electroencephalography)

All BEAM data are collected via a series of electrodes attached according to the International Ten-Twenty Electrode Placement System. Precise placement of the 18 electrodes is necessary. All electrodes are measured and located with a precision of 2 mm. Movement is minimized by attachment of the electrodes with collodion or with the use of the electrocap system. All electrophysiological data are collected with a linked ear reference. BEAM has the capability of digitally remontaging all collected data and playing it on the penwriter. Electrodes are used for recording electrophysiological data. A number of electrodes is also attached to the patient to monitor for myogenic and eye movement artifact. The electrodes are attached at the following locations: one below each eye, one at each zygomatic arch, and two at the base of the neck. These data channels are essential for identifying potential sources of artifact that can lead to erroneous interpretations.

Accurately calibrated amplifiers are used. The calibration signal is generated internally by the BEAM computer and introduced into the EEG amplifiers at the same point that the signals recorded from a patient are normally introduced into the system. The DC offset in each channel is recorded. A precise 10 Hz sine wave is generated within the main BEAM computer and passed through a precision 12-bit D/A converter. This signal is then sent to each individual channel. This sine wave then passes through the entire BEAM system, being treated exactly as incoming electrophysiological data. BEAM then performs a Fast Fourier Transform (FFT) on the data recorded from each channel. The resulting power spectra are then atomically examined by the system and compared to a known power spectrum of a 10 Hz sine wave. Should any individual channel be found to differ slightly from the calibration standard, this automatically prepares a compensation table which results in all channels being precisely matched.

The computer utilized is the Masscomp Minicomputer with 32-bit virtual memory CPU, 2 Mb ECC memory, 650 Kb floppy disk drive and a 160 Mb Winchester hard disk drive, independent graphics processor, streaming tape with controller, keyboard and 15" monochrome monitor with touch screen, color monitor, real time Unix operating system, 32-channel acquisition system, 26 channel penwriter, evoked potential stimulus system, normative database, and color printer.

Continuous EEG data are collected by the system and stored on a 160 Mb Winchester disk. All EEG records are reviewed on the computer screen prior to further analysis. Artifact is removed prior to processing. A complete paper record with the raw data is produced during data acquisition and is interpreted prior to the BEAM topographic analysis and is often referred to during the topographic analysis. The EEG obtained in this way is obtained from many hours of patient study and provides an extremely comprehensive electroencephalographic evaluation of the patient. This record plays an important part in both the evaluation of the patient and aids in the interpretation of the computerized data.

BEAM Topography
EEG Spectral Analysis

(Computerized EEG)

Spectral analysis by the Fast Fourier Transform (FFT) technique is performed on EEG data recorded from a minimum of 20 (18 plus 2 reference) scalp electrodes. Data in the frequency bands of delta (0.0-3.5 Hz), theta (4.0-7.5 Hz), alpha (8.0-11.5 Hz), beta1 (12.0-15.5 Hz), beta2 (16.0-19.5 Hz), beta3 (20.0-23.5 Hz), and beta4 (24.0-27.5 Hz) are individually evaluated. Topographic maps of spectral analyzed EEG are created under computer control after removal, upon visual inspection, of segments containing artifact. Results are viewed on a color data terminal. For spectral images, data are scaled and displayed in a pseudo color format (rainbow colors). Lowest values are black and highest values are red to white. Deviation from normal is displayed in Significance Probability Maps (SPM) with red-orange indicating values above control group mean values and blue indicating values below control values.

References for BEAM and Nutrition:
How the Brain Waves are Corrected

1. Tucker DM, Penland JG, Sandstead HH, Milne DB, Heck DG, Klevay L. Nutrition status and brain function in aging. *Am J Clin Nutr*, 52-93-102, 1990.

2. Thatcher RW, Cantor DS. Electrophysiological Techniques in the Assessment of Malnutrition. RSDA

3. Peirano P, Fagioli I, Singh BB, Salzarulo. Quiet Sleep and Slow Wave Sleep in Malnourished Infants. *Brain Dysfunct*, 3:80-83, 1990.

4. Riekkinen P, Buzsaki G, Riekkinen Jr., P, Soininen H, Partanen J. The cholinergic system and KEG slow waves. *Electro and Clin Neuro*, 78:89-96, 1991.

5. Christensen L, Bourgeois A, Cockroft R. Dietary Alteration of Somatic Symptoms and Regional Brain Electrical Activity. *Biol Psych*, 29:679-682, 1991.

6. Kirby AW, Wiley RW, Harding TH. Cholinergic Effects on the Visual Evoked Potential. *Evoked Potentials*, 26:296-306, 1986.

7. Zemon V., Kaplan E, Ratliff F. The Role of GABA-Mediated Intracortical Inhibition in the Generation of Visual Evoked Potentials. *Evoked Potentials*, 25:287-295, 1986.

8. Bodis-Wollner I, Onofrj MC, Marx MS, Mylin LH. Visual Evoked Potentials in Parkinson'sDisease: spatial Frequency, Temporal Rate, Contrast, and the Effect of Dopaminergic Drugs. *Evoked Potentials*, 27:307-319, 1986.

9. Begleiter H, Porjesz B. The P300 Component of the Event-Related Brain Potential in Psychiatric Patients. *Evoked Potentials*, 49:529-535, 1986.

10. Thatcher RW, McAlaster R, Lester ML, Cantor DS. Comparisons among KEG, hair Minerals and Diet Predictions of Reading Performance in Children. *Annals of the New York Academy of Science*, vol. 433.

11. Lester ML, Horst RL, Thatcher RW. Protective Effects of Zinc and Calcium Against Heavy Metal Impairment of Children's Cognitive function. *Nutrition and Behavior*, 3:145-161, 1986.

12. Thatcher RW, Lester ML, McAlaster R, Horst R. Effects of Low Levels of Cadmium and Lead on Cognitive Functioning in Children. *Environmental Health*, vol. 37, no. 3:159-166, 1982.

13. Thatcher RW, Walker RA, Guidice S. Human Cerebral Hemispheres Develop at different Rates and Ages. *Am Asso for the Advancement of Sc.*, 236:1110-1113, 1987.

14. Struve FA, Straumanis JJ. Electroencephalographic and Evoked Potential Methods in Human Marihuana Research: Historical Review and Future Trends. *Drug Dev Res*, 09:48:19, 1990.

An Analysis of Consciousness

The brain-mapping device or BEAM is a measurement of consciousness. Normally beta and alpha waves are conscious processes and theta and delta waves are normally unconscious processes. Abnormalities in brain waves indicate problems in the person's consciousness. Consciousness-raising, in some ways, is the proper balance of all levels of consciousness so that it can be raised mutually and jointly. So we now know that in certain conditions medications that relieve anxiety or depression can raise beta waves while antipsychotic drugs decrease them. A person who has an excess of beta waves has a lack of tranquility. Unreality, irritability, hyperactivity, anesthesia, and ischemia produce increases in beta waves.

We also know that an absence of alpha waves, which can be increased by certain techniques that relax the brain, can symbolize a lack of creativity, imagination, etc.

An excess of alpha waves can occur in an overly compulsive person and that overly compulsive person can be helped by several anxiety reduction techniques. Religious rituals may increase alpha waves, as most obsessive compulsive rituals increase alpha waves. An individual with spikes in his consciousness or irregular overconcentrated consciousness needs to defocus his attention or antidote this with an anticonvulsant. Antianxiety medicines also widen out consciousness by decreasing delta and theta and increasing alpha and beta. Since an excess of delta and theta waves usually reflect a low level of arousal, it follows that a deficiency in these waves indicate a lack of tranquility. Both antipsychotic and antidepressant drugs increase delta and theta waves. Thus, brain waves represent various dimensions of our consciousness.

Imaging the Brain

BEAM is a Good Imaging Modality for:

- Seizures
- Ataxia
- Chronic headaches or migraines
- Vertigo
- Hearing loss
- Congenital abnormalities
- Dementia
- Parkinson's disease

- Head trauma
- Visual disturbances
- Progressive and intermittent neurologic defects
- Any psychiatric condition
- Increased intracranial pressure
- Suspected multiple sclerosis
- Acute neurologic defects (stroke)

The BEAM tests the function of the brain while MRI and CAT scans test the anatomy of the brain.

P300 Test

P300 stands for a positive brain wave, generated during brain mapping, that occurs at 300 milliseconds (about 1/3 of second to process information) during an oddball paradigm during which an irregular series of beeps are heard. This can also be done through a visual or auditory stimulus. P300's are low in individuals who have narcolepsy, attention deficit disorders (ADD), schizophrenia, alcohol or cocaine abuse, or chronic organic depression from biochemical imbalance or even Alzheimer's or Parkinson's disease that can develop at any age. Low P300's have been correlated to high risk for developing Alzheimer's disease, as well as a high risk for depression, anxiety, and probably a host of other illnesses including cancer. P300's are also low in the prison population because individuals who cannot concentrate will have trouble coping. Nonetheless, an isolated P300 abnormality with the rest of the BEAM being abnormal is frequently more marked by chronic depression and chronic neuropsychiatric problems than criminal and drug behavior. In drug users, low P300 is more commonly abnormal than the visual, auditory, eyes open/eyes closed stress test portions of the BEAM.

P300 Voltage	Condition
0-3	Cocaine use; and often, brain damaged children
4-5	Severe ADD, narcolepsy, schizophrenia, alcoholism, severe hypoglycemia
5-7	Moderate brain disorders, hypoglycemia, and food addiction
8-9	Food addiction, depression, mild to moderate ADD, hypoglycemia
10-12	Borderline -- probably normal
12-16	Normal

The time of delay in P300 time, i.e., 350-370 msec. (milliseconds), is also common in depression, anxiety, ADD. Neurological conditions (e.g.), Alzheimer's and Parkinson's disease, bypass patients, surgical patients, and head trauma patients have severe delays, e.g., 370-420 msec.

The real meaning of an abnormal P300, like an abnormal cholesterol, must be interpreted in light of the patient's entire health, as shown, for example, in the patient's medical records, BEAM results, and psychological test results.

Variables That Affect
Individual Subject P300 Measurements

VARIABLE	P300 AMPLITUDE		P300 LATENCY	
	Polich	**Braverman**	**Polich**	**Braverman**
Age	yes	yes	yes	yes
Cognitive ability	no	small	yes	small
Gender	small	no	no	no
Menstrual cycle	no	no	no	no
Time-of-day	indirect	small	indirect	small
Recency of food	yes	small	small	no
Body temperature	no	small	yes	small
Season of the year	yes	small	no	no
Personality	yes	small	no	no

See: John Polich, P300 in Clinical Applications: Meaning, Method, and Measurement. *Am. J. EEG Technol.*, 31:201-231, 1991.

P300 Diagnosis Based on Voltage and Time

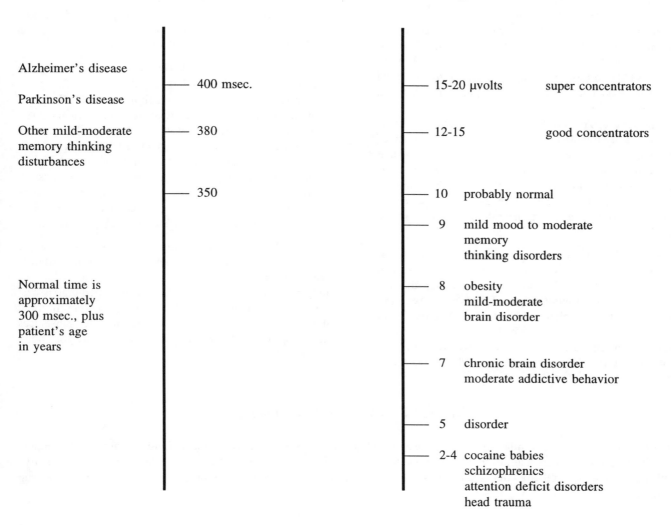

Alzheimer's disease

—— 400 msec.   —— 15-20 μvolts   super concentrators

Parkinson's disease

Other mild-moderate
memory thinking   —— 380   —— 12-15   good concentrators
disturbances

—— 350   —— 10   probably normal

—— 9   mild mood to moderate
memory
thinking disorders

Normal time is
approximately   —— 8   obesity
300 msec., plus   mild-moderate
patient's age   brain disorder
in years

—— 7   chronic brain disorder
moderate addictive behavior

—— 5   disorder

—— 2-4 cocaine babies
schizophrenics
attention deficit disorders
head trauma

Nutrients and Drugs that Can Change P300

Nutrients

- 5-hydroxytryptophan
- Amino Stim (DLPA, methionine, tyrosine)
- Choline
- Phosphoserine
- Thiamine
- N-acetyl-carnitine

Drugs

- Eldepryl
- Anticonvulsants
- Antidepressants
- Benzodiazepines

Hormones and Procedures

- Progesterone
- CES
- Biofeedback

Behavioral Disorders

PATH has pioneered documentation of the information that most serious behavioral disorders can be correlated with brain electrical activity imbalances. We use Harvard Medical School's device, the Brain Electrical Activity Map (BEAM), to discover, diagnose, and study electrical imbalances associated with anxiety, depression, insomnia, and other types of brain disorders ranging from schizophrenia to Alzheimer's disease. These conditions are often easily treatable with anticonvulsants (medicines which stabilize brain activity). We should not assume that just because a person has a brain arrhythmia, or a disorder often called cerebral dysrhythmia, that he or she is having psychological problems, any more than we assume that someone who has a heart arrhythmia is a heartless individual.

Physical disorders of the brain can occur independently or may exist in a mutual dependence with psychological factors. We have found, however, that the so-called anticonvulsants (Dilantin [phenytoin], Tegretol, Klonopin, phenobarbital, Mysoline, Diamox, and Felbamate, among others) have had remarkable success in treating brain disorders of all types and are very safe medications when given with nutrients. Please read and enjoy the two books on Dilantin, keeping in mind that everything said about Dilantin, to a great degree, can apply to the rest of these anticonvulsants.

It is important to know that the brain rhythm approach to brain disorders is also successful using non-drug approaches. For example, Cranial Electrical Stimulation (CES), achieved with a small electrical device, can do what Dilantin does. Additional non-drug approaches are brain exercises, such as biofeedback, which often help regulate brain rhythm, and nutrients that have mild brain-regulating properties, such as GABA, inositol, melatonin, magnesium, B-6, and B-complex. In some cases, the miracle of Dilantin, in our understanding of it, can be duplicated with CES, biofeedback, and nutrients.

It should be noted, however, that some people respond to Dilantin while others respond to different medications; therefore, it is a very complex set of judgments that goes into choosing which medicine is best for you. If you are not on Dilantin, please keep in mind that it is because it was felt that there are other substances more appropriate for you that can help regulate your brain rhythm.

Addiction: Gambling

Gambling addicts are also similar to other people with addictive disorders. Many of the individuals are bipolar, manic depressives, narcissistic personalities that can respond to treatment once we show them the neurological basis of their addictive behavior. It's similar to other addictions, just in some cases more severe than food addiction and less severe than severe drug addiction.

Chronic Lead Poisoning as a Cause of Bulimia: Hair Test and Brain Electrical Activity Mapping as a Diagnostic Aid

The patient, a 24-year-old, nonsmoking female, who had been diagnosed as having an eating disorder, came to PATH for treatment. During the last three years she had worked in a lamp company using lead solder, and had become progressively depressed to the point where now she was bulimic one to two times per day. Her somatic symptoms were moderate bloating, pain in her wrist and ankles, craving for sweets and salt. She also complained of depression, irritability, nervousness, fear of people, fear in general, preference for solitude, and feelings of unimportantance. It was her opinion that her problem was primarily psychological, but her psychologist sent her to me stating that he thought her problem must be biochemical.

She had stress in the last year because of a family member who was having heart problems, and her father was also on an antidepressant. Her mother was also suffering from psychological problems. Recently, she had gone through the stress of the death of a close friend. There were more than enough factors to account for her depression, and a psychiatrist she saw suggested antidepressants which she refused. Her diet was unhealthy; she lived on pastry, salty food, caffeine, and junk foods.

In her history she stated that she had been exposed to lead. She claimed that her blood lead level had been tested at her work place and was found to be normal. Her thyroid and routine blood tests were essentially normal except for a slightly elevated cholesterol level of 244 mg/dl, slightly low white blood count of 3100/cu.mm., and her amino acid test showed that she was deficient in tryptophan. I was interested in looking at the level of zinc in her red blood cells in regard to the existing anorexia, which warranted a red blood cell trace element profile analysis. Her red blood cell lead was 0.36 ppm (normal 0.4). I did not do a blood lead test at this time since the patient reported a normal lead value. However, I did do a hair lead test to see if we could pick up a subacute lead poisoning. Her hair lead was much more than two standard deviations above the mean (96 ppm). On doing her blood lead it turned out that her blood lead was normal at a level of 16 mcg/dl, but her erythrocyte protoporphyrin was elevated at 67 mcg/dl. In fact, on checking the record from her local employer it turned out that three years prior she had an erythrocyte protoporphyrin of 8 mcg/dl and no detectable blood lead. Yet, three years later she had an erythrocyte protoporphyrin of 68 and a blood lead of 28 (our value of 16 was surprisingly lower) even though OSHA's range is 0-40 (Smith Kline's range is 0-20). She was lead poisoned by some standards. She was lead poisoned by solder.

When she was placed on D-penicillamine 250 mg. twice daily, her erythrocyte protoporphyrin fell to 50 in one week and 29 after six weeks. She immediately found relief as she continued with D-penicillamine. She has improved and her depression has lifted significantly. Her bulimic episodes have been reduced to three per week as her erythrocyte protoporphyrin continues to fall. Lead undoubtedly was a significant, if not primary, factor in her psychopathology. This is another example of how hair testing can help pick up subacute and chronic lead poisoning which causes psychiatric disease.

Her psychological inventory was particularly notable. She suffered from severe headaches under tension. Her inventory showed that she experienced the following signs of depression:

- Music did not sound harmonious anymore
- Whatever she was doing she felt she was doing something else
- Quick movements frightened her
- Sunlight seemed dazzling
- Strange ideas came into her head from nowhere
- Letters ran into each other
- Sometimes when she was reading the lines printed zigzaged up and down
- She must always be on her guard
- She would like to escape her body
- People deceived her all the time
- People acted as if she were not there
- Thoughts crowded into her mind too rapidly for discussion

- She had little respect for herself
- Voices of people sounded sharp and hard
- Everyone seems to have changed lately
- Her skin was very sensitive
- Her body was not exactly symmetrical
- She was bothered by murderous ideas
- She had a feeling of pressure and fullness in her skull
- She said she grew up too fast
- She said she was not the person her mother wanted her to be
- She loathed people who touched her
- She felt she had become a burden
- She hated herself
- She could not visualize herself older than she is now
- Without her work she would be nothing
- She felt lonesome most of the time
- She felt lost in unfamiliar places
- When she touched people's bodies they seemed unusually warm
- She dreaded to pass a graveyard
- She said her conscience gave her no rest
- She felt lost in a crowd
- She thought other people's thoughts
- She thought that she usually knew what was going to happen next
- She thought people looked younger than they really were

These are just some of her signs of depression, sensory disperception, and anxiety that disappeared with D-penicillamine treatment. One would have suspected that this would have been a straight case of some form of psychotic depression. It was really lead poisoning. The fact that it was lead poisoning was proven by the result of Brain Electrical Activity Mapping (BEAM), which demonstrated a bitemporal encephalopathy. The brain map documents why this patient did not get a total remission of her bulimia, until four months after lowering her lead level. She now has been free of bulimia for six months.

BEAM Summary

1. Complex EEG is normal. BEAM EEG spectral analysis with eyes open is abnormal due to excessive fast activity (beta two, beta three) in the left frontal pole, possibly due to muscle artifact.
2. BEAM EEG with eyes closed is normal.
3. Cerebral auditory evoked responses are abnormal due to:
    a. excessive negative activation at the vertex and in the left parietal - occipital - temporal regions;
    b. excessive positive activation at the left posterior vertex.
4. Cerebral visual evoked responses are abnormal due to:
    a. excessive positive activation in the left frontal region;
    b. excessive negative activation in the right midtemporal - parietal and right posterior parietal regions.

Conclusion

Lead caused permanent damage (bitemporal encephalopathy shown by brain mapping); hence, total remission of bulimia with antidepressants did not work, but maybe anticonvulsants will. Levels of lead in this patient are high by some labs, i.e., erythrocyte protoporphyrin was over 50, blood lead was over 25. Furthermore, psychopathology correlates perfectly with lead exposure and appearance of bulimia by psychiatric history. Hence, this patient had brain damage, i.e., bitemporal encephalopathy, shown by brain mapping, from low levels of lead over three years. Apparently the brain can recover since she is now relatively free of disease.

Chronic Fatigue Syndrome

Chronic fatigue syndrome (CFS) is not really a disease but describes a symptom for which there are many possible causes. Some of these causes include abnormalities in brain chemistry, which are treated with tyrosine, phenylalanine, and sometimes antidepressants; or seizure disorders, which are treated with anticonvulsants; anxiety disorders, which are treated with CES devices and psychotherapy; immune disorders treated through brain chemistry or allergy treatments; anemia; diabetes; thyroid and endocrinology conditions; abnormalities in the adrenal gland; infectious causes that need to be treated with antibiotics, such as Lyme Disease; rare neurological causes such as M.S. and Alzheimer's disease; or encephalopathy treated with medications. Most chronic fatigue patients tend to have a brain biochemical imbalance, which can be treated through a combination of natural and/or drug therapies. Chronic fatigue is a treatable condition and in most individuals has a primary biochemical basis in which counselling can be helpful as a support, but will not successfully treat the condition. What is CFS? CFS is defined by major, minor and physical criteria. The definition requires (1) both of two major criteria, many of 11 minor criteria, and two or three physical criteria; or, (2) two major criteria and eight minor criteria.

Major criteria are:

1. New onset of persistent or relapsing fatigue, with no previous history, which does not resolve with bed rest and is severe enough to reduce or impair average daily activity to less than 50 percent for six months.

2. Exclusion of other clinical conditions that may produce similar symptoms by a thorough evaluation, including the history, physical examination and appropriate laboratory tests.

Minor criteria (symptoms) are:

1. Mild fever.
2. Sore throat.
3. Painful cervical or axillary lymph nodes.
4. Unexplained generalized muscle weakness.
5. Muscle discomfort or myalgia.
6. Prolonged (24 hours or longer) generalized fatigue after levels of exercise that would have previously been easily tolerated by the patient.
7. Generalized headaches different from those that may have previously occurred.
8. Migratory arthralgia without joint swelling or redness.
9. Neuropsychologic complaints, which may include photophobia, visual scotomata, forgetfulness, irritability, confusion, difficulty in thinking, and depression.
10. Sleep disturbance (hypersomnia or insomnia).
11. Initial development of the main symptom complex over a few hours or a few days.

Physical criteria, which must be documented by a physician on at least two occasions that are at least one month apart, are:

1. Low-grade fever.
2. Nonexudative pharyngitis.
3. Palpable or tender cervical or axillary lymph nodes.

Chocolate Addiction

Chocolate has been used to self-medicate our low moods. Because of this pseudo-elevating effect, it was once known as the food of the gods. It is derived from cocoa beans which are fermented to rid them of their bitterness. They are then dried, cleaned and roasted to develop color, flavor and aroma. Chocolate contains phenylethylamine, known for causing emotional highs and lows associated with mood swings, love, pleasure, and indulgence. Chocolate also contains the chemical theobromine, which triggers the release of endorphins in the brain and works as a natural antidepressant. But in the long run this chemical, with continued intake, will probably deplete endorphins and will not lead to their restoration. So many drugs that enter into the addiction model, although they temporarily release good medicine into the brain, will result in depletion because they do not rebuild. Chocolate is another fermented food and therefore falls in the same category with alcohol and other fermented products which often have negative affects on brain health. Chocolate addiction can be treated like other addictions, with natural techniques such as Cranial Electrical Stimulation and amino acids or drug techniques including anticonvulsants, antidepressants, and any other medications that will affect craving behavior.

Marijuana and Cocaine

Marijuana and cocaine are two illegal drugs that are the most commonly used today among young adults. Marijuana affects the immune system and may cause chromosomal damage. It may affect pregnancy and fetal development. But we see most commonly the psychiatric effects, e.g., chronic schizophrenia and acute paranoid states. Furthermore, marijuana induces violent episodes, lack of motivation, residual movement/coordination problems, and even brain damage. There are other effects such as lung, heart and eye damage, as well as endocrine (glandular) problems.

Although marijuana can be used to alleviate pain in cancer patients as well as to control insomnia, hypertension, migraine, bronchial asthma, appetite, and alcoholism, it can be replaced by other medications that are just as beneficial. The most frightening aspect of marijuana is to see the long-term, psychiatric damage. People who are in the same room with smokers of marijuana can absorb it into their blood system, a process which can be dangerous to their health.

Cocaine is a nervous system stimulant that increases heart rate, blood pressure, and can induce seizures, arrhythmia, heart attacks, and angina. It is an amphetamine-like drug which often causes schizophrenia. Cocaine addiction is marked by paranoia and seizures which can be treated by Haldol and Valium. Interestingly enough, the Fair Oaks hospital staff and other medical doctors have been treating cocaine abusers with L-tyrosine and possibly tryptophan.

The Significance of Having the A1 Allele of the D2 Dopamine Receptor Gene

Do not panic if you have tested positive for this gene. Having this gene does not mean that you or your progeny will become alcoholics or drug abusers. At this time, all we can learn from the presence of this gene is that it increases vulnerability to certain disorders.

There have been multiple studies demonstrating vulnerability to possible alcoholism and attention deficit disorder with the presence of this gene. Multiple confirmations suggest that about 60 to 70 percent of virulent alcoholics may have this gene, while it still may be present in as much as 20 percent of a nonalcoholic prone population although it is possible that 20 percent are actually more prone to more stress disorders than the non-gene carrying population. The gene may even represent a vulnerability to stress, under which individuals might choose to use alcohol or other substances in response to stress. Furthermore, we do not yet know how the expression of this gene might also be modified by simple techniques such as amino acids and other therapies. Expression of the gene might also be modified by environmental and cognitive therapy techniques. It does not mean you have been given any type of prediction or prognosis about your health, but you may have identified an important vulnerability that under guidance you can be directed to correct. Therefore, while presence of this gene indicates high risk, knowledge that you possess this vulnerability can be turned into a strength, since you can then utilize existing modern techniques to overcome it. The gene is found in high prevalence in children of alcoholics. The addition of brain mapping and the identification of the P300 wave and possibly other evoked potentials will indicate further whether or not this gene is being expressed.

Can Brain Biochemical Imbalance be a Causal/Contributory Factor in Homosexuality?

Increasing evidence suggests that sexual choice may be a biological phenomenon related to brain chemistry. In a recent study in *Science* magazine of the brain cells of 41 people, 25 of whom had died of AIDS, the thalamus of heterosexual men was more than twice as large as that in homosexual men. The difference was apparently not caused by AIDS because it was present in the comparison of subgroups of heterosexual and homosexual male AIDS victims. The thalamus of the homosexual male AIDS subgroup was similar in size to the thalamus of woman, according to Dr. Levy of the Salk Institute for Biological Studies.

Being gay or lesbian may not always be a matter of choice, and therefore in such cases homosexuality may be an abnormality that can be modified with chemical treatment.

Case History: A Hispanic bisexual male, age 52, with a long-standing history of both male and female sexual relationships, came to my office in September 1990. He had a diagnosis of dysthymia and major depressive episodes, with significant anxiety and agitation, some impairment in his judgment, impulsive, self-destructive behavior, and insecurity. He claimed he had been raped at age 18 by a man and had been bisexual ever since. In recent years he had been primarily homosexual and had a crush on his heterosexual young male roommate, whom he claimed tortured him by bringing his girl friends to the apartment. He has engaged in numerous acts of unsafe sex, including anal intercourse. After a failed treatment with antidepressants, he underwent a Brain Electrical Activity Map (BEAM). On the brain map, he had a right temporal excess negative to 2.64 standard deviations at 84-100 milliseconds. On the visual evoked response he had left temporal and left posterior frontal excess negative to 2.35 standard deviations, a right central excess negative to 2.58 standard deviations at 212-228 milliseconds, and multiple asymmetries in the temporal and other regions. His EEG was abnormal due to frontally projected arrhythmic sharp activity in theta and alpha ranges. At this point, because he had been treatment-resistant to antidepressants, he was put on tegretol, an anticonvulsant, 200 mg. AM, PM, and bedtime, slowly increased to 800 mg daily.

Approximately one month into the tegretol therapy the patient reported feeling the best he had in years. In addition, he had no sexual interest in men. He reported having had a born again religious experience and became a Jehovah's Witness. At first this was considered a very odd reaction, but on continued observation from November 1990 to September 1991, he has continued with a heterosexual orientation. It would seem conceivable that certain forms of homosexuality are concomitant with psychopathology and have a biological origin of which psychopathology or homosexuality is only a symptom, and that adequate treatment with an organic agent may actually impact the brain chemical abnormality so that homosexuals uncomfortable with their sexuality may become quite comfortable with being strictly heterosexual. In addition, we may look at whether or not religiosity relates to brain chemistry. The relationship between Soviet alcoholism and atheism may be scientifically explored.

Sleep Apnea Syndrome

Many people may have sleep apnea, during which they have periods of sleep when they are not breathing normally. This condition is basically a clue to the presence of an imbalance in brain electrical activity. The whole body is unbalanced, when the brain is imbalanced, and so sleep disorder is common. Typically, during REM (Rapid Eye Movement) sleep and dream sleep, all individuals will have periods where they do not breathe. But when the periods extend to ten seconds, this can be a serious problem. Many individuals tend to put themselves on an incline to create positive pressure, like C-pap which is available as a machine. Individuals paradoxically present as experiencing daytime sleepiness or fatigue and also at night they can be

difficult to arouse between the apneic episodes because they are either tired or retaining CO_2.

Typically, treatments are non-sedating antidepressants like Vivactil, Prozac and Wellbutrin. Medroxy, or natural, progesterone, has also been thought to be helpful. Sleep apnea is a brain electrical activity imbalance and really not a disease but another presentation of brain irregularities. More than 9 percent of men stop breathing at least 15 times per hour during a night's sleep. Because they are seldom fully awake, the only clue comes from a bed partner whose own rest is disturbed by the breathing fits and starts. Apnea can contribute to car and job accidents and may be a factor in stroke and heart attack.

A Cause of National Drug Abuse

The cause of national drug abuse is in part rooted in the parent as drug model. When the parents in this country have fatigue they use coffee; when they have anxiety they use alcohol; for pain and headaches they use aspirin; for premenstrual symptoms they use Ibuprofen and for colds, antihistamines. There is a drug for every symptom and for every problem! Actually, sometimes drugs *are* necessary. This pattern of healing basically states that if you have a

problem take a drug or pill to solve it. The poor and confused, the bored and lost individuals who have brain rhythm disorders also address their problems with the same pattern. They use illegal drugs instead of legal drugs because their problems are often ethical and moral problems. The drug model must be replaced with brain/biochemical, nutritionally preventive and spiritual models.

The Path to Live Again: Nutritional Detoxification from Drugs

PATH Medical makes use of both nutritional and medical approaches for detoxifying drug use. We will not hesitate to use Librium, Tegretol, antidepressants, Parlodel, Prolixin, and many other drugs to take care of symptoms. Many individuals with severe anxiety will temporarily respond to benzodiazepines, and many individuals with substance abuse history will require anticonvulsants for seizure-like activity. Many individuals with drug problems will have deep underlying depression for which an appropriate antidepressant can be chosen based on the needs of the patient, and some will even require antipsychotic medication.

What is distinctive about PATH is that we offer a complete nutritional, natural electrical detox program which includes several grams of niacinamide, B-complex, antioxidants, multivitamins, melatonin, as well as important amino acids, particularly DL-phenylalanine, methionine,

and tyrosine. For cocaine addicts, tyrosine might be emphasized more than for alcoholics. An important element of the PATH detox program is CES (Cranial Electrical Stimulation), a natural electrical therapy which helps restore the brain's normal rhythm. We believe PATH has the most outstanding nutritional detox regimen and we hope eventually to make intravenous vitamin therapy available for more severe cases of patients being detoxified from drugs. Amino acids with B-complex help to build up the proper neurotransmitters in the brain. CES therapy helps to adjust the brain rhythm while melatonin may be a good tryptophan replacement, but should be used sparingly. The daily ritual of vitamins and CES is in itself beneficial in that it helps provide structure and quiet time. All this should be done in conjunction with counselling and the basic 12-step program. Nutritional detox as well as medications are never a replacement for the psychosocial and higher power approaches to addiction.

Classification of Common Tremors

1. **Tremor at rest**

   Parkinson's disease

2. **Postural tremors**

   Physiological tremor
   Exaggerated physiological tremor
   Essential tremor
   Tremor with basal ganglia disease

   > Parkinson's disease
   > Dystonia
   > Wilson's disease

   Cerebellar postural tremor
   Tremor with peripheral neuropathy

   Post-traumatic tremor
   Alcoholic tremor

3. **Kinetic tremor**

   Cerebellar kinetic (intention) tremor

4. **Task-specific tremors**

   Primary writing tremor
   Vocal tremor
   Orthostatic tremor

5. **Hysterical tremor**

   Hereditary peripheral neuropathy
   Acquired neuropathy

Factors Increasing Physiological Tremor

Emotion

> E.g., anxiety, stress, fear

Exercise, fatigue

Hypoglycemia

Thyrotoxicosis

Pheochromocytoma

Hypothermia

Withdrawal from alcohol

Drugs

- B-Adrenergic (isoproterenol, amphetamine)
- Dopaminergics
- Anticonvulsant (Valproate)
- Lithium
- Neuroleptics
- Tricyclics
- Methylxanthine (caffeine, theophylline)

Minor and Severe Head Injuries

Minor head injuries can occur ranging from brief loss of consciousness to lacerations on the scalp and face. Until recently, it was generally assumed that patients who sustained a concussion or were rendered unconscious for several minutes did not sustain any brain injury; yet these patients frequently complained of headaches, memory loss, psychosocial difficulties, and were often called neurotic. They received EEGs and CT scans which were frequently normal. Recent studies challenge the assumption of good health following minor and/or severe head injuries. Approximately 79 percent of the patients who have concussions complain of and show persistent headaches, 59 percent describe problems with memory, 34 percent have trouble with employment. Between 75 and 90 percent of the patients will have an abnormal Brain Electrical Activity Map.

Neuropsychological testing is also very sensitive to sequelae of minor (and severe) head injury. Microscopic examination of monkeys that underwent minor head injuries suggests that micro hemorrhages occur in the brain stem and possibly other areas of the brain. The brain stem is used for regulating the roles of concentration and memory, and also serves to filter out various irrelevant information from the external world, such as bright lights and loud sounds. In contrast are the severe head injuries of those who sustained head injuries and reported a period of post-traumatic amnesia for 24 hours or longer. They frequently sustained brain injuries which are relatively permanent unless treated. These injuries seriously impair intellectual, cognitive, emotional, and social functioning for many years. Initially, these patients deny having any difficulties in the face of even severe disorientation, memory difficulties, and confusion. Later on, they recover and recognize; and when they recognize they often have symptoms of depression and can benefit significantly from antidepressant medication.

Neuropsychological tests can be extremely accurate, even more so than standard psychological tests because they analyze the neurological dimension. Although neurological examination, EEG, and CT scan are frequently normal, the BEAM test has greater sensitivity than any of these tests, as does neuropsychological testing, and can provide documentation of the exact details of the injury, as well as new insights into the medical treatment. As we now recognize the brain's vulnerability to injury, we have come to recognize the brain's vulnerability to healing and treatment.

Head injury can have widespread and complex impact on a person's life and daily functioning, which not only affects the patient, but the family of the patient in many ways. Psychological problems are frequently observed not only in individuals who have had brain injury but also in their families. The former exhibit symptoms such as agitation, denial, anxiety, attention difficulties, concrete thinking difficulties, confusion, decreased initiative and ambition, dependency, depression, disorientation, dizziness, egocentricity, fatigue, fine motor coordination difficulties, headache, impaired judgment, impatience, inflexibility, memory difficulties, motor slowness, pain, paranoia, poor self-esteem, sexual difficulties, social difficulties, somatic complaints, temper tantrums, and tendency to complain. The families frequently exhibit acting out, ambivalence, fantasies of spontaneous recovery, financial insecurity, overcritical attitude, role reversals, problems with guilt, frustration, depression, and denial of deficits -- all the result of compensation to the injured individual. So family therapy can also be an important component.

References for BEAM and Head Injury

1.   Radanov BO, Valach L, Wittlieb-Verpport E, Dvorak J. Neuropsychologische Befunde nach Schleuderverletzung der Halswirbelsaule. *Schweiz. Med. Wschr.* 120:Nr. 19, 1990.

2.   Ruijs MBM, Keyser A, Gabreels FJM. Long-term sequelae of brain damage from closed head injury in children and adolescents. *Clin Neurol Neurosurg*, vol. 92-4, 1990.

3.   Deacon D, Campbell KB. Effects of performance feedback on P300 and reaction time in closed head-injured outpatients. *Electroen and Clin Neurophy* 78:133-141, 1991.

4.   Temkin NR, Dikmen SS, Wilensky AJ, Keihm J, Chabal S, Winn R. A Randomized, Double-Blind Study of Phenytoin for the Prevention of Post-Traumatic Seizures. *New England J of Med* 323:497-502, 1990.

5.   Berget J, Salcmanova. EEF findings after closed cerebral injuries. *Czechoslovak EEG Society.*

6. Walker SH, Patton ES. Brain Electrical Activity Mapping (BEAM) in the Evaluation of Traumatic Brain Injury, *Nicolet*, 1988.

7. Dacey R, Dikmen S, Temkin N, McLean A, Armsden G, Rinn R. Relative Effects of Brain and Non-Brain Injuries on Neurophsychological and Psychosocial Outcome. *The Jour of Trauma*, vol. 31 no. 2:217-222, 1991.

8. Zeitlhofer J, Steiner M, Oder W, Obergottsberger S, Mayr N, Deecke L. Prognostische Wertigekeit evozierter Potentiale in der neurologischen Fruhrehabilitation bei Patienten apallischen Syndrom, Z. EEG-EMG22, 10-14, 1991.

9. Levin HS, et. al. Neurobehavioral Outcome One Year After Severe Head Injury: Experience of the Traumatic Coma Data Bank. *J Neurosurg* 73:699-709, 1990.

A recent study in sports medicine said that injuries to the head may result in headaches as long as five months after trauma.

Head Trauma and Heart Trauma

We should come to recognize that the medical principles controlling the treatment of brain and heart trauma, respectively, are similar in that for post-heart attack treatment we use a beta-blocker to give the heart a quiescent period, and we use anticonvulsants for post-head trauma to create a quiescent period. Both of these methods facilitate healing.

Whiplash and Head Trauma

A study in the Archives of Neurology (January 1993) reported that when older patients suffer whiplash they have more symptoms, including a higher intensity of pain and greater subjective cognitive impairment. Even following common whiplash, most of us will require at least six months to recuperate from even minor car accidents where whiplash occurs. Brain Electrical Activity Mapping and neuropsychological testing can now document the severity of these deficits that occur after common whiplash.

We have been treating whiplash and head trauma at PATH for years and there is a growing body of documentation for the benefits of medication, nutrition and CES (Cranial Electrical Stimulation) to speed recovery and reverse brain injury. We have patients with repeated brain electrical activity maps with a healing transformation of large percentages of their prior abnormality based on these treatment approaches.

Emotional Trauma Damages the Immune System

Dr. Frank Putman of the National Institute of Mental Health and Dr. Marvin Teicher of Harvard Medical School presented their findings at the APA Psychiatric Association meeting in Philadelphia. A study following 170 girls, ages 6 to 15 years old, half sexually abused, showed abnormally high stress hormones which kill neurons in brain areas crucial to thinking and memory.

In addition, high levels of an antibody that weakens the human immune system. Many have been sexually and physically abused. In addition, it hampered development of language and logic and caused damage to the left hemisphere.

Brain wave differences between the abused and non-abused are significant as between normal people and those who have Alzheimer's disease or schizophrenia. The abused should not feel they are doomed, but we do know that emotional trauma damages the immune system and that brain rehabilitation is necessary. The brain controls the body.

Attention Deficit Disorder (ADD) in Adults

(Technically called "Residual Type" -- sometimes called "Undifferentiated")

An important recent development is the recognition that ADD continues into the adult years in a significant percentage of cases. The symptoms can be very disruptive, but researchers are finding that ADD in adults is treatable. It is very important to locate adults with the condition, because they are probably not aware that they have a treatable condition.

To date, most cases have been found as a result of a child's evaluation. Since there is a hereditary component to many of these cases, we always ask if anyone else in the family has the same symptoms. Frequently, the answer is yes, and we proceed to evaluate the adult. Treatment is usually with Tofranil (imipramine) or Cylert. Drugs such as Ritalin or Dexedrine are very effective, but have other problems related to their use.

Making the Diagnosis

Some of the current research is being done by Paul Wender, M.D., Professor of Psychiatry and Director of Psychiatric Research at the University of Utah College of Medicine. The following is the "Modified Utah Criteria" for ADD, Residual Type.

In order to diagnose the condition as an adult disorder, the individual must fulfill criteria one and two, and two out of the remaining five items. Diagnosis is not made on the basis of a check list alone, but the presence of a positive preliminary screen makes it imperative to take the next step to evaluate the problem further.

1. Persistent hyperactivity shown by restlessness; the inability to relax; being "always on the go."

2. Attention problems as shown by easy distractibility, inability to keep the mind on reading material, difficulty keeping the mind on the job, and forgetfulness.

3. Mood Swings shift from normal to down, to mildly up. The moods usually last a few hours. When down, they describe feeling bored or discontent.

4. Inability to complete tasks: the subject reports lack of organization in job, running the household, or doing school work. Tasks frequently not completed, disorganization in activities, problem solving, and organizing time.

5. Explosive temper, easily provoked with short lived outbursts.

6. Impulsivity: decisions made hastily, without reflection, often to the disadvantage of the individual.

7. Stress intolerance: subject cannot take ordinary stresses in stride and reacts excessively or inappropriately.

With this condition there are often associated features. These would include marital instability, academic and vocational success less than expected on the basis of intelligence and education, alcohol or drug abuse, and/or problems in interpersonal relationships.

As more is learned about the physiological causes of ADD in children and adults, new treatments will be developed. At this time the diagnosis is made by observation and a recognition of what we see. There are no laboratory tests to help us out, and it is therefore essential that we be aware of the condition, methods of diagnosis, and current treatments.

BEAM®

Brain Electrical Activity Mapping

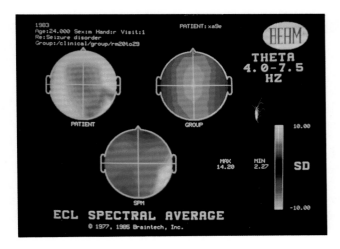

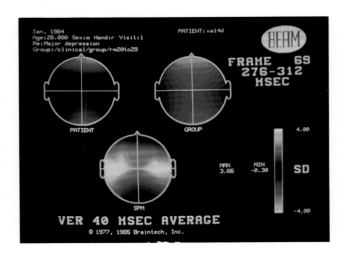

These EEG maps were obtained from a 24 year old male with a seizure disorder. They were generated from the spectral average in the theta band from data obtained during the eyes closed (ECL) condition. The patient's map shows increased right posterior-temporal theta activity which is not present in the map of age-matched controls. The SPM map illustrates that the greatest statistical difference between the patient and the control group is slightly more anterior than suggested by the patient map alone.

These topographic maps were generated from visual evoked potentials recorded from a 26 year old depressed male. The patient's activity was relatively symmetrically distributed over this 40 millisecond time frame, as was the group's activity over the same epoch. However, the SPM map indicates that there is a pronounced difference between the patient's and the group's activity bilaterally and that in these areas the difference exceeds three standard deviations.

As illustrated in the above examples, reliable electrophysiological data concerning a patient's neurological or psychiatric condition can be obtained using the revolutionary BEAM system. This totally non-invasive technique provides the clinician with a functional image of brain activity which is compared to a rigorously defined, age-matched control group. The BEAM system then automatically compares the patient with the appropriate control group and constructs a Statistical Probability Map (SPM) which clearly indicates the degree of deviation from the norm.

BEAM is a useful adjunct to other imaging techniques. However, by itself the BEAM technique is clinically relevant in distinguishing a variety of disorders such as epilepsy, learning disabilities, depression, schizophrenia, dementia, head trauma and organic brain disease.

For further information, patient appointments or a demonstration, contact:

The Place for Achieving Total Health (PATH)
274 Madison Avenue, Suite 402
New York, NY 10016
(888) 231-PATH

® Nicolet Instrument Corporation

The Treatment of
Substance Abuse Withdrawal Syndrome, Anxiety, and Depression by Cranial Electrotherapy Stimulation (CES) as Validated by Brain Electrical Activity Mapping (BEAM®)

CES

Typical P300 wave.

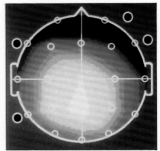

Positive (P) wave at 300 ms after cognitive stimulus.

CES, or cranial electrotherapy stimulation, is an FDA registered treatment modality in which micro-electric impulses are applied to the head. The standard CES configuration is 100 hz (100 pulses of alternating current per second) with a maximum current output of 1.5 milliamperes, current amplitude similar to that in the human body. The primary indications for use of CES are stress and stress-related disorders, primarily anxiety, depression, and insomnia. CES has shown itself to be particularly effective in addressing those symptoms in the context of a variety of illnesses, including substance withdrawal syndrome, chronic fatigue syndrome, attention deficit disorder syndrome, and generalized anxiety and panic disorders.

CES and the BEAM

Chronic Alcoholic, P300 wave, pre CES.

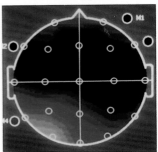

P300 virtually absent.

Dr. Eric Braverman, M. D., of Princeton Associates for Total Health (PATH) of Princeton, New Jersey, employs CES extensively in his practice in conjunction with the BEAM (Brain Electrical Activity Mapping) as a means of monitoring patient brainwave activity and of validating the effect of CES treatment. Using the BEAM machine which records brain wave activity, Dr. Braverman evaluates the brain's electrical activity and identifies those areas that have increased or decreased function. After these electrical deviations are identified -- many of which are associated with drug and alcohol abuse, depression, and other medical conditions -- he then treats the patient with gentle cranial electrotherapy stimulation (CES) -- to alter the activity and treat the drug craving or underlying organic disease.

CES, the P300, and Cognitive Functioning

Chronic Alcoholic, P300 wave, post CES.

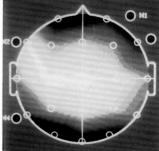

Bright yellow P300 burst occurring after 40 minute CES treatment.

A particularly significant measure in his work is the P300 wave. The P300 wave is so named because it occurs at 300 milliseconds after a cognitive auditory evoked potential. Research indicates the P300 to be a biological marker of alcoholism and drug abuse and substance addiction causing a significant reduction in P300 voltage. Alcoholics frequently have P300 waves of 5.0 - 6.5 microvolts with an average of 6.0 - 7.5 microvolts. A CES treatment can raise this voltage to the normal level of about 8 microvolts. Voltage is directly correlated to cognitive functioning. Enhanced cognitive functioning is often a by-product of CES treatment for anxiety, depression, or insomnia.

® Nicolet Instrument Corp.

Cranial ElectroTherapy Stimulation (CES)
and Normalization of Brainwave Activity
as Validated by
Brain Electrical Activity Mapping (BEAM®)

Normalization of Brainwave Activity

Pre CES   *Post CES*

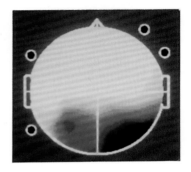   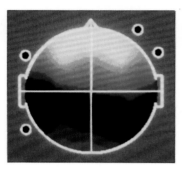

Anxiety Patient: Normalization of Theta Following 40 Miutes of CES.

Pre CES   *Post CES*

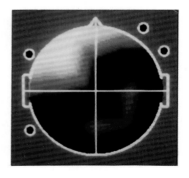   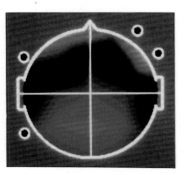

Depression Patient: Normalization of Delta Following 40 Minutes of CES.

® *Nicolet Instrument Corp.*

Typical Brainmaps

P300 Wave

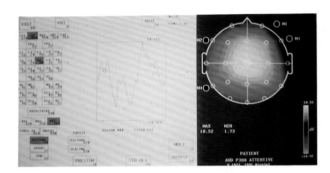

Normal P300 wave at 10.52 microvolts with graph.

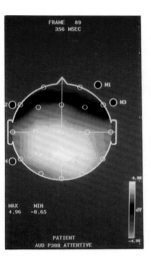

Abnormal P300 because of low voltage of 4.96 microvolts.

Patient/Group (Harvard Control Group) Comparison

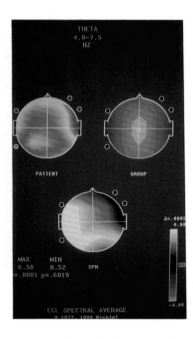

Patient/group comparison during eyes closed which shows typical increased theta at left temporal site -- associated with aging, drug abuse and head trauma.

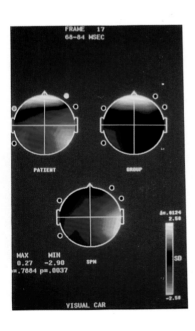

Patient/group comparison showing right temporal excess negative can be typical of mood swings, depression, and even drug abuse.

Typical Brainmaps

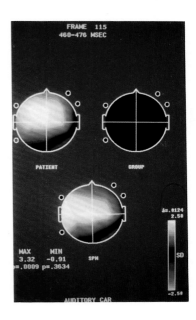

Left temporal excess positive
on auditory evoked response,
late at 460-480 msec.

Potential Temporal Lobe Dysfunction Symptoms

Head injury
Bruise easily
Cold hands, feet
Seasonal
Deja vu
ADD history
Ritualistic behavior
headaches
Synthesis
Time loss, moments or more
Elevator plummeting feeling,
   stomach rise (halo)

Color blind (not a symptom)
Smell hallucinations
Taste hallucinations
Sexual drives
Religiosity
Compulsive behavior
Obsessive behavior
Floating spots, rims, flashes
Out of body experiences
Space perception aberrations
Reaction to red and red-like
   wave lengths

Exacerbation of BEAM Abnormality with Drug Use

Visual evoked response.

Visual evoked response.

Visual evoked response.

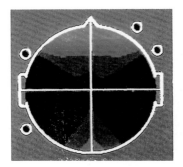

Control

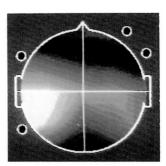

Left temporal excess negative
associated with mood swings,
depression and anxiety is very
common in non-drug users with
these symptoms.

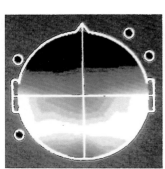

Excess negative bitemporal (both
sides), near the ear area, is typically
found in people with mood swings
and concomitant drug use;   also
typical of individuals who have
violent episodes with or without
drug use.

Diagnosis and Treatment of Substance Abusers
with the Brain Electrical Activity Mapping (BEAM®) Machine
and Cranial Electrical Stimulation (CES)

Using the BEAM machine, which records brain waves, physicians can evaluate the brain's electrical activity and identity those areas that have increased or decreased function. After these electrical deviations are identified -- many of which are associated with drug and alcohol abuse, depression and other medical conditions -- it is possible to treat the patient with gentle, electrical stimulation -- such as Cranial Electrical Stimulation (CES) -- to alter the activity in the brain and treat the drug craving or underlying organic disease.

Eric R. Braverman, M. D., of Princeton Associates for Total Health (PATH), has had dramatic patients with CES, as illustrated by the following case studies:

Substance Abuse

I. The BEAM machine records left temporal lobe abnormality (white area) in the brain of a 30-year-old abuser of alcohol, valium and cocaine. This deviation, indicating decreased brain activity, is characteristic of multi-drug abusers.

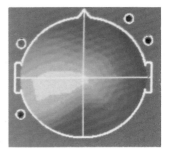 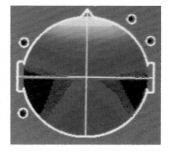 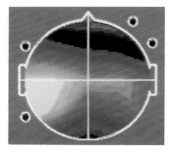

Recorded brain activity of a 31-year-old substance abuser. The white area on left shows decreased electrical activity characteristic of multi-drug abusers.

Recorded Brain activity from a group of normal 30- to 39-year-olds.

By comparing the two images, BEAM indicates the deviation in brain activity of the 31-year-old substance abuser. With gentle electrical stimulation, such as CES treatment, the brain activity deviation can be corrected and the drug craving controlled.

II. The BEAM machine records the changes in electrical brain activity in a patient with a 10-year history of drug abuse after just three months of nightly CES treatment with electrodes pasted to the forehead and wrist.

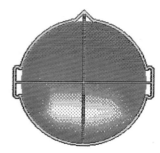 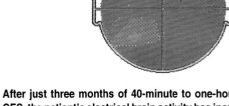

Initial record of the patients electrical brain activity, white region -- which indicates decreased electrical activity -- extends to the posterior temporal lobe. This pattern is characteristic of substance abusers.

After just three months of 40-minute to one-hour treatments with CES, the patient's electrical brain activity has increased; the patient remained free of drugs during that period.

® Nicolet Instrument Corp.

B186ST1

Clinical Patient
143 Maple Street
Anytown, Wisconsin USA 53711
Age: 52
Visit: 1
Mon Dec 22 1986
SS#: 123-456-7890
Reason: Recovered from brain trauma of 3 yrs ago; recent new symptoms
Sensory Deficit: Left-sided numbness
PRP: Recent onset of tingling on left side; mood disturbances
Protocol: basic

Referring MD:

Analysis Location:

General Hospital

ECL SPECTRAL AVERAGE

PATIENT

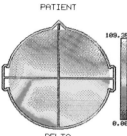
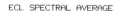

DELTA

GROUP
1m50to59

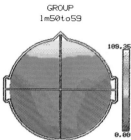

DELTA

SPM

DELTA

Multiple areas of excessive delta. Maximum deviation 4.69 SD.

ECL SPECTRAL AVERAGE

PATIENT

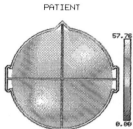

THETA

GROUP
1m50to59

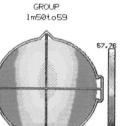

THETA

SPM

THETA

Multiple areas of excessive theta activity. Maximum deviation
of 3.35 SD.

ECL SPECTRAL AVERAGE

PATIENT

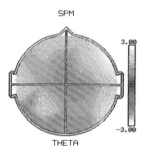

ALPHA

GROUP
1m50to59

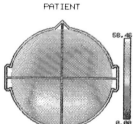

ALPHA

Alpha activity WNL.

SPM

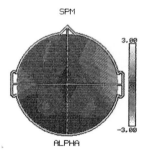

ALPHA

ECL SPECTRAL AVERAGE

PATIENT

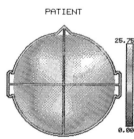

BETA1

GROUP
1m50to59

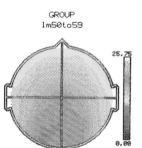

BETA1

SPM

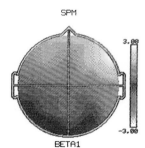

BETA1

Right frontal theta larger than normal by 3.00 SD.

Impression: Multiple areas of slowing with right frontal high amplitude beta. Abnormal VER morphology and scalp
           distribution. Late AER abnormalities noted.
Collection Location: BEAM Laboratory, General Hospital

       Collected by: BEAM Certified Technologist

Insurance: Indemnity General of Des Moines
           062580
           Patient
Meds: None
Notes:

Reader:
_____

BEAM Certified Physician

Obesity is a heterogeneous and prevalent disorder having both inheritable and environmental components. The relationship between macroselection of various foods and familial polysubstance abuse has been documented throughout the literature. Neurochemical studies have supported the commonality of reinforcement through dopaminergic systems by alcohol, cocaine, and carbohydrates. Moreover, a Taq Al polymorphism, as well as other variants, of the dopamine D2 receptor gene (DRD2) was found to associate with a number of addictive behaviors (alcoholism, cocaine dependence, nicotine abuse, and carbohydrate bingeing). While a number of studies demonstrated P3 changes in alcohol and drug dependent subjects, two recent studies found association of P3 latency in children of active alcoholic fathers (Noble et al, 1994) with the Al allele of the DRD2 gene and in a psychiatric population having two copies of the Al allele of the DRD2 gene (Blum, et al., 1994). A total of 53 white obese females and males having a mean body mass index (BMI) of 34.6 ± 8.2 were brain electrical activity mapped and compared with 15 controls with a mean BMI of 22.3 ± 3.0 (p<.001). The P3 amplitude and average P3 time in obese and control subjects were 7.07 ± 2.3 uV (microvolts) and 320 ± 28.8 msec, and 10.9 ± 4.4 uV and 306 ± 27.0 msec, respectively. The P3 amplitude was significantly different (two-tailed; t = 3.24, dF = 16.2, p = .005), whereas P3 latency was not significant. Preliminarily we found a significant correlation of prolongation of P3 latency correlated with the three risk factors of parental substance abuse, chemical dependency, and carbohydrate bingeing (p<.03), and decreased P3 amplitude correlated with family history of alcoholism and drug abuse (p<.049). This work represents the first electrophysiological data to implicate P3 abnormalities in a subtype of obesity.

Brain electrical activity map as a function of risk factors (e.g., parental chemical dependency, Proband chemical dependency, carbohydrate bingeing) in obese patients.

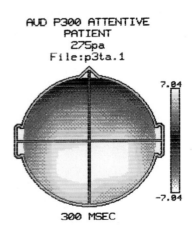

**Obese patient with
no risk factors**

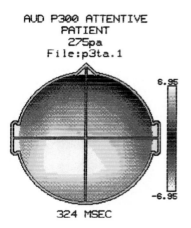

**Obese patient with
any of three risk factors**

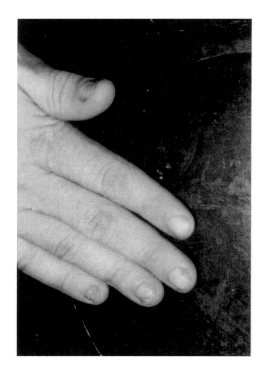

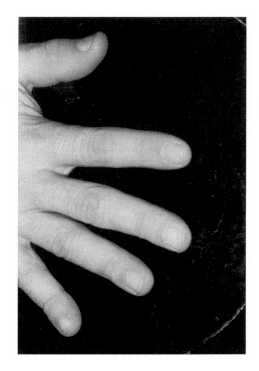

Nail Fungus
Before Treatment
especially note the thumb and pinky

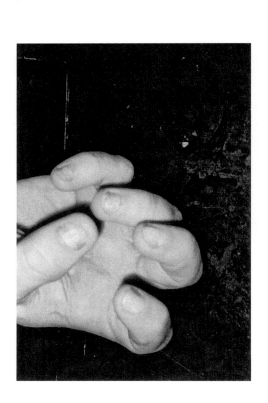

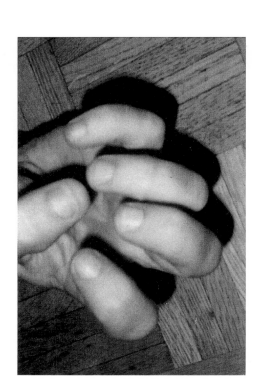

After Treatment
with Sporonox

PET Scan

Pet Scanning Shows Increase in Coronary Collateral Circulation with Cardiac Reversal Therapy: Nutrition, Drugs and Chelation

Pre-treatment

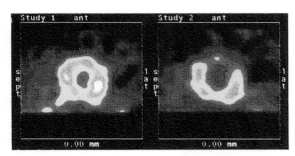

Before persantine   **After persantine**

IMPRESSIONS: Abnormal dipyridamole PET study. These findings are consistent with severe coronary flow reserve abnormalities in the region of the left ventricular anterior, apical and anterolateral walls which correlates with severe obstructive coronary disease. There is also a moderate to severe restriction of flow reserve of the vessel supplying the lateral wall. A decrease in absolute counts during stress suggests collateral circulation supplying the left ventricular anterior wall and apex.

After Cardiovascular Reversal Program

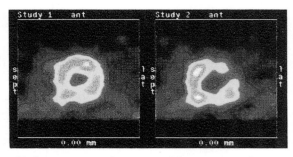

Before persantine   **After persantine**

IMPRESSION: Abnormal Dipyridamole PET study. These findings are consistent with:

1. Severe flow reserve abnormalities of the vessels supplying the anterior, anterolateral, apical and inferoapical walls consistent with severe coronary artery disease.

2. Collateralization of the anterior, anterolateral, apical and inferoapical walls.

Note: The reduction of the yellow color in the "After persantine" frames is indicative of loss of circulation in the heart due to the stress caused by persantine. In the "After Cardiovascular Reversal Program" frames, the increased amount of yellow color indicates improved blood flow in the heart.

Attention Deficit Disorder Resources

Books for Attention Deficit Disorder patients include:

1. *Attention Deficit Disorder in Adults -- A Practical Help for Sufferers and their Spouses*, by Dr. Lynn Weiss, Taylor Publishing Company: Dallas.

2. *You Mean I'm Not Lazy, Stupid or Crazy -- A Self-help Book for Adults with Attention Deficit Disorder*, by Kate Kelly and Peggy Rumondo, Tyrell and Jerem Press.

3. *Total Concentration -- How to Understand Attention Deficit Disorders, with Treatment Guidelines for you and your Doctor*, by Harold N. Levinson, M.D.

4. "Attention Deficit Disorder Can't be Ignored," *Wall Street Journal*, Sept. 27, 1994.

5. "Life In Overdrive," by C. Wallis, *Time*, July 18, 1994.

6. *Why Won't My Child Pay Attention? -- A complete Guide to ADD for parents, teachers and community agencies*, Goldstein, S., and Goldstein, M., John Wiley and Sons.

7. *Driven to Distraction -- Recognizing and Coping with Attention Deficit Disorder from Childhood Through Adulthood*, Hallowell, Edward M., and Ratey, John J.

Temporal Lobe Abnormalities

Temporal lobe abnormalities are quite common in our society, causing mood problems and neurological dysfunction. Risk factors are described in J. A. French, et al., "Characteristics of Medical Temporal Lobe Epilepsy: I. Results of History and Physical Examination," *Annals of Neurology* 34(6):774-780, and include infections, birth events, etc. Very few have no identifiable risk factors. Furthermore, virtually all patients (96 percent) have some type of aura.

Table 1: Risk Factors

Seizures during infancy or early childhood	54
Febrile illness	52
Bacterial meningitis	5
Viral encephalitis	2
No recognized CNS infection	45
Nonfebrile illness	2
Head trauma	10
With loss of consciousness	7
No loss of consciousness	3
Birth trauma	6
Significant birth trauma	2
Other	4
Preeclampsia in mother	1
Toxemia in patient	1
Severe anaphylactic reaction	1
Mumps meningitis (no seizures)	1
Combinations of risk factors	8
Febrile seizures and head trauma	4
Febrile seizures and birth trauma	2
Febrile seizures and mumps meningitis	1
Head trauma and birth trauma	1
No risk factors	5

Table 2: Auras

Patients with auras	(96%)	64
Patients without auras	(4%)	3
Type of aura		
Abdominal visceral sensation		39
Only aura		13
Combined with other symptoms		26
Fear		6
Light-headed		6
Feeling of warmth		3
Gustatory		2
Olfactory		2
Urge to micturate		2
Micropsia		2
Indescribable		2
Vertigo		1
Euphoria		1
Compulsive thoughts		1
Generalized numbness		1
Depersonalization		1
Feeling of having to sneeze		1
Auras not including visceral sensations		25
Fear		5
Olfactory		5
Light-headed		3
Deja vu		3
Generalized somatosensory		3
Indescribable		3
Feeling of warmth		2
Gustatory		2
Urge to micturate		2
Intellectual (spiritual darkness)		1
Breathless		1
Disorientation		1
Vertigo		1
Elementary auditory		1
Elementary visual		1

Head Trauma BEAM Bibliography

Bricklin M, New Respect for Nutritional Healing, *Prevention*, February 1992, 31-32.

Brown DJ, Phytotherapy Review and Commentary, *Townsend Letter for Doctors*, December 1991, 1041-1042.

Crooks DA, Scholtz CL, Vowles G, Greenwald S, Axonal Injury In Closed Head Injury by Assault: A Quantitative Study, *Med. Sci. Law*, 1992, 32(2):109-118.

Dikmen SS, Temkin NR, Miller B, Machamer J, Winn HR, Neurobehavioral Effects of Phenytoin Prophylaxis of Posttraumatic Seizures, *JAMA*, March 13, 1991, 265(10):1250-1271.

Dinan TG, Mobayed M, Treatment Resistance of Depression After Head Injury: A Preliminary Study of Amitriptyline Response, *APS* 1991, 1745,1-3.

Eames P, Hysteria Following Brain Injury, *Journal of Neurology, Neurosurgery*, and Psychiatry, 1992, 55:1046-1053.

Fleming BE, Wilson DR, Pendergast, A Portable, Easily Performed Muscle Power Test and Its Association With Falls by Elderly Persons, *Arch Phys Med Rehabil*, October 1991, 72:886-889

Garber JH, Weilburg JB, Duffy FH, Manschreck TC, Clinical Use of Topographic Brain Electrical Activity Mapping in Psychiatry, *The Journal of Clinical Psychiatry*, June 1989, 50(6):205-211.

Hans P, Franssen C, Pincemail J, Bertrand Y, Hannique G, Damas P, Lamy M, Plasma Myeloperoxidase and Vitamin E Levels in Head Injury: Preliminary Results Related to Outcome, *Journal of Neurosurgical Anesthesiology*, 1992, 4(1):26-30

Haydon M, Handicapping Effects of Brain Injury and Psychological Disorders Resulting From Traumatic Experiences.

Heilbronner RL, Henry GK, Carson-Brewer M, Neuropsychologic Test Performance In Amateur Boxers, *The American Journal of Sports Medicine*, 1991, 19(4):376-380.

Koren T, *Accidents, Injuries and Chiropractic*, Koren Publications, 1991.

Lonsdale D, Allithiamine and its Synthetic Derivatives: A Review, *Journal of Nutritional Medicine*, 1991, 2:305-311.

Marshall LF, Evoked Potentials: A Decade Later, *Critical Care Medicine*, 1991, 19(11):1337.

Mittenberg W, DiGiulio DV, Perrin S, Bass AE, Symptoms following mild head injury: Expectation as Aetiology, *Journal of Neurology, Neurosurgery, and Psychiatry*, 1992, 55:200-204.

Oder W, Goldenberg G, Podreka I, Deecke L, HM-PAO SPECT in Persistent Vegetative State After Head Injury: Prognostic Indicator of the Likelihood of Recovery? *Intensive Care Med*, 1991, 17:149-153.

Oppenheim EB, Losing Sight of the Whole Patient -- A Case With A Fatal Outcome, *Medical Malpractice Prevention*, September 1991, pp. 7-8.

Parkinson D, Concussion is Completely Reversible: an Hypothesis, *Medical Hypotheses*, 1992, 37:37-39.

Pechadre JC, et al., Prevention of Late Post-traumatic Epilepsy by Phenytoin in Severe Brain Injuries: 2 Years' Follow-up, *Presse Med*, 1991, 20:841-845.

Ruddock LA, Impacts: Effects of Whiplash, Advance for Physical Therapists, May 27, 1991, 13-14.

Salzman SK, Puniak MA, Liu Z, Maitland-Heriot RP, Freeman GM, Agresta CA, The Serotonin Antagonist Mianserin Improves Functional Recovery Following Experimental Spinal Trauma, *Annals of Neurology*, October 1991, 30(4):534-541.

Talan J, Absence of Fragile Cells Linked To Epilepsy Spells, *Discovery* NY, 49.

Thatcher RW, Walker RA, Gerson I, Geisler FH, EEG Discriminant Analyses (BEAM) of Mild Head Trauma, *Electroencephalography and Clinical Neurophysiology*, 1989, 73:94-106.

Walker SH, Patton ES, *Brain Electrical Activity Mapping (BEAM) In The Evaluation of Traumatic Brain Injury*, Nicolet Ins Inc., 1988.

3. Brain -- General, and Eye Health

Alpha Waves

Alpha waves are very important waves in the brain, an area associated with creativity and clear thinking processes. They are often deficient in certain individuals, such as in alcoholics and their children, and individuals with a history of alcohol abuse and their children. Alpha waves can also be deficient in individuals with depression or anxiety. Moreover, alpha waves can be lowered by various drugs such as anticonvulsants and antipsychotics. On the other hand, many antidepressants, such as Hydergine and oxiracetam, increase alpha waves. Alpha waves are lowered by numerous medical conditions such as hypothyroidism, hypoglycemia, renal and hepatic disorders.

Alpha rhythms are probably deficient on the right side in a large number of individuals with drug abuse, depression, and Parkinson's and Alzheimer's diseases. This right-sided brain dysfunction can be picked up by brain mapping or psychodiagnostic screening and may be corrected by amino acids and Cranial Electrical Stimulation. It is well known that amino acids such as methionine, phenylalanine, tyrosine, L-dopa, and tryptophan have the potential to stimulate normal alpha rhythms in the brain. Normal conscious processes are beta and alpha. Normally unconscious processes are theta and delta. Wakefulness is beta, reverie is between alpha and theta, and sleep is delta.

Alzheimer's Disease and Change in Mental Status

Alzheimer's disease is not really a disease but a description of symptoms. Alzheimer's is a cognitive or memory deterioration, and although some individuals will have neurofibrillary tangles in the brain, a particular sign of Alzheimer's, in general there really are multiple etiologies, causes, and physiological changes that occur in the brain associated with the loss of memory and mental deterioration. The list of possible causes is extremely long, and although treatment of the condition once it has occurred is almost always very low in success, remarkable reversals do occur. The most common cause of Alzheimer's disease is probably cerebral vascular disease or poor circulation to the brain due to smoking or small strokes. The most common reversible causes of change in mental state and so-called Alzheimer's are depression, B-12 deficiency, and Parkinson's disease. Below is a list of the known medical etiologies of how one might develop Alzheimer's, pseudo-Alzheimer's, pseudodementia, or just change in mental status.

1. **Intoxication by drugs and poisons**

    a. Drugs: anticholinergic agents, sedative-hypnotics, digitalis derivatives, opiates, corticosteroids, salicylates, antibiotics, anticonvulsants, antiarrhythmic and antihypertensive drugs, antineoplastic agents, cimetidine, lithium, antiparkinsonian agents, disulfiram, indomethacin, bismuth salts, phencyclidine
    b. Alcohol: ethyl and methyl
    c. Addictive inhalants: gasoline, glue, ether, nitrous oxide, nitrites
    d. Industrial poisons: carbon disulphide, organic solvents, methyl chloride and bromide, heavy metals, organophosphorus insecticides, carbon monoxide
    e. Snakebite
    f. Poisonous plants and mushrooms

2. Withdrawal syndromes

   a. Alcohol: delirium tremens

   b. Sedatives and hypnotics: barbiturates, chloral hydrate, chlordiazepoxide, diazepam, ethchlorvynol, glutethimide, meprobamate, methyprylon, paraldehyde

   c. Amphetamines

3. Nutritional, hormonal, and metabolic disorders

   a. Hypoxia

   b. Hypoglycemia

   c. Hepatic, renal, pancreatic, and pulmonary insufficiency (encephalopathy)

   d. Avitaminosis: nicotinic acid, thiamine, cyanocobalamin (vitamin B12), folate

   e. Hypervitaminosis: intoxication by vitamins A and D

   f. Hormonal disorders: hyperinsulinism, hyperthyroidism, hypothyroidism, hypopituitarism, Addison's disease, Cushing's syndrome, hypoparathyroidism, hyperparathyroidism

   g. Disorders of fluid and electrolyte metabolism

- Dehydration, water intoxication
- Alkalosis, acidosis
- Hypernatremia, hyponatremia, hyperkalemia, hypokalemia, hypercalcemia, hypocalcemia, hypermagnesemia, hypomagnesemia

   h. Errors of metabolism

- Porphyria
- Carcinoid syndrome
- Hepatolenticular degeneration (Wilson's disease)

4. Infections

   a. Systemic: pneumonia, typhoid, typhus, acute rheumatic fever, malaria, influenza, mumps, diphtheria, brucellosis, infectious mononucleosis, infectious hepatitis, malaria, subacute bacterial endocarditis, bacteremia, septicemia, Rocky Mountain spotted fever, legionnaires' disease, Lyme disease, relapsing fever

   b. Intracranial: acute, subacute, and chronic

- Viral encephalitis, aseptic meningitis, rabies
- Bacterial meningitis-meningococcal, pneumococcal, Hemophilus influenza, etc.
- Postinfectious and postvaccinial encephalomyelitis
- Tuberculous meningitis
- Neurosyphilis
- Fungal infections: cryptococcoses, coccidioidomycosis, histoplasmosis, moniliasis, mucormycosis
- Protozoal infections: Toxoplasma encephalitis, cerebral malaria
- Trichinosis

5. Head trauma: concussion, contusion

6. Epilepsy: ictal and postictal automatism, cerebral dysrhythmia

7. Vascular disorders

   a. Cerebrovascular disorders

- Transient ischemic attacks
- Hypertensive encephalopathy
- Thrombosis, embolism
- Polyarteritis nodosa
- Systemic lupus erythematosus

- ■ Rheumatoid vasculitis
- ■ Temporal arteritis
- ■ Subarachnoid hemorrhage
- ■ Wegener's granulomatosis
- ■ Neuro-Behcet's disease
- ■ Pulseless disease

b. Cardiovascular disorders

- ■ Myocardial infarction
- ■ Congestive heart failure
- ■ Cardiac arrhythmias

c. Migraine

8. Intracranial space-occupying lesions

a. Tumor
b. Abscess
c. Subdural hematoma
d. Aneurysm
e. Parasitic cyst

9. Cerebral degenerative disorders

a. Multiple sclerosis
b. Alzheimer's disease and senile dementia
c. Parkinson's disease
d. Pick's disease
e. AIDS

10. Extracranial neoplasm, e.g., bronchogenic carcinoma

11. Disorders of the hematopoietic system

a. Pernicious anemia
b. Polycythemia vera
c. Thrombotic thrombocytopenic purpura

12. Injury by physical agents

a. Heatstroke
b. Radiation
c. Electrocution or electric shock

13. Disorders due to hypersensitivity

a. Serum sickness
b. Food allergy

Psychiatry and the
Doctor-Patient Relationship

Approximately 50% of our patients have an Axis 1 disorder such as: major anxiety, depression, mood swings, etc. Approximately 80 - 90% have a major problem regarding personality, such as compulsive, shy, withdrawn, self-defeating, borderline, social, egocentric, etc. These types of diagnoses greatly impact the way in which individuals will experience medical problems. The type of personality and its disorders are reflective of the patient's ability to withstand pressure and therefore may influence one's prognosis regarding heart disease, cancer, etc. Knowing one's personality type is essential for the proper medical management of our patients. Many individuals just have personality preferences which affects their health as well as their ability to utilize the doctor's advice.

Biological Psychiatry: Ideal Testing to
Uncover Medical Basis in the Brain of Mood Problems

- RBC or WBC trace elements - R/O trace metal deficiency
- Hair testing - R/O heavy metals
- T-cell Immune profile ratios - R/O autoimmune or infectious disease, e.g., Epstein Barr Virus, Multiple Sclerosis, or Lupus
- Amino Acids - Identifies genetic disease, neurotransmitter precursor deficiency
- Urine MHPG, 5 - HIAA, VMA, HVA metanephrines - helps understand neurotransmitter
- IgE - Basic Allergy screen along with RAST testing can be helpful in balance
- Routine Blood testing often reveals other secondary diseases
- Hypothyroid profile TSH, T3 and thyroid stress test reveals subtle thyroid imbalances
- Glycohemoglobin - identifies hidden diabetes, a person's blood sugar over the past 3 months
- Histamine polyamine - identifies early cancer allergies, etc.
- Cryptopyrroles - identifies stress, B-6 deficiency
- Platelet neurotransmitter - deeper knowledge of biochemical imbalances of the brain
- Further immune evaluation: ESR, Streptozyme, ANA, LE Prep, Rheumatoid factor-can identify further medical contributions to so-called psychosis disease
- BEAM (Brain Electrical Activity Mapping) study - identifies electrical abnormalities in the brain
- MRI with gadolinium identifies anatomical and structural injuries
- Neuropsychological and psychodiagnostic tests identify neurologic and psychologic components

Healing Your Abnormal Brain Maps

References: How Vitamins and
Medication Correct Abnormal BEAMs

1. Kirby, A. W., Wiley, R. W., Harding, T. H., "Cholinergic Effects on the Visual Evoked Potential," *Evoked Potential*, 26:296-306, 1986.
2. Lester, M. L., Horst, R. L., Thatcher, R. W., "Protective Effects of Zinc and Calcium Against Heavy Metal Impairment of Children's Cognitive Function," *Nutrition and Behavior*, 3:145-161, 1986.

3. Gerez M., Tello, A., "Clinical Significance of Focal Topographic Changes in the Electroencephalogram (EEG) and Evoked Potentials (EP) of Psychiatric Patients," *Brain Topography*, 5(1):3-10, 1992.

4. Araki, S. A., Muata, K., Yokoyama, K., Uchida, E., "Auditory Event-Related Potential (P300) in Relation to Peripheral Nerve Conduction in Workers Exposed to Lead, Zinc, and Copper: Effects of Lead on Cognitive Function and Central Nervous System," *Am Jour of Industrial Med.*, 21:539-547, 1992.

5. Halliday, R., Rosenthai, J. H., Naylor, H., Callaway, E., "Averaged Evoked Potential Predictors of Clinical Improvement in Hyperactive Children Treated with Methylphenidate: An Initial Study and Replication," *The Soc for Psychophysiological Res.*, 13(5):429-440, 1976.

6. Prichep, L. S., Sutton, S., Hakerem, G., "Evoked Potentials in Hyperkinetic and Normal Children Under Certainty and Uncertainty: A Placebo and Methylphenidate Study," *The Soc for Psychophysiological Res.*, 13(5):419-420, 1976.

7. Christensen, L., Bourgeois, A., Cockroft, R., "Dietary Alteration of Somatic Symptoms and Regional Brain Electrical Activity," *Biol Psychiatry*, 29:679-682, 1991.

8. Thatcher, R. W., Fishbein, D. H., "Computerized EEG, Nutrition and Behavior," *Jour of Applied Nutrition*, 36(2):81-92, 1984.

9. Sloan, E. P., Fenton, G. W., Standage, K. P., "Anticholinergic Drug Quantitative Electroencephalogram, Visual Evoked and Verbal Memory," *Biol Psychiatry*, 31:600-606, 1992.

10. Maurer, K., Dierks, T., Strik, W. K., Frolich, L., "P300 Topography in Psychiatry and Psychopharmacology," *Brain Topography*, 3(1):79-84, 1990.

11. Fukuda, M., Hiramatsu, K., Honda, M., Niwa, S., Sasaki, T., Hata, A., Nakagome, K., Iwanami, A., Honda, H., Hayashida S., Itoh, K., "Shortening of Nl and P300 Latencies in Event-Related Potentials Observed Coincidentally with Clinical Improvement during Nootropic Medication in a Demented Patient: Specific Effect of Nicergoline," *Jpn J Psychiatry and Neurol*, 46(4)919-925, 1992.

12. Maurer, K., Dierks, T., Laux, G., Rupprecht, R., "Topographic Mapping of EEG and Auditory Evoked P300 in Neuropsychopharmacology (Typographic Pharmaco-EEG and Pharmaco-AEP 300)," *Pharmacopsychiat.*, 21:338-342, 1988.

13. Buchsbaum, M., Wender, P., "Average Evoked Responses in Normal and Minimally Brain Dysfunctioned Children Treated With Amphetamine," *Arch Gen Psychiatry*, 29:764-770, 1973.

14. Prichep, L. S., Sutton, S., Hakerem, G., "Evoked Potentials in Hyperkinetic and Normal Children Under Certainty and Uncertainty: A Placebo and Methylphenidate Study," *Soc Psychophysio Res*, 13(5):419-428, 1976.

15. Pockberger, H., Rappelsberger, P., Petsche, H., Thau, K., Kufferle, B., "Computer-assisted EEG-Topography as a Tool in the Evaluation of Actions of Psychoactive Druqs in Patients," *Neuropsychobiol.*, 12:183-187, 1984.

16. Rockstroh, B., Elbert, T., Lutzenberger, W., Altenmuller, E., "Effects of the Anticonvulsants Benzodiazepine Clonazepam on Event-related Brain Potentials in Humans," *Electroence Clin Neurophysiol*, 78:142-149, 1991.

17. Epstein, C. M., Trotter, J. F., Averbook, A., Freeman, S., Kutner, M. H., Elsas, L. J., "EEG Mean Frequencies are Sensitive Indices of Phenylalanine Effects on Normal Brain," *Electroence Clin Neurophysiol*, 72:133-139, 1989.

18. Itil, T. M., Eralp, E., Itil, K. Z., Mzanco, A., Akman, A., "CEEG Dynamic Brain Mapping, A New Method to Evaluate Brain Function in Different Psychological and Drug Conditions," *Symposium Electric and Magnetic Activity of the CNS; Research and Clinical Application in Aerospace Medicine.* Advisory Group for Aerospace Research and Development, 1987.

19. Peniston, E. G., Kulkosky, P. J., "A-Θ Brainwave Training and B-Endorphin Levels in Alcoholics," *Alcoholism: Clin Exp Res*, 13(2):271-279, 1989.

20. Braverman E., Smith, R., Smayda, R., Blum, K., "Modification of P300 Amplitude and Other Electrophysiological Parameters of Drug Abuse by Cranial Electrical Stimulation," *Curr Therapeutic Res.*, 48(4):586-596, 1990.

21. Trachtenberg, M. C., DeFrance, J. F, Hymel, C., Loeblich, L. A., Ginsberg L, Blume, J., Sharma, A., Sharma, S., "The Effects of Tropamine+ On Attention Processing," *Neurogenesis*, 2-22.

22. Thatcher R. W., Fishbein, D. H., "Computerized EEG, Nutrition and Behavior," *Jour of App Nutr.*, 36(2):81-90, 1984.

23. Pfeiffer, C. C., Goldstein, L., "Assay of Anti-Anxiety Druqs by Quantitative Electroencephalography," *Arch Gen Psychiatry*, 10(5):446, 1964.

24. Bartel, P., Blom, M., Robinson, E., Van de Meyden, C., Sommers, DeK., Becker, P., "Effects of Chlorpromazine on Pattern and Flash ERGs and VEPs Compared to Oxazepam and to Placebo in Normal Subjects," *Electroencephalography and Clin Neurophysiology*, 77-330-339, 1990.

Biological Rhythms

Plants can tell time -- they are very sensitive to how long a day is. Leaves fall when the days shorten, and flowers usually bloom when the days lengthen. A plant in shade will grow spindly and tall, while one in full sunlight will grow more robust and shorter. Plants, like humans, tell time by distinguishing between light and dark. Light is perceived by plant pigments, which are very similar to our hemoglobin pigments.

Our bodies also tell time. They are reactive to light which is mediated by our own pigment center, one of its substances being the chemical hormone melatonin, a derivative of melanin from the pineal gland, which is associated with biological rhythms. Many individuals experience seasonal affective disorder, which can be a neurobiochemical imbalance associated with imbalances of tryptophan, melatonin, phenylalanine, and tyrosine. Some renowned researchers suggest that white light can be useful in seasonal disorders. Others are even looking at different colored lights such as green, blue, and red to modify mood swings. Green and blue lights are supposed to be relaxing, while red light may be stimulating (adequate documentation of these effects is not available yet). We do know that fluorescent lighting can cause fatigue and hyperactivity, and full spectrum lighting can affect our moods positively.

Electromagnetic pollution varies throughout our environment in the forms of video screens, electric blankets, power lines, etc., which may affect behavior in a variety of ways; e.g., by causing anxiety associated with depression. Like air and electromagnetic fields, light is another "nutrient" which affects our total health. Those who are affected by changes in light should put full spectrum lighting in their homes and become informed of the nutrients which may be beneficial for modification of mood swings associated with changes in light, such as melatonin (chronoset).

The benefits of chronoset may extend further than the biological rhythms associated with changes in light and darkness; chronoset also may benefit the individual who suffers from jet lag and PMS. Some people with fluctuating biological rhythms have neurological conditions on BEAM which respond to anticonvulsants and even medicines for manic depressive illness. Other natural agents which may improve the brain's rhythm problems are GABA, taurine, melatonin, manganese, and possibly adenosine. See also discussion of light in Section 19, pp. 334.

Brain Stimulants

Brain stimulants like Fastin, Tenuate, Pondimin, and Adiplex are sympathometic and alternative antidepressants. Just like Ritalin, an amphetamine substance, they can be used for treatment-resistant depression or treatment-resistant chronic fatigue disorder. Brain stimulants are used for treatment-resistant chronic fatigue disorder and not for weight loss. Over 70 percent of all medications currently used by doctors are used for purposes other than what the Physicians Desk Reference suggests. Advil is used for PMS, yet it is approved for arthritis. Aspirin is used for heart disease and not just fever. Antibiotics are recommended for viral illness and not just bacterial infections. Drugs like Verapamil, which is approved for cardiac spasms, are also used for blood pressure. Therefore we know that the *Physicians Desk Reference* statement of use for a drug is not always what the doctors use it for, and brain stimulants are useful not only for weight loss but also for fatigue, depression, and attention deficit.

Eldepryl:
An Anti-Aging Compound

Eldepryl, an anti-aging compound, helps the aging brain build its dopamine, slowing down the natural Parkinson's, and delays latency associated with a delayed P300 wave in brain mapping.

Feel Good Response (FGR)

FGR is conjectured to be a brain state. With the right balance of serotonergic, opioidergic, gabbaergic, dopaminergic, and various amino acid balances in the brain, this creates the synchronous rhythm of peace. The CES device, biofeedback, nutritional supplementation, proper brain chemical and genetic states all seem to help.

Brain Waves and States of Consciousness

BETA *ACTIVITY*	**ALPHA** *ACTIVITY*	**THETA** *ACTIVITY*
Conscious processes	Normal conscious	Normally unconscious
External focus	Internal focus	Internal focus
Active, attached	Relaxed wakefulness	Inactive, detached
Rational-analytical	Calm, quiet, "witnessing"	Receptive-observing
Thinking, concentrating	Dreamily thoughtful	Intuitive, experiencing

FREQUENCY
(HERTZ)
⇐ 20   19   18   17   16   15   14   13   12   11   10   9   8   7   6   5   4   3   2   1   0

BETA   **ALPHA**   **THETA**   **DELTA**

NORMALLY CONSCIOUS PROCESSES   NORMALLY UNCONSCIOUS PROCESSES

WAKEFULNESS   REVERIE   SLEEP

Neurotransmitter-Associated Symptoms and Signs

NEUROTRANSMITTERS	SYMPTOMS AND SYNDROMES ASSOCIATED WITH	
	Deficiency	*Excess*
Acetylcholine	memory deficits	hypervigilance
	flaccidity	hypermotility
	hypoarousal	seizures
	REM [1] sleep deficit	REM sleep enhancement
	desynchronization	synchronization
	xerostomia/dry mouth	excess salivation
		asthma
Histamine	> 8 hrs sleep	< 6 hrs sleep
	easy fatigue	high stamina
	high pain threshold	low pain threshold
	hallucinations/paranoia	asthma, atrophy, allergies
	carefree	obsessions
	drug reactive	compulsions/phobias
	anesthetic sensitive	drug resistant
	thoughts overlap	anesthetic resistant
	suicidal thoughts	ruminate/"blank mind"
	flight of ideas	suicidal actions
	low libido	migraine headache
		high libido
Epinephrine/norepinephrine (adrenaline)	narcolepsy	insomnia
	depression	mania
	hypotension	hypertension
	satiety	hyperphagia
	caffeinism	migraine
Dopamine	Parkinsonism	chorea
	cholinergic	anticholinergic
	agitation	schizophrenia
	sexual disinterest	sexual arousal
Serotonin	insomnia/anxiety	narcolepsy
	impulsiveness	
Glutamine/glutamate	fatigue	endurance
	hypertension	hypotension
	depression	agitation
	seizures	schizophrenia

1. REM = Rapid eye movement

INHIBITORY OR ANTAGONISTIC NEUROTRANSMITTERS	SYMPTOMS AND SYNDROMES ASSOCIATED WITH	
Gamma-amino butyric acid (GABA)	excitation	withdrawn serenity
	action tremors	flaccidity
	multiple sclerosis	excitoneurotoxin
	hyperphagia	satiety
Glycine/taurine/alanine	agitation	sedation
	acetylcholine antagonist	acetylcholine agonist

Neurotransmitters: Sources and Major Metabolites

Amino Acids	Neurotransmitters	Metabolites	
Serine/choline	Acetylcholine	CO_2, bile acids	
Histidine	Histamine	Imidazole	
Tyrosine/tyramine	Epinephrine	Metanephrines	VMA
Phenylalanine	Norepinephrine	Normetanephrines	VMA
Phenylalanine	Dopamine	HVA	
Tryptophan	Serotonin	5-HIAA	Kynurenate
Glutamate	Gamma-amino butyrate	Succinate	
Glycine	Glycine	Acetate	

VMA = vanilmandelic acid; HVA = homovanillic acid; HIAA = hydroxyindoleacetic acid

Neurotransmitter production is regulated by enzymes that are dependent upon specific essential nutrient cofactor. These cofactor and the regulating enzymes responsible for neurotransmitter synthesis and metabolism are shown in the following table. Modulation of regulating cofactor can improve the functional performance of regulating enzymes.

Neurotransmitters: Regulating Cofactor and Enzymes

NEUROTRANSMITTERS	REGULATING COFACTOR(S)	REGULATING ENZYME(S)
Acetylcholine	Coa, choline	ACS
Histamine	Cu, Zn, Mn, B-6	MAO
Epinephrine	Cu, Mg, B-3, B-6, AA, FA	COMT, MAO
Norepinephrine	Cu, Mg, B-3, B-6, AA, FA	COMT, MAO
Dopamine	Fe, B-6, biotin	DD, MAO
Serotonin	Fe, B-3, B-6	TH, MAO
Gamma-amino butyric acid	B-6, biotin	GD
Glycine	Lipoate (Coa)	MAO

ACS = acetylcholine synthetase; COMT = catechol-o-methyl transferase; MAO = monoamine oxidase;
DD = dopamine decarboxylase; TH = tryptophan hydroxylase; GD = glutamine decarboxylase

Core Laboratory Studies for Clinical Management of Mood Disorders Such as the Schizophrenias

The most important neurotransmitters, cofactor, and immunoreactive triggers can now be measured through functional assays that reflect clinical status more accurately than older serum concentration assays. This means that both improved diagnostic precision, therapeutic differentiation, and outcome monitoring are now possible. Such studies, with the usual range (often mistakenly referred to as 'normal range') and suggested healthy laboratory ranges, are shown in the following table:

LABORATORY STUDIES FOR MOOD DISORDERS

NEUROTRANSMITTERS	LABORATORY RESULTS RANGE		
Acetylcholine	40-80	60-70	mg/dl serum
Histamine	25-70	40-50	ng/ml plasma
Epinephrine (platelets)	3-27	8-16	ng/10^8 platelets
Metanephrine (platelets)	4-40	10-20	ng/10^8 platelets
Vanilmandelic acid (VMA, urine)			urine
Norepinephrine (platelets)	3-11	5-9	ng/10^8 platelets
Normetanephrine (platelets)	4-40	10-20	ng/10^8 platelets
Dopamine (platelets)	1-11	4-6	ng/10^8 platelets
Homovanillic acid (HVA, urine)			urine
Serotonin (platelets)	15-300	70-300	ng/10^8 platelets
Hydroxyindole acetic acid (HIAA, urine)			urine
Gamma-amino butyric acid (GABA)	.52-3.00	1-2	umol/dl plasma
Glycine	17-31	22-26	umol/dl plasma

ESSENTIAL ENZYME COFACTOR
(by functional measurements, where known)

Thiamine (B-1) [ETK]	100 ± 10%	100 ± 5%	comparative activity
Riboflavin (B-2) [EGR]	100 ± 10%	100 ± 5%	comparative activity
Niacin (B-3) [1NMethylnicotinamide = 1NMN]	3-17	8-12	mg/D urinary excretion
Pyridoxine (B-6) [EGOT]	<125	<110%	comparative activity
Cobalamin [B-12/B-12 binding capacity]	>60%	>80%	% saturation
Biotin [carboxylase]	200-500	300-400	pg/ml plasma
Ascorbate (C) [WBC ascorbate]	20-50 ug	30-40 ug	per 10^8 WBCs
Folate [FIGLU]	3-7.5	0-3	mg/D urinary excretion

Handicapping Effects of Brain Injury and Psychological Disorders Resulting from Traumatic Experiences [1]

1. About 80% of concussions produce Mild Traumatic Brain Injury (MTBI).

2. Most brain injuries either heal completely within a few months, or develop compensating functions to some degree.

3. A subsequent insult to the brain, not necessarily severe, can escalate the first MTBI into a massive organic breakdown. Every survivor of MTBI is at risk for such a magnified, destructive effect.

4. Most serious automobile accidents and other life-threatening experiences (e.g., rape,war, being mugged with a deadly weapon) cause some degree of post-traumatic stress, marked by severe depression and anxiety.

5. Traumatic psychological conditions can disrupt and degrade cognitive processes (e.g., memory, logical thinking, learning, verbal and spatial perception) as effectively as brain injuries can (lesions, infarcts, hematomas, etc.). In fact, as the lifelong problems of many Vietnam veterans demonstrate, traumatic stress disorders can handicap and destroy lives.

6. The crucial issue is the determination of the degree and nature of a psychological handicap in each case. An impaired numerical ability is an incapacitating handicap for a bookkeeper or accountant, but of little consequence for a truck driver or dentist.

7. Even if there is organic brain damage, the psychological component can be the more handicapping factor. The organic condition often heals or abates, but the psychological disorder may persist for life.

8. Psychological disorders can quickly become habituated if not effectively and promptly treated. Habituation sets distorted perceptions into fixed personality styles, which are highly resistant to change. Such abnormal personality styles limit career potential and disrupt social and family relationships (loss of job, divorce).

9. Psychological impairment can be corrected or mitigated. Cognitive impairments can be improved with new remediation technologies (sometimes above premorbid functioning). Tests are available for determining potential for improvement.

10. The keys to determination of compensability of cerebral dysfunction, both organic and psychological, are (a) immediate and/or permanent impairment of mental processes, (b) transitory or permanent handicapping effects of such impairments for the particular claimant, and (c) potential for progressive mental deterioration or improvement.

11. The patient's clinical interviews are limited in their validity and are not conclusive in themselves. Tests are necessary to provide data for differential diagnosis and for distinguishing specific mental functions (e.g., different kinds of memory). *No single test battery can satisfy those requirements.*

---

1. Used by permission from Martin Haydon, Ph.D

Neuropsychological Evaluation [1]

What It Is

A neuropsychological examination consists of a battery of tests that measure the various functions of the brain. The functions include:

- Perceptual functions
- Attention / Concentration
- Memory functions
- Intellectual functions
- Motor / Tactile functions
- Verbal / Speech functions
- Spatial organization
- Personality functions
- Emotional states

The test battery comprises questions and mental tasks that reveal the degree of efficiency or deficiency in the brain's performance of those functions.

What It Does

The information provided by the responses to the questions and tasks is technically analyzed to determine the nature of the injury or dysfunction of parts of the brain resulting from concussion, emotional disturbance, tumor, or deterioration of the cerebral nerves or biochemical processes that enable you to feel, think, remember, and behave.

Since emotional reactions directly affect the thinking functions, the full battery of neuropsychological tests includes inventories of emotional states like anxiety and depression that can disrupt the cognitive (thinking) functions of the brain. Such emotional states can strongly affect perception and thinking in ways that are just as dysfunctional as injury to the brain structure. It is not necessary for the brain tissue to be damaged for there to be functional deficiencies. Stress and shock can create *organic* impairment of mental processes just as definitely as an injury to the nerves.

Benefits of Proper Diagnosis

The sheer complexity of brain structures and functions makes diagnosis difficult and time-consuming. A careful and skillful analysis of the test results can determine the nature and location of possible defects. It also measures the degree of deficiency in the performance of various mental functions.

The brain, made of billions of neurons, has a lot of what we call redundancy built into its structures. Signals are transmitted through bundles of neurons, or nerves, and processed in various centers that are also masses of neurons. Damage to parts of the brain may cause more or less deficient performance. We now have an arsenal of cognitive remediation and retraining exercises and procedures that can use the brain's redundant mechanisms to compensate for impaired functions. The neuropsychological examination enables us to determine exactly which parts of each process have been impaired -- for example, one impaired function might be the short-term memory for procedures used on the job or in the home.

With a clear determination of which particular mental processes need to be enhanced or reinforced, we can design a program of cognitive remediation, combined with psychotherapy for any emotional factors, that will improve cognitive functioning, with corresponding improvement in intellectual performance. We now know, too, that a well exercised mind will hold its mental skills much better and longer into advanced age.

When Should An Evaluation Be Performed?

Most people go to their physician for regular checkups. They want to catch problems early, to improve their chances of successful treatment. Although the brain is the most important organ in the body, we tend to take it for granted until an accident occurs or some internal problem develops. Just as your physician can help you more if he or she knows your "baseline" organ functioning levels before problems occur, your neuropsychologist can help you more if he or she knows your "baseline" cognitive levels before problems arise.

---

1. Used by permission of Martin Haydon, Ph.D.

How Long Does it Take?

Typically, the comprehensive test battery takes about six hours to administer. This may take one or more sessions. The neuropsychologist may add or substitute tests according to observation of patient's performance. After the interpretation of results, and preparation of the report, a post-test consultation is scheduled with you to discuss evaluation findings and recommended therapy, if needed. The cost of the neuropsychological evaluation depends on the kind and number of tests administered and the time required for completion. An estimate can be provided when previous records and the patient's problems are reviewed. The baseline data enables us to deter mine how serious a mental deficit is when you have had an accident, disease, or age-related loss of function. You should have at least one neuropsychological evaluation when you have reached maturity. You would certainly want to have one in the event of head injury or traumatic disorder or severe disease.

Neuropsychological Screening [1]

It is now possible to administer a short battery of NP tests that will detect structural or functional organicity with adequate, statistical certainty. The short-form test battery provides sufficient information to determine the likelihood of certain types of organic brain impairment based on the various cognitive and emotional signs of such dysfunctions. A negative finding provides a statistically reliable indication of nonorganic status. A positive finding suggests high likelihood of brain impairment, with some indication of specific mental deficits. The positive result does not enable localization of focal site(s) where damage is centered nor does it support decisive differential diagnosis. The latter requires the full battery NP evaluation.

Thus, a positive finding calls for a full battery test evaluation, while a negative finding makes a full battery evaluation unnecessary, except in cases where there is either a pathological family history or symptomatic evidence of psychopathology. In the latter two cases, the screening test may be skipped, going directly to the full battery NP evaluation.

The screening battery takes less than an hour to administer, plus about two hours of analysis and reporting. Total fee of $500 is, of course, about 1/5 of the full battery cost.

Neuropsych screening is useful for some patients who are either intimidated by the full-day test procedure or cannot afford the latter's price. It is also useful as a periodic mental checkup, corresponding to regular physical checkups.

Neurological and Psychometric Techniques

PATH Medical has state-of-the-art neurological and psychometric computerized techniques which help the selected PATH staff to diagnose the vast array of symptoms which help in understanding the biochemical, neurological, and physical diseases.

- The TOVA tests detect attention deficit disorders using standardized objective techniques.

- The neuro-psych test is used for educational evaluations and predicts dementia through memory testing. This test includes cognitive rehabilitation.

- Personality testing, career testing, behavior testing, personality type, and Myers-Briggs testing are all performed at PATH Medical.

PATH Medical can tell you more about your long-term behavior and how it interrelates to your total health and physical well-

---

1. Used by permission of Martin Haydon, Ph.D.

being than ever before. Take care of your mental, emotional and neurological health and you will be taking care of your total health and life.

Advanced Cognitive Remediation System

Cognitive remediation can now be accomplished with newly developed techniques that can improve, and may restore, premorbid operation of various brain functions or enhance complementary abilities that perform equivalent functions. This process enables the improvement of memory and other cognitive functions that have been impaired by traumatic accidents.

Advances in computer technology and neuroscience have made possible the development of computer-based exercises designed for recovery (in some cases rapid) of memory, language, and numerical, visuospatial, and intellectual processes. These are some of the advantages of the new computerized exercise programs:

MORE EFFECTIVE

The interactive computer display programs engage the interest and concentration of patients, and intensify the beneficial effects of the exercises.

VERSATILITY

The computer permits presentation of all types of exercise material, precisely designed, with exact exposure timing and immediate scoring. The instantaneous scoring allows changes to be made in the choice of exercises and difficulty levels during the session.

MEASURABLE RESULTS

The patient's responses to the computer stimuli are automatically evaluated and scored, providing a measured indication of progress and remaining distance to premorbid levels, along with a prognosis of potential for further improvement in functioning.

GRADED DIFFICULTY LEVELS

Remediation for each of the cognitive skills is graded so that difficulty of the various exercises can be matched to each patient's improving ability at every stage of the remediation program.

DESIGN AND CONTENT OF THE REMEDIATION PROGRAM:

The neuropsychological test batteries provide detailed information on measurements of specific cognitive deficits. This information is used in selecting the exercises designed to correct those deficits, starting at the ability level indicated by the test results. The selected exercises are then arranged in a program that produces the optimum results without taxing the patient's capacity. Continuous measurement provides for close monitoring of the patient's performance of the various cognitive functions, enabling exact grading of difficulty to advance his/her targeted abilities to higher levels.

Patients who do neuropsychological tests are often found to have very diverse deficits, including deficits in attention and concentration, memory, hand-eye coordination, categorization, learning strategies, etc. New computer techniques, as well as new exercise techniques, have been shown to result in repair or recovery of these deficits, somewhat like rehabilitation -- one can engage in brain rehabilitation. A cognitive remediation program is now available on computer or in take-home form.

Brain Biofeedback Exercises and Training: How to Heal, Rebuild, and Maximize Brain Potential

Increasing evidence shows that the aging brain slows down and has excess theta waves. Alpha/theta brain wave biofeedback training is a technique which will help maximize brain development and improve brain functioning, increasing stimulation to the brain and the ability to focus and concentrate. Techniques such as eye exercises and cognitive remediation can help rebuild the brain. With the development of neuropsychological tests new strategies for learning can help the individual who has neuropsychological and brain deficits to rehabilitate. Biofeedback can be used to maximize and help develop injured parts of the brain in trauma patients, etc. Brain exercise holds a great future for antiaging and relaxation effects. See Natural Steroid Therapy and What is Aging, pp. 184.

Properly speaking, the procedure is *Biofeedback Training*, not merely exercises. The patient is supposed to master the skill, so that he/she can do it on demand, when necessary, without biofeedback instruments. You learn how to tune in to your autonomic nervous system as naturally as your voluntary system. Making the patient come to the office whenever relaxation is needed is not what biofeedback is all about.

The Brain Beats on the Path

The heart beats one time per second. The electrical rhythm of the brain beats eight times per second or 480 times per minute. Is it any wonder we can all go out of rhythm frequently, especially when bombarded by electromagnetic radiation?

Eye Health

The eyes are the lamp of the body, the extension of the brain, and therefore they are noticed in this section of this book. Macular degeneration is thought to be slowed down by zinc supplements and vitamin E. Nutrients can be used for glaucoma and some nutrients may slow down hemorrhages of the eye as described in the section below.

Hemorrhage of the Eye

Eye hemorrhage is not easy to treat. Some people think that collections of hemorrhages in the eye can be treated with potassium iodide, 5 drops, twice a day. The FDA took the pill form of potassium iodide off the market because they did not think it was effective. Other treatments for hemorrhage are oral enzymes such as bromelin and pancreatin, although none of these have been proven effective.

Nutrition: Glaucoma And Other Eye Diseases

There are very few studies that suggest that individuals with glaucoma may have vitamin deficiencies. Some studies suggest that low levels of vitamin C deficiency may be associated with higher intraocular pressure and that higher dosages of vitamin C may reduce eye pressure.

The same has also been said of rutin. Possibly other bioflavonoids and, on rare occasions, food allergies have been associated with glaucoma. None of this is strong evidence at this time for a relationship between nutrition and glaucoma. Other eye diseases may respond to a variety of natural approaches. For example, abnormalities in taurine metabolism result in an increase in the cataract crystals in lenses of retinitis pigmentosa. Glaucoma may begin with different losses of chromatic color vision. GPC, giant papillary conjunctivitis, which occurs with contact lenses, and probably many other irritants, can be treated with vitamin A drops. Vitamin E may be helpful in retinitis pigmentosa. N-acetyl-cysteine may be helpful for chronic macular edema in retinitis pigmentosa. Antioxidants protect the brain against optic neuritis. Eye drops may help superior limbic keratocon junctivitis. Recent studies show that eye exercise and long-term physical training can help reduce the risk of glaucoma. Myopia can predispose an individual to glaucoma. Eyebright may help glaucoma.

Glaucoma is high pressure in the eye that leads to death of optic nerve cells. Death of cells leads to a loss of vision. Peripheral vision is lost first. Central vision can remain until the late stage, when 90 percent of the optic nerve is already destroyed. Glaucoma usually has no symptoms aside from silent painless loss of vision beginning peripherally. Glaucoma is the second leading cause of blindness in the United States and the leading cause in virtually every other country in the world. Over 70,000 people in the U.S. are blind from glaucoma -- 200,000 are blind in one eye, 2 million or more have some degree of visual damage and 8 million more are susceptible. Glaucoma is more common than diabetes and hypertension, probably because of abnormalities in blood sugar and blood pressure. Therefore it is extremely important to control these abnormalities. Risk factors are being black, myopia, diabetes, family history, hypertension, smoking, alcohol and other drugs, thyroid disease, arteriosclerosis, steroids, and eye drops. Glaucoma is very often missed. Routine eye examinations are extremely important. Sometimes, glaucoma may occur with a low tension. Diurnal variations may be a factor, and therefore pressure must be checked extremely carefully.

Glaucoma is not one disease but a number of different diseases affecting the conditions of the eye and producing high pressure. There are two types of glaucoma -- angle closure and open glaucoma. Angle closure glaucoma is most common in Asians, least common in blacks and affects farsighted people. With an acute attack there is pain, red eye, blurred vision, nausea. It is a medical emergency and can be cured with laser treatment, the primary definitive treatment. Open angle glaucoma is

most common in blacks, least common in Asians. Exfoliation syndrome occurs in 20 percent of all glaucoma. The drain of the eye gets clogged by pigment, much like coffee grounds clogging a kitchen drain.

Pigmentary glaucoma may be more common than we realize, affecting maybe 250,000 people. Hereditary glaucoma affects young people 20-30 years old. It is, therefore, important to check family members. Over 1,000 current patients at New York Eye and Ear who have glaucoma are under age 35. There is congenital glaucoma and infectious glaucoma. The goal of therapy is to minimize side effects of medication, lower the pressure, turn the so-called faucet down, and open the angle up and let things drain. Miotic drops such as pilocarpine and carbachol can be used. But side effects are very prominent in younger patients, including possible retinal detachment. Beta-blockers, Timoptic, Betoptic, and Betagan have few local side effects but could lower your pressure and cause other problems which might affect exercise tolerance, exacerbate asthma, congestive heart failure, memory loss, insomnia, depression, and hallucinations. Carbonic anhydrase inhibitors or pills (e.g., Diamox or Neptazane) turn the faucet down. There are many new medications being tested. Nonsteroidal drugs may be helpful. Laser, surgical treatment, ultrasound, and cyclodestructive procedures, e.g., laser sclerostomy, are being developed.

Drugs that worsen glaucoma are numerous, e.g., antipsychotics, antidepressants, inhibitors, antihistamines, anti-Parkinson's agents, anti-spasmolytic agents, and a variety of other agents that can cause idiopathic lens swelling, as well as sympathomimetic agents. As a rule, these are not prominent problems. Antioxidants are most useful in the prevention of cataracts, maybe they will someday be shown to benefit glaucoma. Antioxidants work to prevent cataracts probably by preventing damage by UV light. They also protect the aging macula.

Glaucoma also occurs frequently with increased sympathetic tone. It is possible that CES device can reduce vagal tone. Forced unilateral nostril breathing induces selective contralateral hemispheric stimulation as measured by relative increases in EEG amplitude and the contralateral hemispheres alternating lateralization of plasma catecholamines. Forced right nostril breathing produces a functional vagotomy which leads to a bilateral decrease in intraocular pressure.

4. Cancer and Oncology -- Hematology

Cancer: Diagnosing Gastrointestinal Malignancies

Increasing evidence now suggests that we have increased ability to diagnose pancreatic, stomach, and other intestinal malignancies through the blood. There are tests such as the antimalignant antibodies screening (AMAS) test, the T-helper/T-suppressor ratio, cancer antigen CA19-9, and now the testosterone to dihydrotestosterone ratio. This is a useful marker for pancreatic cancer in males. Androgen metabolisms are characterized by the synthesis of testosterone from androstenedione in the testes and its conversion to its reduced metabolite 5 alpha dihydro-testosterone and 17 beta estradiol in extragonadal tissues. Both normal and malignant pancreatic tissue are involved in the metabolism of androgens, and derangements in these pancreatic and android enzymes are associated with cancer. Increased androstenedione levels have been found in these patients, indicating enhanced conversion of testosterone into this metabolite by the pancreatic tumor. Yet, measurement of testosterone androstenedione alone has not been sufficient to predict cancer. The ratio of testosterone (T) to dihydrotestosterone (DHT) is maintained at 10 in healthy males and is found to be significantly lower in men with pancreatic cancer. A ratio of 5 or less was seen in 91 percent of patients with this disease, whereas only 1 in 40 controls had it. The only other clinical situation where an altered T to DHT ratio can be found is deficiency in five alpha reductase. Thus the T to DHT ratio is proposed as a potentially useful mark for pancreatic cancer. One of the drawbacks of CA 19-9 is that it is frequently negative in the early stages of disease, and there is a greater sensitivity of the T to DHT ratio in stage 1 pancreatic carcinoma. The findings in a recent study suggest that the T-DHT ratio and CA 19-9 determinations, especially when combined with the AMAS and T-cells, will be particularly useful in cancer screening.

Idiopathic Thrombocytopenic Purpura (ITP)

ITP is often an acute disorder, which usually occurs in adults and rarely resolves itself spontaneously. It is most common in immune hemolytic anemia and can occur for a number of reasons. One cause for occurrence is when platelet counts fall to the 80-90,000 range, which might also lead to death. Some other causes of ITP are sarcoidosis, lymphoma, leukemia, lupus, thyroiditis, carcinoma, scleroderma, myasthenia gravis, hemolytic anemia, and pregnancy. Almost any drug can cause ITP, but the worst offenders are the quinines.

ITP is probably found most often in drinkers and smokers even though its presence is not documented.

The wide variety of treatments include: Vitamin C, intravenous gamma globulin, anti-idiotype antibodies, therapeutic plasmapheresis and immune suppressants such as azathioprine and prednisone. Dannzol and testosterone may also be helpful.

Some ITP patients respond to alpha-interferon and 79% improve after a splenectomy. Unfortunately there are no methods to tell if a patient will benefit from a splenectomy and there is an increased risk of infection after a splenectomy has been performed.

There might also be a genetic predisposition to ITP in some patients, which can be identified by using such antigens as HLA/B-8/B-12.

ITP is also considered a malignancy to some degree given, e.g., its association with proliferation.

ITP can be found in blood cells themselves rather than in the platelet elements of blood. Hormone imbalance may be a factor since it is found in post-puberty, premenopausal women.

Polycythemia

Polycythemia is an increased proliferation of the elements of the blood. This can include red blood cells, platelets, and even white blood cells. The causes are many, e.g., high altitude, chronic pulmonary disease, cardiovascular shunt, massive obesity, smoking, congenital decreased red cell DPG, cerebellar hemangioblastomas, fibroids, cysts, Barter's Syndrome, and other familial conditions.

The real worry concerning polycythemia is an increased risk for stroke and clotting. Typical treatment includes phlebotomy, chemotherapy, and/or nutrient therapy (fish oil (EPA) -- which can decrease clotting and reduce risk of stroke -- beta-carotene, selenium, cysteine and vitamin E, all of which are excellent antioxidants for this precancerous condition). Since polycythemia is much like a cancer, antioxidants must be used.

The use of zinc (150 mg twice a day) may produce a copper anemia, which may reduce the red and white blood count as well as platelets. Interestingly, an extract of grapefruit may be helpful in polycythemia.

Anti-Cancer Diet & Nutrients

Cancer accounts for at least 10-25% of our national health costs. The cause of cancer and forms of cancer are multiple. All people are at risk because carcinogens, like nitrates, hydrogenated oils, cigarette smoke, radiation, saturated fat, caffeine, Valium, estrogens (hormones), aflatoxin (peanut butter), food additives, air pollutants, radon, etc., are so prevalent. One out of three Americans will develop cancer.

Data are overwhelmingly in favor of the benefits of diet and vitamins in cancer prevention. Not surprisingly, obesity and immune deficiency are risks for cancer. Evidence suggests that various nutrients can inhibit growth of tumors in man and in experimental animals, that a deficiency of these nutrients is a risk factor, that higher levels of these nutrients in the blood give protection against cancer, and that the nutrients can be used to treat cancer. This is far less established than prevention. The nutrients that have been shown to be especially protective are vitamin A, beta-carotene, vitamin C, vitamin E, cysteine, and selenium. These nutrients are found in pigmented vegetables (green, yellow or orange), vegetable oils, eggs, whole grains and cereals, fruits and vegetables, seafood, liver, and meat (selenium). Hence, a high vegetable, high whole grain diet with some fish and meat is the general anti-cancer diet. Each cancer patient may need a unique diet, e.g., sarcoma patients generally need a high protein diet. Vegetables, because of the anti-cancer properties of fiber, plant sterol, and dithiolthiones (broccoli, cabbage, cauliflower) are usually the most important part of the diet. Whole grains, because of the fiber, are the next most important food group to protect against cancer. Many other nutrients may have a role in cancer, particularly cysteine. Furthermore, some nutrients, especially cysteine and selenium, can reduce the side effects of chemotherapy. Several other nutrients may have a role in cancer prevention and treatment (e.g., calcium -- colon cancer), arginine, folic acid, vitamin B-12, primrose oil, bioflavonoids, riboflavin, vitamin B-6, zinc, manganese, and molybdenum. Probably any nutrient missing for a long period of time can lead to a cell deficiency injury. This is well documented in cases of B-12 and folic acid deficiency where early cancers have occurred.

See McGinnis, JM, and Foege, WH, Actual Causes of Death in the United States, *JAMA* 270:18 p. 2207ff., 1993.

Potential Cancer Fighters in Foods

Although no food or food combination has yet been clinically proven to prevent or retard cancer in people, animal and test-tube research strongly suggest that many components have specific biological actions that may prove helpful. Scientists suspect that to treat tumors, compounds would have to be extracted or synthesized and given in larger doses than those found naturally; on the other hand, extracts or synthesis might overlook protective compounds in a healthy, varied diet.

COMPONENT	POSSIBLE DISEASE-FIGHTING PROPERTIES	FOOD SOURCES
Allelic sulfides	May protect against carcinogens by stimulating production of a detoxification enzyme, glutathione S-transferase.	Garlic and onions
Carotenoids (Vitamin A precursors)	Antioxidants and cell differentiation agents (cancer cells are nondifferentiated).	Parsley, carrots, winter squash, sweet potatoes, yams, cantaloupe, apricots, spinach, kale, turnip greens, citrus fruits
Catechins	Antioxidants, linked to lower rates of gastrointestinal cancer, mechanisms not understood.	Green tea berries
Flavonoids	Block receptor sites for certain hormones that promote cancers.	Most fruits and vegetables, including parsley, carrots, citrus fruits, broccoli, cabbage, cucumbers, squash, yams, tomatoes, eggplants, peppers, soy products, berries
Genistein	In test tubes, blocks angiogenesis, growth of new blood vessels essential for some tumors to grow and spread, and deters proliferation of cancer cells.	Found in urine of people with diets rich in soy beans and to a lesser extent in cabbage family vegetables
Fiber	Dilutes carcinogenic compounds in colon and speeds them through digestive system, thus discourages growth of harmful bacteria while bolstering healthful ones; may encourage production of healthier form of estrogen.	Whole grains and many vegetables.
Indoles	Induce protective enzymes.	Cabbage, Brussels sprouts, kale
Isothiocyanates	Induce protective enzymes.	Mustard, horseradish, radishes
Limonoids	Induce protective enzymes.	Citrus fruits
Linolenic acid	Regulates prostaglandin production.	Many leafy vegetables and seeds, especially flaxseed.
Lycopene	Antioxidants.	Tomatoes, red grapefruit
Monoterpenes	Some antioxidant properties; inhibit cholesterol production in tumors; aid protective enzyme activity.	Parsley, carrots, broccoli, cabbage, cucumbers, squash, yams, tomatoes, eggplant, peppers, mint, basil, citrus fruits
Phenolic Acids (tannins)	Some antioxidant properties; inhibit formation of nitrosamine, a carcinogen, and effect enzyme activity.	Parsley, carrots, broccoli, cabbage, tomatoes, eggplant, peppers, citrus fruits, whole grains, berries

Plant sterols (Vitamin D precursors)	Differentiation agents.	Broccoli, cabbage, cucumbers, squash, yams, tomatoes, eggplant, peppers, soy products, whole grains.
Vitamin C	Antioxidant, inhibits creation of nitrosamine, a potentially dangerous carcinogen in the stomach.	Citrus fruits, tomatoes, green leafy vegetables, potatoes
Vitamin E	Antioxidant.	Wheat-germ, oatmeal, peanuts, nuts, brown rice

Source: Dr. Christopher W. W. Beedner, *Eating Well Magazine.*

Anti-Cancer Polyamine Diet

Low polyamines have been linked to senility, hypoglycemia, deterioration, and aging. On the other hand, high polyamines have been linked to psoriasis, cancerous processes, and other growth processes. Polyamines are ubiquitous molecules made primarily from putrescine, cadaverine, spermidine, and spermine. Now they are primarily made from arginine and ornithine, the amino acids, and so these things promote growth. Foods such as cheddar cheese, tomatoes and oranges contain much putrescine. The food that contains the most polyamines

and can cause serious problems is mushrooms. We generally do not recommend mushrooms because of their potential side effects. Spermadine is probably the most toxic polyamine and is found in cheddar cheese and aged cheese, which probably have carcinogenic dimensions. Blockers of polyamine synthesis DMFO (ditluoremethyl-ornithine) have some promise as anti-cancer agents. It will require time to see if polyamines can impact health. (Source: Bardocz, S., The Role of Dietary Polyamines, *European Journal of Clinical Nutrition* 47:683-690, 1993.)

Cancer: New Treatments and Notes on Nutritional Deficiencies

It is now known that cancer is not a localized phenomenon but a systemic disease symbolized by and reflected in the numerous imbalances both in our society and in our individual biochemistry. Cancer is related to psychological dynamics, increased depression, and personality disturbances, etc., which are associated with its development and possibly even its premorbid state. The origin of these problems could be biochemical, even caused by toxins, imbalances in nutrition such as antioxidants, folic acid, B-12, zinc, and many other nutri-

ents which can predispose an individual to cancer. Management of cancer with hormone manipulations such as tamoxifen, Megace, Taxol, interferons, and retinoids has opened up a whole new vista of treatment combining natural and drug therapies. Cancer treatment, properly, should be done in a complete medical/psychological setting. Most cancers still relate back to addictive behaviors, e.g., dependence on food fats, cigarettes, caffeine, etc.

Natural Cancer Therapies

Much has been written about laetrile as a natural cancer therapy. The theory is that nitrilosides (laetrile) may have natural anti-cancer properties, and that once entering the body, the beta-glucosidase of cancer cells synthesizes hydrogen cyanide from nitriloside, while rhodanese from normal cells synthesizes nutritional agents, and the hydrogen cyanide actually destroys the cancer cell. Attached is a list of foods that have this natural anti-cancer property, if it truly does exist. One thing for certain is that these types of foods have been associated with lower rates of cancer because grains, berries, beans, seeds, and fruits have other anti-cancer nutrients. Additional cancer tests are serum sialic acid which helps the measurement of tumor growths.

Probable Natural Sources of Nitrilosides

Kernels or Seeds of Fruits

Apple
Apricot
Cherry
Nectarine
Peach
Plum
Pear
Prune

Beans

Broad
Burma
Chick peas
Lentils
Lima
Mung
Scarlet runner

Grasses

Acacia
Alfalfa
Aquatic
Johnson
Milkweed
Sudan
Tunus
Velvet
Wheat grass
White clover

Miscellaneous

Bamboo shoots
Fuschia plant
Sorghum
Wild hydrangea
Yew tree (needles, fresh leaves)

Nuts

Bitter almond
Cashew
Macadamia

Berries

Blackberry
Chokeberry
Christmas berry
Elderberry
Raspberry
Strawberry

Seeds

Chia
Flax
Rangoon
Sesame

Grains

Barley
Brown rice
Buckwheat groats
Flax
Millet
Oat groats
Rye
Vetch
Wheat berry

Tamoxifen and Megace:

Hormonal Manipulation for Treatment of Cancer

Tamoxifen is a soybean-like compound which protects against cancer. It is a synthetic antiestrogen substance, and therefore has the anti-cancer property of fighting the pro-cancer effects of estrogen. It also has some estrogen effects, and therefore it can treat osteoporosis. It can probably help many other cancers such as ovary, pancreas, and bowel, as can a new compound from yew trees called taxol. Taxol is also used for ovarian and now breast cancer. Megace, in contrast, is an anti-progesterone. These drugs have the effect of increasing weight gain, and eye exams may be necessary regularly during these therapies (except for tamoxifen). Blood clotting can be a problem with tamoxifen, but can be antidoted by fish oil or aspirin.

Cancer Treatments -- Shark Cartilage

New studies suggest that shark cartilage can be a potential therapy for cancer. Shark cartilage is an excellent source of calcium and mucopolysaccharides, and it is thought that it slows, or interrupts, the development of blood vessel growth in cancer, a process known as angiogenesis. Without a continuous source of blood nourishment, tumors cannot grow or metastasize. The Chinese have been aware of shark cartilage for centuries; they make shark fin soup. It is by no means a proven treatment, but it is an interesting new avenue of research. Most likely what will happen is that the chemical property of shark cartilage that is useful will be extracted so that eventually we will not need to administer ridiculously high dosages of 10-70 grams. Cartilade is a good brand of shark cartilage. To order shark cartilage (Cartilade) call 914-939-9000, or write to 222 Grace and Church Streets, Port Chester, NY, 10573.

Screening for Testicular Cancer

There is an approximate 50 percent, five-year survival rate for the most common type of testicular cancer, but it approaches 100 percent with early detection. The first signs of testicular cancer are 1) enlargement of one of the testes and change in consistency; 2) dull ache in abdomen and groin; 3) sensation of dragging and heaviness.

A three-minute monthly self-examination is advisable after a warm bath or shower when the scrotal skin is most relaxed. Roll each testicle gently between the thumb and the first two fingers. If you find any lumps, see your doctor immediately. It may not be malignant, but only a doctor can distinguish malignancy from a benign growth.

Reversal of Preleukemia with Antioxidants: [1]
A Case Report

With recent advances in analytical technology and blood analysis doctors are now able to make earlier diagnoses of precancers as well as identify early stages of cancer. As technology continues to advance, it will lead us to more and more preventive and early intervention oncology. A 25-year-old male in good health with preleukemia is described with reversal of preleukemia and normalization of his low white count neutrophils and platelets with the use of high dosages of antioxidant nutrients and amino acids. The new ways of identifying premalignancies and early malignancies can lead to significant reversal of preleukemia. Nutritional medicine's role is particularly relevant in the treatment period following these new, early diagnoses of malignancies.

CASE REPORT

A 25-year-old male with a negative medical history complained of a two to three year period of progressive malaise and fatigue in association, during the past several months, with headache. There also was some muscle weakness, but he denied experiencing any fevers, chills, night sweats, abdominal pain, hematuria, rash, or adenopathy. There was no history of risk factors for mononucleosis or HIV. This patient was an environmental educator and walked 5-6 miles a day on his job. He was found to have a significant leukopenia and low platelets. On 7 June 1989 his white count was 3.5×10^3 mm^{-3} (normal $n = 3.8$-10.1), and on 17 June 1989 it was 2.8 with a differential of 35% ($n = 40$-75%) neutrophils. His physical examination was unremarkable. He was ruled out for viral illnesses, e.g., Epstein Barr Virus, CMV, and toxoplasmosis. On 5 July 1989 his platelet count fell to 145 ($n = 150$-400). The workup on 27 July 1989 showed he was negative for ANA, PT/PTT (prothrombin and partial thromboplastin), rheumatoid arthritis, erythrocyte sedimentation rate (ESR) and routine bloodwork. He had bone marrow showing myelodysplasia and megaloblastoid features and ringed sideroblasts in July 1989. He had normal chromosome studies. His oncologist was certain he would progress to leukemia.

His blood tests in August also showed a low normal T-helper/T-suppressor ratio of 1.21 ($n = 1.2$-2.4) with high normal T-suppressor cells at 33% ($n = 13$-38). The T-helper cells were 40% ($n = 32$-50). He also had a urine MHPG which was low at 1.8 ($n = 2.4$). He also showed an elevated red blood cell copper at 0.794 ppm ($n = 0.62$-0.79). At that time he was placed on a regimen which included large daily doses of antioxidants -- 50 mg of beta-carotene, 400 mcg of selenium, 2 g of cysteine, 1 g of vitamin C, 800 IU of vitamin E, 3 g of tyrosine, 3 g of phenylalanine -- as well as one multivitamin, 25 mg of vitamin A, 30 mg of zinc, 3 g of N-acetyl-cysteine, and 1 mg of folic acid. A diagnosis of depression was made based on fatigue, sadness, and the urine MHPG, but antidepressants could not be used at this time because of the leukopenia.

He had a tremendous response to this regimen in three months, i.e., a normal full blood count (FBC) resulted. The oncologist stated he had never seen this type of recovery and it was very unusual that he had a normal FBC with a white count of 6.5×10^3 mm^{-3}. Six months after the initial bone marrow biopsy, in January of 1990, he had normal bone marrow. None of his consultants had seen a reversal of this type in bone marrow which normally advances to further disease. This patient initially was told that he would eventually progress to leukemia, probably within the next six months to a year and now had a complete reversal. This patient is greatly improved and has gained 8 pounds (from 137 pounds to 145 pounds, height 5' 7"). It was also noted that his total T-cells went up from 72% to 82% ($n = 56$-78%) and his T-helper cells increased to 46% (up from 40%). The suppressor cells only dropped to 32% from 33%. Possibly, antioxidants or zinc improved the T-helper ratio. It cannot be said with certainty why he improved; but possibly the repair of a leak in carbon monoxide exhaust in his car was a factor.

Preleukemic states, like other precancer -- cervical, bronchial, dermal, and colonic -- may be reversible by modified vitamins (e.g., synthetic retinoids) or meganutrients, once again highlighting the importance of early diagnosis of all precancerous lesions wherever they occur in the body, and the possibility of successful aggressive meganutrient treatment. Early bone marrow testing may identify early cancers which can be treated by antioxidants.

---

1. Braverman, E., M.D., *Journal of Nutritional Medicine* 2:313-315, 1991.

References

[1] Braverman ER., T-cell ratios: Modulation by nutrition: case report. J Ortho Med 1987; 2,1: 1.

[2] Lippman SM, Meyskens FL., Vitamin A derivatives in the prevention and treatment of human cancer. JACN 1988; 7,4:269.

[3] Braverman ER, Pfeiffer CC., Essential trace elements and cancer. J Ortho Med 1982, 11: 28.

[4] Mortensen PB, Abildgaard K, Fallingborg J., Serum selenium concentration in patients with ulcerative colitis. Dan Med Bul 1989; 36(6): 568.

[5] Horrobih DF., The reversibility of cancer the relevance of cyclic AMP, calcium, essential fatty acids and prostaglandin E. Med Hypo 1980; 6: 469.

[6] Risch HA, Burch JD, Miller AB, et al., Dietary factors and the incidence of cancer of the urinary bladder. Amer J Epid 1988, 127,6: 1179.

[7] Meyshens, FL, Prevention and Therapy of Human Cancer with Vitamin A Derivatives. JAN 1989: 452.

[8] Schneider A, Shah K., The role of vitamins in the etiology of cervical neoplasia: an epidemiological review. Arch Gynecol Obstet 1989, 246: 1.

[9] Rozen P., et al., Oral calcium suppresses increased rectal epithelial proliferation of persons at risk of colorectal cancer. JAMA 1989, 262,18: 2526.

[10] Edwards L, Meyskens F, Levine N., Effect of oral isotretinoin on dysplastic nevi. J Amer Derm 1989,20,2,257.

[11] Heimberger DC., Improvement of bronchial squamous metaplasia in smokers treated with folate and vitamin B12. JAMA 1988; 259: 1525.

New Era in Cancer Diagnosis and Prevention

We are entering a new era in cancer diagnosis and prevention. Many types of cancers can be identified in their early stages and could well be prevented by very simple procedures. For example, skin cancers -- basal cell, melanomas, and actinokeratoses -- can be identified early in the precancerous state. In the case of basal cell and the actinokeratoses and other precancerous lesions of the skin, they can be treated with a modified version of Retin-A or they can be excised. Melanomas need to be excised but they could be adjunctively treated by nutritional methods, such as reduction of phenylalanine and tyrosine in the diet or adjunctive treatment with antioxidants and other nutrients. Precancers in the mouth, such as leukoplakia, have also been treated with Retin-A cream, beta-carotene (90 mg), steroids, or surgical removal. They, too, can be treated more successfully if caught early enough [2].

Cancers of the lungs have been diagnosed early by various tests. Early dysplasias or metaplasias, that is, early changes in the cells (the 'missing link' between the normal cell and the cancerous cell) can be diagnosed early via sputum examination. Some of these cancers have been shown to remit with high dosages of B12 and folic acid [11]. Furthermore, various types of cancers of the lungs are being treated with vitamin A derivatives (retinoic acid) and/or antioxidants.

There are also various tests which can indicate early liver cancers: the conventional blood tests or liver enzymes, alkaline phosphatase, 5'-nucleotidase, SGPT, SGOT, direct and indirect bilirubin. These tests and their isoenzymes can help distinguish between bone and liver cancers as well as metastatic prostate cancers.

There are new breakthroughs in the early diagnosis of prostate cancers with tests such as prostate-specific antigen and prostatic acid phosphatase, as well as ultrasound screening of the prostate.

There are breakthroughs in colon cancer monitoring besides the carcinoembryonic antigen. Total sialic acid protein levels can reveal early colon cancers. Furthermore, studies such as proctosigmoidoscopes, hemoccults, barium enemas, colonoscopies, and upper GI studies are all helpful in catching early cancers. Individuals with a family history of colon cancer should have colonoscopies or barium enemas done every three years after reaching 40-50 years of age. Hemoccults probably should be done yearly on virtually everyone over 35. Rectal exams are also an important part of cancer detection.

Colon cancers do not respond well to traditional treatment. Nutritional approaches such as antioxidants, calcium, and acidophilus may prevent colon cancer.

There are new breakthroughs in early identification of breast, ovarian and endometrial cancers with cancer antigens. Cancer antigen 15-3, cancer antigen 125, cancer antigen 19-9, and the usual screening procedure of T-helper/T-suppressor ratios (killer cell screening also) may give insight into the immune system in the early stages of cancer.

Cystic breasts are precancerous lesions but respond extremely well to antioxidants, a low fat, high fiber diet without caffeine and alcohol. The screening mammogram is also a superb procedure for early detection. I think that the consequences of radiation can be antidoted successfully through nutritional approaches, e.g., cysteine. It is to be hoped that improved ultrasound techniques will replace the mammogram.

Early stages of cervical cancer are easy to diagnose with the conventional Pap smear, and now there are investigational treatments such as Retin-A creams and other treatments which may have the potential to reverse the cervical precancerous state. Oral antioxidant vitamins may also be helpful.

Early leukemias and hematological cancers are often picked up routinely by the CBC and bone marrow tests. Additionally, some of these cancers also may be reversible through nutritional means. Our patient is the first reported example, to my knowledge, of a reversal of preleukemia. In general, T-cells and polyamines are probably the most general and basic cancer screening tests while many other tests have specific cancer screening purposes.

Other cancer tests include:

- CA125-Ovary
- Prostate Specific Antigen-Prostate
- Prostate Acid Phosphatase-Prostate
- CA-15-3
- Alpha-Beta Protein-Embryonic Tumors
- Human Chorionic Gonadotrophin-Embryonic Tumors
- Dihydrotestosterone-Pancreatic Tumors
- Anti-Malignant Antibodies Screening-All Tumors

In summary, we have entered a new era through a variety of testing procedures, enabling the catching of cancers at very early stages and in such a way that they can be reversed and treated successfully. This is a new and exciting approach to preventive medicine.

Prostate Cancer

Prostate cancer and benign prostatic hypertrophy are easy to diagnose by PSA (Prostatic Specific Antigen) and PAP (Prostate Acid Phosphatase) in blood or by ultrasound. Zinc, saw palmetto herb, and Proscar, Doxycycline, or Bactrim are all thought to be helpful in treating enlarged prostate. Many new drugs treat prostate cancer, such as Lupron and Flutamide, and surgery is frequently done too quickly.

Cancer Information

The best book on cancer is Dr. Charles Simone's book, *Nutrition and Cancer* (Avery Publishing, 1992). His book is a comprehensive guide to the effects of environment and nutritional substances on cancer. Dr. Simone is an oncology consultant to PATH.

Cancer Referrals:
Where to Check the Promises

Until quite recently, consumers had no way to evaluate the promises for effective treatment published in brochures, or the testimonials of people who had used alternative methods. But their growing popularity has prompted several groups to evaluate many of them:

1. The American Cancer Society has prepared evaluations of 26 commonly used unproven methods. Call 800/ACS-2345.

2. The 312-page book, *Unconventional Cancer Treatments*, published by the Congressional Office of Technology Assessment, has exhaustive evaluations of dozens of therapies. To order, send a check for $14 to: Superintendent of Documents, Government Printing Office, Washington, DC 20402-9325. Specify GPO stock number 052-003-01207-3.

3. A database on unproven, untested therapies for children's cancers is available from Candlelighters Childhood Cancer Foundation. Candlelighters was established as a support and information group for families of children with cancer. Call 800/366-2223. A new database for adult cancers is planned. Until then, for information write to Grace Monaco, 124 Street SE, Washington, DC 20003.

Whole Body PET Scan

Whole body PET scanning is a new breakthrough technique that finds cancers throughout the body better than any other technique currently available. Although there are certain areas where PET scanning may not be the best choice, PET scan seems to be outstanding for ovarian cancer, colon cancer, lung cancer, musculoskeletal cancers, and staging of a wide variety of tumors.

Without invading the body and without any significant radiations, a PET scanner can find all the hot spots in the body from bone to soft tissues. One test can tell you whether or not you have a malignancy, where it is, and how much. Whole body PET scanning is available from my colleague, Dr. Abass Alavi, Department of Radiology, Hospital of the University of Pennsylvania, 3400 Spruce Street, Philadelphia, PA 19104 (215) 642-0248.

All patients participating in the early research protocols will be required to pay only the 20 percent copayment to have this procedure done.

One of the great benefits is PET's ability to evaluate the internal mammary nodes (important for diagnosing breast cancer). These are neglected by most surgeons. PET is accurate except for differentiating malignant cells from fibrous tissue, inflamed tissue, or necrotic debris. However, the PET scan will identify an abnormal latent mass which can later be biopsied to determine its malignant potential.

A PET scanner can identify cancer due to its increased uptake of glucose and increased level of 2,3DPG metabolism. Patients who are about to undergo PET scanning are to be kept N.P.O. (do not eat) for four hours prior to this exam. Furthermore, no alcohol, coffee, nicotine, or nitrates should be ingested for 11 hours prior to the scan.

5. *Childhood Disorders*

Hyperactivity

There are alternatives to Ritalin and Cylert for the treatment of childhood hyperactivity. In an article published by the American College of Nutrition, I showed that high dosages of tryptophan (as high as three to six grams) can replace Ritalin in cases of hyperactivity. Although tryptophan has been removed from the market, 5-hydroxytryptophan can serve as a replacement to some degree at even lower doses. Another article, in the *Journal of the American Academy of Child Psychiatry,* describing a study conducted at Ohio University, stated that a dose as low as 100 mg of tryptophan could improve a child's behavior.

Five-hydroxytryptophan is an excellent approach to the treatment of hyperactivity, although the appropriate dose may vary greatly with each child. The function of 5-hydroxytryptophan can be improved by the addition of niacinamide, vitamin B-6, and possibly niacin. In cases of hyperactivity resistant to the use of tryptophan, a low dose of antidepressants, anticonvulsants, or lithium, rather than the amphetamines, may be a safer approach. Wellbutrin may be the most effective of these. The amino acid, tyrosine, is also an alternative treatment. Melatonin holds promise as well. Thyroid deficiency may also be a factor in hyperactivity.

Attention Deficit Disorder With Hyperactivity Symptoms [1]

A. Inattention.

(1) often fails to finish things he or she starts

(2) often doesn't seem to listen

(3) easily distracted

(4) has difficulty concentrating on schoolwork or other tasks requiring sustained attention

(5) has difficulty sticking to a play activity

B. Impulsivity.

(1) often acts before thinking

(2) shifts excessively from one activity to another

(3) has difficulty organizing work (this not being due to cognitive impairment)

(4) needs a lot of supervision

(5) frequently calls out in class

(6) has difficulty awaiting turn in games or group situations

---

1. In addition to my own clinical experience, some of which has been cited above, and some bibliographical material, also cited in part, the following source has provided some information supplementing my own observations: *Diagnostic and Statistical Manual of Mental Disorders*, Washington, D. C.: American Psychiatric Association, third edition, revised, 1987.

C.   Hyperactivity.

(1) excessively runs about or climbs on things

(2) has difficulty sitting still or fidgets excessively

(3) has difficulty staying seated

(4) moves about excessively during sleep

(5) is always "on the go" or acts as if "driven by a motor"

Children and Childhood Diseases and Nutrition: Notes on Autism, Attention Deficit, and Depression

Many serious children's diseases are a result of head injury and head trauma, which result in malfunctioning of the brain in such a way that the neurotransmitters operate in an imbalanced or incomplete fashion. Hence, typical treatments for Attention Deficit Disorder, autism, and depression include neurotransmitter boosting methods from antidepressants to anticonvulsants, as well as the use, for example, of magnesium, zinc, vitamin B-6, hydroxy-tryptophan and tyrosine, etc. Nutritional deficiencies are often contributing factors, as are toxin exposures, but because of the brain injury, there is often insufficient success in treating childhood problems with nutrition alone and medication often has to be instituted.

Nutritional testing gives clues on the treatment of neurotransmitter imbalances but may not identify a malabsorption problem. For example, nutrients either do not cross the blood-brain barrier or are not held adequately in the brain and therefore neurotransmitters are not synthesized sufficiently. Sometimes the testing still leaves the physician with decisions to make based more on art and experience than on science.

6. Dentistry

Periodontal Disease (Gum Health) and Dental Care

Periodontal disease is one of the most prevalent health problems in the world and is the major cause of tooth loss in the adult population. Its two major categories are gingivitis where disease is confined to the gingiva (gums), and periodontitis where disease is present both in the gingiva and the supporting periodontal tissues. During the first stage there is inflammation of blood vessels (treated by vitamin C, bioflavonoids, and proper brushing). Symptoms are red and swollen gums, halitosis, gum bleeding when brushing teeth, sensitivity to hot, cold or sweet foods or liquids, and loose teeth.

Ascorbic acid deficiency has been shown to be an important factor in the development of gingivitis. When humans are placed on ascorbic acid deficient diets there is increased edema, redness and swelling of the gingiva. This vitamin, like methionine, may act directly to detoxify histamine (related to inflammation) or effect a change in the level of enzymes responsible for histamine metabolism (inflammatory response).

Treatment consists of brushing teeth daily, paying particular attention to removing plaque and bits of food between teeth and along the gum line. Use a toothpaste that contains fluoride. Control oral bacteria with a mild antiseptic mouthwash or hydrogen peroxide solution.

Floss teeth daily to remove plaque. Visit your dentist every six months for professional cleaning.

The diet for optimum gum health is high in fruit and fiber and low in fat. Fruit contains vitamin C and bioflavonoids and fiber roughage, while fat contains promoters of inflammation. A diet high in calcium and low in phosphorus (junk foods) protects against dental caries and gum diseases. Betel nut chewing and bioflavonoids also may be helpful in preventing caries. Lithium, fluoride, molybdenum, strontium, and vanadium in water may also prevent caries, while high copper in water increases caries. The healing of bleeding gums can be accomplished with meganutrients, e.g., 1-5 grams of vitamin C, 30-120 mg of zinc, 2-5 grams of bioflavonoids, and supporting nutrients, especially vitamins A and E.

Other essentials for dental health are:

- Water pick
- Interplak -- a plaque-removing device
- Rotodent -- a plaque-removing device
- Viadent -- an herbal sanguinaire root mouthwash known to help remove plaque and treat periodontal disease.

Temporal-Mandibular Joint Dysfunction (TMJ)

This is a common condition in which there is present a grinding of the teeth and in which the jaw frequently cracks. These symptoms occur primarily during extreme stress periods and often begin as a symptom of extreme anxiety. As the condition persists, actual damage may occur to the joints requiring a wide variety of techniques from balancing the teeth, to surgery, or bite plates. But, as a rule, TMJ begins as anxiety and stress. The source of the brain chemical imbalance associated with that

anxiety and stress or medical condition must be identified. After having lectured on this topic at the University of New Jersey Medicine and Dentistry School, I have come to understand that there are nutrients such as tryptophan and hydroxytryptophan, and medications such as prozac, that can reduce the pain of this condition as well as reduce the pain of surgery (which is rarely necessary) related to this condition.

7. Dermatology and Skin Disease

Acne

Acne can often be controlled by dietary restriction of all sugar, chocolate, alcohol, caffeine, oil, fat, cream, fried foods, shellfish, cigarettes, and drugs. Traditional treatment of acne focuses upon topical creams or antibiotics, e.g., benzoyl peroxide, Retin-A, Cleocin, erythromycin, or tetracycline. Oral antibiotics which can produce yeast overgrowth and stomach upset are often prescribed, e.g., clindamycin, erythromycin, and most commonly, tetracycline or doxycycline.

Acne that is resistant to these treatments often will respond to an oral vitamin A drug, Accutane, but this medication has many side effects (even infertility) when taken in large doses. Various nutrients such as zinc, garlic (tetracycline-like effect), and vitamin A and beta-carotene (Accutane-like effect) are useful in treating acne and augment the benefits of antibiotics. Boron, which has an estrogen effect, may benefit acne. Niacin, due to its flushing action, may clean out pores and is helpful. Lecithin, primrose oil, and even fish oil (EPA) can worsen acne. Some recommend omega-3 for dry acne. Most acne can be controlled through diet, nutrition, or drugs. Don't worry about scarring. Dermabrasion, phenol, trichloracetic acid, and Zyderm injections (collagen) by a plastic surgeon can correct most problems.

Medical causes of acne, e.g., liver disease, hyper-hyroidism, etc. should be ruled out in all patients. Acne rosacea and possibly other forms of acne may respond to the anti-parasite, anti-yeast medicine called Flagyl (MetroGel .075%).

Acne Treatments

Category I agents: (Safe and effective for nonprescription use)

- Benzoyl peroxide
- Salicylic acid (0.5-2.0% strengths)
- Sulfur
- Sulfur - Resorcinol

Category II agents: (Ineffective and/or unsafe for nonprescription use)

- Aluminum salts, e.g., aluminum hydroxide
- Benzocaine
- Benzoic acid
- Borates, e.g., boric acid, sodium borate
- Phenolates, e.g., phenol, sodium phenolate
- Resorcinol
- Sodium thiosulfate
- Zinc salts, e.g., oxide, stearate, sulfide
- Benzoyl peroxide-sulfur

Category III agents: (Safe, but more information about effectiveness is needed)

- Povidone-iodine
- Salicylic acid (2-5% strengths)
- Thymol

Combinations: (May be more effective than individual ingredients)

- Sulfur/resorcinol
- Sulfur/resorcinol/thymol/zinc oxide
- Sulfur/salicylic acid
- Salicylic acid/resorcinol
- Salicylic acid/resorcinol/sodium thiosulfate
- Benzoic acid/boric acid/zinc oxide/zinc stearate

Risk Factors for Acne

Premenstrual flare-ups.

Emotional upset.

Oils in cosmetics and soaps, e.g., Tone, Caress, Oil of Olay, Keri Lotion.

Infrequent cleansing of skin and hair.

Use of oily products on the skin and hair. Avoid comedogenic cosmetics, e.g., lanolins, petroleum bases, cocoa butter. Avoid topical products containing oils such as isopropyl myristate, octyl palmitate, mineral oil.

Systematically administered drugs reported to cause or aggravate acne:

Androgens	Lithium
Bromides	Iodides
Corticosteroids	Isoniazid
Haloperidol	Oral contraceptives

Acne mechanica or acne developing at friction points, e.g., chin straps, shaving. Acne also results from occupational exposure to industrial chemicals or air contamination, e.g., "McDonald's acne."

Acne Rosacea

Acne Rosacea is commonly known as W. C. Fields disease. Clusters of papules and pustules; red, swollen spots of the skin, "spiders" on cheeks and foreheads, or it may be just a mild case with a bit of acne around the nose and cheek area. People in their 30's, 40's, and 50's are often afflicted. Acne rosacea can be worsened by sun, alcohol, caffeine, food allergies, hot drinks. It is most common in people of Celtic origin, and is frequently chronic, lasting for years, sometimes accompanied by oily skin and edema of the cheeks and nose. Irreversible hypertrophy occurs in some cases and is called rhinophyma. It can also occur on the eye, with conjunctivitis, soreness, redness, large infections, corneal vascularization, and thinning. The most common problem is red eye and red face. Treatment is usually very successful. The first treatment line of defense is MetroGel 0.075% which is an antifungal agent. Another choice is doxycycline or tetracycline and then erythromycin. Resistant cases are treated with metronidazole, 200 mg twice a day. In rare cases we use Accutane. We can also use flesh-colored lotion. Patients who do not respond to antibiotics may have mite infestations or tinea, which should be looked at. In most cases potassium hydroxide examination can aid in the diagnosis of acne rosacea, making a dermatology visit unnecessary.

Atopic Dermatitis

Atopic dermatitis is usually marked by itching, facial and extremity involvement in infants and children, dermatitis with itching of the skin and chronic relapse irritation, and a family history of asthma, allergic rhinitis, and atopic rhinitis. Some of the minor features of atopic dermatitis are higher risk of cataracts, irritation around the mouth, conjunctiva, eczema with peeling, facial paleness or redness, food intolerance, itching hands, fishlike hands called ichthyosis, allergies on IGE, hardening of the skin texture, darkening around the eyes, increased lines on the palms, dermatographism on the hands, wool intolerance, etc. Atopic dermatitis is worse when widespread on the body, associated with allergic rhinitis or bronchial asthma, and has a higher frequency of occurrence in females. Late in life it is less severe. Exacerbating factors are temperature change, decreased humidity, excessive washing, contact with irritants (including gloves), emotional stress. The condition may even be related to a variety of brain chemical imbalances from head trauma to depression.

Therapy includes high doses of topical steroids, creams, bath oils, antibiotics, antihistamines, hydroxyzine. For severe cases, ultraviolet light, intramuscular steroids, or a course of prednisone is necessary. It is important to protect the skin from moisture, various foods, rough clothing, scratching, temperature, humidity, airborne allergens, aerosol, cigarettes, ragweed, and dander. It is also important to reduce stress and control diet. Diets high in polyunsaturated oils are particularly helpful. Hospitalization treatments of the hands could include bland diet, a low temperature environment, cotton bed clothes, tepid bath with bath oil twice a day for 20 minutes, applying steroid cream to the body lesions. Systematic therapy with antihistamines, antibiotics, etc. can be used if needed.

Nutritional treatments for atopic dermatitis include polyunsaturated oils, safflower oil, sunflower oil, linseed oil, borage oil, and fish oil. Zinc and antioxidants can also be extremely helpful. For the emotional dimension, cranial electrical stimulation (CES), amino acids, and other nutritional approaches may reduce exacerbation.

Contact Dermatitis

Contact dermatitis is characterized by itchy skin, red rashes, flaking skin, blistering skin, oozing skin blisters. Most likely it is allergy. Avoid various soaps, detergents, cleaning compounds, nickel jewelry, perfumes, cosmetics, shaving lotions, chemicals used in the hair, dyes, furs, dyes in chemicals, using paints, leather processing, plants, poison ivy, oak or sumac, rubber compounds, chemicals used in ink, paper, and insecticides.

Dermatology and Nutrition

There are numerous nutritional concepts related to the development of healthy skin. The concept of using vitamin A modified or vitamin D and C with modifications is a new concept in the development of healthy skin. Retin-A is one example. Other examples of natural product development include various placentas and omexins, and, recently, fruit acid creams (alphahydroxy-acids, etc.) have been particularly helpful. These products may have benefits to skin health development. Drinking lots of water and good nutrition are both critical dimensions.

Dermatology and Diet Update

New studies suggest that beta-carotene is thought to help non-melanoma skin cancer. This is not completely proven, but there seems to be a benefit. You may need at least 100 mg of beta-carotene daily to protect yourself from photosensitive and/or erythropoietic protoporphyria reactions. Fifty milligrams of beta-carotene may be sufficient for other types of problems. It has been suggested, although not proven, that beta-carotene or additional vitamin A may prevent basal cell carcinoma. Topical selenium has been shown to protect against UV-induced erythema, and it decreased the incidence of non-melanoma skin cancers induced by UVB irradiation. Toxicity is usually seen with doses greater than 1600 mcg of selenium. Serum selenium levels have been found to be low with various types of squamous cell carcinomas. Just as topical selenium has been shown to be a photo protector, topical vitamin C has been shown to protect skin from UVB and UVA toxic reactions.

New studies have shown the benefits of zinc for wound healing. Zinc is thought to be helpful in acne. Vitamin E has been shown to be helpful in accelerating wound healing. Ten to 20 percent of patients with atopic dermatitis have food allergies as a trigger as well as nutritional problems. Food allergy testing is important. Fish oil, as much as 1.8 gm has also been shown to be beneficial, as has borage oil and primrose oil. Chinese herbal tea is also thought to be beneficial. In the treatment of psoriasis, fish oil is thought to be helpful and to augment the benefits of certain steroids. Fish oil also prevents the side effects of Accutane and reduces the toxicity of Cyclosporine. Dermatitis herpetiformis is also worsened by wheat, iodides, and milk. Acanthosis nigricans has been thought to improve with fish oil, particularly when associated with diabetes. Allergic contact dermatitis has been helped by chelation with disulfiram. Supplemental nutrition is thought to help with dystropic epidermal lysis bullosa. Various food additives have been associated with urticaria. Elimination diets have been helpful.

Reference: Rackett SC, et al., Diet and Dermatology: The Role of Dietary Manipulation in the Prevention and Treatment of Cutaneous Disorders, *J AM Acad Dermatol* 29:447-61, 1993.

New Studies in Dermatology

1. Research has documented the fact that zinc in combination with erythromycin is more effective than either alone in the control of acne.

2. The fact that doxycycline works for acne on a long-term basis has been attributed to its antioxidant properties. Hence, all the research on antioxidants suggests that high dosages of antioxidants, as much as 50 mg of beta -carotene, 800 mg of dry E, 2 gm of vitamin C, 1-2 gm of cystine, and 200-600 mcg of selenium are important, plus avoiding foods that act as oxidizers. The number one oxidizer in the diet is fat, such as peanut oil, peanut butter, etc. Acne is an antioxidant deficiency disease in which doxycycline is really a supplement and not just an antibiotic treatment.

Retin-A: Instruction Information

Retin-A is a useful substance because it is a derivative of vitamin A. It can be applied to the skin in four doses, 0.01%, 0.05%, .025%, and 0.1%, as cream or gel. It is put on at night and taken off in the morning -- otherwise, the skin can become sensitized to light. Retin-A is useful in treating acne, fine wrinkles, sun damaged skin, reducing incidence of and treating basal cell carcinoma, and treating early stages of dysplasia that may be progressing to melanoma. Retin-A can cause redness and abrasion of the skin. The more redness and abrasion that is tolerated by the patient, the faster the resolution of your wrinkles and other skin problems.

Apply about a pea size amount to your finger and rub into one area initially. Later on spread it to all the desired areas of treatment. Increase the dose as tolerated. If the dose is too irritating use every other or every third day. For maximum benefit, Retin-A should be applied to the skin immediately after the skin has been washed and dried. This helps the Retin-A to penetrate into the skin.

Moles

Non-harmful moles are often symmetrical and round or oval in shape. Their borders are sharp and well-defined, and they have a uniform color of tan, brown, or natural skin color. They are usually smaller than 1/4 inch and uniform in that the moles on the body are similar. These moles are harmless and very rarely turn into skin cancer. Harmful moles are asymmetric; one-half looks different -- the borders are irregular or hazy, and the mole blends into the normal skin. Moles are of varied colors and have haphazard speckles and are generally larger than a pencil eraser in size. The surface may be flat or raised. They are often greater than six millimeters in their elevation. Moles are evaluated with the **A, B, C, D, E** system: **Asymmetry,** **B**order, **C**olor, **D**iameter (greater than six millimeters -- larger than a pencil eraser) and **E**levation.

Hair

Hair quality can be a sign of overall health or genetic makeup. Most male pattern baldness is due to human imbalances which are best corrected by hair transplants and possibly steroids or topical Minoxidil. Alopecia areata is severe hair loss, frequently the size of a quarter. Hair loss of this kind is frequently associated with autoimmune diseases, i.e., hypothyroidism, pernicious anemia, exfoliative dermatitis. Radiation exposure, or chemotherapy can result in hair loss. Frequently nutrient deficiency can be found in Alopecia, especially cysteine and zinc deficiency. Large doses, up to 7 gm of cysteine, and up to 150 mg daily of zinc, may be needed. Vitamin A, C, EPA, lecithin (makes hair more oily), may be useful. Other sulfur amino acids (methionine, taurine) may make hair more curly. Arginine has been deficient in some patients with coarse hair. Hair loss due to vegetarianism (B-6 deficiency) can occur, and this may be very dangerous. Minoxidil may be helpful in Alopecia areata. Selenium also may have a role as well as Accutane, the vitamin A drug. Eczema and dandruff respond to dandruff shampoos (selenium and zinc are active ingredients). Occasionally, a coal tar (psoriasis) shampoo is necessary. Thyroid and estrogen deficiency are common in hair loss. A full endocrinological workup is necessary in hair loss. Usually, removal of sugar, caffeine, fat or nuts, and shellfish will stop dandruff and drying up of the scalp.

Reference: James, MB, Hair Growth Benefits from Dietary Cystine-gelatin Supplementation, *J. Appl. Cosmetol.*, 2:15-27, 1984.

Eczema

Atopic eczema is a common skin disorder, often caused by contact with a skin allergen, i.e., antibiotics, balsams, soaps, dyes, jewelry, plants, rubber, etc. Many foods can cause eczema; and hence these patients are placed on an oligoallergenic diet (1 protein, vegetable, and whole grain product per meal with no fruit, nuts, or fat).

Frequently patients with eczema have deficiency in fatty acids, particularly omega-3 oils (primrose, safflower, linseed, linoleic) as well as omega-6 oils (fish oil). Zinc is also a common deficiency. Most adult discord eczema will go away with nutrients and diet. Antioxidants and magnesium also have an important role in eczema. Aloe vera may reduce inflammation in eczema.

Oligoallergenic Diet

Turkey or Rabbit	**plus**	Rice or Sago or Potato	**plus**	Cabbage or Carrots or Leeks	**plus**	Stewed apple or Rhubarb

plus kosher margarine, calcium, vitamins, and sunflower seed oil.

References:

Essential fatty acids and maintenance of the epidermal water barrier, *Nutrition Reviews*, 44(4):151, 1986.

Galland, L, Increased requirements for essential fatty acids in atopic individuals: a review with clinical descriptions. *J Amer. Coll. Nutr.* 5:213-228, 1986.

Hass, PJ, Antiallergic effect of oral calcium. A clinical-experimental study. *Fortschrltte der Nedizin.* 103(12):328, 1985.

Hattevig, G, Kjellman, B, Johansson, SGO, and Bjorksten, B, Clinical symptoms and IgE responses to common food proteins in atopic and healthy children, *Clin. Allergy* 14:551-559, 1984.

Natow, AJ, Aloe vera, fiction or fact. N. Y. University Medical Center, skin and cancer unit, New York, NY, 1986.

Psoriasis

Psoriasis is a red, scratchy, itchy, skin disease which usually occurs at pressure points, i.e., elbows, knees, ankles, etc. It is often seasonal, disappearing in summer in response to ultraviolet light. Conventional treatment, i.e., steroids may be useful in short term for psoriasis. Other topical creams used for psoriasis are coal tars and other hydrocarbon products. Seleniun sulfite, Retin A, zinc oxide, and vitamins A and D, may be useful in some cases. Traditional treatments use immunosuppressive therapies, i.e., azathioprine, even chemotherapy, e.g., methotrexate.

Nutritional treatment of psoriasis emphasizes zinc which is often deficient. Antioxidants (particularly sulfur amino acids) and oils, e.g., lecithin and especially fish oil have anti-inflammatory properties. Beta-carotene and vitamin A may be useful, as is the vitamin A drug, Accutane, which may be effective in pustular psoriasis and possibly plaque psoriasis. Elevated polyamines may be the predictor of psoriasis that will respond to Accutane.

Various drugs can cause or worsen psoriasis, e.g., lithium, progesterone, and possibly aspirin, as well as long-term steroid therapy, sugar, caffeine, nuts, vegetable oil, and shellfish. The nutrients, folic acid, arginine, ornithine, and copper may worsen psoriasis by elevating polyamines.

Reference: Moy, RL., et al., Isotretinoin vs Etretinate Therapy in Generalized Pustular and Chronic Psoriasis. *Arch Dermatol*, 121:1297-1301, 1985.

8. *Diabetes and Hypoglycemia*

Diabetes

Diabetes, or elevated blood sugar, is the most common, serious metabolic disease of humans and affects one percent of the population. Most doctors define diabetics as having fasting blood sugars of greater than 140 milligrams per deciliter (mg/dl). Diabetes can be classified as primary, or insulin-dependent diabetes (type 1), which occurs in juveniles, or non-insulin-dependent diabetes (type 2). Many individuals who have pancreatic disease or hormone abnormalities and take drugs such as Lasix, or other diuretics or steroids, can develop elevated blood sugar. Milk allergy, insulin receptor abnormalities, genetic abnormalities, or other diseases such as cancer, can also cause elevated blood sugar.

Complications with diabetes are intense and serious and include diabetic foot ulcers, circulatory abnormalities, coma, silent heart attacks, and heart disease. Diabetic side effects such as neuropathy (nerve pain) can be treated with many brain-chemical altering medicines, from Prozac to amino acids and even natural substances such as B-vitamins.

Fortunately, the total health approach has now been established as helpful in diabetes, particularly type 2 adult onset. In fact, most adult onset diabetes is a result of refined carbohydrate addiction and obesity. Additionally, individuals with diabetes tend to develop hypertension concomitantly with insulin resistance. Many diabetic individuals have tremendous response to nutritional therapies as long as they use such therapies along with Cranial Electrical Stimulation (CES) to break their addiction to carbohydrates. An average individual with adult onset diabetes frequently benefits from zinc, fish oil for circulation, magnesium, increases in selenium, diets high in fiber, B-6, olive oil and other polyunsaturated oils, such as safflower, with high amounts of linoleic acid. Today, doctors can measure all of these nutrients in the blood and therefore come up with more accurate nutritional regimens. New studies suggest that other fibers, such as guar gum, can also be extremely valuable. Side effects with guar gum include gas and diarrhea, and patients frequently need to adjust their dose carefully. Some studies suggest that adult onset diabetes will also respond to a teaspoon of aloe vera, 500 mg twice daily,

and that foot ulcers can respond to atypical therapies such as Dilantin. Monosaturated fats can be an important part of the diet in diabetics. Potassium can also be deficient in diabetes, as well as magnesium and zinc, and nutrients such as thiamine, niacinamide, and tyrosine have been thought to be beneficial in the prevention of diabetes. Some people believe that certain teas may be beneficial to diabetics. One of those teas is Syzygium Jambos. Another tea that may be beneficial is Devil Club, or Oplopanax Horridum. Niacin can actually exacerbate non-insulin dependent diabetes, so it is usually not recommended as a medication. Fish oil, zinc, and B-6 can prevent the cardiovascular effects of diabetes. Research is being done on the relationship between abnormalities in inositol metabolism and diabetes. New breakthroughs have now shown that inositol may help diabetic neuropathy. Topical capsaicin, or red pepper extract, which is FDA approved, can be enormously helpful in treating diabetic neuropathy by releasing substance P (an amino acid peptide associated with pain). Numerous studies document that chronic magnesium supplementation can contribute to an improvement in islet (pancreas cells) beta cell response to insulin. Exercise is also helpful in diabetes.

New tests document numerous ways to identify the severity of diabetes and predict whether or not diabetes is developing. One can measure blood sugar response with a glucose tolerance test and detect disposition for diabetes at a very early stage. Hemoglobin A1c is useful, and measures the blood sugar over the last three months. Fructosamine is able to measure the blood sugar over the last 2-4 weeks, and fasting blood sugars can be done for an immediate checkup. Diabetes often develops gradually and can be identified very early through proper testing. The immune system can often be compromised in diabetic patients and frequently should be studied. It is extremely important for diabetics to have regular eye exams. Sed rates (ESR or erythrocyte sedimentation rate) and fasting blood sugars can also be useful measurements. Frequently, diabetics develop kidney failure and anemia, another area in which monitoring must be done. New treatments for this aspect of the disease include genetically manufactured Erythropoietin (trade name Epogen) or a natural peptide for increasing blood count.

Diabetes incidence is low in countries with high-carbohydrate diets if the carbohydrates are unrefined.

Since diabetes in adults is usually an outcome of refined carbohydrate addiction, one has to break the cycles of addiction to sugar or carbohydrates. If an individual breaks the addiction to sugar and/or carbohydrates and then goes back to it, he or she will have even more problems with addiction with each subsequent return to addiction.

Insulin-dependent diabetes, or juvenile diabetes, can now be treated with human forms of insulin, and eventually science hopes to do transplantation of various parts of the pancreas. Oral hypoglycemic agents have benefits but can cause even more problems with side effects, e.g., stroke, fatigue, etc. Carnitine is often thought to be deficient in these patients, and immune-suppressant drugs like cyclosporin show promise. In all forms of diabetes, stress is a factor and will exacerbate blood sugar control, while exercise will help. Coffee consumption is known to exacerbate diabetes significantly.

The epidemic of diabetes in our society is probably due in part to the high refined sugar content of so many foods. Most people do not realize that foods like Jello are as much as 80 percent sugar. Hershey bars are 50 percent sugar. Salad dressings frequently consist of as much as 30 percent sugar; barbecue sauces, 50 percent sugar; ketchup, as much as 25 percent sugar; fruit yogurts, as much as 15 percent sugar; and Coca Cola, 10 percent sugar. We are in a society that is addicted to sugar as well as empty carbohydrates.

It is extremely common that type 2 (adult onset) diabetics have biochemical depressions and need neuro-transmitter treatments either with CES and amino acids or medication, e.g., Prozac and Wellbutrin.

We should remember that diabetes has been around for a long time. Ancient doctors, even in the time of Jesus, simply would taste the diabetic sweetness in the urine of a patient. Jesus may have confronted diabetes in Jairus's daughter in Mark, chapter 5. It was said that the daughter was dead. But Jesus said she was sleeping or in a coma. He roused her and immediately gave her some food to eat. Possibly she had been in a hypoglycemic or diabetic coma.

There is considerable debate about the role of diet in diabetes. Some individuals have pointed to the salutary effects of high protein diets, others to high fiber. Both can be useful; yet when individuals are severely overweight, high protein needs to be emphasized. In individuals with more normal weight, high fiber is better. Individuals with glucose tolerance problems are subject to alcohol abuse. This has been seen in the Pima Indians and individuals with severe hypoglycemia. Some people that have hypoglycemia as adolescents and young adults develop diabetes due to poor diet. It may be helpful to consult a blood sugar index on how foods compare to elevating glucose. Some foods can actually impair glucose more than one realizes. Fruit and carrots, which have a high sugar content, and certain vegetables that are high in sugar may need to be eliminated. Corn flakes, raisins, peas, and brown rice can elevate blood sugar. Many diabetics also need a lot of chromium, along with tryptophan, which may be another method of cutting the appetite for sugar.

In sum, diabetes is a diverse disease but most cases of adult onset respond remarkably to nutrition, natural supplements and/or plant substances and diet. (See Diabetic Diet, p. 137.)

Glycemic Index of Foods [1]

The glycemic index of foods (next page) sets forth the hyperglycemic effect of individual foods. This index is widely accepted as a source which states the glucose response to individual foods, although the improvement of metabolic control expected from its use is modest. Its major use (and, therefore, its major effect) is probably during snack times to aid the diabetic patient with glucose self-monitoring. By informing the diabetic patient of high sweet tasting, but low glycemic index, carbohydrate foods that safely can be consumed, the quality of life for diabetics can be enhanced.

---

1. Derived from LeFloch, J. P., and Perlmutter, L. *Index Glycemique des Alimentes*, La Presse Medicale, 21:43, Dec. 12, 1992.

Blood Sugar Index

(how foods compare to glucose in
raising blood sugar when eaten alone)

sugars and candy		water	fruits	
maltose	105	0%	raisins	64
glucose	100	0%	bananas	62
honey	87	0%	orange juice	46
Mars bar	68	0%	oranges	40
sucrose	59	0%	apples	39
fructose	20	0%		

breakfast cereals

vegetables			corn flakes	80
			shredded wheat	67
parsnips	97	80%	Swiss musli	66
carrots	92	88%	all-bran	51
instant mashed potatoes	80	5%		
rutabaga	72	87%	**legumes**	
white potatoes	70	80%		
potato chips	51	2%	peas	51
sweet potatoes	48	71%	baked beans	40
			lima beans	36
grain foods			chickpeas	36
			black-eyed peas	33
white rice	72		kidney beans	29
whole-wheat bread	72		lentils	29
millet	71		soybeans	15
white bread	69			
brown rice	66		**dairy foods**	
sweet corn	59			
pastry	59		yogurt	36
Rich tea biscuits	55		ice cream	36
buckwheat (kasha)	51		whole milk	34
white spaghetti	50		skim milk	32
sponge cake	46			

Index derived from Trusswell, A. S., Glycaemic Index of Foods, *European J. of Nutrition*, 46 (Supp. 2): S91-S101 (1992).

We have added to the above table the water content of some items. Many of the good foods are 80% water and we do not want to mislead anyone into thinking that carrot carbohydrates are worse, or equal to, candy bar carbohydrates. The above calculations are based on constant body weight. So you have to eat an enormous amount of vegetable carbohydrates to have a significant impact on blood sugar.

Glucose Tolerance Test

You are about to receive a medical test which will help your doctors to determine your ability to handle a dose of sugar (or glucose). This test can help to determine whether or not you may have a tendency to develop diabetes, also known as hyperglycemia. In addition, hypoglycemia, or an abnormally low blood sugar, can also be detected by this test.

Procedure:

In order to perform this test properly you must be fasting. At the start of the test you will be given a glass of a sugar (glucose) water solution to drink. You will then refrain from eating for the next 5 or 6 hours! Every half-hour or hour, a drop of blood will be taken from your finger or arm and the level of glucose and/or insulin will be measured. You will be asked to tell the nurse any symptoms you are feeling throughout the test. Typical reactions might include hunger, sleepiness, dizziness, or an inability to concentrate. Near the end of the test a tube of blood may be drawn to test for the hormone Adrenalin and for insulin to measure how the adrenal gland is managing under the stress.

Purpose:

Inability to regulate sugar properly is a major cause of medical disease in today's modern society. People who are overweight run the risk of diabetes as do people who have diabetes in their family. The abundance of food low in fiber in our diet is toxic to our body and prevents us from absorbing sugar gradually from our intestines. As a result, we absorb too much sugar too fast and overburden our pancreas and our adrenal glands. Eventually, we may end up with our blood sugars staying elevated (diabetes) or we may produce too much insulin and may get the opposite result: hypoglycemia. In either case, the essential task is to diagnose the problem by a glucose tolerance test. Then proper medical treatment, e.g., diet, exercise, supplements, and even medication, can be started.

Results:

When your test is complete you will be able to receive a graph of your glucose levels. This test needs to be interpreted by the doctor at your next office visit. However, the nurse will give you an idea of where you fall in the following ranges: Hypoglycemic-Normal - Hyperglycemic - Diabetes, etc.

It is important to note that the symptoms of hypoglycemia on a long-term basis and on a short-term basis are identical to the symptoms listed for anxiety and depression in this book. Therefore, hypoglycemia is one of the great psychiatric mimickers of pseudo-psychological disease. The test can be useful in identifying how much of the anxiety or depression may be coming from hypoglycemia rather than psychological factors.

Guar Gum - The Most Valuable Fiber

Guar gum is an extremely valuable fiber, possibly seven times stronger than oat bran in reducing cholesterol absorption and lowering cholesterol. Frequently, individuals using guar gum may reduce their cholesterol as much as 25 points with a 28 percent drop in LDL cholesterol, while oat bran might produce only a 10 percent drop. Guar gum also increases serum zinc and magnesium concentration in diabetics and, as an adjunct, is associated with an excellent modification in patients with non-insulin dependent diabetes mellitus because it helps regulate blood sugar. Since guar gum is a blood sugar regulator, it might even be beneficial for a hypoglycemic. Side effects with guar gum include gas and diarrhea, and each patient needs to adjust to his or her toleration. If possible, guar gum probably should not be taken with your vitamins because it may block the absorption of some of the oils.

Sugar Content in Certain Manufactured Foods

(calculations based on dry weight)

Jello	82.6 %
Coffee-Mate	65.0 %
Cremora	56.9 %
Hershey Bar	51.4 %
Shake'n Bake Barbecue Style	51.0 %
Sara Lee Chocolate Cake	35.9 %
Wishbone Russian Dressing	30.0 %
Heinz Tomato Ketchup	28.9 %
Quaker 100% Natural Cereal	23.9 %
Sealtest Chocolate Ice Cream	21.4 %
Hamburger Helper	23.0 %
Wishbone French Dressing	23.0 %
Libby's Peaches	17.9 %
Wyler's Beef Boullion Cubes	14.8 %
Dannon Fruit Yogurt	13.7 %
Ritz Crackers	12.0 %
Del Monte Whole Kernel Corn	10.7 %
Skippy Peanut Butter	9.2 %
Coca Cola	8.8 %
Wishbone Italian Dressing	7.3 %

Is it any wonder that so many Americans are sugar addicts?

Foods and Insulin Control

A study by Richard Anderson, Ph.D., Beldsville Human Nutrition Research Center, published in *Food and Nutrition Briefs*, April/June 1993, states that certain foods actually help insulin control blood sugar two to four times better than normal. This could be cinnamon, dandelion, sweet bay, birch, cops, lavender, and beer berry. There is scientific data backing some of the uses of herbal plant therapeutics.

The Use of Nutrient Supplements for Diabetes

Numerous articles have been published linking nutritional imbalances with diabetes. Exacerbation of nutritional imbalances occurs with stress. As kidney disease can be protected against by Vasotec or other ergosterol inhibitors; and as tyrosine supplementation has been shown to protect dopamine deficits in the retina and other eye problems, so essential fatty acids have been shown to be beneficial in diabetes in numerous studies, although there has been some controversy. This benefit has been demonstrated primarily in non-insulin dependent diabetics, and dosages have been as high as 7.5 grams. Insulin resistance, of course, has been the big killer, and that is what diabetics have. In fact, you can predict obesity by comparing insulin to growth hormone level. Glucagon has been shown in a Saudi Arabian study to reverse juvenile diabetes as has niacinamide. This raises the question that endocrinologists, some day in the future, may be able to manipulate insulin resistance in the juvenile diabetic with either glucagon, growth hormone and/or nutrients. Cure is just a postulation, and, unfortunately, frustration occurs because everyone keeps hoping for this so-called cure. All these years of diabetes research have yet to make a large change in the general course of the disease, although human insulin has been a good breakthrough.

More and more tests for fine tuning diabetes have been developed -- like checking for glycohemoglobin, fructosamine, C-peptide and microalbuminerin in the urine. Notable recent studies by the National Institutes of Health show that diabetic neuropathy is responsive to a serotonin reuptake inhibitor, Paxil. Although Prozac was not effective, Elavil and Norpramin were effective in diabetic neuropathy. In the past, inositol, taken for insulin-dependent diabetes, has been shown to help diabetic neuropathy. Probably all caffeine consumption is harmful.

Recently, there has been a lot of interest in the effect of a tea called Sishium Jampos as well as Devils Club tea. Whether or not these are really helpful is not clear. On the herbal side, fenugreek seeds have been shown to be beneficial for type 1 diabetes. Early changes in diabetics and electrophysiologic changes in juvenile diabetics have been picked up with retinal studies. Brain Electrical Activity Mapping and brain stem mapping may pick up early changes (a lowering of the P300) in the diabetic brain, since all blood sugar abnormalities have been shown to affect the P300.

Recent studies have shown that carnitine insufficiency in juvenile diabetics has been associated with weakening, fatigue, and disturbances in trace elements. Zinc and selenium deficiencies and increases in copper have been associated with diabetes. On the issue of B-vitamins, there have been numerous studies on B-6 deficiency, B-2 deficiency, and B-12 deficiency in diabetics. Supplements for nutritional deficiency are worthwhile. Guar gum has been the most recently studied fiber. Unfortunately, guar gum can cause flatus, but it has been shown to be an extremely beneficial fiber and is used in Saudi Arabia and countries with a tremendous number of juvenile diabetics. Stress has been shown to greatly impact diabetes. Chromium and nicotinic acid have been thought to be beneficial in diabetes although there have been some equivocal studies about niacin -- that it protected the diabetic, but in high dosages worsened blood sugar control. Cyclosporin, an immune suppressor drug, has been used recently for control and treatment of juvenile diabetes. Whether or not that can be done in adults is difficult to determine. Notable is the control of diabetes with the oral hypoglycemic sulfonamide drugs. Frequently, however, some individuals have developed a high risk of arteriosclerosis with those drugs. Some people feel that you are better off with insulin than with the use of oral drugs. Needless to say, many drugs -- from Dilantin to MAO inhibitors, to fenfluramines, to alcohol, to Klonopin, to hypertensive drugs -- can interact with these diabetic medications, impairing their efficacy. Virtually all drugs can impact oral hypoglycemics.

Much has been written about essential oils: benefits of cod liver oil have been shown in a *New England Journal of Medicine* study; and certain diabetics have benefited from dietary linoleic acid and olive oil. All saturated fats should be avoided. It also has been suggested that a total vegetarian diet that eliminates oil can be greatly beneficial with diabetics. We have seen blood sugar levels drop by as much as 70 points during such a regimen.

Paying attention to the glycemic index of foods can be important for a diabetic. Fructose does not raise blood sugar but raisins can, and, in some cases, so can carrots and other vegetables high in sugar content. Certainly sucrose should not be used as a first-line treatment for hypoglycemic attacks in diabetics, but it should be kept on hand. It would be better to use fructose obtained by fruit-sweetened types of foods.

It is notable that chronic hyperinsulinemia (diabetes) will cause hypertension and other problems if untreated. The proper diets for diabetics can vary. The high protein, low carbohydrate diet probably will help the non-insulin dependent diabetic. But there is increasing evidence that the complex carbohydrate diet is now the diet of choice; but, again, that depends on the individual. Red pepper extract, topical capsaicin, has been shown to help diabetic neuropathy in a recent *New England Journal of Medicine* study.

Vitamin C and magnesium supplements have been associated with getting rid of low levels of diabetic blood pressure and microvascular disease. A great deal of impaired glucose tolerance occurs in diabetic Pima Indians, as well as high amounts of alcoholism and problems with the brain.

Clearly blood sugar will impact the brain because of cerebral vascular disease. A study has shown that tryptophan reduces depression and aggression in diabetics, which is why tryptophan is frequently prescribed. Klonopin may also do the same. Prozac has been tried with diabetics, with anecdotal success. In other cases Elavil has been more successful. A study in *Diabetology* showed the prevention and delay of type 1 insulin diabetes in children using nicotinamide. Vitamin E has also been shown to be deficient in diabetics. Additionally, plasma homocystine levels may indicate a need for vitamin B-6, which has been found to be helpful in treating diabetes. Neuropsychological performance is affected in diabetics in that there are deficits in concentration and attention associated with low blood sugar. Cognitive remediation can be achieved for diabetics through biofeedback exercises. The possibility that cow's milk is another trigger of juvenile diabetes has sparked interest. It may very well turn out that the lack of breast milk feeding in our society, coupled with the use of soy and cow's milk, may trigger autoimmune diseases. This has been shown to be the case in thyroid disease.

9. Dieting, Weight Loss, and Eating Disorders

Anorexia

Causes and Origin. Anorexia can be the result of heavy exercise as well as chronic exposure to lead. Symptoms of lead poisoning are: depression, constipation, and abdominal pain. Other causes of anorexia may be depression or having a poor self-image (chronic dieting to lose weight). This condition starts out as something small, but can become an avalanche if it is not treated. Alcoholics and cancer patients can also become vitamin-deficient, which in turn can lead to anorexia. Most anorexia has an organic brain disease basis. The excessive use of birth control pills (causing depression first and leading to anorexia), as well as caffeine and alcohol can cause anorexia. Adolescents, who are the most common group to become anorexic (often after drug abuse), should not be exposed to any kind of drug, sometimes not even aspirin or Tylenol. In many cases, psychiatric help may be necessary in addition to medication, nutrients, and natural electrical therapies, such as CES.

Symptoms. Women who suffer from anorexia can stop menstruating, contract osteoporosis (loss of calcium), become depressed, suffer from constipation and anemia, develop arrhythmias, such as slow heart-rate, which may ultimately cause sudden death. Holter monitoring may be essential to detecting heart arrhythmias.

Treatment. Nutrition plays an important role in the treatment of anorexia. Zinc, vitamin E, fish oil, vitamin A, and a high protein diet are all important. Tryptophan, isoleucine, leucine, and valine may also be deficient, and can be administered intravenously. Antidepressants, antipsychotics, and lithium are often beneficial forms of treatment. Normally, a patient taking lithium, Stelazine, Mellaril, or many other antidepressants gains weight, which can be extremely helpful.

Anti-Hyperactivity Diet

Artificial additives, preservatives, and salicylates may contribute to childhood hyperactivity. Some fruits and vegetables containing salicylates should be avoided. Essentially, all manufactured baked goods, luncheon meats, ice cream, powdered puddings, candies, soft drinks, punches, teas, coffee, margarine, colored butter, and most commercially produced condiments are eliminated from the diet. These dietary restrictions make it practically impossible to eat in a school cafeteria or restaurant. In addition, many nonfood items such as mouthwash, toothpaste, cough drops, perfume, and some over-the-counter and prescription drugs are prohibited. Mild to moderate results are the best one can expect from dietary change in hyperactive kids.

Obesity

Obesity is one of the number one health risk factors. It is an epidemic in America, affecting 25 to 50 percent of Americans. What most people do not realize is that biochemical factors and genetics play a dominant role in obesity. Most cases of obesity can be treated through brain chemistry manipulation. There are an enormous number of agents that can alter appetite, all of which work on major neurotransmitters. Typical agents such as Prozac, Wellbutrin, Nardil, Desyrel, Ritalin, and hormone manipulations have been associated with reducing appetite. The brain is the area in which the battle for weight control is won because most obesity is really nothing more than carbohydrate addiction, and addictions are destructive, repetitive behaviors which can be replaced by constructive, repetitive behaviors. Addiction can be defeated by strictly following the principles and programs of the PATH for Achieving Total Health. (See Obesity Diet, p. 144.)

The Fast Path to Weight Loss

The PATH Medical weight loss program includes:

- nutritional counseling
- Nutritionist 3 evaluation of diet
- eating for a healthy heart
- learning the basics of low fat and low cholesterol
- food recipes
- specialized diets for all medical conditions e.g.,
    diabetes
        heart disease
        gastrointestinal problems
- information on vegetarianism
- low fat living on high fiber diet for prevention of
    cancer
- general nutritional information
- individual nutritional counseling

- individual behavioral and psychological
    counseling for those who cannot maintain a
    specific diet
- body composition analysis
- high risk weight management programs for those
    who need extremely low calorie diets with high
    protein
- new shape/new life exercise regimens
- 12-step programs
- brain chemical and neurological obesity programs
- treating medicine -- the biological origin of
    obesity
- staying on track programs
- long-term maintenance regimens
- Fast Path supplements -- high protein amino acids
    which decrease appetite while providing
    brain fuel

Appetite Suppressants that May Alter Brain Chemistry

- Alpha-adrenergic antagonists
- Amino acids: Methionine, D, L-phenylalanine,
    hydroxytryptophan, tryptophan, tyrosine
- Beta-adrenergic agonist (amphetamines)
- Bombesin
- Calcitonin (thyrocalcitonin)
- Cayenne
- Cerulean
- Cholecystokinin
- CES (Cranial Electrical Stimulation)
- D-Fenfluramine

- Enterogastrone
- Ephedrine
- Estrogen
- Fiber
- Gastrin-releasing peptide
- Glucagon
- Glycerol
- Guar gum
- Lactate
- Melatonin
- Naloxone

Avoiding Fungus

FAMILY: Fungi

Molds and yeast are the chief source of food spoilage. They feed on the same food that we do. They are in the air that we breathe. Refrigeration and freezing slow down their growth and high temperatures will destroy them. On the other hand, their growth rate under favorable conditions (room temperature, sitting on the counter) is quite high.

Although baker's yeast and brewer's yeast have different metabolic characteristics, people sensitive to any form of yeast should avoid all forms of yeast, mold, moldy cheeses, and other forms of fungi in their foods and environment. Foods high in carbohydrates (fruits, fruit juices, root vegetables, and grains) tend to be yeasty in nature, since yeasts have accelerated growth on these foods. Cooked foods also tend to attract yeast, especially when left out at room temperature. For these reasons, you must handle all foods carefully, and freeze any leftovers that you do not plan to eat within 24 hours. Avoid eating any leftovers that have been in the refrigerator more than 24 hours.

Wash all produce well by soaking in a sink filled with water and 1/4 cup 20 Mule Team Borax or Clean Greens. They will kill the yeast on the surface of the foods. Grapes and the rinds of cantaloupes and other melons are covered with yeast. Eating food without killing the yeast could give you a reaction. Be sure to *rinse well* in clear water before serving.

Processed foods (hot dogs, processed meats, frozen concentrated fruit juice, canned fruit juices, sausages, and other man-made food combinations) tend to be yeasty in nature due to long exposure of the food to air during processing.

WHAT TO AVOID

Avoid ALL ALCOHOLIC BEVERAGES (fermented food and drinks, cider, sauerkraut, beer, malts, ales, soy sauce, vinegar, etc.); MOLDY AND AGED CHEESES (bleu, gorgonzola, roquefort, stilton, brie, camembert, brick, limburger, muenster, port de salut, processed cheese food, and cheeses with mold growing on them); BREADS [except those made without yeast] (as well as buns, coffee cakes and breakfast rolls made with yeast); CAKES, cake mixes, crackers, cookies, flour enriched with malted barley; FORTIFIED FOODS (they either contain malt or yeast); FROZEN FRUIT JUICE concentrate or juices made from concentrate; MILK fortified with vitamins from yeast, buttermilk, and malted products.

The Yeast Connection

Many individuals have symptoms of anxiety and depression that they attribute to yeast infection or hypoglycemia. There are several problems with this approach:

a)   There is a problem with diagnosis in virtually every case because almost all patients who take these tests are positive, including well-functioning adults.

b)   Primary symptoms frequently do not go away permanently with treatments such as Diflucan or Nizoral or nystatin.

c)   The religious practice of doing without yeast products at Passover may be a sufficient way of dealing with yeast overgrowth for those observing this ritual. Others can try a weekly yeast elimination diet from time to time and see if it produces any improvement in health. (See Yeast Diet, p. 150.)

Basic Health and Diet Rules

1.   READ ALL LABELS! Ask questions in restaurants about how the food was prepared. Foods that you may think are pure may contain unsuspected ingredients.

2.   If you are sensitive to a food, the raw state may cause you more problems than the cooked. Fresh food is more potent than foods (e.g., produce) several days old.

3.   DO NOT EAT a combination of foods that you have reacted to. If one food causes you problems, two problem foods combined could cause you multiple problems.

4.   Prepare simple meals of four or five foods. Try to eat fresh vegetables whenever possible and avoid processed foods with chemicals added.

5.   Cook meats medium to medium-rare, poultry until done, and fish until it flakes. Do not overcook!!

6.   Vitamin and mineral supplements need to be examined to see if they contain or are derived from foods to which you are sensitive. Beef, corn, wheat, liver, and yeast are often the sources used.

7.   Purchase pure food, not food that has been loaded with chemical additives. This means routinely picking up fresh produce, meats, poultry, and fish.

8.   Select high quality fresh vegetables; wash and wrap before refrigerating; then keep covered. Eat within two or four days. Frozen food should be kept frozen and stored no longer than two to three months. Steaming and possibly microwaving (five to seven minutes per lb.) with little or no water is best.

9. Drink lots of water in between meals. Do NOT drink alcoholic beverages. Alcohol interferes with the healing process and may make matters worse.

10. Avoid all sugar. The stress caused by sugar in your diet not only feeds the Candida but also overworks your adrenal gland, which is of great importance in resistance to an attack on the body.

Breaking Your Bad Addictive Habits

To break a bad habit, replace it with good habits. Usually, the best of all good habits is to have joy in your life. Joy is the source of happiness, pleasure, satisfaction, and peace. It can be found, for example, in dance, song, friendship, love, and faith. Unless a person can find more joy and peace in his life, the ability to break a bad habit is almost impossible. For the Lord is the rock that stabilizes the person who wishes to grow more healthy.

Bad habits in eating are extremely common. Many people use food and drugs as a form of addictive behavior to treat frequently occurring unwanted emotions. Some individuals overeat fruit, others overeat whole grains, thereby gaining weight. Other people overeat saturated fat and salt, increasing their risk for hypertension and heart disease, while others overeat white flour and sugar, thus gaining weight and providing a cause for nervousness, anxiety and depression. Some people are addicted to caffeine and cigarettes, thereby becoming vulnerable to panic attacks, heart disease, and even psychosis, while others are addicted to alcohol, sometimes becoming schizophrenic or emotionally disabled and disturbed. And still others are addicted to marijuana and Qualudes and become permanent schizophrenics due to brain injury. Cocaine, heroin, and LSD users can have a worse fate and can actually die. This is the hierarchy of addiction: fruit, whole grains, meat, saturated fat, salt, white flour, sugar, caffeine, cigarettes, alcohol, marijuana, cocaine, quaaludes, LSD, heroin and methadone. Other lesser addictions can include T. V. and diets.

It's interesting that addictions can begin even with fruit, as it began in the Garden of Eden. In some ways fruits are the first of all cravings, which can lead to other cravings and destructive habits. The unsophisticated say that a habit is just an unhealthy activity, while others call it a sin. Bad habits are both unhealthy and unholy.

What kind of psychological and spiritual factors must we be aware of to change?

1. First, we must confess our sin or habit, i.e., I confess I have a bad habit. Most people today choose to see a doctor to confess their illness. They recognize that they have an illness, but most do not recognize the importance of the discovery that most illness has its origin in bad habits.

2. The second thing to do is to identify what part of the illness is a result of bad habits or some type of sin.

3. Thirdly, we must try to understand why we commit wrong actions, looking carefully at what motivates us to do these things. From a religious point of view, people give in to evil when they give in to bad habits. From a medical point of view, people are exhibiting destructive behavior as a result of either depression, anxiety, or unhappiness. Bad habits can also be a result of distancing ourselves from our Creator (as we move away from the Creator we get closer to the destroyer). God is the source of all creativity.

4. Fourth, we must realize that there are ways to break bad habits. No matter how bad our habits are, we can break them! The power of the Lord destroys evil, i.e., bad habits and addiction. Modern medicine has techniques which can give us the power to change, e.g., Nicorette (cigarettes), lithium (alcohol), and behavior modification. CES and vitamin-taking substitute health building daily rituals that make war with developing bad habits. Habits can be broken if the resolve and interest is there. We must admit our habits, thus recognizing the source of the illness, and search out the source of the habit, which is usually in the brain chemistry.

5. Fifth, to have the resolution to break a habit, we must be convinced that breaking it will lead to healthiness and holiness.

6. Sixth, the goal is to stop the habit and fault the negative behavior, not the person. The 12-step program can be helpful in this regard.

7. Seventh, stop the negative substances, e.g., caffeine, cigarettes. Use nutrients and lesser addictions during the weaning process. Many people need a slow withdrawal from bad habits. It is impossible, due to human nature, for many individuals to withdraw completely from a bad habit all at once. The less dangerous the habit, the easier it is to withdraw. In the case of sugar addiction, Nutrasweet, chromium, tryptophan, glucose tolerance factor, etc. can be used. In the case of saturated fat, more salad oil, olive oil and fattier meats can be substituted. In the case of

white flour, the use of fruit can be beneficial for weaning. One can be weaned off cigarettes by the use of nutrients, nicotine patches and chewing gum. Alcohol withdrawal can be assisted by the use of amino acids, Librium and lithium. One can be weaned off marijuana and the strong addictions, like heroin, by the use of other medications, like tranquilizers, antidepressants and anticonvulsants. Some individuals can break bad habits cold turkey.

These basic approaches can be applied to all bad habits: medical, nutritive, psychological, and spiritual. Yet, in all cases, nutritional evaluation of the bad habit is needed. The final step in breaking all habits is to be sorry and to repent. Without this step, no one will break a bad habit forever. To reach this point one must develop joy in the worship of the Lord. To accomplish this, repentance of the bad habit is necessary.

Other Techniques for Breaking a Bad Dietary Habit

One of the best ways to break a bad dietary habit is to bless the Lord when eating, thanking Him for the food received. This focuses your energy on the creative, peaceful aspects of food as sustenance and nourishment. It is also important to pray at the table to control appetite. A typical blessing is: "I bless this food and drink for building my body as a temple in the service of the Lord." This may be repeated, and it is also important to thank the Lord after eating.

Earnest seeking of the Lord's will, with repentance, is the basic step for long-term weight control. You must recognize that you must not sin against your physical self. It affects both your physical and psychological well-being. Keep these basic scriptures in mind. For example, "Man does not live by bread alone but by every word that

proceeds out of the mouth of the Lord. The Lord is the bread of life. He who comes to Him shall not hunger."

It is important to set your mind on things that are heavenly and spiritual, finding peace, knowing that God is God. Also, it is important to follow your diet and perform your healthful activities without murmuring and questioning. Keep faithful with the disciplined health approach.

Faith is not easy; it is a vigil that must be worked at. Faith in the Lord, repentance, and joy are substantial resources of strength when dieting or changing a bad habit. Of course, they will not help as much if you are working with inadequate nutrition or medical advice. That which is flesh is flesh; that which is spiritual is spiritual. (See also Peace and Well-being Diet, p. 144.)

Addiction: The Most Critical Dimension of Nutrition and Preventative Medicine

Learning to break addictive patterns is the most critical dimension of nutrition and preventive medicine. Addictive patterns of behavior always lead to poor nutrition and diseases that could have been prevented. How is this so? It is because of our new understanding of what addiction is. Addiction is not just limited to dangerous drugs such as heroin, LSD, crack, cocaine and amphetamines, but addiction is also found to occur in less serious substances such as alcohol, cigarettes and caffeine, and even less serious substances than these, such as carbohydrates, sugar, fat, junk food and even with people in codependent and addictive relationships. Addiction by our definition is any behavior that a person does repetitively that they know is dangerous for them or destructive or unhealthy but for a variety of reasons are unable, by will power, to stop that behavior.

When we understand addiction as repetitive, compulsive, destructive behavior that a person cannot willfully stop, addiction then becomes the root of most of our chronic diseases. We all know now that the search for higher consciousness in the 60's led to lower consciousness and brain injury. The strong drugs, from LSD to heroin, all cause brain damage, as does alcohol, and even cigarette smoking puts an individual at the highest risk for developing Alzheimer's disease, due to microvascular blockage and cerebral vascular dementias. We also know that caffeine causes pancreatic cancer and alcohol may be linked to breast cancer and many other chronic diseases. It is eating addiction that indirectly produces obesity, diabetes, hypertension and therefore virtually all the major killers in our society are linked to repetitive, destructive, addictive behavior and obesity and a high fat diet, leads to cancer and more heart diseases. There is nothing more critical in our society for nutrition and preventive medicine than to be able to do the techniques that will break the addictive cycle.

In the field of preventive medicine, all of us are trying to get our patients to increase their fiber intake, stop smoking, give up caffeine and alcohol, remove refined sugars and carbohydrates, exercise regularly, to have positive and productive relationships with their loved ones, to get appropriate amounts of rest, to avoid fried foods and salty foods, excessive spicy foods, and to transform their healthy emotional life-style into a diet of lean protein, high fiber, low fat, regular, balanced and other appropriate health goals.

It appears that most patients fall off the band wagon of diet relatively quickly and the pattern of life-style often returns to its previous functioning. Attempts to restructure a person's health away from addiction is difficult. Therapy has been tried, antidepressants have been tried. Medications to motivate the individual from Pondimin to Tenuate, from Prozac to wellbutrin can be used to certain degrees, but most patients still tend to return to bad habits, particularly their addictive bad habits with food, drugs, relationships; anything, from ice cream to LSD.

What is the source of this repetitive destructive behavior? Sigmund Freud called it the death instinct, the compulsion to repeat. Others call it the quest and desire for ritual. What is it in the body that causes this cycling?

Historically we have learned from plagues. Scurvy

taught us the value of vitamin C, Beri-Beri taught us the value of B-1, and Pellagra taught us the miracle of niacin. **The plague of drug abuse has taught us something about repetitive, destructive behavior that affects every individual.** Although fewer people are becoming addicted to the dangerous drugs, a great majority, if not all Americans have repetitive, destructive behaviors that they can not break. The technique of Cranial Electrical Stimulation (CES) has been so helpful in helping drug abusers withdraw from drugs, break their addictive patterns, and has even greater consequences for the average neurotic and health-oriented patient. The average severe drug abuser frequently needs medication along with CES because of the advanced brain disease that has occurred either as a result of preexisting brain disease or as a result of drug abuse. The wider applications of CES are on a day-to-day preventive nature for treating drug abuse in adolescents and bad habits of white flour, junk food, sugar, coffee, and cigarette addiction for a large group of Americans.

Any health practitioner that has ever dealt with a patient that cannot execute his/her good advice for the patient must now recognize that patients have addictive behavioral patterns which can be dealt with on a psychotherapeutic, spiritual, and emotional level. We have come to recognize that the medical and electrophysiological component has been identified with BEAM testing and is treatable with CES, or CES with medication depending on severity. As the Lord has provided Christ to light the world, He has given us His BEAM to light the path of healing. He has given us new rituals which are spiritual because they are filled with the spirit and aid health.

Carbohydratism and Alcoholism

Carbohydratism (carbohydrate addiction) is probably one of America's most prevalent diseases. It is an addiction to empty carbohydrates such as sugar and white flour. This can result in cravings, weight gain, and anxiety, as well as most of the symptoms associated with alcoholism. Sugar addiction is just one step away from alcoholism. Alcoholism is usually treated by nutrients (zinc, niacin, etc.), lithium, and Librium and by trying to reduce or eliminate the addictive behavior.

The same approach is necessary for carbohydratism. To live on sugar and white flour is to increase the risk of heart disease, cancer, anxiety, schizophrenia, etc. People who are addicted to carbohydrates must realize that they

are helpless before them, and that they should avoid them for all practical purposes. The same principle holds true for alcoholism: an alcoholic should never touch a drink again. If a person starts to eat ice cream, white flour, etc., after being off them, a dangerous situation may result, because he may become addicted again unless he stops short. Junk food leads to more junk food, as sin leads to more sin.

Carbohydrate addicts are usually overusers of other stimulants such as salt, caffeine, and saturated fat. Carbohydratism is one of the primary causes of many diseases in our society.

Fiber

Diet is a factor in five of the ten leading causes of death in the United States, these being heart disease, cancer, stroke, and diabetes mellitus, which we see and treat at PATH every day of the year. Due to overprocessing of our grains, most if not all of the beneficial fiber is removed.

Fiber is a necessary component to a healthy diet, involved in maintaining the motility and increasing transit time within the gastrointestinal system, thus preventing constipation, decreasing the absorption of toxic substances that may be in our foods, and lowering LDL cholesterol levels in the blood. The tables below set forth additional benefits:

Table 1:

Disease States For Which Fiber May Be Beneficial

WATER-INSOLUBLE FIBER	WATER-SOLUBLE FIBER
Constipation*	Atherosclerosis*
Diverticulosis	Hypercholesterolemia
Appendicitis	Hypertriglyceridemia
Colon polyps	Diabetes mellitus*
Colon cancer	Obesity*
Hemorrhoids	Hypertension*
Varicose veins	Dumping syndrome*
Irritable bowel syndrome+	Gall stones*
Crohn's disease+	
Hiatal hernia*	
Peptic ulcer disease*	

*Beneficial effect.
+Possible detrimental effect.

Fiber is optimally obtained from the diet and can also be taken in supplement form. Ideally, if possible, foods containing water-soluble and water-insoluble forms of fiber should be balanced at each meal.

Table 2:

Types of Fiber

TYPE OF FIBER	EXAMPLES	HIGH-FIBER FOODS
Water-soluble	Pectins, gums, mucilage	Fruits, oats, barley, legumes, psyllium
Water-insoluble	Lignin, cellulose	Vegetables, wheat, whole grains, cereal, hemicellulose

Reference: Gabel, L. L., Fahey, P. J., Gallagher-Alred, C., Ricer, R. E. and Sickles R. T., *Supplement to American Family*, November 1992; 41S-48S.

Fiber for a Healthier You

Did you know?

Thirty-five percent of all cancer deaths may be related to diet.

Diets high in fiber and low in fat may reduce the risk of certain types of cancer.

Most Americans eat only about half the amount of fiber suggested for good health and fitness.

Because of its relevance to general health and well-being, fiber is no longer simply a topic of conversation among dieticians, nutritionists, and health care practitioners. Today, more than ever, experts agree that it is important for us to eat fiber every day. In fact, the National Cancer Institute tells us that a regular fiber intake of 25 to 35 grams daily may reduce the risk of developing some chronic diseases and health problems. The preferred way to include fiber in your diet is simply to eat the right foods in the right quantities. You'll get the suggested 25 to 35 grams of fiber per day if you eat approximately six servings of breads and cereals and four servings of fruits and vegetables.

There are five components of dietary fiber: celluloses, hemicelluloses, lignins, pectins, and gums. They are found in vegetables, fruits, legumes, grains, and nuts. It is important to eat a variety of foods from each of the above sources, since many foods don't contain all five types of fiber.

Important Note: Rapid increases in dietary fiber intake may result in gastrointestinal discomfort (such as gas, bowel distention, burping, etc.) in some individuals. Therefore, fiber intake should be increased gradually to 25 to 35 grams daily. Excessive intakes of dietary fiber (50 grams or more daily) may really upset your intestines, i.e., diarrhea.

How Fiber Can Help Reduce Health Problems

Increasing the fiber in your diet can be an important step toward better health and a longer life. Among other things, fiber can help prevent constipation, lower cholesterol levels,! and may reduce the risk of colon cancer. Here are a few examples of how fiber works:

Fiber is beneficial in preventing constipation because it helps move food through the digestive tract quickly. Fiber also increases the amount of stool. Thus, the concentration of potentially carcinogenic substances is appreciably diluted. Fiber may lower the cholesterol count by binding bile acids.

Some research suggests that fiber may help with weight control because it fills you up not out. Guar gum is especially helpful fiber to fill you up. The feeling of fullness that comes with eating high-fiber foods may actually help you to eat less.

All people need fiber, which is best taken at several meals or times throughout the day.

Trimming the Fat

Substitute the following low-fat foods for high-fat ones.

High-Fat Food	*Low-Fat Food*
Whole or condensed milk	Skim milk, buttermilk, nonfat powdered milk
Bacon	Chicken (or Canadian bacon)
Bologna, frankfurter, sausage	Chicken or turkey, lean, thinly sliced
Avocado	Cucumber, zucchini, lettuce
Creamy or high-fat cheeses	Low-fat cheese, cottage cheese
Ice cream	Ice milk, frozen low-fat yogurt
Nuts	Fruits or vegetable snack
Hot fudge sundae	Frozen yogurt or ice milk with sliced or crushed fruit
Ground beef	Lean beef with all fat trimmed
Fatty pork (spare ribs, ground pork)	Well-trimmed lean pork (leg, ham, picnic)
Sour cream	Low-fat yogurt, imitation sour cream
Regular salad dressing	Reduced calorie salad dressing, vinegar, lemon juice
Cream	Skim milk
Egg fried in fat	Poached, boiled or baked eggs
Liver	Lean meat, chicken, fish

Dietary Information for
Meats, Fish, and Poultry

Data is for four ounces of the item.

ITEM per 4 ounces	CALORIES amount	SATURATED FAT grams	CHOLEST-EROL mg
Skinless Chicken Meat - Roasted	215	2.32	101
Skinless Chicken Thigh - Roasted	238	3.45	108
Chicken Thigh - Roasted	280	4.92	106
Chicken Breast - Roasted	223	2.50	95.20
Skinless White Turkey Meat - Roasted	159	0.43	97.20
Skinless Dark Turkey Meat - Roasted	212	2.75	96.40
Turkey - White - Roasted	223	2.67	86.20
Turkey - Dark - Roasted	251	3.98	101
Ground Turkey Patty - Cooked	267	3.85	116
Beef Filet Mignon Steak - Roasted	239	4.25	95.20
Beef Sirloin Steak - Choice	229	3.54	101
Ground Beef - Extra Lean - Broiled, well done	311	7.13	121
Beef Chuck Arm Pot Roast - Baked	245	3.43	114
Lamb Shoulder Roast Trimmed - Baked	231	4.64	98.70
Atlantic Salmon Fillet - Baked	206	1.43	80.30
White Tuna in Water - Drained	154	0.74	47.60
Cod - Steamed/Poached	116	0.19	61
Sole/Flounder Fillet - Baked	133	0.41	77.10
Swordfish - Baked/Broiled	175	1.59	56.70
Prawns/Large Shrimp - Steamed	112	0.33	221
Snapper Fillet - Baked/Broiled	145	0.41	53.30
Pork Spareribs - Braised	450	12.60	137
Pork Loin Cop - Broiled	274	5.93	90.70
Whole Ham - Roasted	275	6.78	70.30

Dietary Information
for Salad Dressings [1]

Data is for one tablespoon.

ITEM per 1 tbs	CALORIES		SATURATED FAT	
	amount	%	grams	%
Olive Oil	119	11	13.5	13
Blue Cheese Dressing	77.1	7	8	8
Russian Dressing	75.6	7	7.75	8
Oil and Vinegar Dressing	71.8	7	8.02	8
Creamy Italian salad Dressing	71.4	7	7.74	8
Italian Salad Dressing	70.1	7	7.25	7
Italian Dressing	68.6	6	7.13	7
French Dressing	67.2	6	6.44	6
1000 Island Dressing	58.9	5	5.58	6
Mayonnaise Type Dressing	57.3	5	4.91	5
Ranch Salad Dressing	54.5	5	5.64	6
Caesar's Salad Dressing	52.2	5	5.16	5
Honey Mustard Dressing	50.4	5	2.81	3
LoCal Ranch Dressing	30.6	3	3.06	3
Kraft Fat Free Ranch Dressing	25	2	0	0
7 Seas Italian Olive Oil	25	2	2.5	5
LoCal 1000 Island Dressing	24.4	2	1.64	2
LoCal Russian Salad Dressing	23	2	0.65	1
LoCal French Dressing	21.8	2	0.944	1
LoCal Caesar Dressing	16.5	2	0.66	1
LoCal Blue Cheese Salad	15.1	1	1.1	1
Nakano Natural Rice Vinegar	0	0	0	0

1. The two Dietary Information tables were contributed by Kathleen Esposito, M.S., Nutrition/Fitness Consultant at PATH.

Body Composition Analysis

Body composition analysis is one good measure of your muscle and body fitness. Knowing your percentage of body fat is an important tool in evaluating your total health because an excess of body fat has been associated with a multitude of health risks including heart disease, diabetes, back problems, sleep disorders, cirrhosis of the liver, hypertension, gall bladder disease, arthritis, depression, hernias, intestinal problems, lack of endurance, being generally more at risk for injury, and more at risk during surgery.

To find out your lean body mass to fat ratio and how to get it in better balance, make an appointment with Kathleen Esposito, M.S., Nutrition/Fitness Consultant. She will go over your nutritional and fitness status and help you to make changes that will fit into your life-style so that you can achieve your goals for health, weight, appearance, and general well being.

STANDARD VALUES FOR PERCENT BODY FAT

Rating	20-29	30-39	40-49	50-59	60+	Age
Men						
Excellent	<10	<11	<13	<14	<15	
Good	11-13	12-14	14-16	15-17	16-18	
Average	14-20	15-21	17-23	18-24	19-25	
Fair	21-23	22-24	24-26	25-27	26-28	
Poor	>24	>25	>27	>28	>29	
Women						
Excellent	<15	<16	<17	<18	<19	
Good	16-19	17-20	18-21	19-22	20-23	
Average	20-28	21-29	22-30	23-31	24-32	
Fair	29-31	30-32	31-33	32-34	33-35	
Poor	>32	>33	>34	>35	>36	

Dietary Fats

My favorite fats are canola oil, safflower oil, sunflower oil, olive oil, corn oil, and soybean oil, to some degree.

Fat	Saturated Fat (%)	Polyunsaturated Fat (%)	Monounsaturated Fat (%)
Canola Oil	6	62	62
Safflower Oil	10	77	213
Sunflower Oil	11	69	20
Corn Oil	13	61	25
Olive Oil	14	8	77
Soy Bean Oil	15	54	
Margarine	17	32	
Peanut Oil	18	33	
Chicken Fat	31		
Lard	41		
Beef Fat	52		
Butter Fat	66		

Nutritional Facts and Fancies

By Easy A. Clean [2]

Many food myths are dispelled and other food facts are spelled out in "The Wellness Encyclopedia of Food and Nutrition."

Grapefruit is popular with dieters because of the belief that it burns away fat. But no food can cause fat to be burned away. Grapefruit is filling, tasty, low in calories, and virtually fat-free, but it does not digest calories or diminish appetite.

White potatoes should be eaten with the skin whenever possible. Ounce for ounce, the skin is fiber, iron, calcium, phosphorus, and potassium. However, don't eat the skin if it has a greenish tinge, which may signal a high concentration of an alkaloid called solanine.

Carrots. As children most of us learned that carrots were good for our eyes -- a claim that's only partially true. The beta carotene in carrots is converted to vitamin A, essential for the functioning of the retina.

Oranges. The white membrane under the skin of an orange -- called the albedo -- holds more vitamin C than the flesh. It also contains much of the pectin, the type of soluble fiber thought to help lower cholesterol levels.

Pears. Much of the vitamin C is concentrated in the skin. Canned pears, therefore, are low in vitamin C not only because canning undermines the vitamin, but because the pears are peeled.

Avocados are high in fat -- especially when compared with other fruits and vegetables. They derive 71% to 88% of calories from fat. But the fat is monosaturated -- the same type found in olive oil -- which has been shown in studies to lower blood cholesterol.

Legumes. Despite the long cooking time needed by some, don't worry about nutrient loss. Analysis by the FDA has found that beans requiring up to 75 minutes of cooking retained from 70% to 90% of most vitamins and minerals.

---

2. USA TODAY, Dec. 10, 1992.

Sugar Cravings

Sugar cravings in individuals suffering from, hypoglycemia, diabetes, and depressions, have multiple origins. One biochemical study of sugar cravings suggests that decreases in the brain content of serotonin causes us to crave sugar. Serotonin is made from the amino acid tryptophan, and tryptophan supplementations frequently decrease sugar craving. High protein diets with high tryptophan to carbohydrate ratio also reduce sugar cravings.

GTF (glucose tolerance factor) has been reported to help regulate blood sugar. This compound is beneficial for both diabetics and hypoglycemics. GTF contains chromium, which is frequently reduced in the plasma of patients with sugar cravings as well as in patients with cardiovascular disease.

Glutamine has been suggested to be useful in treating sugar cravings. This is because glutamine is converted into sugar rapidly. Glutamine may reduce sugar cravings because it's like eating sugar.

In sum, sugar cravings are treated with tryptophan and GTF as well as evaluation of depression. Supportive nutrients in carbohydrate cravings include B-vitamins, zinc, inositol, and even lithium therapy when this impulse disorder becomes unmanageable.

Mastering Desserts

The natural way to master the desire for deserts is to use creativity in making them. Sorbet is very good. Fresh fruit such as banana, ice cubes, and orange juice mixed in a blender can make wonderful fruit desserts. Combining cantaloupe, pineapple, and ice cubes in a blender makes a delicious treat.

Yogurt can be a tasty dessert with your own fresh fruit spread added. Try a dessert of low sugar, low fat carrot cake and fresh berries with a small amount of natural whipped cream, made out of egg white and NutraSweet. Fruit of course is the best dessert!

Some New Ideas on Weight Loss

Our new weight loss programs begin with an assessment of brain abnormalcies in persons with an addiction to carbohydrates and treatment with some of the new appetite suppressants. These, when coupled with a good nutrition program and CES (Cranial Electrical Simulation) have been very effective. We believe that many individuals need to be on these medicines for several years to redress long standing weight problems because of metabolic abnormalities. A program of long term, successful weight loss requires recognition of the severe chemical imbalances in the brain of persons who are carbohydrate addicted, as well as the need for medication support.

Feingold Anti-Hyperactivity Diet

Today, artificial additives and preservatives receive the major emphasis while the possible role of salicylates in hyperkinesis commands less attention. This change is very clear in Feingold's most recent publication on this subject, a cookbook. Here, Feingold includes BHA and BHT, two antioxidants commonly added to foods in the United States.

Adherence to the Feingold diet, sometimes referred to as the K-P diet, results in an abrupt change in eating patterns. Most fruits and many vegetables are forbidden, at least for the first several weeks. Essentially all manufactured baked goods, luncheon meats, ice cream, powdered puddings, candies, soft drinks, and punches are eliminated. Teas, coffee, margarine, colored butter, and most commercially produced condiments are also excluded. These dietary restrictions make it practically impossible to eat in a school cafeteria or restaurant. In addition, many nonfood items such as mouthwash, toothpaste, cough drops, perfume, and some over-the-counter and prescription drugs are prohibited.

Oxy-Cholesterol in Food [1]

Years ago the discussion around cholesterol in food began. Cholesterol was viewed as causing arteriosclerosis and being responsible for the formation of plaques. In the sixties and seventies cardiologists recommended that their patients eat low cholesterol foods and more polyunsaturated fatty acids. Linoleic acid became famous. The sales of products rich in this essential acid -- especially diet margarines -- were staggering.

Animal experiments were done with rabbits in which pure cholesterol as well as oxy-cholesterols were given. After 45 days, thickening of the intima of the aorta was observed in the oxy-cholesterol group. No thickening was observed in the rabbits which got the pure cholesterol. The same experiment has been done with monkeys. The results were the same. Radioactive, labeled oxy-cholesterols showed that they were notably connected to the LDL's and VLDL's. There was practically no affinity towards the high density lipoproteins.

Oxy-Cholesterol Foods

Bacon
Brains
Butter
Cheese (grated)
Chips fried in animal fat
Egg products
Fast foods (containing butter and eggs)

Lard
Whole milk powder
Parmesan cheese
Pork
Radiated food (gamma-radiation)
Salami

---

1. *Journal of Orthomolecular Medicine*, vol. 3, No. 4, 1988.

Bone Spurs

Bone spurs are commonly found in people with alkaloses, arthritis, neuritis, and tendonitis. They may be helped by eating foods with a low pH. Low pH foods are acidic and help restore the disturbed acid-alkaline balance of the body indicated by the above problems. Examples of some low Ph foods which may be helpful are:

Food	pH	Food	pH
Limes	1.9	Carrots	5.1
Vinegar	2.9	Potatoes	5.8
Oranges	3.5	Butter	6.3
Beer	4.5	Salt	7.5

Of course, taking pressure off the irritated area is very important. Additionally, insufficient stomach acid may be another factor.

The PATH High Protein (Protein Sparing), Low Carbohydrate, High Fiber Diet

This is a therapeutic diet. In many cases, it is short term. Your doctor may adjust it according to your needs. The amounts are adult one-day limits unless otherwise noted.

Unlimited

Fish (broiled or baked; no fried food)

Chicken or turkey (cooked without skin). Lean beef, veal, shellfish, and pork can be used if this is the only way to keep the diet, but it is usually best to eat these as little as possible.

Abundant

2 cups salad per day

Try a variety of vegetables (but not as much iceberg lettuce). More colorful ones are high in vitamins and minerals. Try romaine and red leaf, bean sprouts, red cabbage, zucchini, peppers, celery, mushrooms, radishes, onion, spinach (unless restricted due to oxalates). Max., 1 med. tomato or carrot a day.

6-8 oz. cooked vegetables

Steaming is preferred method of cooking vegetables (5-8 mins. for most vegetables; 12-18, for tougher ones). Baking is okay. Do not eat starchy ones such as corn, potatoes, beans, peas, winter squash. (Green beans OK.) Broccoli and cabbage are especially nutritious and thought to help prevent cancer. Try new foods and recipes: try steaming kale or collard greens for only 12 mins. and adding vinegar. Bake a head of cauliflower with grated cheese on it.

Moderate

Diet Jello -- as you wish. (Must have no carbohydrate content.)
Seven tbsp. lemon juice plus addition of Nutrasweet to make lemonade.

Seven eggs per week (depending on your cholesterol level).
Herbs and salt-free seasonings (Mrs. Dash is okay. Garlic Pritikin No-oil dressings especially healthful. Roll leafy herbs between fingers to release flavor).

Very Little

2 tbsp. safflower oil

Olive oil or Paul Newman dressings are OK for people who don't have high blood pressure. Turn plain oil into a dressing by adding herbs and vinegar.

2 oz. hard cheese

Hoop, farmer, and pot cheese are best. Next best, Gruyere, Swiss, and Cheddar.

2 oz. low-fat yogurt or cottage cheese or tofu
1 handful of raw sunflower seeds

Melons. Pectin lowers cholesterol

Use primarily pectin fruits, bananas, grapefruits, apples, pears

Salt substitutes

For example, No-Salt (potassium chloride)

1 tbsp. mayonnaise -- sugar free

Safflower oil mayo two or fewer times per week is the ideal. (Check your health food store or make it.)

2-4 oz. lean red meat only
1 tbsp. vinegar

Beverages

Spring water is good; no-salt seltzer water; diet caffeine-free soda; decaffeinated tea; Crystal light lemonade; herb teas (but see restrictions below); tomato or other vegetable juice ___ oz./day (no carrot juice); 1/3 cup unfiltered fruit juice in place of 1/2 cup fruit is okay. (Decaffeinated coffee generally is not advised because it has a harmful oil in it.) Nutrasweet may be used to sweeten beverages.

Not Permitted

Sugar (includes cane and brown sugar, honey, corn syrup, jams, other syrups, fructose, dextrose, sucrose, maltodextrin, etc.)
Nuts; salt (including monosodium glutamate and soy sauce)
Milk, ice cream, butter, cream; fried food
Canned food (except fish, turkey or chicken in water; olive oil is okay if one's blood pressure is normal)
Margarine (1 tbsp./day is okay if first ingredient is safflower oil, e.g., Hain brand in health store.)
Grain products -- pasta, pizza, bread, cake, crackers, pastry, cereal, etc.
Alcohol -- check over-the-counter remedies; caffeine -- check diet sodas
All starchy vegetables, including potato, sweet potato, beans, winter squash
Sausage, bacon, cold cuts, hot dogs; salty food, e.g., pickles and olives
Regular mayonnaise; herb tea that is aromatic or has fruit extracts
Fats and oils, except safflower, EPA-GLA, fish oil. Olive oil is okay if blood pressure is normal

Helpful Tips

Later, when you have reached your therapeutic goals, complex carbohydrates (i.e. whole grains, potatoes, more fruit) will be reintroduced to your diet in moderation. You will do well to permanently avoid excessive eating of red meat, and fruit, any fried or fatty foods, refined flour or sugar (including sweeteners listed above), most canned foods, and cold cuts. *Always read labels.* Avoid highly processed foods; generally, try to eat foods as close to the natural state as possible. Wash produce well.

Avoid frying. For stove-top cooking, use a nonstick pan. Saute vegetables in water. Poach eggs if possible. Limited use of PAM to grease pans is okay, but may raise cholesterol. Bake, broil or stir-fry meats. It is best to steam vegetables in a steamer basket (5-8 mins. for most veggies; 12-18 mins. for tougher ones). Boiling destroys vitamins. Refrigerate all oils (including therapeutic ones, e.g., fish oil). *Cook without oils* if possible; cooking oils, even healthful ones, will transform them into fats which clog arteries. Add oil after cooking.

Sample Menus for General High Protein Diet

Note: Good fish for the diet high in EPA -- mackerel, bluefish, herring, chinook salmon, and tuna.

#1 (For hard-working people)

Breakfast: Cheese omelet (2 eggs, chopped onion, celery, pepper, 2 oz. cheese)
5 oz. tomato juice

Lunch: Large piece of baked chicken
Spinach salad with a dressing made of 2 tbsp.
olive oil, basil, dill, a splash of vinegar

Dinner: 4-6 oz. broiled salmon steak or other fish
Steamed broccoli
No-salt seltzer with lemon
1/2 apple

#2 (Lighter - low to moderate activity)

Breakfast: 1/2 grapefruit
2 oz. of cottage cheese

Lunch: 6 oz. canned salmon with herbs, salt
substitute 1 cup of salad vegetables with lemon juice

Dinner: Caesar salad with 1 boiled egg, spinach,
2 oz. hard cheese, celery, carrots, etc.
Easy olive oil dressing (as above)

#3

Breakfast: 1/2 pear, sliced
1-egg omelet with 2 oz. cheese (veggies of your choice)
cup of herb tea

Lunch: 1 bowl chicken soup (made with fat-free broth and
vegetables; without rice, grains, potatoes, or fat)
2 oz. cottage cheese or yogurt
1 Nutrasweet soft drink (water is preferable)

Dinner: 4-6 oz. lean steak
4 oz. steamed green beans
1-2 cups of salad vegetables with a dressing
of 2 tbsp. safflower oil and a dash of garlic and parmesan cheese

#4

Breakfast: Smoked salmon
1/2 baked apple
1 warm drink (decaf. coffee or tea)

Lunch: 4-6 oz. turkey (no nitrates)
1 cup steamed vegetables

Dinner: 1 1/2 c vegetable casserole (chopped broccoli,
cauliflower, onions, topped with grated cheese and baked -- see recipes)
Diet ginger ale

#5

Breakfast: 1/2 banana with 2 oz. low fat yogurt
1 handful sunflower seeds

Lunch: Salmon steak, "blackened" or broiled
Lemon wedge
Steamed broccoli
No-salt seltzer water

Dinner: Small lean steak
Asparagus spears (steamed)
Romaine salad with scallions (olive oil, dash of vinegar and garlic)

#6

Breakfast: Chicken salad (made with celery, scallions and
1 tbsp. of Hain safflower mayonnaise)

Lunch: Caesar salad with safflower oil/vinegar dressing

Dinner: Gazpacho (cold vegetable soup)
Tuna kabobs
1/2 c cubed melon

#7

Breakfast: 2-egg omelette (with celery, scallions, and pepper,
dash of pepper and garlic)

Lunch: Can of sardines packed in water
Celery and carrot sticks

Dinner: Broccoli and cauliflower steamed
1 lean lamb chop
1/2 grapefruit

#8

Breakfast: Smoked salmon and sauteed onions

Lunch: Greek salad (romaine, tomato, 4 black olives,
cucumber, 2 oz. feta cheese)

Dinner: Baked chicken breast (cooked without skin)
6 oz. steamed string beans with handful of sunflower seeds sprinkled, plus 1/2 apple cubed.

#9

Breakfast: 1/2 grapefruit
2 oz. pot cheese

Lunch: Mahi-mahi (fish) broiled with paprika
Lemon wedge
Spinach salad with Pritikin no-oil dressing

Dinner: Chicken soup (made with low-starch vegetables, no grain or fat)
Add 1 tbsp. olive oil to bowl before eating
2 oz. yogurt
6 oz. steamed spinach with 1 tbsp. olive oil, dash of garlic

#10

Breakfast: 1 poached egg
2 baked tomato halves topped with melted cheddar cheese and oregano
1/2 pear or grapefruit

Lunch: Chicken salad (2 chopped vegetables and 2 tbsp. safflower
mayo) on a bed of spinach

Dinner: Medley: carrot, celery, relish, onion, pepper, etc.
Steamed 6 oz. canned salmon seasoned with allowed seasoning

#11

Breakfast: Chicken soup
2 oz. hard cheese

Lunch: 2/3 can tuna on bed of Boston lettuce and other
greens
1-2 tbsp. safflower or olive oil dressing

Dinner: Baked scrod
Steamed okra

#12

Breakfast: Tuna or egg salad

Lunch: 2 hard-boiled eggs (easy to take to work)
1 stalk celery
1 small carrot
2 oz. hard cheese

Dinner: Small baked quail (okay 1x/per 3 weeks)
2 stalks steamed broccoli

#13

Breakfast: 1-egg omelette. 2 oz. Swiss cheese, chopped onion and pepper
6 oz. tomato juice

Lunch   3-4 slices low-salt turkey (easy to take to work)
1/2 apple
2 celery stalks

Dinner: Broccoli and lean beef stir-fry (you can stir fry in water, using a nonstick pan)

#14

Breakfast: 2-egg omelette with chopped smoked salmon and sauteed onion

Lunch: Sole broiled with parsley; (basted with olive oil and
lemon just after removing from oven)

Dinner: Salad of celery hearts, sunflower seeds, scallions, 3-4 black olives, radishes and cucumbers.
Pritikin no-oil dressing

#15

Breakfast: Eggs Benedict: 2 poached eggs topped with melted Monterey Jack
cheese on bed of steamed spinach (no hollandaise sauce)

Lunch: Fish soup
Steamed cabbage
2 oz. yogurt

Dinner: Chicken/vegetables stir fry (use low sodium soy sauce
or other herbs)
1/2 grapefruit

#16

Breakfast: Tuna fish and vegetables with 1 tbsp. olive oil and garlic

Lunch: Large piece baked chicken
Cole slaw (made with Hain Mayo)
1/2 pear

Dinner: 1/2 c "The I can't take it anymore!" spaghetti squash
topped with 3-4 lean beef meatballs.
1/4 c homemade sugar-free tomato sauce (okay 1x per 3 weeks)

#17

Breakfast: 2 oz. yogurt and a handful of sunflower seeds
1/2 grapefruit

Lunch: Salad (endives or escarole, 3-4 black olives,
cucumbers, tomato, 2 tb olive oil dressing, 4 to 8 oz. of tuna fish)

Dinner: Flounder souffle
Stir-fry green peppers and zucchini

#18

Breakfast: 6 oz. tomato juice
4-6 oz. canned tuna

Lunch: Salad of spinach, 3 oz. tofu, tomato, celery, handful sunflower seeds, 1-2 tbsp. olive or safflower oil dressing
(easy to take to work in a plastic container)

Dinner: Lean sliced roast beef
2 oz. cheese of your choice
Horseradish
6-8 oz. steamed cauliflower
1/2 baked apple

#19

Breakfast: 1/2 banana sliced into
2 oz. low fat yogurt

Lunch: Eggplant parmesan (made with no-sugar tomato sauce;
not breaded)
4 oz. steamed carrots

Dinner: Bluefish scampi (broiled with water in casserole, but
               basted at end with olive oil/garlic mixture, topped with tomato)
               Lemon wedge
               Steamed broccoli

#20

Breakfast: Lean beef patty
               1 scrambled egg -- no-stick pan, no oil

Lunch: "Sea Legs" (make sure these are all 100% fish, pressed to look like
               lobster legs). Watch for salt content if high blood pressure is present
               (easy to take for lunch if you have a refrigerator at the office)
               2 oz. cheese
               cucumber sticks

Dinner: Roast turkey
               Spinach (steamed); 2 oz. yogurt and herbs added after cooking
               String beans
               1/2 grapefruit

#21

Breakfast: Lean turkey sausage (no salt) (best in winter)
               1-egg omelette
               1/2 grapefruit

Lunch: Baked sole stuffed with mixture: 1/4 cup mushrooms,
               chopped scallions, 2 oz. yogurt, dash of garlic, other herbs

Dinner: Casserole with tuna, veggies, spices

Additional Menu Ideas

BREAKFAST

alternating:
fresh squeezed orange or grapefruit juice
whole grain muffins or bread
eggs (any style)
fruit
cereal -- whole grain (hot or cold)
rice cake with nut butter

LUNCH

choice of (alternating):
chicken, salmon, halibut, sole, tuna (baked or broiled)
large garden salad with at least 3 vegetables
lemon, olive oil, herbs & spices

DINNER (week 1)

Saturday: (large salad accompanying each dinner)
lamb shank (natural seasonings, e.g., herbamare)
sauted vegetable medley, potatoes, carrots, celery (cooked with lamb)

Sunday: vegetarian meal, e.g., eggplant parmigiana with tofu, broccoli, cauliflower, carrots, cabbage, rice
or couscous, quinoa pasta with pesto or tomato sauce

Monday: salmon steaks (broiled)
spinach -- steamed
quinoa

Tuesday: roast chicken
cauliflower, broccoli florets, and carrot strips
couscous

Wednesday: turkey meat balls (ground turkey, wheat germ, whole wheat bread crumbs, eggs & water)
whole grain or soba pasta sauce made with crushed tomatoes, basil, garlic, olive oil
simmered 2 hours

Thursday: scrod -- baked with lemon
corn on the cob
couscous

Friday: halibut steak
kale
sweet potato or baked/mashed potato

DINNER (week 2)

Saturday: London broil, baked potato, broccoli & carrots

Sunday: vegetarian meal (see week 1)

Monday: whole grain crust pizza with vegetable toppings

Tuesday: turkey cutlets marinated in soy and ginger root dressing, brussels sprouts, couscous

Wednesday: salmon, spinach souffle (eggs, whole wheat flour, herbamare, olive oil), quinoa

Thursday: baked chicken (whole) with potatoes, carrots, tomatoes, celery and onion, brown or wild rice

Friday: grey sole, pasta with pesto sauce (whole grain or soba), peas and carrots

DINNER (week 3)

Saturday: old fashioned stew with zucchini, onion, celery, red potatoes, and carrots

Sunday: vegetarian meal (see week 1)

Monday: turkey tetrazzini over pasta

Tuesday: scrod, cauliflower, kale, couscous curry style

Wednesday: vegetable lasagna with eggplant, whole grain pasta (layer and bake with ricotta, egg, tofu, herbamare mixture) sauce, mozzarella on top

Thursday: chicken tarragon, quinoa, vegetable medley

Friday: grilled tuna, wild rice, succotash (tomato, zucchini, onion, stewed)

Health Spa

PATH plans eventually to build a health spa in a country setting for the promotion of your health. Special diets and fasting programs will be tailored to your needs. The 12-step program, psychotherapy, addiction counseling, interfaith counseling, biofeedback, meditation, and massage will be available when necessary.

The Fast PATH to Dieting

The supplement Fast PATH has been developed by Dr. Braverman to speed up dieting success. The best concept in dieting is to be able to burn body fat while preserving lean muscle. Lean muscle is made up of higher amounts of essential amino acids, and the preservation of lean muscle depends on taking essential amino acids which preserve muscle mass. For doing work the body needs to process essential amino acids.

Therefore, protein sources high in essential amino acids are higher quality forms of protein. High quality protein, like an egg, has a higher proportion of essential amino acids than nonessential amino acids, and therefore a more favorable distribution of amino acids. The essential amino acids are the ones the body cannot make, and the nonessential are made from the essential. Substances like CoQ10, and occasionally other nutrients, can be made from the essential, or in this case, vitamin E. Hence vitamin E is the more critical nutrient. The Fast PATH in dieting is to ingest this high quality protein (essential amino acids) not the cheap high protein found in Medifast and Optifast and all the other cheap diet supplements. These diet supplements are high in protein, which is actually poor quality protein, probably leading ultimately to depletion of neurotransmitters in the brain. The essential amino acids, however, build neurotransmitters (they are the precursors) in the brain. The Fast PATH to dieting is to supplement with high quality essential amino acids to be combined with low fat and low carbohydrate diets. Such a diet is lean to the body and streamlined to build up the brain's neurotransmitters. Fast PATH is ideal as a nutritional booster with vegetarian diets.

The processing and digesting of essential amino acids is much easier than that of nonessential amino acids, because when only, or chiefly, nonessential amino acids are consumed, the body's own muscle must be broken down and used as a source to make the essential amino acids. Therefore, the higher the percent of intake of essential amino acids, the greater the preservation of muscle mass and the less the strain on the kidneys, which is why this approach has been taken with predialysis patients in order to preserve their kidney function.

Depression Diet:

The Mood Foods

Use these foods to fine-tune your moods to a mild degree. If you find yourself becoming irritable and tense during the day on the high-protein diet, reduce your consumption of foods rich in tyrosine. For an even more calming effect, include some tryptophan-rich foods. Reverse the process if the problem is low energy levels or mild depression. Armed with all the information you need, you can custom design your diet to meet your unique needs.

TYROSINE FOODS
(during the day)

- Eggs
- Green beans
- Lean meat
- Natural aged cheese
- Peas
- Seafood
- Seaweed
- Skim milk
- Tofu (bean curd)
- Whole wheat bread
- Yogurt

TRYPTOPHAN FOODS
(during the evening)

- Bananas
- Beef
- Cookies
- Dates
- Figs
- Pastas
- Peanuts
- Pineapples
- Processed cheese
- Sweets
- Turkey

An Explanation of The Low Carbohydrate Diet:

With Individualized Portions for Hypertension, Obesity, Anxiety, Depression, and Hypoglycemia

If a furnace is loaded with paper, cardboard, or wood, what burns first? Obviously, paper, then cardboard, then wood. The same is true when the body ingests carbohydrates, fat, and protein. Carbohydrates burn first. Hence, since fats burn next (second), foods like sausage and butter keep a person warm in the winter. Finally, protein burns third -- a good steak is slow to give energy but can maintain energy for the longest period.

Hence, a high protein diet, when combined with low carbohydrates, results in the body selecting its own fats to burn. This ketosis (a fat-burning state) diet can be dangerous without medical supervision. (Consult Dr. Atkins' books for recipes, yet avoid his high fat foods.) Dangers with the diet can usually be eliminated by adding fruit or carbohydrates to the diet. The diet has advantages in that high protein results in diuresis (water removal). We can all remember protein-starved Biafrans, whose bodies swelled up with water. In contrast, a high protein diet leads to dehydration. This helps weight loss slightly and diminishes the chance of heart failure and lowers blood pressure. Side effects can be prevented by vitamins. Hence, you must take supplements on this diet.

The diet is also useful for control of anxiety, hypoglycemia, and depression, because the lack of stimulants and the high amino acid content may lead to steadier nerves and better neurotransmission in the brain.

The Low Carbohydrate and High Blood Pressure Diet

This diet is not your permanent diet, but is a corrective diet to lower your blood pressure and, in some cases, cholesterol and triglycerides; and to raise your HDL, as well as to heal angina and other heart problems. It is important that you bring this program with you every time you visit the doctor.

The high blood pressure diet includes the Basic Diet, as well as some very specific dietary restrictions, which may also be necessary in your case.

Protein or Animal Foods: Fish, chicken, turkey, beef, veal, and pork are allowed unless sugar, MSG, corn syrup, corn starch, flour, pickling nitrates, or other preservatives are used in preparation. You are to emphasize fish daily or even twice daily. The best fish include mackerel, sardines, salmon, herring, and trout. Omit shellfish, which is a major cause of hepatitis, plus it contains less omega-3 fish oil and is high in cholesterol.

Grains: If you do not need to lose weight, the doctor can give you whole grains or cereals. White flours or refined carbohydrates are like sugar and have to be avoided as well as bread, crackers, and pasta. Whole grain can be used, including matzoh, kasha, oats, brown rice, and millet. You may have _____oz. per day. The amount depends on your need for weight loss.

Cheese: Hard or semisoft aged yellow cheese. Examples are: Swiss, Cheddar, Brie, Camembert, Blue, Mozzarella, Gruyere, and Goat. Avoid all diet cheeses, cheese spreads, cheese food substitutes, or Velveeta.

Fresh Cheeses: Cottage, Farmer, Pot, Ricotta, Tofu, and Monterey Jack. You may have ____ oz. per day.

Beverages: It is important when you have high blood pressure not to drink excessive amounts of water. Spring water and mineral water are preferred to tap water. Tangy club soda or herbal teas can be helpful. All herbal teas should be free of caffeine, sugar, or barley. Decaffeinated coffee, which is ulcerogenic, is permitted (up to 3 cups). All caffeine sources are prohibited, e.g., tea, regular coffee, etc., which raise blood pressure. Diet soda use is necessary but only temporarily. A glass of fruit juice can be substituted for a piece of fruit, if weight loss is not a problem. Vegetable juices can be made fresh.

Lemon and lime juice (up to __ tsp.) can be used with seltzer and Nutrasweet to make a good lemonade.

Eggs: You are not to eat more than seven eggs per week if your cholesterol is not low, or has not been lowered by vitamins.

Fruits: Restricting fruit can be useful in a low carbohydrate diet for weight loss, yet not for long. Fruit is high in potassium, can prevent strokes, night cramps, and heart arrhythmias. Melons result in the least amount of weight gain. A banana, pear, and orange are high in potassium. Other potassium sources include parsley and sunflower seeds. You may have __ fruits or ____ glasses of fruit juice per day. Salt substitute is a good source of potassium.

General Consideration of Foods Permitted: Your diet must be made up of exclusively wholesome foods, 100% pure, contain no additives, sugar, starch, fillers and, if possible, no preservatives.

Salad Vegetables: Leafy greens, lettuce, escarole, romaine, parsley, collards, endive, spinach, mushrooms, cucumber, celery, radishes, peppers, and bean sprouts, up to ____ cupsful per day.

Permissible Vegetables: e.g., asparagus, broccoli, string or wax beans, cabbage, beet greens, cauliflower, chard, eggplant, kale, kohlrabi,mushrooms, tomato, onion, spinach, peppers, summer squash, zucchini, squash, okra, pumpkin, turnips, avocado, bamboo shoots, bean sprouts, water chestnuts, snow pea pods, and sauerkraut. You may have ____ oz. per day.

Nuts and Seeds: Nuts and seeds generally are to be avoided by the hypertensive, although sunflower seeds (unsalted), almonds, English walnuts, and pecans are less fatty and somewhat tolerable, while pistachios and cashews are very poor choices. You may have __ oz. daily.

Other Dairy Products contain a lot of carbohydrates, e.g., yogurt, buttermilk, and milk. You may have __ oz. per day.

Spring Water: Use only spring water because your water supply may be contaminated by lead, and may have excess copper from your plumbing.

Salt Substitute: Use only salt substitutes (not "light salt") -- i.e., use salt substitutes that contain only potassium chloride or, in some cases, magnesium chloride.

Alcohol: No more than one drink a day ever, but preferably none at all.

Fats and Oils: Because cholesterol and triglycerides are fats, good fats and oils have a particular role in cleaning out the bad fats and oils. For those who have high blood pressure, safflower, sunflower and linseed oils (this is probably the best) lower blood pressure best and may work as a diuretic. Some individuals benefit from as much as four to six tablespoons per day of these oils. You need __ tbsp. per day. If you have high cholesterol as well, you may need to use olive oil which lowers cholesterol better but may slightly raise blood pressure. You need ____ oz. per day. You are to generally avoid saturated fat which includes cream, butter, etc. You may use your oil with vinegar, adding grated cheese and mustard (contains salt) in small quantities.

Program for Hypertension

Dr. Braverman treats hypertension with a two-part program of diet and nutrients. He describes the first part as "the best of Pritikin and Atkins." The second part is an orthomolecular approach -- using megadoses of nutrients to treat disease.

Accompanying the diet program Dr. Braverman prescribes the following regimens:

1. **Stop smoking** -- Tobacco smoke contains harmful cadmium that can harden arteries and damage the heart.

2. **Eliminate caffeine** -- Drinking two cups of coffee a day can raise your blood pressure five or 10 points.

3. **Lose weight** -- This is the key factor in lowering blood pressure and increasing your life span. By losing 30 pounds you can lower your blood pressure at least four points.

To lose weight initially, Dr. Braverman advises eating a low-carbohydrate diet -- not the Pritikin diet, which is about 85% complex carbohydrates (vegetables, starches, fruit). Since carbohydrates cause fluid retention, Dr. Braverman recommends a diet high in protein, which acts as a diuretic. For example, Dr. Braverman suggests a diet of fish, fresh vegetables (not starchy ones: potatoes, corn, peas, and carrots), small amount of cheese and salad.

This diet, which restricts salt and fried food, is called Plan A. Once the patient has lost weight, he is switched to Plan B -- a complex carbohydrate, Pritikin-type diet of fish, chicken, whole grains, salads, vegetables, and fruit. Patients are also advised to increase their intake of polyunsaturated oils (safflower, sunflower), which have a diuretic effect, lower cholesterol, and eliminate saturated fats (e.g., butter).

Plan B does not work for everybody; many obese hypertensives have biochemical imbalances and gain weight on a complex carbohydrate diet, even one restricted to 1500 to 1800 calories. In such a case, Dr. Braverman would design a tailor-made diet.

Part two of Dr. Braverman's program for hypertension consists of megadoses of nutrients to treat the brain's biochemical imbalances. High on the list of essential nutrients is fish oil, which contains the fatty acid, omega-3, to lower elevated triglycerides and raise low HDL levels. Dosage depends on the individual; a patient with extremely elevated triglycerides and reduced HDL might need 12 to 15 capsules of fish oil a day.

Other nutrients found to be particularly beneficial are linoleic acid (5-15 grams), magnesium (500-1500 mg), vitamin B-6 (200-1000 mg), taurine (1-3 grams), and zinc (15-60 mg).

Additional nutrients may be prescribed: CoQ10, calcium, and potassium (as salt substitute or in fruit). Ginger, garlic, and onions also lower blood pressure and are valuable for their anticlotting properties.

Excellent results are achieved by treating patients with this diet and nutrient program, even though the patient may be taking one or two drugs when he starts the program. Once the number exceeds two, it's harder to eliminate all medications, but it can be done.

See, Jane Heimlich, *What Your Doctor Won't Tell You*, New York: Harper Collins, 1990.

Hypertension Diet

Recipe: Fresh-Start Tomato Juice

See Recipes, p. 151.

Recipe: Better Butter

See Recipes, p. 152.

Herpes Diet

Eat meats like red meats, salmon, and tuna, as well as dairy products, barley, corn meal, and root vegetables. Try to restrict nuts and white flour. If necessary, cut down on fruits. (Increase lysine; reduce arginine. See *Healing Nutrients Within* by E. Braverman, M.D.)

Low Tyramine Diet (Low Headache Diet)

(Diet # 1)

FOODS EXCLUDED

* Aged Cheese (General rule of thumb - all cheeses, except cottage cheese and cream cheese)
  Bananas and any food product made with bananas
* Beer, Ale, Wines (Especially Chianti)
  Broad Beans and Pods - lima beans, Italian broad beans, lentils, snowpeas
  Livers
  Chocolate in any form
  Cultured Dairy Products - buttermilk, yogurt, sour cream
  Figs - canned
  Legumes
  Nitrates - any food containing preservative
  Nuts - and any food product which contains nuts
  Pickled Herring and salted dry fish
  Pineapple - and any food product which contains pineapple
  Pork - all forms, e.g., bacon, ham
  Prunes
  Raisins - and any food product which contains raisins
  Soy Sauce
  Wine and any food product made from wine
  Vanilla extracts and any food product which contains vanilla
  Yeast Extracts
  Monosodium Glutamate - additive in many foods (read labels), particularly Chinese food

* Primary offending agents. (See Headache (Low Tyramine) Diet, p. 139.)

Low Monamine Diet

(Tyramine Diet # 2)

There are specific foods that are high in substances, e.g., tyramine, that elevate the levels of brain monamines, that is, amino acids that contain only one amino. Enkephalin, endorphin, and opiates all inhibit the activity of these monamines. Much of what one experiences during drug withdrawal is due to a rapid increase in monamines when opiate levels suddenly drop off. In addition, there are some indications that a natural excess of monamines is present in those persons vulnerable to opiate abuse. The following foods should be avoided if you are adhering to this diet in strict fashion.

- aged cheese (all cheese except for cottage cheese, cream cheese, and American processed cheese)
- alcohol (including wind and beer)
- avocado
- bacon
- bananas
- broad beans (pods)
- brains
- canned figs
- chicken livers
- Chinese food (or any food with monosodium glutamate - MSG)
- chocolate and cocoa
- cola
- citrus fruits and juices (orange, lime, lemon, grapefruit)
- coffee and decaffeinated coffee
- eggplant
- fermented sausage (bologna, salami, pepperoni, summer sausage)
- herring
- hot dogs
- nuts
- meat tenderizer
- oatmeal
- onions (also large amounts of garlic)
- pineapple
- plums
- prunes
- raisins
- sour cream
- soy sauce
- smoked fish
- tomatoes
- yogurt

It is crucial that these foods be kept to a minimum during periods of cravings or withdrawal. In addition, it may be a good idea to reduce intake of these foods at all times if opiate abuse is a problem.

Foods with Monamine Oxidase Inhibitors to be Avoided

(Tyramine Diet # 3)

Foods definitely to be avoided:

- beer, red wine
- aged cheese
- dry sausages
- fava Italian green beans
- brewer's yeast
- smoked fish
- liver (beef or chicken)

Foods that may cause problems in large amounts but are otherwise less problematic:

- alcohol
- ripe avocado
- yogurt
- bananas (ripe)
- soy sauce

Foods that were thought to be problems but are probably not problematic in usual moderate quantities:

- chocolate
- figs
- meat tenderizers
- caffeine-containing beverages
- raisins

Source: based on McCabe, B., and Tsuang, M. T., Dietary Considerations in MAO Inhibitor Regimens, *J. Clin. Psychiatry*, 43:178-181, 1982.

The Princeton Plan Diet

The Princeton Plan Diet was developed by Edwin Heleniak, M.D., and Barbara Aston, M.S. The diet is basically a combination of a high-protein diet with a complex carbohydrate diet on alternating days. The purpose of the alternating days is to utilize brown fat. Brown fat is the fat that actually increases the number of calories you burn and can be activated by eating certain foods, including special fats. The Princeton Plan Diet basically has you eat certain foods that activate brown fat or brown adipose tissue. It usually takes only 24-48 hours of dieting for the body to adjust and slow the body's natural calorie burning fires. The purpose of the alternating plan is to keep a high metabolic rate and avoid dietary plateaus. Snacking on the wrong sugars and fats leads to insulin resistance, but a high fiber diet restores insulin sensitivity.

High protein diets with high fiber pull extra fluids out of body tissues and works like a diuretic. You don't have to give up red meat, eggs, or oils to lose weight because you can have these in the high-protein diet section of the Princeton Plan Diet. Fatty oils and fatty acids found in certain vegetable oils can be used as natural appetite suppressants as can calcium and other nutritional approaches (Bioguar, capsilum, etc.). Exercise only accounts for 12% of the calories we burn while the other 88% is a matter of metabolism. The purpose of the Princeton Plan is to activate your metabolic rate and in many cases it can be successful for weight loss and a good maintenance diet.

Moderate Protein, Moderate Complex Carbohydrate High Fiber Diet

Note: These are guidelines for a maintenance diet only for those adults without serious medical conditions. Adjust portions to avoid over or underweight condition. Avoid foods which are strong allergens. Amounts are reasonable *per day* limits unless otherwise noted or doctor adjusted. The doctor may adjust your diet to meet your health needs or suggest a different diet.

ABUNDANT

Up to 3 cups salad per day	Try to use vegetables with color (e.g., not iceberg lettuce) -- they contain more vitamins and minerals.
6-10 oz. steamed vegetables	Try a variety of vegetables. For starchy ones, use amounts listed in "Moderate" category, unless they are nutritious and thought to help prevent cancer, then use more.
Fish or Poultry	Cook without the skin; bake, broil, boil or stir-fry; *do not fry*. (Lean beef, veal, shellfish, or pork can be used if this is easier; however, it is best to limit these as much as possible.)

MODERATE

7 eggs per week -- adjust, based on the individual's need
2 small carrots/day OK
2/3 c. whole grain (incl. corn, whole wheat pasta)
    or 2 1/2 slices whole grain bread
1-2 fruits (Usually have banana, grapefruit, apple,
    pear, or 1/2 c. melon)
(2/3 c. unfiltered juice in place of 1 fruit)
1 med. potato or 1/2 c. beans
4 oz. low fat milk, yogurt, cottage cheese, soy milk or tofu
Diet Jello - as you wish (make sure it has no carbohydrate content)
7 tbsp. lemon juice and 2 tbsp. vinegar
Herbs and salt-free seasonings as you wish (e.g., garlic,
    oregano, cayenne)
Roll leafy herbs between your fingers to release the flavor
Pritikin no-oil dressings

VERY LITTLE

2 tbsp. safflower oil	Olive oil is also fine for people who do not have high blood pressure. Turn this into a dressing for vegetables (raw or steamed) by adding vinegar or lemon juice and herbs. Hoop, farmer, and pot cheese are best. Next best are gruyere, swiss and cheddar.
2 oz. hard cheese or 3 oz. tofu	
1 handful of raw sunflower seeds	
4 oz. lean red meat up to 3x/week maximum (best to avoid)	
1 tbsp. mayonnaise/day	Only a sugar-free safflower oil mayo; at your health food store or make it.
Very small amounts of salt	Best to use salt substitutes like Mrs. Dash or no salt. Do not use table salt (sodium chloride) if history of high blood pressure.

BEVERAGES

Spring water is best; also okay are: no-salt seltzer water; Crystal light lemonade (with Nutrasweet); diet caffeine-free soda; herb tea; decaffeinated tea. Tomato or other vegetable juice - 6 oz/day; low fat milk - 4 oz/day; 2/3 c. unfiltered fruit juice, all count as one fruit. (Decaffeinated coffee is generally not advised because it has an unhealthful oil in it.)

NOT PERMITTED

Nuts (Even peanut butter has unhealthful oil)
Sugar (Avoid cane and brown sugar, corn syrup, other syrups, jams, honey, sucrose, maltodextrin, dextrose, etc.)
    (1/2 tbsp./day all-fruit spread OK. Rare use of fruit juice sweetened, whole-grain cookies OK. Occasional use of barley malt, brown rice syrup or molasses OK. Fructose may be used as sweetener
Ice cream, butter, cream; canned food (but canned fish is OK)
Margarine (1 tbsp./day OK if liquid safflower oil is listed first, e.g., Hain brand at health store)
Fried food; highly processed foods in general
White flour in any form (bread, pasta, pizza, crackers, etc.)
Good news: 100% whole wheat versions of the above exist -- check your health food store
Alcohol -- check over-the counter-remedies; caffeine -- check diet sodas
Sausage, bacon (but occasional use of turkey sausage is okay)
Cold cuts (unless low salt, without fat, nitrites, or preservatives)
Salty foods such as pickles and olives should be used very sparingly

HELPFUL TIPS

You will do well to permanently avoid any fried, fatty foods, refined flour, cold cuts, very salty or sugary foods. Always read labels. It is best to limit red meat. To prepare foods healthfully, avoid frying. Use a nonstick frying pan for stove-top use. You can saute vegetables in water. Preferably, broil or bake meats. Steam veggies (5-8 minutes for most, 12-18 for tougher vegetables, using a steamer basket) or bake vegetables or eat them raw. Boiling destroys vitamins. Popcorn can be made in an air-popper and enjoyed with simply a salt substitute.

Note: If you are on a weight gain diet, add more carbohydrates and fruit, and drink a weight gain shake at least once a day. You might whip up this shake in your blender:

    1 med. ripe banana or other fruit (e.g., 2/3 c. frozen strawberries); 2-3 tbsp. safflower oil; 6 oz. low-fat milk or soy milk; vanilla extract (non-alcohol type); Nutrasweet to taste; 2-3 tbsp. Nature's Plus Weight Gainer (or another brand) is advised.

The Benefits of Fasting

Fasting has some very great potential benefits. In America we diet, but in biblical times fasting for spiritual development, changing your life and changing the course of your behavior was typical. Today, a revolution in American dieting was started by Dr. Atkins' high protein diet, which also included high fat. Now high protein diets are low fat, high fiber and are very successful, occurring in several forms, e.g., Optifast, Medifast, Slim-Fast, Nutri-Fast, and Fast-PATH. Probably the best medically documented ones are, Optifast and Fast-Path. Fasting is important because we need to keep our weight at the optimum. Twenty-five percent of Americans are overweight. This is probably the single greatest disease in our society. The primary benefits of high protein, low calorie diets are the rapid weight loss, diuretic effect, lowering of blood pressure, help for idiopathic edema and congestive heart failure, lowering of blood sugar, etc. High protein diets are toxic, however, for patients already in or approaching kidney failure. Blood clotting can also increase with all dieting unless fish oil is given. Dieting or fasting increases one's need for all nutrients, particularly iron.

It should be pointed out that when animals are put on low calorie diets there is an increase in their life spans of 15 days to 26 days: water fleas have an increased life span of 42 days to 61 days; guppies have an increased life span of 1550 days compared to 707 days; rats increase their life span from 1000 days to 1500 days. Many individuals feel that low calorie diets have substantially contributed to the prolongation of their lives. We also believe the approach towards fasting, as long as it is done under medical supervision and is properly nutritionally supplemented, may actually contribute to longevity.

Options for fasting are: the carbohydrate fast or a high protein diet, the carbohydrate and fat fast, daytime fast with one meal at night, total fast with water (in some cases distilled) for a maximum three to 21 days under medical supervision.

Therapeutic Fasting

Therapeutic fasting is used to dramatically accelerate the healing process. This occurs under conditions of complete physiologic rest when the individual abstains from all forms of food or drink except pure water. Resting allows the body to conserve energy that would normally be spent on the activities of daily living, to be used in the healing process. After the third day, fat is burned.

Fasting should not be undertaken on your own. It is essential that fasting be supervised by a physician who specializes in this type of therapy.

Joel Fuhrman, M.D. is our consultant in therapeutic fasting. He has supervised hundreds of therapeutic fasts achieving remarkable recoveries, particularly with patients with autoimmune diseases. He is on the board of governors of the International Association of Professional Hygienists, the physician body involved in research and training of physicians utilizing this modality. Besides supervising hundreds of successful fasts, Dr. Fuhrman has compiled and analyzed all 1200 scientific studies from the medical literature on therapeutic fasting. A bibliography is available on fasting.

Fasting is an effective treatment for autoimmune diseases such as rheumatoid arthritis and lupus. It allows the body to detoxify and the immune system to normalize itself. Those who have been suffering from allergies, sinusitis and other immune sensitivities can rapidly recover. Fasting can also be extremely effective at reversing heart diseases and diabetes. It rapidly reverses symptoms of angina (chest pain) and normalizes high blood pressure, allowing patients to discontinue their medication. Fasting has on rare occasions also effectively resolved noncancerous tumors such as ovarian cysts, enabling patients to avoid surgery. Fasting has a long history and it has been used by religious leaders and doctors for millennia.

Food Diaries: Keeping a Food Diary Helps Dietary Compliance

DATE/DAY	BREAKFAST	LUNCH	DINNER	NOTES

Remember, 98 % of all dieters break their diet. Be honest with yourself and let's see how we can learn to walk on the PATH towards wellness.

Supplemental Food Diary

DATE	BREAKFAST	LUNCH	DINNER

Remember: Dr. Braverman maintains that 98% of the people recording their diet fail. Strive to prove him wrong -- stay on the Path!

Eating Out Tips

1. You will need to ask questions about HOW some of the foods were prepared. What thickening and breading agent was used -- corn starch or wheat? Are any spices, sugars, or food additives added that you should avoid?

2. Choose a restaurant with a large variety of foods so you will have many choices. Call before going, and ask about the food and preparation methods.

3. You may need to bring your own salad dressing, crackers or bread.

4. Fast food restaurants need to be chosen carefully to avoid hidden additives and hidden sources of ingredients as well. It is difficult to get them to reveal a list of ingredients for the prepared dishes you choose.

5. Cafeterias may be a solution to eating out, but they may use sulfating agents, sugar, and MSG on the foods to improve taste.

6. A la carte eating can give flexibility in choosing the items of food to eat.

7. Select meats, fish, and poultry cooked simply, accompanied by steamed vegetables to be safe. A salad bar allows you to select the foods you can eat. Ask about sulfating agents.

8. When going out to a cocktail or a dinner party, contact your host and ask what's being served. You may need to bring some munchies of your own. This is especially important for children's birthday parties. Make a small cake or suitable treat with a candle in it for your child to bring along.

The Problem of Vegetarianism

Many people throughout the world adopt a vegetarian diet for a variety of reasons, avoiding meat and, in some cases, all animal products such as eggs and milk. It is beyond the compass of this book to address the religious and ethical considerations involved in vegetarianism, but we feel that some comment on its adoption for reasons of health is relevant here, as it presents problems with respect to an adequately balanced intake of amino acids.

Epidemiologists have suggested that true vegetarian societies cannot adapt to stress adequately. Rechig (1983) pointed out that most vegetable proteins have amino acid deficiencies and are thus unsatisfactory as a sole source of protein; usually, lysine, methionine, tryptophan, and threonine are deficient. These deficiencies can be overcome in part by the addition to the diet of other proteins rich in these amino acids. Although the essential amino acids may be adequate in a vegetarian diet, many other protein products may be deficient, e.g., essential peptides.

Many vegetables are toxic, such as cabbage and beans, which have an antithyroid effect. Part of the problem in a vegetarian diet is not in the toxins in the vegetables, but in the deficiencies they induce. If inadequately cooked, many legumes, including soybeans, lima beans, navy beans, and peanuts, contain trypsin inhibitors. These interfere with the digestion of the protein and availability of the limiting amino acid, methionine. Hellebostad (1985) has reviewed problems of vitamin B-12 deficiency and vitamin D-deficiency rickets in vegetarianism. *Nutrition Reviews* (1979) suggests that children less than two years old, on a vegetarian diet, are shorter and lighter than other children. Several studies suggest that reduced growth is due to zinc and calcium deficiencies. Calkins, *et. al.*, (1984) have established that vegan (pure vegetarian) diets are well below recommended calcium requirements for females. Lacto-ovo-vegetarians, who eat eggs and milk, seem to have less deficiency in zinc, calcium, and vitamin D.

Meat, fish, fowl, and liver are concentrated sources of vitamins E, A, and B complex. Furthermore, animal foods are loaded with iron, zinc, and other nutrients. Harris (1986) suggests that for the lack of these nutritional advantages vegetarians throughout history have not coped with stress as well as meat eaters.

The advantages of a high-vegetable diet are due to increased fiber and beta carotene, which protect against cancer, particularly colon cancer. A high-vegetable diet is undoubtedly healthful, but probably should not exclude meat and other proteins. Kurup (1989) showed that the ability to degrade fiber increases in high meat diets. It has been shown that beef protein, even when present in up to 55 percent of a diet (Wiebe, et al., 1984), will not raise cholesterol levels in normal men. Ingram, et al., (1985) suggest that the real danger of high-protein, high-meat diets is that they are frequently accompanied by high consumption of refined carbohydrates. A diet high in vegetables, whole grains, and lean meat may be the best.

The great contribution of vegetarianism is that it has made us aware of the need to eat more vegetables and fruit and less refined carbohydrates and junk foods.

Braverman, E., M.D., *The Healing Nutrients Within: Amino Acids*, App. A., p. 366.

B-6 and Zinc Deficiency and Vegetarianism

Zinc is an important nutrient that may be lacking in a vegetarian diet. Most vegetarians not only avoid meat, a good source of zinc, but increase their consumption of foods rich in phytates (beans, legumes and grains) which cause the elimination of zinc, calcium, and other minerals in the digestive system; this can become a major problem. However, the addition of leaven or yeast to grains, as in leavened bread, destroys the phytates by fermentation; sprouting also destroys phytates. Sprouted grains, beans, and seeds are most nutritious and should be a part of everyone's diet.

One patient from a southern city found that she could not eat any protein food such as fish, chicken, or red meat without developing unreality, dizziness and even hallucinations. Without fail she was unduly suspicious of her companions whenever she ate meat -- she had paranoia.

She thought she had an allergy to all proteins. She came to the Brain Bio Center for food allergy testing, but on the initial tests we found her to be pyroluric, with a high cryptopyrrole level in her urine. We next found her to be deficient in zinc, manganese, and vitamin B-6, as are most pyroluric patients. Manganese, zinc, and B-6 are needed by the body to handle protein foods. With administration of these nutrients she found that she could tolerate proteins for the first time in many years. She also started losing her excess body fluids and fat, dropping fifteen pounds in two months; her old dresses began to fit again.

We bring up this case because it is similar to those of many disperceptive teenagers, who when stressed find that paranoid symptoms increase after a protein meal. They feel better on an all-vegetable diet and so may not only eat as vegetarians but also join one of the many cults which espouse vegetarianism. A less drastic answer to their protein intolerance is typically zinc, 15 to 30 mg per day; vitamin B-6 to the point of dream recall (often 1 g); and manganese, 50 mg each morning (of course, after consulting a physician). With these supplements they can again tolerate and enjoy protein foods.

Reducing Allergy to Protein

We have become extremely limited in the kinds of meat we eat. Most eat beef, lamb, pork, chicken, and turkey. Overuse of one protein can produce allergies to that protein.

When we eat different kinds of fish as a main source of protein, knowing that each fish protein is antigenically unique, we have an unlimited source of varied proteins if we are allergic to animal protein. Occasionally, kosher meat helps the meat-allergic individual. The koshering process removes blood in which the hemoglobin is antigenic and may cause immune complexes to form after absorption by the body (Hemmings, 1976).

The Healthiest Choice

If sufficient vegetables, whole grains, and fish are eaten, the hazards of meat (produced organically) are probably canceled out. Some meat is necessary for resistance to stress. But excess meat and fat are to be avoided since they are implicated in cancer and heart disease. The threats to our meat and fish supply such as steroids, PCBs, antibiotics, or hormones should be reduced or eliminated.

But until that goal is reached the nutrients such as cysteine that protect us against those hazards should be increased in our diets. In sum, meat diets should be high in vegetables, whole grains, fish, and supplemental nutrients. We think that this combination is the one that leads to optimum health for most people.

Problems With Vegetarianism

Problems with vegetarianism are:

1. Inadequate warming of the body in some cases.

2. Inadequate in essential amino acids for the brain.

3. Second and third generations of vegetarians may have lower intellectual functioning and possibly impaired immune system functioning

4. B12 deficiency in strict (ovo non-lacto) vegetarians (vegans)

(See Vegetarian Diet, p. 149.)

Cardiac Patients and a Vegetarian Diet

Some cardiac patients, however, probably would do well on a strict vegetarian diet. By following such an eating regimen they would not have to make determinations about cholesterol intake or saturated fats -- no gram counting, no choices, no opportunity to "cheat."

Dr. Joel Fuhrman, mentioned earlier as our consultant in therapeutic fasting, has designed just such a vegetarian diet which could meet the needs of cardiac patients:

Dr. Fuhrman's Strict Vegetarian Diet

BREAKFAST: 2 grapefruit or melon

LUNCH: Whole grapefruit, orange or melon

Large green salad	--	lettuce, snow peas, tomato, cucumber, string bean, shredded carrot, red pepper
Vegetable soup	--	all vegetables
More fruit	--	apple, kiwi, pears, banana, strawberries

DINNER:

Steamed vegetables	--	green string beans, broccoli, zucchini, asparagus, artichoke
Starchy vegetables	--	potato, sweet potato, butternut, acorn squash
Brown rice		
Carrots and peas		
Whole grain cereal/lentils		

No dairy, milk, chicken, turkey, meat, oils or fats of any kind, nuts or seeds, sweets except for fresh fruit, fruit juices.

Dr. Braverman would prescribe a regimen of nutritive supplements for any patient following this diet.

The Much Maligned Egg:

The Best Amino Acid Food

Heart disease often involves obstruction of the coronary arteries by fatty plaques which consist mainly of cholesterol. Cholesterol combines with calcium to become hard, hence the term "hardening of the arteries" The plaque which accumulates on the walls reduces arterial volume and results in higher blood pressure and harder work for the heart.

A well-proven strategy to prevent heart disease is to reduce indigenous cholesterol synthesis. Reducing dietary cholesterol has little, or no, effect on this and an indigenous cholesterol synthesis diet has made little, or no, contribution. The overall rate of cholesterol intake in this country has dropped from 800 mg/day to less than 500 mg/day in the last ten years. At the same time, consumption of the "good" unsaturated fats and olive oil has increased by 60 percent. These changes in diet may have done more to reduce heart disease than all medical procedures combined, according to Robert Levy of Columbia University.

Changes in cholesterol consumption have come mainly from reduction in meat intake, which is 40 percent less than ten years ago. Egg consumption has dropped only 12 percent, so it is apparent that the reduction in eggs has made little, or no, contribution to the decrease in heart attacks. In spite of the almost universal advice to limit their consumption because of their high cholesterol content, we think it is good to eat eggs, because the egg is a nearly perfect amino acid food. Furthermore, the egg, because of its high lecithin content and other nutrients, does not raise blood cholesterol levels by more than 2 percent. In one study, three eggs did not raise cholesterol

significantly. To consider cholesterol content only is misleading, because the ratio of cholesterol to other nutrients is what is important. This is the reason why Dr. John Yudkin was able to show that sugar and junk foods raised blood cholesterol levels, despite their low cholesterol content.

Most foods are of lower quality as protein sources than the egg, which is proportionally the most balanced and best source of the essential amino acids. In each food, only one or two essential amino acids are deficient or totally lacking, and these are called the "limiting amino acids" for that food. The protein in that particular food will be utilized by the body only to the extent that the limiting amino acid is present in another food being ingested at the same time. The egg's superior balance makes its proteins more utilizable than those of most other foods.

Careful study of the effect of egg proteins on plasma amino acids shows that egg, like steak, raises lysine, valine, threonine, and leucine to extremely high levels. Yet, the ratio to other amino acids is slightly better balanced with the egg than with steak. For example, steak increases the plasma valine-to-plasma methionine ratio to more than five to one, while for egg it is only four to one. The egg is slightly better balanced, but not perfectly balanced. Amino acid formulas are now being studied, which may suggest ways to achieve a more balanced rise in plasma amino acids than food itself can provide. At present, the egg is probably the best amino acid food source.

Braverman, E., M.D., *The Healing Nutrients Within: Amino Acids*, App. B., p. 340 (1986).

Lactobacillus for Antibiotic Side Effects and for Indigestion

What is Lactobacillus Acidophilus?

It is a therapeutic means of equalizing the flora of the intestinal tract. L. Acidophilus is well established as a normal, desirable inhabitant of the lower intestines. Its exact mode of action is not entirely known but may depend upon one or more of the following factors:

1. It promotes a mildly acid reaction which stimulates peristalsis and a favorable environment for normal metabolism.

2. The lactic acid which it produces has a bacteriostatic effect on many undesirable organisms.

3. The possibility exists that it may produce an antibiotic of some comparable substance antagonistic to many enteric organisms.

L. Acidophilus is the organism most readily employed in intestinal bacterial therapy. L. Acidophilus is known to be able to retain its viability throughout the intestinal tract and thus afford a means of implantation in the lower intestine. This ability to survive is one of the chief identifying characteristics of L. Acidophilus. (Kline and Sabine, 1963) This fact differentiates it from L. Bifidus.

L. Bifidus is the organism found to be predominant in the intestines of breast-fed infants. It is more fastidious in its growth requirements than L. Acidophilus, therefore more difficult to grow in vitro.

What is the recommended dosage?

In practice, the administration of L. Acidophilus Liquid is uncomplicated. When an existing condition is to be treated, the maximum rate of dosage should be employed first, decreasing the amount as symptoms subside. In many cases, particularly diarrhea, relief is experienced overnight. Other conditions may require therapy for several weeks. There are no harmful results or side effects from overdosage or excessive use. No single

recommendation will fit all individuals, however. The organism, which is a normal inhabitant of the intestines, is desirable and there are no harmful side effects associated with its presence. It is nonpathogenic and non-toxigenic. At best, it can do much good. At worst, it can do no harm.

What are some conditions that require L. Acidophilus therapy?

An imbalance of the intestinal flora may manifest itself in many ways such as diarrhea, constipation, flatulence, colitis, pruritus, enteritis, bloating, or as a general gastrointestinal discomfort. It is toward such symptoms that the use of L. Acidophilus has been most directed in an attempt to gain relief through the establishment of normal flora.

The use of antibiotics destroys the equilibrium of the intestinal flora and L. Acidophilus has proven to be beneficial in correcting this condition and reestablishing equilibrium.

Greater weight gains in breast-fed infants than in comparable bottle-fed infants have been reported. However, in a study of approximately 800 subjects by Robinson and Thomas (1952), it was reported that bottle-fed infants on formulas supplemented with L. Acidophilus showed significantly larger weight gains than the control groups. Other studies have reported a lower incidence of gastroenteritis in infants receiving L. Acidophilus in their diet.

L. Acidophilus is believed to be a normal vaginal inhabitant. It is considered desirable since it promotes a mild acid reaction which is antagonistic to Candida yeast and other undesirable microorganisms.

Some other symptoms of metabolic disorders may yield to acidophilus therapy, such as acne and its various forms, as well as constipation.

The Diet Almanac:
Finding the Diet for Life,
Health and Combating Disease:
There is a Diet for All Occasions

Introduction

There are many diet books written every day, and, most of the time, they are books devoted to one diet. Each diet book often contains one diet which an author may write about for 200 pages. Usually this diet is condensable to several pages but here it is condensed to just a few. To give the basics, references are available on request.

It is wonderful that we have so many diets, since every disease requires a specific diet. There is a diet for osteoporosis, a diet for hypertension, a diet for obesity, a diet for arthritis, a diet for heart disease, a diet for diabetes, a diet for virtually every disease. Often there are several valuable diets for one disease.

This section seeks to be a catalogue of all the general diet suggestions and diet information for diseases, and for general health. It is my hope that this catalogue of diets will help lay people and doctors choose a diet for every disease, for diet therapy is almost always a key consideration. Furthermore, I hope this educates the public in the science of diet, so that they may reject fad diets and choose and adapt a basic diet as their health needs.

Basic Health Diet Guidance

There are some basic fundamental rules for the generally healthy person to follow. These rules make up the Basic Health Diet, which is the diet of which all other diets are a variation. (See Basic Health and Diet Rules, p. 89.)

ADDITIVES AVOIDED

It eliminates simple sugars, MSG, corn syrup, corn starch, white flour, pickling, nitrates, or other preservatives used in food preparation.

PROTEIN FOODS

Concerning protein foods, it emphasizes fish first, for its great cardiovascular preventive benefits. Secondly, it emphasizes chicken, turkey, and other fowl. Thirdly, it includes at a very reduced rate, either beef or veal once a week. Pork and shellfish are the least valuable protein sources. Pork is frequently fatty and filled with nitrates and preservatives and it contains too much serine and histidine. Shellfish is relatively high in cholesterol and low in cardiovascular protective fish oils. Shellfish also contains hepatitis A virus as well as toxins that scavengers collect or accumulate.

EGGS

Eggs are permitted, but generally no more than seven per week. If cholesterol is a problem, this is because, although blood cholesterol levels are not necessarily related to cholesterol intake, there is for some people a relationship between too much cholesterol intake and high serum cholesterol. High cholesterol intake, when combined with other poor eating habits, will definitely lead to serum cholesterol buildup. Carbohydrateholics (addicted to junk food) usually have high cholesterol.

NUTS

Nuts are permitted on the diet as a basic snack, including nut butters, if they are without simple sugars like glucose. So are soy flour and textured soy products permitted. The type of nuts that need to be emphasized, however, are high in polyunsaturated oils and low in saturated fats. These include English walnuts, almonds, pecans, and sunflower seeds, while nuts that are high in saturated fats, such as macadamia and cashews may be less healthful, except in the case of a weight-gain diet.

DAIRY PRODUCTS

For most people, dairy products are permitted, particularly milk, except in the case of lactose-intolerant individuals or individuals on a low-estrogen diet. Cheeses can be permitted, with less of the aged, salty cheeses, and more of the fresh cheeses, such as cottage cheese, ricotta, farmer cheese, etc. being emphasized. Avoid diet cheeses, cheese spreads, or cheese foods such as Velveeta, because they are generally high in carbohydrates or have additives. Cream and butter should be used at a complete minimum, since they promote cancer and heart disease. Nondairy lighteners or creamers are completely forbidden, due to the high saturated oil and toxic aluminum content.

When using oils and fats, most individuals should emphasize either polyunsaturated oils (sunflower, safflower) or monosaturated fat (olive oil). Polyunsaturated oil content is highest in safflower, then sunflower, walnut, soybean, and sesame. These oils are especially good for individuals with heart disease and hypertension. Yet, olive oil is better for cholesterol lowering. Linseed oil may also serve this same purpose. Mayonnaise is usually not a saturated fat, and is to be avoided. Fried oils as well as hydrogenated oils are all dangerous fats.

CARBOHYDRATES: VEGETABLES

Complex carbohydrates are the goal. All vegetables steamed and cooked can be taken freely. Generally, there should be less use of starchy vegetables (see Obesity Diet, p. 144), which increase weight gain, and may increase craving for sweets. These include peas, corn, carrots, beets, etc.

CARBOHYDRATES: GRAINS

Grains should be emphasized. Fiber is an extremely important component of grains, because it lowers cholesterol which reduces heart disease as well as the risk of a variety of cancers (speeds elimination of toxins), and treats irritable bowel syndrome and constipation. All grains are allowed as whole-grains or cereals. White flour, white rice, white bread, or other refined carbohydrates must be avoided. Whole grain breads, crackers, and sourdough bread are made with yeast, and they are allowed depending on the person's diet. (Matzoh and pasta are examples of no-yeast products.) Spinach pasta may substitute for a white pasta.

Some vegetables and grains with high carbohydrate content include brown rice, kasha, oats, corn, cracked wheat, millet, peas, lentil beans, parsnips, and acorn squash. These are acceptable if you are not trying to lose weight.

FRUIT

Fruit is excellent under most conditions, because its high water content is good for the skin, and it has many valuable nutrients. Excessive fruit juice-drinking can lead to sugar cravings and mood instability. Fruit is valuable, particularly in the case of bananas and apples, for lowering cholesterol, or in the case of other high-potassium fruits, which are important in heart arrhythmia, stroke prevention, or in bowel regularity.

OTHER CATEGORIES

Lemon, lime, vegetable juice, and olives are allowed, although olives need to be removed on the low salt diet, and avocados may need to be eliminated on the low fat diet.

SPICES

Seasonings are generally healthy. There is a particularly useful benefit to onion, garlic, and ginger, which make cells called platelets stick less easily; their properties reduce the risk of blood clots, stroke, heart attack, etc. Other seasonings, such as pepper, thyme, and cumin have a lot of trace nutrients, which are healthy.

Unfortunately, most condiments, such as catsup and mustards must be watched carefully, since they frequently have quite a bit of added sugar, salt, and non-nutritious contents. Avoid clear broth and consommes, unless not on salt restricted diets.

DESSERTS AND SWEETENERS

Desserts are not on the general diet, because they are filled with sweets which raise cholesterol, weight, and cause tooth decay. Therefore, the individuals need to be weaned off such desserts. They can use instead noncarbohydrate sweeteners, such as Aspartame (Equal, Nutrasweet), which is simply a combination of two amino acids. Saccharine and cyclamates, which are available in Canada and Europe, are not recommended, because they have been linked to cancer in epidemiological studies.

SUGAR

Sugars, or hexitols called sorbitol, honey, fructose, lactose, maltose (which is in barley malt), and dextrose (which is corn sugar), and other simple sugars are generally not healthful. Of these, fructose would probably be the best, since it produces the lowest glycemic index change (see Diabetes, Section 8, pp. 79).

BEVERAGES

Vegetable juices are extremely good, but all caffeinated beverages are to be avoided, since high caffeine ingestion has been associated with hypertension, high cholesterol, and heart disease. Even one cup a day of caffeine has been associated with ovarian cancer, pancreatic cancer, breast cysts, and other cancer-like problems.

Because they have less heart disease and cancer risk, decaffeinated beverages are allowed. But such beverages may contribute more to ulcers. Diet sodas, caffeine-free, are allowed, although not for a prolonged periods of time, because they are filled with chemicals that may be carcinogenic.

Herbal teas are allowed, but we need to get a better understanding of their content. There is certainly a variety of medicinal values to herbal teas which can be used to enhance our diet and our health (e.g., possibly fenugreek to eliminate mucus, chamomile to lessen anxiety). After all, the great drug digoxin was isolated from foxglove herbal tea!

Spring and mineral waters are preferred to tap water, because tap water is filled with copper (from plumbing) in most cities or iron or polluted hydrocarbons from the ground. Spring and mineral waters generally have a higher trace element content of some rare but some essential trace nutrients (e.g., lithium, molybdenum).

Alcohol is not generally emphasized on the diet, except up to one or two drinks per day (1 oz. of alcohol of any kind), which, according to some studies, may reduce the incidence of heart disease and raise the HDLs, the good form of the cholesterol complexes. If a person is trying to lose weight, alcohol would not be permitted.

QUANTITIES AND FREQUENCY

The general rule is to eat slightly less than you desire, or to leave the table slightly hungry, for your appetite will diminish in a few minutes. Frequent small snacks are generally not advised, except in the case of hypoglycemics or individuals who tend to have symptoms (anxiety) without eating frequently.

A sizable breakfast is important, particularly with protein in the breakfast when energy levels frequently fall before lunch. Protein includes primarily eggs, fish, meat, and cheese. Those who wish to lose weight will have to restrict carbohydrates, which will be discussed in other diets.

EXERCISE

Exercise is an important part of every health plan (exceptions include strenuous activity), and it is better to exercise before eating. Aerobic exercise, particularly swimming, may have some benefit in heart conditioning. Limbering and stretching exercises for everyone, especially arthritis sufferers, are important.

Types of Diets

ACNE ROSACEA DIET (middle-aged acne around the nose)

No hot drinks, spiced foods, alcohol, caffeine, sugar, or white flour! Follow the Well Being diet if appropriate.

ADRENOLEUKODYSTROPHY DIET

This genetic, neurologic disorder can be marked by increased motor, cognitive, and affective disturbances. Restriction of very long chain fatty acids (VLFA), particularly hexcosonoic (26:0), and administering glyceryl trioleate oil may also be helpful.

ANTI-AGGRESSION DIET

This diet, in particular, looks for sources of poisoning by heavy metals that could be in the blood. It also looks for foods that contain uric acid. The use of tryptophan, B-6, zinc, and potassium in the diet is beneficial. Basically, the Anti-Aggression Diet is a combination of the gout, B-6, zinc, and tryptophan diets.

ALLERGY OR LOW HISTAMINE DIET

Allergy diets emphasize foods high in vitamin C, quercetin (citrus), calcium (osteoporosis), and methionine (sulfur) and elimination of a diet high in histamines. Foods high in histamines are wines, alcoholic beverages, artificial sweeteners, ice cream, sweets, commercially available desserts, colored toothpaste, colored cosmetics. Processed foods tend to be higher in histamine content and need to be eliminated.

To reduce allergy, some patients may find it beneficial to reduce or entirely eliminate additives and high histamine foods. (See Allergic Disorders, p. 1, and Allergy: Low Histamine Diet, p. 132.)

ANXIETY DIET

The antianxiety diet requires the elimination of all foods that affect the sympathetic nervous system such as caffeine, sugar, and MSG. These particular foods can produce anxiety-like reactions. Certain nutrients, like tyrosine and phenylalanine, can worsen anxiety, while foods that have a high amount of niacin, tryptophan, or inositol, can reduce anxiety. Excess sugar, alcohol, or carbohydrates frequently promote anxiety. Alcoholism, sugarholism, and carbohydratism., e.g., addiction to carbohydrates, sugar or alcohol, increase the need for protein in diets. This can be accomplished by following the Basic Diet with a reduction of stimulants. (See Basic Health and Diet Rules, p. 89.)

ARTHRITIS DIET

See Osteoarthritis Diet, p. 144.

APPENDICITIS DIET

Diets high in vegetables protect against appendicitis. Diets high in sugar, potatoes, and fruit have caused appendicitis, and they also cause gastrointestinal and respiratory infections.

BEAUTY DIET

The Beauty Diet is mostly the Basic Health and Diet Rules, p. 89, with an emphasis on vegetables, liver and fruit. The reason for the emphasis on liver is that it contains a lot of iron and copper which can lead to a nice glow in hair and skin. The reason for the emphasis on vegetables is, of course, the large amount of vitamin A. Vitamin A keeps the skin clear and beautiful. The emphasis on fruit is for vitamin C for collagen buildup but also the high water content. The more you drink fluids, the better your skin looks.

Fluids may cleanse the skin. Other factors that are important to beauty are: the use of tofu which is a nice lean protein to prevent you from gaining too much weight. Fish products may help your hair shine due to fish oils (Omega-3). Whole grains are beneficial in that they are loaded with B complex. Spinach contains a form of vitamin A and vitamin C, and legumes which are loaded with trace elements are to be emphasized. Turkey which has a good content of potassium and tryptophan, may be thought of as a beauty protein.

BEZOARS DIET

The Bezoars Diet is basically a low-fiber diet, one that is not very restrictive but eliminates those foods most likely to cause bezoars. These foods include citrus fruits and pulpy fruits such as pears and persimmons. For recurrent bezoars, a modified low-fiber diet can be used, eliminating many fresh fruits and vegetables with moderate (>2 g per serving) fiber content.

BILIARY ATRESIA DIET

This diet counters a condition marked by low zinc levels; possibly an increase in the amount of zinc foods to your diet will be helpful.

BODY BUILDER'S DIET

The body builder's diet emphasizes foods which increase growth hormone stimulation. High protein foods are best, especially those high in the branch chain amino acids (BCAA) which are in very high proportion in muscle. BCAA help substitute as fuel for the body giving the liver a bit of rest, as the liver breaks down glycogen and fuels your workout needs. Hence, it is the branch chain amino acids that you need more of. BCAA need to be supplemented or increased in total content. The fascinating thing about amino acids is that the more you take of them, the more other amino acids can elevate. Another way to continue to body build is basically to go on an amino acid diet -- i.e., a high protein, low complex carbohydrate diet.

You do need complex carbohydrates though; otherwise, you will not have any short term fuel with which to body build. Tyrosine, phenylalanine and methionine may also help body build because they raise branch chain amino acids in the blood indirectly. Concentrate on the branch chain amino acids in your diet in between workouts. Complex carbohydrates are good prior to exercise. Prior to a big event an individual should increase his/her branch chain amino acids by following a ketogenic diet for a week, then switch for a few days to complex carbohydrates only.

BREAKING BAD HABITS DIET

There are seven major barriers to successful dieting. Since dieting's essential to every disease and to general health, these barriers must be overcome by all of us for optimal health.

1. Emotional eating; that is eating when you're bored, angry, sad, or happy.

2. Freedom eating; eating because someone says you shouldn't.

3. Friendship eating; eating food you're offered so you will not insult somebody.

4. Social eating; overeating at parties and restaurants.

5. Binge eating; where one bite leads to another and another and another.

6. Poor self image; when eating makes you look as bad as you feel.

7. Spiritual hollowness; eating to fill yourself up physically, but you are spiritually empty. (See the spiritual distress section of the *PATH Wellness Manual* to cope with these problems.)

Your diet must be oriented toward spiritual revival or you will be doomed to failure.

BUERGERS DISEASE DIET

Stop smoking. Use the Thrombosis Diet (which refers to Embolus Diet, p. 137) and emphasize a diet rich in fish, fish oil, garlic, niacin, and primrose oil. Use lots of polyunsaturated oils, especially safflower oil. If you suffer from obesity, use a low carbohydrate and low fat diet. (See High Protein, Low Carbohydrate, High Fiber Diet, pp. 102.) Don't forget -- lots of aerobic exercise!

(CHRONIC) BRONCHITIS DIET

This is a modified form of the Allergy Diet (see Allergy or Low Histamine Diet, p. 132). Increase sulfur foods and use N-acetyl-cysteine supplements. Diets high in vitamin C, garlic, magnesium, zinc, and B-6 may also be helpful.

(ANTI)CANCER & NUTRIENTS DIET

Cancer accounts for 10-25% of our national health costs. The cause of cancer and forms of cancer are multiple. All people are at risk because of the prevalence of various carcinogens, e.g., nitrates, hydrogenated oils, cigarette smoke, alcohol, radiation, saturated fat, caffeine, Valium, estrogens (hormones), aflatoxins (peanuts), potatoes, mustards, black pepper, shellfish, food additives, air pollutants, radon, water pollutants, etc.

Data are overwhelmingly in favor of the benefits of diet and vitamins in cancer prevention. Not surprisingly, obesity and immune deficiency are risks for cancer. Evidence suggests that various nutrients can inhibit growth of tumors in man and experimental animals, that a deficiency of these nutrients is a risk factor, that higher levels of these nutrients in blood is protective against cancer, and that the nutrients can be used to treat cancer. The nutrients that have been shown to be especially protective are vitamins A, C, E, beta carotene and selenium. These nutrients are found in pigmented vegetables (green, yellow or orange), vegetable oils, eggs, whole grains and cereals, fruits and vegetables, seafood, liver, and meat (vitamin E and selenium). Fruits and vegetables contain a lot of vitamin C. Hence, a high vegetable, high whole grain diet with some fish is the general anticancer diet. Each cancer patient may need a unique diet, e.g., sarcoma patients may need a high protein diet. Vegetables, because of the anticancer properties of fiber, beta carotene, plant sterols, and dithiolthiones (broccoli, Brussels sprouts, cabbage, cauliflower) are usually the most important part of the diet. Whole grains, because of the fiber, are the next most important food group.

Many other nutrients may have a role in cancer, particularly cysteine. Furthermore, some nutrients, especially cysteine, vitamin C, and selenium, can reduce the risk of chemotherapy's side-effects. N-acetyl-cysteine, rather than glutathione, is probably the best form and can be used up to 7 grams in cancer prevention. Several other nutrients may have a role in cancer prevention and treatment, e.g., calcium (for colon cancer), arginine, folic acid, vitamin B-12, primrose oil, bioflavonoids, riboflavin, vitamin B-6, zinc, manganese, and molybdenum. These nutrients are prevalent in whole grains and the macrobiotic diet.

It is important to increase consumption of garlic and onion and to decrease eggs, fried foods, olive oil, sugar, hydrogenated oils, pickled and cured foods.

CARDIOMYOPATHY DIET

Avoid all alcohol and increase B-complex vitamins.

CARDIOVASCULAR DIET

The Cardiovascular Diet is basically the Cholesterol-Lowering Diet (see below, this page). Soy and fish are very good sources of protein in these diets.

CARPAL TUNNEL DIET

Many studies suggest foods high in vitamin B-6 may help this condition. (Studies used 50-200 mg a day, usually not available in food.)

CATARACT DIET

Follow a low sugar diet, and it is especially important to follow the Basic Health and Diet Rules, p. 89. Supplements including vitamins C and E are needed.

CHOLESTEROL-LOWERING DIET

To lower cholesterol, emphasize lots of fish, vegetables, fruit, and whole grains. Avoid all sugar and saturated fat as well as excessive amounts of foods which lower thyroid functions, e.g., cabbage, cauliflower, Brussels sprouts, and broccoli. Emphasize olive oil, lecithin (only highly purified forms), primrose oil, fish oil, and safflower oil (very high in omega-6), all of which can lower cholesterol. Emphasize vegetables to a very high degree, and in some cases, no meat, chicken, nor turkey is necessary. Amino acids which can help lower cholesterol may include arginine, methionine, and taurine. Beware of hydrogenated oils as well.

CIRRHOSIS DIET

Eat a low protein diet with supplemental branched chain amino acids as well as lots of fruits, vegetables, fiber, and magnesium foods. (Magnesium will keep the bowel movements soft but formed, not loose or liquid). Emphasize high zinc and niacin foods. Take extensive multivitamin but be careful of too many fat-soluble vitamins.

CLAUDICATION DIET

See Embolus Diet, p. 137. Eat enough fish until you grow gills, and eat garlic until everyone runs for cover! Take supplemental niacin, fish oils, garlic, and vitamin E at mega dosages under medical supervision. Lots of exercise to tolerance level.

COLD AND CITRUS DIET

Drink large quantities of diluted lemon or lime juice. Pink grapefruits and oranges should be used until slightly loose bowels occur. Extra vitamin C and zinc lozenges can also be helpful. Use decongestants if necessary.

COLITIS DIET

In the colitis diet, one especially needs to avoid nuts, seeds, corn, and peas. Furthermore, one should increase the foods which are high in antioxidants -- for example, sulfa foods such as eggs, vegetables, and whole grains. Reducing the amount of meat intake is recommended. Bran, in particular, is very important. High protein diets, with the removal of fruit, usually quickly eliminate the frequency of bowel movements.

CONSTIPATION DIET

Bowel motility is easy to control by diet and nutrients. Those who have constipation or diarrhea need more bulk or bran in their diet (either pure bran or whole grains). Those who have a serious constipation problem need to ingest a high magnesium and high Vitamin C diet. It means using a lot of fruit (citrus and dried fruits), roughage, vegetables, bran, and fluids. You may drink up to eight glasses of water a day. Don't underestimate grandma's favorite prune juice, an osmotic catharsis. Acidophilus foods, e.g., buttermilk and yogurt, can also help constipation.

CRAVINGS DIET

Eating foods abundant with spices may reduce cravings for salt, sugar, fat, etc. Spices contain known trace elements and probably some unknown elements as well. High protein may also reduce cravings for carbohydrates.

CROHN'S DISEASE DIET

Crohn's disease is a disease characterized by inflammation of the small intestine. It's often marked by potassium, magnesium, zinc, vitamin A, and thiamine, deficiency. Eat foods that are high in these nutrients. Crohn's disease patients need to eliminate saturated fat and refined carbohydrates from their diet. Both these categories of nutrients can increase the frequency of bowel movements. Crohn's disease patients also need more fat soluble vitamins, particularly vitamin A. They should try to increase, if possible, the amount of vegetables ingested -- both uncooked and those cooked in polyunsaturated vegetable oils. Calcium in high doses contributes to constipation in Crohn's patients. Nuts, corn, peas, seeds, and large amounts of fruit must be avoided.

CYSTITIS DIET

Drinking plenty of water is of the utmost importance. Fruit is a food high in water content. Hence, the cystitis diet requires an extremely high fruit content as well as the drinking of large quantities of water. There is great debate as to whether or not the acidic foods, e.g., vitamin C or cranberry juice, will lessen your symptoms. Tomato juice, cranberry juice, lemon juice, and orange juice may be helpful in cystitis. But increase the fruit content in the Basic Health and Diet Rules, p. 89, possibly as many as five fruits a day, and drink water.

DEPRESSION DIET

During depression, individuals often retain water and are under more stress; their neurotransmitters, which are made up of amino acids, become depleted. Hence, the Depression Diet generally emphasizes the Basic Health and Diet Rules, (see p. 89), but with higher protein, since these are the sources of the neurotransmitters. See table below. Avoid constipation during depression. (See Depression Diet -- The Mood Foods, p. 111.)

Amino Acids as Precursors of Neurotransmitters	
Amino Acid	**Neurotransmitter (s)**
Cysteine	Cysteic Acid
Glutamine	GABA, Glutamic Acid
Histidine	Histamine
Lysine	Pipecolic Acid
Phenylalanine	Phenylethylamine plus same as Tyrosine
Tyrosine	Dopamine, Norepinephrine, Tyramine
Tryptophan	Serotonin, Melatonin, Tryptamines

Amino Acids as Neurotransmitters	
Amino Acid	**Function**
Alanine	inhibitory or calming
GABA	inhibitory or calming
Glycine	inhibitory or calming
Taurine	inhibitory or calming
Glutamic Acid	excitatory
Aspartic Acid	excitatory

For those who have a sad (i.e., monopolar) depression, foods emphasizing tyrosine, phenylalanine, and methionine in the diet may be helpful. Treatment with tyrosine, phenylalanine, and methionine may be necessary.

For those who have a bipolar depression, and/or suicidal tendencies, foods emphasizing tryptophan, niacin, and possibly vanadium, molybdenum, lithium, and vitamin B-6 are the most beneficial. For example, high tryptophan sources include a cup of low-fat cottage cheese (300 mg), a pound of chicken or turkey (600 mg), and wheat germ (400 mg per cup). The metabolism of tryptophan also requires intake of a significant amount of vitamin B-6. (See Sleep Diet, below.)

DIABETIC DIET

There is great debate about which diet is the best for diabetes. Some say the basic diet should emphasize more protein; others say, more complex carbohydrates. It is certainly clear that it depends on the patient's diabetes. There are some patients whose insulin requirements go down as their intake of carbohydrates go down, while others need more fiber to reduce their insulin requirements. Therefore, you may not benefit as much from the high protein diet. Another approach is to eliminate foods that have a high glycemic index, that is, foods that raise blood sugar as much as glucose does. (See Glycemic Index of Foods, p. 80.) Certain foods that you might not think raise blood sugar do; e.g., corn flakes raise blood sugar 80% of what glucose does, parsnips and carrots 90%, instant mashed potatoes 80%, white potatoes 70%, beets 60%, honey 87%, and Mars bars 68%. All simple sugar must be eliminated from a diabetic diet and all refined carbohydrates as well. After that, it's trial and error to see whether or not a high fiber diet and/or a high protein diet is the best for each diabetic. Adult onset diabetics generally do better with a high protein, low carbohydrate diet with grain and fiber supplements. Juvenile diabetics should be started on the Basic Health and Diet Rules (see p. 89).

DIARRHEA DIET

Eat lots of whole grains and cheese and take calcium supplements. Avoid vitamin C, magnesium, and fruit.

Those who have diarrhea need a high calcium diet. Calcium has natural binding qualities. Foods high in pectin may help treat diarrhea. Hence, bananas and apples may help some individuals. Niacin, niacinamide, B-complex, and potassium are needed in surplus with diarrhea. Also follow the Colitis Diet, p. 116, to appropriate degree to reduce stool frequency.

DIVERTICULOSIS DIET

An avoidance of seeds, nuts and corn is critical, but coupling such avoidance with a high intake of grains is equally critical. Also, reduce your fruit. Increased use of garlic and foods high in antioxidants is good.

EDEMA DIET

Use special, low carbohydrate, ketogenic Obesity Diet, below. If you have heart risk, use low fat, low carbohydrate diet and discuss potassium supplements with your doctor. Parsley is a good low carbohydrate, high fiber source of potassium.

EMBOLUS DIET

Becoming a vegetarian might be helpful. Eat fish twice a day as well as lots of garlic, onion, ginger, fish oil, and primrose oil. Use lots of polyunsaturated oils with mega dosages of fish oil, garlic, and vitamin E under medical supervision.

EPILEPSY DIET

Use the ketogenic Obesity Diet, below, and keep in mind that the true ketogenic diet for epilepsy is used only for children for intractable seizures. In adults this may also be used. These ketogenic diets, unlike high protein diets, derive 75% of calories from fat and only 25% from protein or carbohydrates. This has been shown to be useful in childhood seizures of various types. Its use in adults may be of value. Avoid foods that are high in folic acids and eat foods that are high in manganese, vitamin B-6, vitamin E, magnesium, and taurine.

ETHNICITY DIET

Most of the health problems that are associated with ethnic groups require that they eat the complete opposite of the ethnic group they grew up in. For instance, the high degree of rheumatoid arthritis among the Irish should force them away from their typical high nightshade diet to low nightshade diet. The Italians, who frequently have a weight problem, need to go far away from a diet high in pasta to a diet low in carbohydrates. Jews, who have a diet usually high in salt and fat, need to go more towards a vegetarian type diet. Whatever your ethnic background is, whatever diet you've grown up on, go opposite to the excesses of that diet and you'll usually find greater health.

FAST-EATING DIET

Many people are fast food addicts, because they're always trying to eat fast. Unfortunately, most fast food in our culture is high in salt, sugar, refined flour, and saturated fat. It's probably some of the most unhealthy food that anyone could ever eat. The way in which we can eat a fast food diet without getting sick is to eat just two health foods per meal in high quantity. Therefore, for breakfast have soft-boiled eggs and milk, for lunch have tuna fish and lettuce, for dinner have sardines and celery. This is a quick way to eat for yourself if time is really a factor. Even though this may be a boring way to eat it certainly is the fastest way to eat for a bachelor or medical intern! It is preferable to eat limited types of food than to be a fast food addict, which will do nothing but raise your blood pressure and cholesterol, promote cancer, and may eventually kill you! Two food groups per meal is also an excellent allergy diet.

(LOW) FAT DIET

The Low Fat Diet is basic to anti-cancer, anti-heart disease diets because saturated fat raises cholesterol levels and promotes cancer growth. Elimination of all high-fat foods is often necessary. Elimination of whole milk or condensed milk, bacon, bologna, frankfurters, sausage, creamy or high fat cheeses, ice cream, sugar, and hot-fudge sundaes (as well as all refined sugar) is necessary. Elimination of ground beef, pork and spareribs, as well as ground pork, sour cream, cream, fried eggs, and liver may also be necessary. The Low Fat Diet substitutes skim milk, buttermilk, chicken, turkey, cucumbers, zucchini, and lettuce, a high-vegetable diet with low-fat yogurt and polyunsaturated or monounsaturated oils (olive oil, linoleic acid and sunflower oil). Vinegar, lemon juice, poached or baked eggs, lean meat, chicken, and fish are acceptable. The Low Fat Diet is an essential model for most healthy diets today. (See Section 9, Trimming the Fat, p. 95.)

FLATULENCE OR GAS DIET

Flatulence can be produced by different types of foods: excessive fruit (particularly dried fruit), beans (due to the high amounts of nitrogen which can be converted into gas), high lactose foods (particularly milk or aged cheeses), and junk foods (white flour because of the lack of nutrients and fiber as well as an excess of yeast).

Various medical conditions can also lead to gas, e.g., diverticulosis, colon disease, or aging with a weak colon. Also, some nutrients, etc., can also lead to gas formation: cysteine, methionine, garlic, taurine, magnesium, vitamin C, excess calcium carbonate, or Tums. Eating too quickly (swallowing air) also promotes gas formation.

Treatment for flatulence or gas can be the elimination of harmful foods that cause the condition as well as dealing with the underlying ailment itself. Simethicone and charcoal are natural "gas" relievers that are available in many forms, e.g., Mylicon 80. Tums or if need be Zantac or Tagamet can be prescribed antacids. Librax, an antianxiety medication, can also aid in the treatment of gas. Bland diets, in which acid and spicy foods are eliminated, may also be helpful.

FOOD ALLERGY DIET

Choice of Elimination or Rotation Diets. See Allergy and Fast Eating Diets, pp. 132 and 138, respectively.

FUTURE DIET

Diets of the future most likely will include ways of avoiding eating all together. Hence, we will no longer have to kill plants or animals to live. We will synthesize carbohydrates, amino acids, and essential fats. Ways in which we can be fed either intravenously or by manufactured food are already developing. Diets of the future will be something like total parental nutrition where all the trace elements, amino acids, essential oils, and vitamins will be included in three oral feedings per day. We hope it doesn't disappoint you that the future holds the end of taste. We will all become less destructive in terms of our own daily lives with the end of eating. As we stop destroying the land, plants, and animals, we will stop destroying each other. Hence, the future diets are peace diets.

GALL BLADDER DIET

Gallstones are a common occurrence in fat, feminine and fertile 40-year-old women with a predisposition to high estrogens. A low estrogen diet is essential. Hence, dairy and meat products should be reduced since beef cattle frequently receive estrogen injections. Estrogen supplements must be avoided. Patients who have gall bladder risk must reduce their fat intake and lose weight. A low cholesterol diet, high in olive oil, may also help to reduce the size of the gallstones (See Cholesterol-Lowering Diet, p. 134.) A diet high in vegetables probably reduces gall bladder disease. Taurine, methionine, and glycine may reduce cholestasis in some patients. A diet high in these amino acids may be helpful.

GASTROINTESTINAL ALLERGY

This is a condition of malabsorption, protein-wasting enteropathy. Stopping milk, wheat, cheese, and nuts in children may be necessary. Meat and fish may be the problem in adults. Use lots of foods containing calcium. Eat a low fat diet. (See Low Fat Diet, p. 138, Trimming the Fat, p. 95, and Fats in the Subject Index.)

GOUT DIET

Gout is a disease in which uric acid, a breakdown product of DNA, builds up in the blood and tissues, causing acute inflammatory joint pain particularly in the big toes. Arthritis sometimes occurs with deposits of uric acid crystals, often called Tophi. Chronic gout patients and possibly all high uric acid patients frequently have a risk for kidney stones and an increased incidence of heart disease. About 20% of elderly patients may progress to gout when they have elevated uric acid levels. Hence, a low purine diet with less red meat is the first approach. High purine foods, such as anchovies, asparagus, brains, kidney, liver, meat extracts, mincemeat, mushrooms, sardines, sweetbreads, all red wines, and possibly all alcohol, must be eliminated. Nicotinic acid (niacin) and tartaric acid, found in red wines, may increase the gout attacks. A diet that is low in niacin is recommended. Diets high in vitamin C foods reduce uric acid. Bicarbonate also may reduce uric acid. There are of course various drugs that can treat elevated uric acid such as: allopurinol, probenecid, and aspirin. Immediate gout attacks may be treated with nonsteroidal drugs or colchicine.

HAIR DIET

Hair quality can be a sign of overall health, although most male pattern baldness is due to hormone imbalances. Hair loss is frequently associated with autoimmune diseases such as hyperthyroidism, pernicious anemia, exfoliative dermatitis, as well as radiation exposure, and chemotherapy. Large doses of zinc, cysteine, and possibly arginine may be useful. Hence, foods high in cysteine, zinc, and arginine are recommended. Topical Vitamin A drugs have been used in some cases to help promote hair growth. A high vegetable diet, high in vitamin A and beta carotene, is recommended.

Hair loss can be exacerbated by dry scalp and dandruff. Avoidance of high fat diet, sugar, caffeine, and shellfish usually stop most dandruff while liberal use of polyunsaturated oils and monosaturated oils tend to prevent the drying of the scalp.

HEADACHE (LOW TYRAMINE) DIET

Frequently, sinus and migraine headaches are due to a chemical called tyramine in a diet. Headaches which are above the eyes, or one-sided cluster headaches (which occur on the eye and one side of the face), or migraine headaches, which are usually proceeded by an aura or lights, and/or nausea, often respond to the low tyramine diet.

Foods high in tyramine are basically all cheeses (especially aged cheeses) except the fresh cheeses, cottage cheese, cream cheese, ricotta cheese, farmer cheese, and tofu. Very ripe bananas need to be avoided, as well as all beer, ales, and wine, especially Chianti, which contain a lot of tyramine. Broad beans, pods, lima beans, Italian broad beans, lentils, and snow peas also contain tyramine, as does liver. All chocolate should be excluded from the diet, as well as all cultured dairy products, such as buttermilk, yogurt, and sour cream. All figs, especially canned ones, nitrates, and any food with this preservative should be avoided. All nuts contain tyramine and should be eliminated. All pickled herring and salted, dried fish should be avoided. Pineapple and any food product which contains pineapple, pork in all forms, bacon, ham, etc., prunes, raisins, soy sauce, any food sauce with wine, vanilla extracts, yeast extracts, and MSG produce headaches and should be avoided.

These foods with tyramine also need to be excluded in some individuals with hypertension, or patients who are on the antidepressant drugs called MAO monoamine-oxidase inhibitors, since they can cause hypertension crisis in individuals taking these drugs.

The low tyramine diet is extremely effective in reducing headaches in many individuals. Also excluded is the use of all caffeine beverages. Smoking also must be stopped for it is a big factor in headache production. Many headaches are psychological in origin. (See also Low Tyramine Diet #1, p. 139.)

HEART ARRHYTHMIA DIET

The Heart Arrhythmia Diet is the Basic Health and Diet Rules (see p. 89), but high in sources of potassium and magnesium which prevent various arrhythmias. A high fruit, high potassium diet is important. Peaches, raisins, dates, apricots, figs, prune juice, watermelon, and bananas are extremely high in potassium, as well as orange juice and cantaloupe. Dried fruit is loaded with sugar and should be used less. Beef has its share of potassium as well as does milk.

Also, foods high in magnesium are needed in this diet. Preventricular contractions and paroxysmal atrial tachycardia can respond to magnesium and potassium therapy, and there are certainly a number of arrhythmias that can respond to this diet. Elimination of caffeinated beverages (the biggest culprit), alcohol, sugar, etc., is also necessary. An evaluation of heart size and other heart tests are essential. Lower blood pressure may reduce arrhythmia. (See Hypertension Diet below; also Program for Hypertension and Hypertension Diet, pp. 114.)

HEART ATTACKS -- DIET TO PREVENT

Diets used to prevent heart attacks emphasize fish and vegetables. Vegetarians tend to have fewer heart attacks and heart disease than meat eaters. I believe fish-eating vegetarians will have even better success. Rural people have less heart disease than urban dwellers because hard water is better than soft city water (metals from plumbing, e.g., copper pipes). Several other nutrients are important to emphasize in the heart prevention diet. Large amounts of polyunsaturated oils, e.g., linoleic acid, linseed oil, and safflower oil, are important. Olive oil, which lowers cholesterol and raises HDL, is also good. Liberal use of foods high in fiber keep cholesterol down. High pectin fruits such as apples and bananas lower cholesterol. Various nutrients may help prevent heart attacks, such as EPA, niacin, magnesium, antioxidants, vitamin B-6, chromium, and selenium, all of which can be found deficient in some patients who have had heart attacks.

HEMORRHOID DIET

Keep bowels loose with fruit, vegetables, water, and high magnesium foods. Keep on low calcium diet if response is still not adequate.

HEPATITIS DIET

See Cirrhosis Diet, p. 135.

HERPES DIET

See Herpes Diet, p. 115.

HIVES DIET

No nuts, refined carbohydrates, shellfish, chocolate, fruit, or food additives. Citrus can oftentimes be the culprit.

HYPERTENSION OR HIGH BLOOD PRESSURE DIET

Diet and nutritional treatment of high blood pressure is very successful. Traditional treatments have side effects, e.g., diuretics can raise cholesterol and the chance of sudden death. Beta blockers can increase depression, promote heart attacks, and decrease sexual function. Hypertensive patients benefit from a low carbohydrate diet, weight loss, limited use of sodium, and a reduction in the amount of fried foods. Hypertensive patients frequently have decreases in plasma sulfur amino acids. We treat hypertensive patients with taurine (up to 3 grams) and occasionally cysteine and methionine. Studies in Japan have shown that taurine alone can lower blood pressure.

Hypertensive patients usually have arteriosclerosis, which can be partially reversed by a diet high in polyunsaturated oils (safflower or sunflower), because they have a diuretic effect and can lower blood pressure. All saturated fat must be eliminated from the diet (e.g., butter, fried food, mayonnaise, animal meats, nuts, and high fat cheeses).

Large doses of mega-EPA, a fish oil (4-15 grams per day), have an anti-clotting function, reduce the risk of stroke and lower blood pressure. Eat an abundance of fish, i.e., eat until you sprout gills is the proper approach! Evening primrose oil is also useful as a diuretic and lowers blood pressure. Vitamin B-6 (500-1000 mg) is a mild diuretic and may potentiate the effect of primrose oil and the sulfur amino acids. Avoid all refined carbohydrates. Fruit is good if weight loss (ketosis diet) is not needed.

Magnesium is also useful in the treatment of hypertension, especially in pregnant women, because drugs are too dangerous for the fetus. Although magnesium is difficult to supplement, chelated magnesium (500-1000 mg) or magnesium oxide or carbonate are the best forms of supplementation. Calcium may also have a role, particularly for hypertensive women. High potassium is also important in the diet of patients (as light salt or fruit). Herbs (ginger, garlic, and onion) lower blood pressure as well as provide valuable anti-clotting functions. All caffeine and alcohol must be avoided. (See Hypertension Diet and Program for Hypertension, p. 114.)

HYPERTHYROID DIET

Certain vegetables may help lower thyroid activity over prolonged periods of time. These are the goitrogens which include kale, cauliflower, broccoli, and brussels sprouts. The trace element, lithium, also has antithyroid effects but is not very abundant in food. Eat a diet low in iodide foods.

HYPOGLYCEMIC DIET

The Hypoglycemic Diet is the Basic Health and Diet Rules (see p. 89) with more emphasis on protein, particularly fish, since fish is the healthiest of the protein sources. Frequent meals, maybe as many as six meals a day of protein foods may be necessary to control hypoglycemic symptoms. Nutrient supplementation is also necessary.

ICHTHYOSIS DIET

Ichthyosis is a disease of the decreased amount of sweat and oil in the skin. Increase vegetables and use of safflower oil. Eat foods high in vitamin A and EPA. Consider taking retinoic acid (Accutane) under the supervision of a dermatologist.

IMMUNE-BUILDING/ANTI-INFECTION DIET

It is extremely important to build the immune system. All diseases attack the defenses of the immune system, particularly AIDS, herpes, and general infections. The immune system's failure is also implicated in causing cancer, and its hyperactivity is implicated in diseases such as arthritis, myasthenia gravis, lupus, and other so-called autoimmune diseases.

Those who have deficient immune systems, particularly patients who suffer from vital illnesses, and cancer, need to follow the Basic Diet. (See Basic Health and Diet Rules, p. 89.) Increase in zinc and vitamin A foods is especially important. Selenium and other nutrients have important roles as well.

To increase the intake of vitamin A, one should especially increase vegetables with beta carotene, e.g., green, yellow, and orange vegetables such as carrots, squash, and zucchini. The vitamin A drug, Accutane, may be helpful under a doctor's supervision. Many drugs can boost the immune system, e.g., Tagamet and Trexan, but must be followed under the supervision of an experienced physician.

To increase the amount of zinc in the diet, certain foods such as wheat bran, whole oatmeal, herring, whole oysters, carrots, peas, nuts, and milk can be increased. Zinc supplements may be necessary to build the immune system. Other nutrients that are important to immune system-building are foods high in vitamin C, e.g., citrus fruits.

Branched chain amino acids help heavily-infected (sepsis) and trauma patients survive the stress on the liver. They may also help cancer patients when the liver is involved.

In contrast, foods high in copper and folic acid are important to those who have autoimmune diseases. Foods high in folic acid include foods like spinach and leafy greens.

Foods high in copper are generally the same foods that are high in zinc. Cancer patients need to avoid excess copper and folic acid. Ironically, high doses of folic acid (5-10 mg) may help to prevent early forms of lung cancer.

INFECTION AND HEPATITIS DIET

Diets high in branched chain amino acids give the liver a rest by providing an alternative. Antioxidants, sulfur amino acids, zinc, and vitamin C can help many infections.

(ANTI-)INFLAMMATION DIET

The Anti-Inflammation Diet avoids all nightshade foods which include peppers, tomatoes, white potatoes, eggplant, and paprika. Also avoid all fried foods because they contain the inflammatory intermediate arachidonic acid. For this same reason, monosaturated oil (olive oil or walnut oil) may be better than polyunsaturated oil. Fish oil is especially good. Inflammation may be reduced by copper, antioxidants, fish oil, histidine, and vitamin C. Hence, this diet emphasizes the principles of the Basic Health and Dietary Rules (see p. 89) as well as the foods that contain high quantities of these nutrients.

KELOID DIET

Keloids are hypertrophic, topical scars. Since zinc and vitamin A may be helpful, increase foods that are high in these nutrients.

KIDNEY STONE DIET

The kidneys are located on both sides of the lower back, and they are filled with millions of cells that filter the ocean of life. Kidneys clean out our blood, getting rid of waste products. Each person has an enormous amount of kidney nephrons, which are made up of millions of tubules with filters attached to them. They don't fail until you lose about 98% of the functioning cells; there is a lot of surplus.

The most common causes of kidney malfunction are due to kidney stones (early in life) or renal failure (later in life). Kidney stones form into the shape and texture of rock candy. The stones grow on top of one another on the inside of the kidney. They pass down through the tubule, which is the pain people feel when they have kidney stones; it is like a stone passing through a straw.

Kidney stones are primarily composed of calcium oxalate, which is a chemical found in foods that contain oxalic acid, e.g., spinach, rhubarb, celery, tea, coffee, and nuts. Foods that contain the highest concentration of oxalates (e.g., 25 mg/100 mg) are beans, cocoa, instant coffee, parsley, spinach, rhubarb, and tea. Other frequently eaten foods containing oxalates are beet tops, carrots, celery, chocolate, cucumber, grapefruit, kale, peanuts, peppers, and sweet potatoes. Vitamin B-6 and magnesium deficiencies can also cause oxalate stones. If the stones block the kidneys, they can cause kidney failure or uremia, which fills the body with toxins. When the kidney stones are made of uric acid, they are gout-related stones. This kind of stone is related to stress and a diet rich in asparagus, anchovies, sardines, and mushrooms. Nutrition can prevent the formation of these stones.

Once you have had kidney stones, it is highly probable (about 70%) that they will occur again in the future. Once you're a stone-former, you will usually continue to be a stone-former.

The use of magnesium is an excellent therapy for calcium oxalate-type stones. The tendency to get stones with calcium in them occurs with magnesium deficiency. Magnesium raises the calcium/magnesium ratio, and it keeps calcium soluble in the urine, thus preventing stones. Magnesium (500-1000 mg) as well as vitamin B-6 (100 mg) and/or potassium citrate (75 mg daily) prevent oxalate stones in adults. The use of bran is important in binding calcium. Ten grams of bran (several tablespoons a day) is used to treat people with stones.

Calcium supplementation can reduce other nutrient absorption. Women, who are now taking more and more calcium for osteoporosis, should watch the dosage. 1000 mg is the recommended dosage for a woman who is premenopausal and 1500 mg, postmenopausal. If calcium is taken with magnesium, vitamin B-6, vitamin D, and bran, the risk for stone formation will be reduced.

Low sodium diets and low fat diets also protect against stone formation. A low sugar diet is also essential. Too much magnesium or cysteine can cause magnesium stones. Remember, the first sign of kidney failure can be discovered through a blood test.

LICHEN PLANUS DIET

Eat lots of vegetables and consider including extra beta carotene in your diet. Vitamin A or steroids may help, but should be given under the guidance of a qualified dermatologist.

LIVER FAILURE DIET

See Cirrhosis Diet, p. 135.

MEMORY LOSS DIET

Foods rich in choline may be helpful. This includes eggs, caviar, and other young animal life. Foods rich in antioxidants (grains, vegetables), taurine (eggs), and vitamin B-6 (grains) may also be helpful.

MIGRAINE HEADACHE DIET

See the Headache (Low Tyramine) Diet, p. 139, and consider as well the Allergy Diet, pp. 132.

MOTION SICKNESS AND NAUSEA DIET

Ginger may be useful; try ginger cookies to reduce nausea, or better, ginger capsules or 1/2 teaspoon from a spice can. Foods high in B-6 may also reduce nausea, while foods high in zinc will increase nausea. Antihistamines also help; hence, bioflavonoids, particularly quercetin and vitamin C, may have use since they both have antihistamine qualities. (See Allergy: Low Histamine Diet, p. 132.) Dietary oleic acid may also help.

MULTIPLE SCLEROSIS (MS) DIET

There are several diets proposed for multiple sclerosis patients. The best of these includes a very high content of polyunsaturated oils, particularly safflower oil (high in polyunsaturated linoleic acid). Some patients use as many as four to five tablespoons of safflower or sunflower oil daily to get a large amount of polyunsaturated fats. This is all that's needed in addition to the Basic Health and Diet Rules, p. 89. Dr. Nieper of Germany suggests reducing dairy products, and even stopping them. In addition, he suggests eliminating or reducing shell fish, cereals, red meat, white flour, sugar, caffeine, food additives, hydrogenated fats, fried foods, peanut butter, alcohol, tobacco, and salt. MS patients are encouraged to eat more raw fruit and vegetables than in my Basic Health and Diet Rules. They are encouraged to stay away from tap water, fluoridated tooth pastes, and an excessive number of eggs. A high roughage diet is good.

NEPHROTIC SYNDROME DIET

If kidney failure is not present, then use a high protein, low fat, low carbohydrate diet. Also follow the Cholesterol-Lowering

Diet, p. 134. (See High Protein, Low Carbohydrate Diet, pp. 102.)

OBESITY DIET

There are generally two approaches towards losing weight: the low calorie (starvation) diet or the ketogenic (fat-burning) diet. The ketogenic diet is not a healthful one in the long run, but short run (3 months - 1 year) weight loss on this diet is the fastest.

Ketogenic diets work on the principle of burning fat, which is why one can smell ketones on a dieter's breath. If you eliminate carbohydrate from your diet, your body will burn fat next. Therefore, virtual elimination of carbohydrates is necessary for the ketogenic weight-loss diet, e.g., starchy vegetables, grains, fruits, nuts, and dairy, except cheese. This diet often causes a large water diuresis. (See Obesity in the Subject Index for more references.)

In the case of the low-calorie diet, one should reduce the starchy vegetables and fatty foods. Essentially, follow the Basic Diet and exercise a lot. Beware, if you are a severe underburner with slow metabolism, this diet won't work.

The ketogenic diet needs a lot more nutrients than the low calorie diet because it is a metabolic marathon. The ketogenic diet is best followed under a doctor's supervision. Low calorie diets also need some supplementation of nutrients. The ketogenic diet frequently produces leg cramps, which could lead to heart cramps, even fatalities, if not under the management of a physician. Potassium, calcium, and magnesium supplementation is often necessary.

OSTEOPOROSIS DIET

This includes eating foods that are particularly high in estrogen, calcium, vitamin D, and manganese. This includes lots of dairy products (meat may slightly leach out calcium, vitamin D, magnesium, and manganese) and green vegetables. Boron and lysine may also be necessary nutrients for calcium absorption. High fiber diets reduce the need for calcium.

OTITIS MEDIA EAR INFECTIONS (CHRONIC) DIET

Consider the Allergy: Low Histamine Diet and the Infection Diet, pp. 132 and 142, respectively.

PANCREATIC CANCER DIET

Pancreatic cancer is frequently associated with alcoholism and caffeine. Stop these drugs and get on the *anticancer* diet. Peptides and antiestrogens might also help this problem.

PARKINSON'S DIET

Follow a vegetarian diet for breakfast and lunch. Emphasize fruit to minimize the blocking of L-dopa, tyrosine, and DLPA absorption. Eat foods high in these amino acids as well as those rich in methionine and octacosanol. See Vegetarian Diet, pp. 149. A recent study found 3200 IU/day of vitamin E and 3 g/day of vitamin C helps prevent progression See *Ann Neurol* 32:S128-S132, 1992.

PEACE AND WELL-BEING DIET

The Peace Diet is designed to bring you peace, which consists of spiritual, psychological, and physical health. Physical peace is achieved through the worship of God and is mediated by exercise, good nutrition, and elimination of foreign chemicals and nutrient-poor foods from your diet. High protein is the most fundamental food since protein is broken down into amino acids. Amino acids are the most important building blocks of the entire body, used for the brain's neurotransmitters, heart and skeletal muscle, connective tissue, antibodies, and most cells. The uses and structures of protein are the most sophisticated of all food groups. A high protein diet helps us to adapt best to stress and will help to develop, with exercise, a lean, muscular body. The hazard of high protein occurs in patients with osteoporosis, kidney disease, and abuse of protein supplements. Fortunately, we will not always have to kill animals to produce these protein sources, but this has been necessary since the time of Noah.

When we return to the Garden of Eden, we will not have to kill to live.

The Peace Diet eliminates all artificial ingredients when possible. It does make use of valuable man-made chemicals when synthesized to work with God's creation in peace. Hence, Nutrasweet and especially nutrient supplements, e.g., tryptophan and niacin, are an essential part of the diet's effectiveness. Nutrient supplements represent working according to God's will, utilizing the natural world scientifically. By avoiding pesticides and all kinds of nutrient-poor foods, we recognize God's domain over man. By using man-made chemicals like Nutrasweet and synthesized vitamins, and even drugs if necessary, we make peaceful use of man's technology, thus fulfilling the Biblical command to have dominion in this world. The Peace Diet combines high levels of tryptophan and is low in fruit because of its high sugar content. Many individuals crave fruit for a "high." We postulate that Adam's hypoglycemia led him to accept Eve's apple! Indeed, the moral of the story is that the quest for pleasure through eating fruit takes a man and a woman out of the Garden of Eden. Fruit will inhibit our metabolism from using fat which we need to burn up thereby helping us into the Garden of Eden and good health.

The mind also influences the body. Your diet is developed to foster the best attitudes toward life. Attitude effects bodily health. Bodily health effects attitude. Positive attitudes help build the immune system, develop proper endocrine secretion, and fight stress all of the time. Emotions such as love and joy are health builders. Studies have shown that immune cells can be increased by positive attitudes or decreased during life stress events. We believe metabolic rate is also affected by the mind. Communication and loving relationships with other human beings are an essential part of the Peace Diet plan.

The Peace Diet's success depends upon spiritual awareness. Spiritual awareness affects bodily and mental health. The fullness of peace implies spiritual riches of prayer, dance, song, charity, a sound view of God, an awe of life, a spiritual community, compassion, and disciplined spirituality. An individual's home, dress, and purpose need to be dedicated to God for the Peace Diet to be the most effective. Weight loss can be obtained through peace in the body, peace in the mind, and peace in the spirit. God's name is peace, and whoever calls upon God shall find what he/she seeks -- a Peace Diet. (See also Other Techniques for Breaking a Bad Dietary Habit, p. 91.)

Foods Permitted

Fruits per day (as bowel movements dictate) (as dessert)

Two cups of dairy products. Low fat products only; Lactaid.

Fish, eggs, fowl, lean beef, lamb, veal, liver (3-4 servings per day) Fish daily (all you desire). Salmon and fresh fish preferable to tuna fish.

Asparagus, broccoli, string or wax beans, cabbage, beet greens, cauliflower, chard, kale, onion, spinach, peppers, summer squash, zucchini squash, okra, pumpkin, turnips, bamboo shoots, bean sprouts, water chestnuts, snow pea pods.

Salad daily -- lettuce, radishes, celery, cucumbers

100% whole wheat bread, spaghetti, oatmeal or whole grain rye bread, macaroni, spaghetti made from spinach or artichoke, breakfast cereals: shredded wheat, grape nuts (from barley), and rolled oats

Herb teas with Nutrasweet, spring water with lemon or lime

Safflower oil -- 2 tbsp. all spices, especially ginger, garlic, onion

Foods to Avoid

Grapes, bananas, persimmons (except ceremonial uses)

Sour cream, cream or buttermilk

Pasta, white flour, spinach pasta

Dried fish, shellfish, monkfish, swordfish, shark

Sugar, sweets, carrots, beets, corn, olives, potatoes, peas, sweet beans,

Condiments, ketchup, mustard, salad dressing

Salt, caffeine or alcohol

"Supermarket" cereals with additives

Raisins, dates, figs, dried fruit

Saccharin, honey, etc.

Decaffeinated beverages

Diet soda

Pork (migraines)

Mushrooms, sardines (gout only), vinegar

Eggplant, tomato, pepper (arthritis)

Frozen, canned foods

Fried foods, rice

PHOTOSENSITIVITY DIET

Eat lots of vegetables and take extra beta carotene.

POLYP DIET

This is simply your Basic Diet, plus the anticancer diet, because any disease which is manifested by polyps may have an increased risk of cancer.

PRAYER AND SALVATION DIET

The Salvation Diet is your Basic Health and Diet Rules, except with prayer before and after each meal. The benefit of prayer surrounding your food is a constant sense of salvation, God's salvation and God's blessings that follows. Certain scripture verses may be useful in supporting all dieters. They are:

Avoid sweets and all wickedness.

Put a knife to your throat, if you be a man given to appetite. Be not desirous of pastries for they are deceitful meat (Prov. 23:2-3).

Set a watch, O Lord, before my mouth; keep the door of my lips. Incline not my heart to any evil thing (unhealthy food), to practice wicked works with men that work iniquity; let me not eat of their pastries (Ps. 141:3-4).

Pray to the Lord for new desires.

O Lord, I beseech, for now, that Your ear be attentive to the prayer of Your servant, and to the prayer of Your servants who desire to revere Your name (Neh. 11:1).

Therefore, I say to you, what things you desire, when you pray, believe that you will receive them and you shall have them (Mark 11:24).

Desire spiritual gifts and you will receive your own desires.

Follow after charity, and desire spiritual gifts (1 Cor. 14:1).

Delight yourself in the Lord, and He shall give you the desires of your heart (Ps. 37:4).

Healing is the forgiveness of sin.

And behold, they brought to him a man sick of the palsy, lying on a bed; and Jesus seeing their faith said unto the man sick of the palsy, son, be of good cheer; your sins are forgiven you. And behold, certain of the scribes said to themselves, this man blasphemeth. And Jesus knowing their thoughts said, why do you think evil in your hearts? Is it easier to say, your sins be forgiven you; or to say, arise and walk? (Matt. 9:2-5).

Dietary indiscretion can be forgiven.

I do not do what I want, but I do the very thing I hate (Romans 7:15).

PREMENSTRUAL TENSION DIET

The Premenstrual Tension Diet is also your Basic Health and Diet Rules, p. 89, with extremely low amounts of carbohydrates (avoid the refined) and fat. Eating a high protein - low carbohydrate diet results in diuresis, or removal of water; it is retention of water which is one of the main problems of premenstrual tension. Premenstrual tension is usually treated by nutrient diuretics, vitamin B-6, primrose oil, and magnesium (even lithium and progesterone may be necessary), which basically remove retained water.

Since fluid retention is the problem, all salt must be avoided (see Hypertension Diet, p. 140), because it can also cause depression. A ketosis diet (see Obesity Diet, p. 144) may be helpful during this period by producing diuresis of fluid. Premenstrual tension patients should make use of linseed, safflower, and sunflower oils (2-4 tbsp. daily), which are the best diuretic foods. Avoid all salt, alcohol, and caffeine; these may effect fluid retention or mood swings.

PROSTATE DIET

High fiber, low fat, and increased polyunsaturates are the best general approach. High zinc foods are also important.

PSEUDOGOUT DIET

See Gout Diet, p. 139.

RECTAL FISSURE DIET

See Colitis Diet, p. 135. Especially avoid spicy foods, nuts, acid foods, e.g., citrus and tomatoes.

RELIGION DIET

The Religion Diet emphasizes fasting. During the fasting period people are more likely to have the experience of rebirth, illumination, moral exaltation, a feeling of being chosen, a sense of immortality. This is because fasting is a "taste" of conquering the natural lusts of eating. Having conquered those lusts, a person becomes more open to the Kingdom of God. This is why Jesus, before he went public, fasted 40 days. Moses, before he received the Ten Commandments, fasted forty days. May dieting bring all Americans greater health and holiness. Dieting is to Americans as fasting is to Israel -- a spiritual experience.

Basically, many diseases are associated with an excess of parasympathetic nervous system stimulation. Many diseases have an excess of sympathetic nervous system Adrenalin, e.g., hypertension, backaches, and nervous tension. Parasympathetic nervous system is the resting system and we need to shift into the parasympathetic system to have a religious experience. In general, the parasympathetic system can be increased by taking foods that are high in choline, egg yolks, meat, fish, cereals. Avoiding foods which stimulate the sympathetic nervous system such as coffee, alcohol, tea, or cola is necessary. Niacin and tryptophan are parasympathetic nutrients. The Greeks thought that their gods ate nectar and ambrosia. The Scandinavians thought their gods ate honey. Interestingly, John the Baptist and Elijah lived on honey. Simple carbohydrates sustain life in a partial fasting state.

RESPIRATORY FAILURE DIET

This diet consists of 20% protein, to 30% carbohydrate -- 50% to 60% fat, and 20% other.

SCHIZOPHRENIA DIET

Use the Peace Diet (see p. 144), and especially avoid coffee, alcohol, white flour, and sugar. All stimulants and depressants may bother schizophrenics significantly.

SEX DIET

The Sex Diet seeks to increase certain foods which have hormonal type agents in them and to avoid antihormonal substances. Thyroid-slowing substances, which include turnips, kale, cabbage, brussels sprouts, and possibly soy beans, may slightly inhibit sexual activity. Foods containing cortisone-like substances may be sexually stimulating include, for example, sasparilla and ginseng. Foods with estrogens may help women increase their sex drive. Foods which have estrogen-like agents are yams, hops, palm kernels, pomegranate seeds, carrots, meat, and dairy products. Foods which are high in zinc, such as oysters, and have a lot of iodine may have some sexual stimulating benefits. Foods that are high in the protein, or acid, tyrosine, such as meat and milk, may have some stimulating effect.

Purely vegetarian diets probably in general decrease sex drive, although vitamin A, which is in some ways a steroid-like substance, sasparilla has a steroid-like substance which may be similar to progesterone. Hormone stews, made of chicken giblets, testicles and ovaries, have been recommended for centuries, but are of doubtful benefit. Alcohol, sugar, and chocolate are possible sex spoilers for men. The more protein you eat and the less vegetables the greater the sex drive. Of course, the greater the sex drive, the less peace, which is why the happiness diet is far higher in whole grains and vegetables!

SJOGREN'S SYNDROME DIET

Antibodies to wheat have been found in persons having this disease; possibly wheat should be eliminated from their diet. Beta carotene and primrose oil (polyunsaturates and high fiber vegetables) may help the dry eyes symptom of this condition.

SLEEP DIET

The Sleep Diet emphasizes foods that are high in tryptophan, niacin, pantothenic acid, and niacinamide. Generally you can get these nutrients in warm milk, turkey, or cheese before bed. The goal of the Sleep Diet is to use the general Basic Health and Diet Rules, p. 89, plus a higher protein content to relax you more at your dinner meal. Avoid all alcohol, caffeine, tobacco, and stimulants as is written in the general diet.

SPICE DIET

Eat an abundance of spices at all time for trace elements. This can reduce your cravings for salt, sugar, fat, etc.

SUGAR CRAVER'S DIET: BREAKING ADDICTION TO SUGAR

Sugar-cravings have multiple origins, such as hypoglycemia, diabetes, and depression (sugar is often a good antidepressant). Many biochemical studies suggest that sugar-cravings result from a decrease in the brain content of serotonin, which is made from the amino acid, tryptophan. (See Sleep Diet, above, for high tryptophan foods.)

Hence, the sugar craver's diet is very similar to the Basic Health and Diet Rules, p. 89, except that it calls for foods high in tryptophan. (See Sleep Diet for high tryptophan foods.) Furthermore, this diet reduces the patient's carbohydrate levels, since carbohydrates act to use up tryptophan metabolic (serotonin) supplies. Because a high protein diet may reduce a carbohydrate appetite, protein should be emphasized in a sugar-craver's diet.

A nutrient called GTF (glucose tolerance factor), made up of the trace element chromium, may help regulate blood sugar. A high chromium diet may also be important in another way, as chromium has been found to be reduced in a variety of cardiovascular diseases.

For those who have an impulse disorder associated with sugar-cravings, other therapy, such as lithium or antidepressant therapy and psychological counseling, may be necessary. The key principle, in conclusion, is to increase the protein ratio, to reduce the amount of fruit and carbohydrate (even complex carbohydrate) sources, and to increase the tryptophan and chromium in the diet.

(LOW) SUGAR DIET

The Low Sugar Diet is essential to the entire population. Sugar is even criticized in the Bible, which says, "Beware of sweet dainties; they are a deceitful food." Sugar, including saturated fat, is probably the main agent in the Western diet responsible for raising cholesterol levels. Sugar is certainly responsible for tooth decay, as well as for much adult-type diabetes, elevated triglycerides and skin diseases, such as eczema and psoriasis. Mood disorders, particularly mood swings, are common in sugar-addicted persons.

Sugarholism is a much less serious disease than alcoholism, yet, like alcoholism, prompt withdrawal seems to be the only effective method of treatment. The substitution of high fruit diet, or a large amount of Nutrasweet or other artificial sweeteners, as well as, in some cases, the use of plenty of vitamin B-complex (especially niacin), and even, in some individuals, the use of lithium and antianxiety drugs, are necessary for complete sugar withdrawal.

For those of you who are slow starters, the first place for you to start is by reducing the sugar content in your purchases of manufactured food. (See the sugar content in certain manufactured foods, p. 81.)

TANNING DIET

Lots of vegetables, vitamin B-6 and beta carotene.

THROMBOSIS DIET

See Embolus Diet, p. 137.

THYROID DIET

Hyperthyroidism requires treatment usually with an antithyroid drug in combination with lithium, diet, and nutrients. Eating foods from the Brassica family can also be helpful. These foods, which slow down the thyroid, are broccoli, cabbage, cauliflower, kale, kohlrabi, rutabaga, brussels sprouts, and turnips. These foods also protect against cancer.

TIC DOULOUREUX DIET

See Herpes Diet, p. 115.

TOURETTES DIET

See Allergy: Low Histamine Diet, pp. 132.

(HIGH) TRIGLYCERIDE DIET

The diabetic diets are helpful for individuals with high triglycerides. In addition, the high triglycerides diet requires an extreme consumption of fish. Fish lowers triglycerides, although you can take the supplement EPA (eicosopentoic acid) to lower them effectively. Daily fish intake or even twice daily fish intake of salmon, tuna, trout, bluefish, haddock and mackerel are important. Another way to lower triglycerides is to consume foods high in niacin and pantetheine. Foods with a high glycemic index generally have to be avoided by patients who have high triglycerides. Exercise lowers triglyceride levels. We know of no patient with high triglycerides who does not completely respond to diet, fish oil, pantetheine, and other nutrients.

TRIGEMINAL NEURALGIA DIET

See Herpes Diet, p. 115.

VEGETARIAN DIET

I don't recommend this "Garden of Eden" diet for now. Although there are possibly good sources of vitamin B-12 (tempeh, spirulina), too many vegetarians may develop psychological problems due to B-12 deficiency. I, therefore, suggest bimonthly vitamin B-12 shots (which are better absorbed than tablets) for all strict vegetarians.

Epidemiologists have suggested that true vegetarian societies cannot adapt to stress adequately. Most vegetable proteins have amino acid deficiencies and are thus unsatisfactory as a sole source of protein; usually lysine, methionine, tryptophan, and threonine are deficient. These deficiencies can be overcome in part by the addition to the vegetarian diet of other proteins rich in these amino acids. Although the essential amino acids may be adequate in a vegetarian diet, many other forms of protein may be deficient in, e.g., peptides. (See The Problem of Vegetarianism, pp. 124, 125.)

WEIGHT GAIN DIET

Eat plenty of whole grains, cashews, pistachios, fish oils, and take low doses of lithium, doxepin, Elavil, or even Stelazine if necessary.

YEAST DIET

Much to do has been made about yeast as an allergen, particularly as the cause of such problems as bowel disorders, gas, bloating, psoriasis, and colitis. Yeast is a common pathogen throughout our entire environment. It is particularly common among women as a cause of vaginal infections, characterized by a white mucus and strong yeast odor.

The Yeast Diet is also called the Passover Diet, since it is the one time of the year that yeast is eliminated from the diet for religious purposes!

Yeast items include cheese, tofu, vinegar, wine, beer, and breads of all kinds, as well as fermented beverages, malted products, and possibly citrus fruit juices. Many vitamin products contain yeast, but usually in an insufficient amount to bother a patient.

Yeast foods also include catsup, mayonnaise, olives, pickles, sauerkraut, horse radish, French dressing, salad dressings in general, barbecue sauce, tomato sauce, chili peppers, mince pie, Gerber's oatmeal, all cookies and cakes, and any other flour foods, such as pretzels, pastries, and crackers (which wouldn't be on the diet anyway unless they were made of whole wheat). Pita bread may have no yeast. All other Basic Diet rules apply. Often, yeast patients need to be treated with nystatin, or nystatin suppositories, either vaginally or rectally. Most individuals allergic to the so-called yeast nutrient also suffer from anxiety and an intolerance to refined carbohydrates.

References

Aipers, D. H., Bezoars following partial gastrectomy. *JAMA* 259(10):1560, 1988.

Christiansen, E. N., Piyasena, C., Aa Bjorneboe, G. F., Nilsson, A. and Wandel, M., Vitamin E deficiency in phrynoderma cases from Sri Lanka. *Amer. J. Clin. Nutr.* 47(2):253-255m 1988.

Goke, B., Richter, G., Grebe, A., Keim, V. and Arnold, R., Tryptophan rich diet as a new approach to study the serotoninergic enteropancreatic axis. *Gut* 28:203-205, 1987.

Macfarlane, B. J., Bezwoda, W. R., Bothwell, T. H., Baynes, R. D., Bothwell, J. E., MacPhail, A. P., Lamparelli, R. D. and Mayet, F., Inhibitory effect of nuts on iron absorption. *Amer. J. Clin. Nutr.* 47:270-274, 1988.

Miller, M. E., Cosgrill, J. M. and Roghmann, K. J., Cord serum bromide concentration: variation and lack of association with pregnancy outcome. *Amer. J. Obstet. Gynecol.* 157(4):826-830, 1987.

Olim, A. G., Diet and respiratory failure. *JAMA* 258(14):1894, 1987.

Science News, The acid test: a way to quit smoking? 115:244, 1988.

Van der Meer, J. B., Zeedjik, N., Poen, H. and van der Putte, S. C. J., Rapid improvement in dermatitis herpetiformis after elemental diet. *Arch. Dermatol. Res.* 271:445-459, 1981.

Werback, M., *Nutritional Effects on Mental Illness*, Tarzan CA: Third Line Press, 1989.

Werback, M., *Nutritional Influences on Illness*, Tarzan CA: Third Line Press, sec. ed., 1993.

Recipes

FRESH-START TOMATO JUICE

(Made from scratch -- near-zero-sodium thirst quencher)

12 large red ripe tomatoes (about 8 lbs. peeled and cored) *

1 celery heart with leaves *

1 small yellow onion, peeled and sliced *

1/4 tsp. dill seed

2 strips carefully scrubbed orange peel

Salt substitute or Tabasco to taste

Freshly ground white or black pepper to taste

Chop tomatoes and celery. Place with their juices in a large nonreactive kettle over high heat. (Porcelain or stainless steel are good; avoid aluminum cookware, as it is toxic.)

Add remaining ingredients and bring to a boil. Reduce heat and simmer 20 minutes, stirring occasionally to prevent scorching.

Strain mixture into a large bowl and puree remaining pulp in a blender or food processor.

Strain puree into bowl with juice. Mix well and transfer everything to a container with spout. Refrigerate, and for maximum nutrition and taste, finish in 5 days.

Makes 2 quarts.

NOTE: Contains less than 20 mg sodium per 6-ounce serving. Commercial canned tomato juice contains 550 mg per serving.

Contains a total of 3 hypertension-breaking ingredients. (*)

BETTER BUTTER	TANGY CUCUMBER DRESSING
Blend 1/2 stick of soft, whipped, no-salt vegetable margarine with 1/2 cup regular or high-oleic* safflower, corn or peanut oil, or pure olive oil.* For additional choline and vitamin E and better spreadability, add the contents of one 400 mg vitamin E capsule* and 1 tablespoon high potency soy lecithin granules. Blend well. Spoon into a butter dish or margarine tub and refrigerate. Contains a total of 3 hypertension-breaker ingredients per serving.	(All-purpose low sodium, high-potassium dressing) 1 12-oz. cucumber, pared, seeded and coarsely chopped * 1/2 cup parsley sprigs * 1/4 cup plain nonfat yogurt 1 scallion with top, sliced * 1 tbsp. tarragon vinegar 1 tbsp. Dijon-style mustard 1 clove garlic, sliced * 1/2 tsp. celery seed 1/2 tsp. dried dillweed * Few drops Worcestershire sauce Place all ingredients in blender container and process until smooth. Refrigerate several hours to blend flavors. Makes 1 cup. Preparation time: 10 minutes plus refrigeration time. A perfect complement to the tanginess of mustard greens, cabbage, as well as fresh spinach and tender greens. May be used as a dip for other vegetable or crackers. NOTE: Refrigerated, keeps one week. 15 calories per 2 tbsp. serving; 2 grams fat (13% of calories); .4 mg cholesterol; 34 mg sodium; 114 mg potassium.
Contains a total of three hypertension-breaking ingredients. (*)	**Contains a total of five hypertension-breaking ingredients. (*)**

CHINESE STEAMED FISH WITH CASHEWS	TUNA KABOBS
12 oz. swordfish (or 16 oz. halibut) steak, 3/4-inch thick *	1 lb. fresh tuna steak cut into 1 x 1 inch squares
2 tsp. reduced-sodium soy sauce 1 tsp. lemon juice	2 tbsp. chopped garlic
1 tsp. safflower or olive oil *	1 tbsp. chopped ginger root
1 clove garlic, minced; 1/8 tsp. red pepper *	1 cup safflower oil
2 green onions with tops, cut into thin 1-inch strips *	1/2 cup Tamari soy sauce,* low sodium
2 tsp. thinly-sliced cashews or almonds	8 cherry tomatoes
2 tbsp. minced cilantro (Chinese parsley) *	1 small onion cut into quarters

CHINESE STEAMED FISH WITH CASHEWS

Rinse fish; pat dry. Cut into serving portions. Combine next 5 ingredients in a small bowl; set aside. Boil water in bottom half of steamer. (A steam cooker is ideal but any deep saucepan (or electric skillet) with a tight fitting lid will work. Improvise by setting a wire rack on empty tuna cans, tops and bottoms removed, inside saucepan.) Arrange fish on top rack of steamer; brush with soy sauce mixture.

Scatter green onions on top of fish.

Position fish over boiling water and cover steamer tightly. Steam 5 to 6 minutes until fish is opaque. Using a spatula, transfer fish to serving platter. Sprinkle with cashews and garnish with cilantro.

Two servings. Preparation time: 15 minutes. Cooking time: 10 minutes.

178 Calories per serving; 25 grams protein (59% of calories); 7 grams fat (35%); 48 mg cholesterol; 253 mg sodium; 470 mg potassium.

Contains a total of five hypertension-breaking ingredients. (*)

TUNA KABOBS

Dice tuna and marinate in remaining ingredients except tomatoes and onion.

Drain and alternate tuna, tomato, onion on skewers.

Cook on hot outdoor grill or indoor hibachi approximately 5 minutes on each side.

Two to three generous servings.

* If you have a wheat allergy, use non-wheat Tamari sauce, available at health food stores.

Variation: Leave tuna in steaks and marinate tuna steak undiced. Grill 7-10 minutes each side.

Any firm-flesh fish may be substituted (e.g., halibut, salmon, swordfish).

Leftovers make tasty tuna salads for lunch.

HAVE-IT-YOUR-WAY FILLET SOUFFLE	**TWO-STEP, TWO-HERB PESTO**
	(50% lower in fat and sodium)

1 lb. sole or flounder, filleted

1/4 cup Monterey Jack cheese, grated 1/4 cup mild cheddar, grated 5 egg whites

2-3 tbsp. poaching liquid 1 cup plain nonfat yogurt

1/4 cup wholewheat bread crumbs (optional)

Poach fish 4 minutes in hot water (not boiling); remove and flake. Reserve 2-3 tbsp. hot liquid.

Beat egg whites until they form stiff peaks; and set aside. Combine grated cheese, yogurt and poaching liquid with flaked fish, then fold into egg white. Pour into baking dish. (Optional: sprinkle 1/4 cup wholewheat bread crumbs on top.) Bake in 350-degree oven for 35 minutes.

Note: If available, use reduced-fat, reduced-sodium cheese. Variation: Substitute turbot or catfish for either the sole or flounder.

---

8 shelled Brazil nuts

1/4 cup grated

or 1/4 cup of Asiago* or low-fat parmesan cheese *

2 cloves garlic, crushed *

1/2 cup pure safflower oil

1 1/2 cups fresh parsley, chopped, stems included *

1/2 cups fresh basil, chopped, stems included *

Tabasco sauce or potassium salt substitute to taste *

1 to 2 tbsp. boiling water

Put nuts, cheese and garlic in blender. Cover and start machine. Add oil in a thin stream, blending until mixture is smooth. Add herbs a few sprigs at a time. Season with Tabasco or potassium substitute.

With blender running, add boiling water to bring mixture to a mayonnaise-like consistency. Makes 4 servings.

Note: change the nut and the cheese and you can put this traditionally high-fat high-sodium sauce back on the menu. Eight Brazil nuts supply half the fat of the usual 1/3 cup of pine nuts. And Asiago (a parmesan-like grating cheese carried by better supermarkets such as the Food Emporium) has 75% less fat than conventional grating cheeses.

Contains a total of six hypertension-breaking ingredients. (*)

JICAMA-CHILI PEPPER RELISH

1 medium jicama, about 1 pound *

1 large carrot *

1 medium zucchini *

1 pickled chilpotle pepper in an adobo sauce with liquid *

1 cup finely chopped onion *

4 garlic cloves, peeled and minced *

1 bay leaf

6 whole black peppercorns

1/2 cup water

1/3 cup olive oil *

1 tbsp. chopped cilantro or parsley *

1 tsp. good quality dried oregano

Using a knife, remove skin from jicama. Cut into half-inch dice. Place in a bowl.

Peel carrot. Steam cook. Cut into half-inch dice. Add to the bowl with jicama.

Scrub and trim the zucchini. Cut into half-inch dice, add it to the bowl.

Drain the chilpotles, reserving the pickling sauce (one chili makes a relatively mild marinade; use 2 if desired). Cut chilies open lengthwise, scrape out the seeds. Finely chop and place in a separate, medium-sized bowl.

Add onion, garlic, bay leaf, peppercorns, vinegar, water, olive oil, and cilantro or parsley to chilpotle in bowl. Blend in the reserved chilpotle sauce. Crumble oregano and add to bowl. Whisk all the ingredients together and pour the marinade over jicama mixture. Toss with the marinade to coat completely.

Boil. Cook 10-12 minutes until tender. Drain.

Return vegetable to pan, add yogurt or ricotta and oil.

Mash ingredients until coarse. Add remaining seasonings, blend thoroughly and serve warm.

Makes 4 servings.

Variation: Substitute carrots or celery root for parsnips; use Jerusalem artichokes in place of potatoes to reduce starch.

Contains a total of three to six hypertension-breaking ingredients. (*)

HEALTHY HEART SPREAD

1 medium size eggplant

1 small onion, finely chopped or grated

3 tbsp. sugar-free salt-free safflower oil mayonnaise

Tabasco to taste

Peel eggplant and slice.

Bake at 375 degrees approximately 30 minutes. Dice and puree by hand or in food processor until smooth. Fold in mayonnaise, onion and tabasco.

Delicious as a pita bread spread or filling; or cracker dip.

Variation: Add 1-2 cloves, mashed, minced garlic, or one finely chopped fresh tomato.

TWO-WAY TOTAL HEALTH SALAD

Salad Base

1/4 cup pure extra-virgin olive oil or 1/4 cup safflower oil

2 tbsp. herb vinegar

Pepper and salt substitute to taste

1/3 cup thinly sliced green onions

2 crushed and diced garlic cloves *

Salad A With Herbs

1/4 cup finely minced fresh parsley

1/4 cup finely minced fresh tarragon

1 tbsp. minced fresh dill

1 tbsp. minced celery leaves

1/2 lb. green snap beans, steamed and cooled in 1-inch lengths

2 hard boiled eggs, coarsely chopped

HYPERTENSION SHAKE

Complex Carbohydrate Diet (Normal)
Plan A

1/2 banana

2-3 tbsp. safflower oil (as directed)

6 oz. low-fat milk or soy milk

Dash of nonalcoholic fruit or vanilla extract (available through health food stores)

Complex Carbohydrate Diet (Underweight)
Plan B

1 large banana

3 tbsp. safflower oil (as directed)

6 oz. low-fat milk; Nutrasweet to taste or soy milk

Dash of nonalcoholic vanilla or fruit extract

BEEF STROGANOFF
(serves four)

1 1/2 lbs. filet or round cut in 1/2" strips
1/4 cup butter
1 tbs. chopped onion
1 tsp. salt
1/2 lb. fresh mushrooms, sliced thin
4 tbs. whole wheat flour
1 3/4 cups canned bouillon
1 cup sour cream

Melt butter, add onion and beef and cook until slightly brown.
Add salt, stir in flour, add bouillon and mushrooms.
Stir.
Transfer to low casserole, cover and bake at 375 degrees approx. 1 hour.
Stir in sour cream just before serving.
Serve with mashed potatoes or over wide noodles.

PATH to Healthier Food Choices [1]

Pizza Recipe

Whole wheat or multi-grain "Za Pit-za Bread" may be ordered by phone, or inquire for closest source, ast 1-800-654-2882 (they also have gift packs).

- spray Za Bread lightly with "Olive Oil Pam" and spread a low fat/no cholesterol pasta sauce like "Healthy Choice," or a no sugar added pasta sauce like "Aunt Millie's Marinara";

- add your favorite cut up fresh vegetables (spinach, broccoli, peppers, onions, garlic, etc.) and top with nonfat "Healthy Choice" shredded mozzarella cheese;

- bake at 400 degrees for 10 minutes or until cheese is melted.

Combine nonfat plain yogurt with prepared horseradish and use as a mayonnaise substitute on sandwiches, as a butter replacement on potatoes, as a raw vegetable dip, and on fish in place of tartar sauce.

Oatbars Recipe

1 cup brown rice syrup (or honey or fructose)
1/2 cup 2 parts Canola oil/1 part Safflower oil
1 cup applesauce -- unsweetened
1/4 cup water
2 eggs
2 tsp. pure vanilla extract
1 1/2 whole wheat flour
1/4 cup wheat germ
1/2 cup unhulled sesame seeds
2 tsp. baking soda
1/2 tsp. light salt (Morton)
1 tsp. cinnamon (optional)
3 cups rolled oats
 	
  ■ Combine all ingredients above;
 	
  ■ spread into 9 by 13 inch pan prepared with Pam;
 	
  ■ bake at 350 degrees for 30 minutes.
	Analysis
	
	One serving equals 1/48th of the recipe above, or 38.1 grams; which is 1.34 oz.

Analysis

One serving equals 1/48th of the recipe above, or 38.1 grams; which is 1.34 oz.

Calories	74
Protein	2 gm
Carbohydrates	8.9 gm
Fat -- total	3.2 gm
Sat. fat	42 gm
Mono fat	1.4 gm
Poly fat	1.3 gm
Cholesterol	8.8 mg
(NOTE: all cholesterol can be removed by using egg whites only)	
Dietary fiber	1.3 gm
Calcium	20 mg
Iron	0.635 mg
Selenium	5.37 mcg

1. Kathleen Esposito, M.S., Nutrition/Fitness Consultant.

Pumpkin Cake Recipe

24 oz. canned pumpkin
1 cup brown rice syrup (up to 1 1/2 cups)
1/2 cup 2 parts Canola oil/1 part safflower oil
1/2 cup applesauce -- unsweetened
4 eggs
3.5 cups whole wheat flour
1/2 cup wheat germ
2 tsp. baking soda
1 tsp. light salt (Morton)
2 tsp. cinnamon
1 tsp. ground ginger
1 tsp. ground nutmeg
1 tbs. dried parsley

- Combine all ingredients above;

- pour into 9 by 13 inch pan prepared with Pam.

- bake at 350 degrees for 60 to 75 minutes;
  until knife comes out clean.

Analysis

One serving equals 1/48th of recipe above or
      38.1 grams; which is 1.34 oz.

Calories	79.6
Protein	2.13 gm
Carbohydrates	11.8 gm
Fat -- total	3.02 gm
Sat. fat	0.386 gm
Mono fat	1.18 gm
Poly fat	1.2 gm
Cholesterol	17.7 mg

(NOTE: all cholesterol can be removed by using
      egg whites only)

Dietary Fiber	2 gm

Brand New High Protein Breakfast

1 cucumber
1 or 2 whole peppers (red, green, orange, yellow)
2 sticks of "Healthy Choice" nonfat string cheese sticks (they are only 45 kcals each).

The whole breakfast is around 100 kcals. Not only is this a good high protein breakfast, but it is a good for the morning after eating out, or breakfast the day of a big feast -- to keep things in check. This is what weight management is all about -- balance.

Contains: 9 gm of protein; 1 gm carbs.; 0 gm fat.

Healthy Choice Shopping List

AT THE GROCERY STORE

Fresh Express Salad, Italian Blend (washed, cutup, ready to eat)

Mann's Broccoli Coleslaw

"Healthy Choice" Nonfat Mozzarella String Cheese

"Healthy Choice" Nonfat Shredded Cheese (mozzarella, cheddar, jack, etc.)

"Crazy Richard's" Peanut Butter

Pam (butter and olive oil flavors)

El Paso Salsa

Butter Buds

Low Sodium V8

"Hodgson Mill" Whole Wheat Pasta

Soft Tofu

Firm Tofu

Wheat Germ

"Apple and Eve" Cranberry Juice (no sugar or corn syrup added)

AT THE HEALTH FOOD STORE

"Lundberg" Brown Rice Syrup

Fructose

"Bragg" Liquid Aminos

Sunflower Butter

Sesame Butter

"Health Valley" Chili

"Health Valley" Soups

Unhulled Sesame Seeds

Whole Wheat Flour

Wheat Bran

Oat Bran

Crispy Brown Rice Cereal

10. *Electromedicine*

What Most Doctors Won't Tell You: The New PATH -- Our PATH -- in Medicine and Science

What most medicine has finally come to recognize is that most diseases relate back to the brain and most visits to doctors relate to brain chemical imbalances. Most doctors do not yet know how to deal with the brain's chemistry, nutritional imbalances, stress, and life-style problems which are the primary expenditures in medicine. The end stage of medicine, generally, has its origin in chronic illnesses, addictive behavior, repetitive, destructive eating, smoking, drinking, etc., all activities which are based fundamentally in brain imbalances. If one wants to deliver health

to people, deliver as you would deliver children: head first! The Brain Electrical Activity Mapping (BEAM) test identifies the exact degree of brain health (based on statistical measurement) and the approaches of nutrition, amino acids, Cranial Electrical Stimulation (CES) devices are the first approaches to maintaining long-term successful preventive medicine. This is *the new PATH* in medicine and science, where the brain is dealt with first, and the bioelectrical and health ritual (daily CES) is the basis of health maintenance.

Electromedicine at PATH

We are now using numerous devices for electrical therapy at PATH. A 3M TENS unit (Transcutaneous Electric Nerve Stimulation) is used for chronic back or neck strains and sprains, joint injuries, degenerative diseases, osteoarthritis and bursitis, and postoperative recovery. TENS can help in the regaining of strength and endurance, and control treatment; it also provides proven pain relief and helps block pain without drugs. Thus TENS can also be helpful for reflex sympathetic dystrophy, multiple sclerosis and other medical conditions of the nervous system. TENS is easy to use and our staff can demonstrate these devices. When used on the head, the

TENS device is called a CES device. These devices can be used for anxiety, depression and insomnia; they also may improve concentration. A device called Alpha Stim can be used for chronic pain. The combination of nutrition with electricity is the optimum natural approach for healing. With the entrance of the large corporation 3M into the electromedicine field we are hoping that new and improved devices will be available, including their recently developed dysmenorrhea PMS device, which I believe is extremely effective and can replace the potential side effects of many strong drugs that are used.

Electromagnetic Pollution:
Is There an Electromagnetic Antidote?

INTRODUCTION

Throughout history there have been many descriptions of the devil seen as working through unseen powers and forces: the occult, drugs, spirits, etc. We have come to recognize that the devil has forces that are unseen, such as pollutants like lead and mercury that affect our environment, and bacteria and viruses like AIDS and herpes. The unseen devil has now taken on a new form with electromagnetic pollution. Thank God that whenever there has been an unseen devil, there has been an antidote that God has provided, whether it is an antibiotic for bacteria, or an antiviral drug for a virus, or good nutrients that antidote toxins. There is now an electromagnetic antidote for electromagnetic pollution, which is a new, unseen devil in our environment.

In recent years, scientific evidence has been mounting to suggest that there is a possible link between extremely low frequency electromagnetic fields (ELF EMF) and a variety of health problems. Individuals who work in an electrical profession may have a 2.6 times greater risk of dying of myeloid leukemia. The incidence of brain cancer in children may almost double in households where the average magnetic field strength is greater than 2 milligauss. Research suggests a direct link between ELF EMF and calcium ion concentration in the human cell, leading to altered hormone production. There are many possible mechanisms by which ELF EMF has an affect on the central nervous system, hemopoietic cells, and pineal gland as well as producing abnormal signal transductions, immune modulator effects, etc.

The legal ramifications of ELF EMF cancer link are dawning. Already the Boeing Company in a highly publicized case agreed to pay $500,000 to an employee who claimed exposure to EMF while testing MX missiles.

ELF EMF milligauss exposure has been associated with cancer and is of critical interest for a variety of reasons:

1) Greater than 2 milligauss ELF EMF is common in our environment (see Table 1).

Table 1

Type of equipment	Distance for 1 mG (Front)	Distance for 1 mG (Back and Sides)
Television set	3-5'	3-6'
Microwave oven	2-4'	3-6'
Clock radio	1-2'	1-3'
Electric range	1-2'	1-2'
Personal computer	2-3'	3-5'
Electric typewriter	1-3'	2-4'
Printer	1-3'	2-4'
Copying machine	2-4'	3-5'

2) ELF EMF is extremely common in a variety of instances as far as 5 and 6 feet away from various objects (see Table 2).

Table 2

ITEM	MAX (MILLIGAUSS)	TYPICAL RANGE OF DISAPPEARANCE
CTX color monitor	29 center 19 side 18 right hand corner 19 all around edge	6 inches 12 inches 22-24 inches
WIN monitor	8 center	4-5 inches 6 inches
Auto. Balancing Sys. and elect. apparatus	400	2 feet
Air conditioning apparatus	4	1-2 feet
Light bulb	0	
Fluorescent lights	70 center 10 sides some as low as 25	2-3 feet
Gold Star turntable microwave	20 at rest 115-200 turn on center	2 feet
Xerox machine	9-10 at waist high	1-2 feet
Garden variety time recorder	4	
Black and white AT&T screen	11 center 7 corners	2 feet 1 feet
Citizen 200 GX printer Solid state vidiomatic B and W TV set	6 42 center 20 edges	6 inches 1 foot 3.5-4 feet
Electric clock	140 dead center 20 edges	3 feet 1 foot
Welch Allen Otoscope	15-20	4 inches 1 foot
TV set at back	1600	41-65 inches

3) A great number of cancer patients deplete endorphins at the end stage and thereby become addicted to opium and other narcotics. This depletion in small degrees may precede the cancer.

4) ELF EMF may not only cause cancer, but also depletes endorphins in the brain, which may be one critical mechanism underlying addiction and other psychiatric disorders.

ELF EMF in a strict technical sense, produces magnetic fields while voltages produce an electric field. It is the magnetic fields that have caused the most concern, and these magnetic fields can be easily measured by milligauss meters that are now commonly available. ELF EMF radiation is generally thought to encompass frequencies between 30 and 300 hertz.

WHERE ELF EMF COMES FROM AND HOW TO AVOID IT

Every electrical device, appliance, and machine using AC power generates ELF since AC power is at approximately 60 hertz. Is ELF EMF toxic? We saw the typical reactions with lead poisoning. First toxicity was 80 parts per million in the blood, then 60, then 40, then 20, and now recently, 10 parts per million. We can all be certain, based not only on the history of lead and of other toxicities, e.g., organic chemicals, and aluminum, etc. that severity is frequently underestimated. Evidence mounts for toxins until effects are established, then the search for antidotes begins. Currently, in the biochemical spectra, the role of antioxidants to antidote our low level, toxic heavy metal organic chemical exposures is now considered a critical part of virtually every medical disease and by every medical theoretician looking at public health problems. The primary antioxidants consist of beta carotene, selenium, vitamin E, niacinamide, ascorbic acid, and L-cysteine.

The data suggests we can count on ELF EMF to be demonstrated to be an increasing public hazard with the 2 milligauss threshold probably not being sufficient in terms of significant effects. We must ask the question where is ELF EMF and how do we avoid it? The answer is *we can not avoid it* (Tables 1, 2, and 3), although utility companies and electronic manufacturers are attempting to make electromagnetic shields. Yet, with the exception of iron and steel, shields such as concrete walls, office dividers and computer monitor screens have little or no effect on reducing magnetic radiation. The most effective and inexpensive way to protect oneself from magnetic radiation is to increase one's distance from the source, which can be difficult at times. In the case of most home appliances and light office equipment and fluorescent lights, if you are close enough to touch it you are probably too close. It seems advisable and prudent that individuals should be restructuring the placement of equipment in their offices, classrooms, and homes so as to minimize the risk.

WHAT IS THE ANTIDOTE FOR THE ELF EMF?

The general principle which we have come to accept in science is that the antidote of psychological problems is psychological treatments. The antidotes for toxic heavy metals such as lead and cadmium are good heavy metals such as zinc, selenium and, of course, chelating agents. The antidotes for organic chemicals such as benzenes and carbon tetrachlorides are beta carotene and cysteine, and N-acetyl-cysteine (an organic amino acid), which antidotes an incredible range of toxic compounds (see Table 3). Organic chemicals antidote organic toxins. We believe CES may be the antidote for a wide variety of ELF EMF effects.

It would seem probable that some type of electrical device at a low level might be the antidote. Recent studies have shown that magnetic fields can effect quantified EEG in the brain. The most probable mechanisms by which electromagnetic fields and pollutants work to affect human health is through the brain. The brain is the key battle place between toxins and antitoxins, whether it be lead, benzenes, organics, etc. Cranial Electrical Stimulation (CES) can normalize numerous types of brain rhythms. We believe strongly that models can be developed showing that the abnormalities induced in spectral analysis and evoked potentials by milligauss ELF EMF exposure can be corrected by daily therapy with Cranial Electrical Stimulation (CES). Recent studies demonstrate that ELF EMF produced by display terminals can increase theta waves. We have demonstrated CES can antidote this effect.

CONCLUSION

Wherever there are toxins, God will provide the antitoxin. In the case of electromagnetic fields, CES is going to become the antidote. Praise God, for He has given us water to antidote fire, and Christ to antidote the anti-Christ. He has given us love to antidote fear. He has given us the Word of God to antidote this world's words of confusion.

Table 3 Some substances rendered less toxic by N-Acetyl-Cysteine, Cysteine, and Glutathione	Table 4 Ten Observed Miscellaneous Sources of ELF-EMF

Table 3
Some substances rendered less toxic by
N-Acetyl-Cysteine, Cysteine, and Glutathione

1. Halogenonitrobenzenes and congeners -- fungicides
2. 2-Chloro-S-triazines and congeners -- herbicides
3. Aryl Nitrocompounds-nitrates, nitrosamines
4. Phenoltetrabrompthaleins -- dyes
5. Aryl & alkyl halides -- solvents, intermediates
6. Aryl alkyl esters -- solvents, flavorings
7. Alkene halides -- plastics (vinyl chloride)
8. Alkyl compounds -- intermediates
9. Alkyl methanesulfonates -- dyes, detergents
10. Organophosphorus compounds -- insecticides
11. Arylhydrocarbon epoxides (arene oxides) -- solvents
12. Arylhalide epoxides -- solvents
13. Other epoxide intermediates -- solvents
14. Alpha, beta-unsaturated compounds
15. Arylamines, arylhydroxylamines, carbamates, and related compounds (phenols)
16. Steroids -- drugs (phenolics)
17. Quinones and catechols -- drugs
18. Isothiocyanates -- such as methylisocaynate
19. Tricloromethylsufonyls -- pesticides
20. Thiocarabamates -- pesticides
21. Heavy metals -- such as lead, mercury, arsenic, cadmium -- found in paints, cans, gasoline, amalgams in teeth, batteries, plating
22. Bacterial toxins -- clostridia difficile
23. Automobile exhaust, cigarettes
24. Many over-the-counter drugs -- substances detoxified by the liver and too numerous to name

Table 4
Ten Observed Miscellaneous
Sources of ELF-EMF

	Approx feet away
1. Under high tension wires on Eisenhower Parkway in Livingston north:	
a. Under wires	55
b. On road near (northbound) lane	20
c. On road far (northbound) lane	10
2. Toy electric train circa 1935	
a. At transformer	112
b. At lock on	50
c. At track	0
d. At lock on with train passing	78
e. At track with train passing	37
3. Old G. E. electric can opener	500
4. Electric wall clock	120
5. Battery operated wall clock	6
6. Small G. E. clock with noisy motor	1510
7. Small Westclox clock with noisy motor	1775
8. Remington electric shaver -- rechargeable	
a. Running not connected to outlet	2
b. Charging not running	250
9. Electric blanket -- high setting	26
10. Bathroom fluorescent fixture	180

References

1. Koch, M., *Electromagnetic fields: a guide to understanding what they are and how to reduce your exposure to them.* Teslatronics, Inc., Alachua, FL 1991.

2. Goldberg, R. B., Creasey, W. A., A review of cancer induction by extremely low frequency electromagnetic fields. Is there a plausible mechanism? *Medical Hypothesis* 35:265-274, 1991.

3. U.S. Congress, Office of Technology Assessment, *Biological effects of power frequency electric and magnetic fields - background paper*, OTA-BPE-53 (Washington, DC: U.S. Government Printing Office, May 1989).

4. Electric Power Research Institute, Technical Publications Department, Palo Alto, CA (415-855-2281).

5. Wertheimer, N., and Leeper, E., Electrical wiring configurations and childhood cancer, *American Journal of Epidemiology*, vol. 109, no. 3, pp. 273-284, 1979.

6. P. Brodeur, P., *Currents of death: power lines, computer terminals and the attempts to cover up their threat to your health*, Simon and Shuster, 1989.

7. Dodge, C. H., *High voltage in extremely low frequency communications systems: Health and Safety concerns.* Congressional Research Service, The Library of Congress, Washington, D. C., 1984.

8. Sheppard, A. R., and Eisenbud, M., *Biological effects of electric and magnetic fields of extremely low frequency*, New York University Press, New York, 1977.

9. Becker, R. O., and Marino, A. A., *Electromagnetism and life*, Pub. State University of New York, New York Press, New York, 1985.

10. Aldrich, Timothy E., and Easterly, Clay E., Electromagnetic fields and public health, *Environmental Health Perspectives*. 75: 159-171, 1987.

11. Meyer, R. E., Aldrich, T. E., and Easterly, Effects of noise and electromagnetic fields on reproductive outcomes. *Environmental Health Perspectives*, vol. 81, 193-200, 1989.

12. Modan, B., Exposure to electromagnetic fields and brain malignancy: a newly discovered menace? *American Journal of Industrial Medicine* 13:625-7, 1988.

13. Bassett, C., Schink-Ascani, M., and Lewis, S. M., Effects of pulsed electromagnetic fields on Steinberg ratings of femoral head osteonecrosis. *Clinical Orthopaedics and Related Research*, no. 246, pp. 172-185, September 1989.

14. Braverman, E., Smith, R., Smayda, R., Blum, K., Modification of P300 amplitude and other electrophysiological parameters of drug abuse by cranial electrical stimulation, *Current Therapeutic Research*, 48:586-596, 1990.

15. Braverman, E., Blum, K., Smayda, R., A commentary on brain mapping in 60 substance abusers: can the potential for drug abuse be predicted and prevented by treatment? *Current Therapeutic Research* 48:569-585, 1990.

Cranial Electrical Therapy Stimulation (CES): A Brief Summary

Cranial Electrotherapy Stimulation (CES) is a therapeutic procedure using minute battery-powered electronic stimulation for the purpose of inducing a relaxed state for the treatment of stress-related disorders: anxiety, depression, and insomnia.

Cranial electrical therapy stimulation (CES) is done with a Transcutaneous Electric Nerve Stimulator (TENS) used on the head. It has been used for healing muscles, and, as an FES, or fine electrical stimulator, it enables stroke patients to open their hands. Electricity can be used for healing heart rhythms and healing bones. A technique developed by Dr. Braverman will change brain rhythms back to normal without the use of drugs. CES is FDA permitted and can be used as a primary treatment in anxiety, depression, and insomnia. Many publications show its benefit in anxiety, depression, insomnia, and even drug abuse in which anxiety and depression are frequently a part. CES is a safe, tested and proven therapy for:

Anxiety: an average improvement of over 50% in test scoring of hospitalized psychiatric patients and inpatient alcoholics with measured anxiety.

Stress Related Withdrawal Syndrome: reduced stress measure, in every instance, by at least 40% for inpatient substance abusers related to withdrawal syndrome.

Depression: an average reduction of 50% in the depression score of: long term psychiatric patients, university counseling center clients, post-withdrawal alcoholic patients and hospitalized para- and quadraplegics.

Insomnia: significant improvement in: sleep onset time, sleep efficiency, percentage of bed time sleep, percentage of sleep time in stages 1 and 4, and percentage of delta sleep.

Additional research by Dr. Braverman with the BEAM machine suggests that CES, when worn on the forehead and left wrist over the radial pulse, is effective for daily use and will change brain rhythm without injuring the brain, like ECT, because it is gentle electrical stimulation.

Why the left wrist? Possibly because of the transportation of electricity through the blood stream to the left vagus nerve where studies suggest implanted CES devices can control brain rhythm.

Why the forehead? Possibly because the right brain is important to brain rhythm. CES is not a replacement for all drugs, but it is another useful medical technique for reducing anxiety when used frequently.

CES is safe and noninvasive. It is nonaddictive and has no pharmaceutical side effects. It is easy to use, and involves the simple nonirritating placement of electrodes. CES is efficient, comfortable, convenient, compact, and portable for easy transport.

Recommended Treatment Regimen

As prescribed and monitored by the health professional: once a day for 30-60 minutes or more depending on physician and treatment goals. Some patients with severe addictions and depression may require 4-8 hours daily.

Contraindicated

Although CES treatment is not known to be harmful to patients with any present disorder, it may be counterindicated in those patients known to be epileptic or pregnant. It should not be used on patients suffering from brain tumor and stroke.

In Conclusion

In conclusion, the forehead-left pulse position cannot be scientifically documented to be absolutely, without a shadow of a doubt, the best way, but we can say that it makes sense because the rhythm of the brain should be in synchrony with the pulse of the body. The CES device is like water on a stone; like a drop of electrical current daily upon the hard stoniness of the human brain, healing it, bending it, welding it into a healthy rhythm. The brain "beats" eight times per second.

Cranial Electrical Stimulation

Cranial Electrical Stimulation has a long history. The use of electricity in therapeutic disorders dates back in scientific history to Mesmer, who tried to use magnetism for a variety of medical problems. Allen Childs, M.D., Assistant Professor of Pharmacy at the University of Texas at Austin, suggests that electrical therapies actually date back to ancient Egypt. Currently acceptable electrical uses include the TENS or Transcutaneous Electrical Nerve Stimulation device, which is an acceptable use for pain, and variations on the TENS (FES or fine electrical stimulators) are used for some stroke patients.

Electrical currents have been experimented with for hard-to-heal bone fractures. There are also now brain or cranial TENS devices (CES) which seem to impact brain chemistry in many significant ways. Cranial Electrical Stimulation (CES) devices are thought to raise alpha waves, raise blood levels of endorphins and increase conversion of amino acids into the brain's neurotransmitters. The FDA has approved CES devices for anxiety, depression, insomnia, and stress. The usual treatment can be 15, 30, or 60 minutes twice daily for stress; often individuals wear it overnight with a timer. At first comfort level may be exceeded after the first ten minutes. A poor connection or too high a dose can be discomforting and should be avoided. Poor electrode placement with reapplication can suddenly give a slight but uncomfortable shock. The device does possess an automatic shut-off valve. The intensity of current should be set at a comfortable level and the electrodes can be placed firmly on the mastoid process, forehead or arm. New studies suggest the best placement of electrodes will be near the left hand over the wrist or the forehead and above the nose. We are collecting data to evaluate precise location. If headache or any side effect occurs the CES is discontinued. Pacemakers are contraindications for use of the device.

Other possible applications of the CES are menstrual cramping, stiff neck, allergic reactions, headache, temporal lobe disorders, etc. The bioelectrical approach may be useful to modulate neurotransmitters in the brain so that they may rebalance the immune system and help with aspects of all depression and anxiety type symptoms. Patients who first use the Cranial Electrical Stimulation device can often experience benefit in the first 30-minute session. Often a good marker of its benefits is that it will produce good relaxation and even improve sleep. For other individuals an appropriate trial may be concurrent use with amino acids or antidepressants, which require at least three weeks to reach their full effect, and sometimes as much as two months to reach the full benefit.

The voltage of the CES device is one milliamp at 100 Hertz (cycles/second) and 20% duty cycle. TENS units are 2-50 milliamps. To put this in perspective, wall sockets have 10 amps, or ten times the voltage, 60 Hertz (cycles/second), 110 volts.

Cranial Electrical Stimulation may be a very useful alternative to drug treatments in individuals who have treatment resistant anxiety and/or depression. Furthermore, CES used in combination with the natural amino acids may convert the amino acids more rapidly to neurotransmitters resulting in greater effectiveness. The TENS device in combination with amino acids is also more effective than amino acid augmentation alone. Therefore, there is hope that this new approach, or brain bioelectrical approach, can be extremely successful and may actually become a first line therapy for psychiatric disorders because of its noninvasiveness and low level of side effects. It should be noted that individuals using this device may initially feel a tingling sensation. This is a good and normal reaction. It has been noted that the device has been experimented with by many other individuals and it has been called by some cerebral electrical therapy or CET, which started in the USSR in 1947. Treatment was done for 30 minutes, and double-blind studies were done. Again, frequency was at 100 cycles per second and pulse duration of 1 millisecond. There were changes in 24-hour urinary free catecholamines and 17 ketosteroid levels. Researchers have experimented with other cranial electrical devices and called them neurotonic therapy or neuroelectrical therapy

(NET). Many researchers all around the country are actively studying the device, and I am sure our ability to use it effectively will continue to grow.

In summary, Cranial Electrotherapy Stimulation (CES) is the FDA's term for any application of 1.5 ma or less of electricity across the head for medical purposes. Its use requires a prescription. Currently, all approved devices give 100 Hertz, 0.5-1 milliamp, on a 20% duty cycle. Having followed recommendations of the National Research Council and after over 20 years of medical experience with CES in America, the FDA now considers the side effects of CES to be nonsignificant. For that reason their policy is not to require an Investigational Device Exemption prior to experimental studies of CES.

CES began in Europe in the 1950s under the rubric, "Electrosleep." Eastern nations soon picked it up as a treatment modality and its use had spread worldwide by the late 1960s when animal studies of CES began in the U.S. at the University of Tennessee and at what is now the University of Wisconsin Medical School. These were soon followed by human clinical trials at the University of Texas Medical School in San Antonio, the University of Mississippi Student Counseling Center, and the University of Wisconsin Medical School. As of April 1990, there were over 100 published CES studies appearing in the American literature.

Open marketing of the CES device began in the early 1970s in the U.S. for the clinical condition of anxiety, depression and insomnia. Under the 1976 Medical Devices Amendment, the FDA grandfathered CES devices, which are currently marketed as previously, but limited to the earlier treatment claims until such time as a Premarket Approval Application is submitted to FDA for these and/or any additional treatment claims.

To date, several thousand Americans are treated with CES annually and more than eleven thousand persons own CES devices, which have been prescribed for their home use. Possibly the most exciting application of the CES is for drug addiction. Further studies are needed to fully document use of the device for these purposes. In this technological age when we are surrounded by electromagnetic fields and currents, CES treatment may be necessary as an antidote and for maintenance of fully optimum health. Electromagnetic "pollution" from video screens, televisions, stereophonic equipment, microwaves, hairdressers and phone lines may be destroying our health and may require a device of this type. In addition, CES also probably incorporates some of the benefits of electroconvulsive shock therapy (ECT) without the damaging effects of high amounts of current. CES probably provides natural levels of supplementary current to keep the brain healthy in the electrical age. It was said years ago, everyone needs to antitox, antitox. Now its in the media every day. The CES device is for counteracting the effects of electromagnetic pollution.

Pulsing Brain Hormones by CES?

A recent reference showed once again that the brain electrically pulses its own hormones. Evidence will increasingly show that electromagnetic fields affect pulsing of the brain's hormones which is affecting the mental health of America. One out of two Americans now are suffering from a mental disorder. So much of this is biochemical and we want people to know that their mood problems, depression problems are greatly physical as a result of our environment. Hormones released by electrical pulse may be aided by the electrical pulses of the CES device.

Reference:

Byrne, KT, and Knobil, E, Electrophysiological approaches to gonadotrophin releasing hormone pulse generator activity in the rhesus monkey. *Human Reproduction*, 8:37-40, 1993.

Cranial Electrotherapy Stimulation

(CES)

INTRODUCTION

Cranial Electrotherapy Stimulation (CES) is a process which utilizes minute electrical stimulation for therapeutic purposes. Low voltage electrical stimulation of the brain has proven to be therapeutically beneficial in the treatment of numerous conditions such as depression, anxiety, substance abuse, withdrawal syndrome, and insomnia (Smith, 1985). Because these symptoms are so widespread in a variety of psychiatric diagnoses, CES is a useful adjunct in treating schizophrenia, learning disability, hyperactivity, even hyperacidity (Kotter 1975).

The most exciting research concerns the effects of CES with alcohol abuse and the withdrawal syndrome. CES has been shown to be one of the best approaches for a faster and safer way to overcome alcoholism (Smith, 1985). The treatment is accomplished simply by the application of small amounts of pulsed electric current to the patient via electrodes applied to the head and wrist (Braverman, *et. al.*, 1990). The sensation felt by the patient is normally one of relaxation and may even cause the patient to fall asleep while being treated.

HISTORY

The first recorded cure attributed to electric stimulation was noted by the physician, Scribonius Largus, in the first century A. D. He made use of a live torpedo fish (electric eel) for the treatment of gout (Jarzembski, 1985), a disease causing inflammation of the joints, especially the toes, knees, and fingers. For almost 2,000 years therapeutic use of electrical stimulation languished, but, in 1747 interest in the subject revived. This was evidenced by some journal accounts which have described how electric current applied over a period of time abated pain.

It appears that the therapeutic use of electricity had languished due to the difficulty of providing a suitable source of electrical potential or current. It was not until the mid-twentieth century that the interdisciplinary elements required for an understanding of electrotherapy began to emerge. The technology to manufacture significant numbers of high quality CES devices also emerged.

Early studies were primarily done in Russia. Interest in the smaller amounts of electric current involved in CES did not begin in earnest until work by Gilyarovski, et al., who in 1953 published a book *Electrosleep*. That work initiated much interest in Europe and work was begun in numerous centers, mainly in the East Bloc European nations, but also in Western Europe, South America, the Orient, and finally, the United States (Boblitt, 1969).

The first paper on CES published in the United States was in 1959. Interest in this country developed slowly because of a lack of translated material and the attitude of the American Medical Association relative to the general use of electrical currents for therapeutic purpose. The fact that we use large amounts of electrical currents for the legal destruction of criminals and for causing convulsion in treatment-resistant depression (ECT) caused an adverse reaction to its use and thus created difficulties for future application of electrical currents in therapy (Jarzembski, 1985). CES is, of course, gentle electrical stimulation (as neck massage is a gentle form of touch, and choking, a dangerous form of touch). Although CES applications to humans had spread rapidly through Europe in the fifties, animal studies began in the U.S. at the University of Tennessee and at the University of Wisconsin Medical School in the sixties. Later, human trials were carried out at the University of Mississippi, the University of Texas at San Antonio, and at the University of Wisconsin Medical School. Smith has noted that as of April 1990, there were over 100 published CES studies in the American literature (Budzynski, 1989).

Today, several thousand Americans are treated with CES annually, and more than 11,000 persons own CES devices which have been prescribed for their home use. From a broad reading of published literature, virtually no negative effects have been found from the use of CES to date. Headache occurs if one is too aggressive with turning up the dial. A burning sensation on the skin occurs if electrodes are damaged or misplaced. If placed on a tendon or otherwise incorrectly positioned, CES causes significant discomfort, yet if properly used CES produces no side effects. In fact, the FDA now considers the side effects of CES to be nonsignificant.

How can a simple CES device produce so much relief in so many different ways? What really happens to the brain when you apply electrical stimulation? How does this help depression? Could many so-called psychiatric conditions really be brain rhythm disorder that can be reset (defibrillated) by a CES device, and can a CES device be like a brain pacemaker?

RESEARCH

Cranial Electrotherapy Stimulation (CES) has proven to be therapeutic in many ways. It reportedly aids in curing insomnia, depression, anxiety, and stress related withdrawal syndrome. The most fascinating and best research with CES has been with alcoholics and substance abusers. This paper will mainly consist of findings and conclusions from patients' substance abuse. It's likely that substance abuse/alcoholism has been a principal area of study for CES because alcoholism, as disease, is strongly correlated with depression, anxiety, and stress -- all of which CES affects.

ALCOHOLISM, THE DISEASE

Alcoholism refers to excessive consumption of alcoholic beverages resulting in persistent social, psychological and medical problems. It is a behavior disorder. The motivation underlying alcoholism is often obscure. When asked to describe why they drink, alcoholics usually attribute it to a particular mood, such as depression or anxiety. The full range of symptoms associated with depression and anxiety neurosis -- insomnia, low mood irritability, and anxiety attacks -- are present. Alcohol temporarily relieves these symptoms, resulting in a vicious cycle of drinking-depression-drinking which ultimately may result in an alcohol withdrawal syndrome.

CES AND DEPRESSION/SUBSTANCE ABUSE

Smith (1985) was one of the first to study the relationship between substance abuse and depression. He notes that codeine (an opiate) stimulates the production of norepinephrine and will produce a high in the presence of endorphins. As a result of codeine abuse an excess of norepinephrine accumulates in the nerve synapse thus causing the brain to temporarily cease production of this neurotransmitter. With this decrease in norepinephrine levels a severe depressive state is produced as the neurochemical levels in the brain are no longer homeostatically balanced (Budzynski, 1990).

According to Smith (1985) and Ostrander (1989), alcohol and Valium bind to the endorphin receptor sites. This results in the brain shutting down its manufacture of the natural endorphin due to a surplus endorphin accumulation in the synapse. Since the natural endorphins inhibit the overproduction of norepinephrine, the lack of a normal true endorphin level allows the norepinephrine to range out of control, causing severe anxiety reaction and panic states. Along with this reaction there are all the other symptoms of the classic withdrawal syndrome or delirium tremors. This situation progressively worsens, in that after several days, a severe chemical depression results from an overproduction of norepinephrine causing a rebound shutdown of its production. CES can prevent this process (Schmitt, 1980; Grinenko, 1988; Braverman, 1990).

Smith (1985) reported on 5 studies which involved depression. Overall, the analysis indicated that there was an average reduction of 50% in the depression scores of alcoholic patients as a result of CES treatment.

CES AND COGNITIVE BRAIN DYSFUNCTION

Very often the serious addictive state is accompanied by an insidious and progressive condition known as Korsakoff's Psychosis. This is an advanced condition which manifests itself as a destruction of normal brain functioning, particularly in the area of recent or short-term memory losses (Smith, 1977), and in the ability to process information dealing with abstract symbols.

Several different psychological scales of cognitive function were used to test brain dysfunction. Resulting statistics showed that CES treatment halts and significantly reverses brain dysfunction in patients as measured on seven different psychological scales of cognitive function, bringing many such functions back to the level of the preaddiction state in the majority of patients studied (Schmitt 1984). Research findings indicated that CES stimulated the production of acetylcholine in the memory channels of the hippocampal gyrus which, in turn, improved cognitive functioning in alcoholics (Smith 1982).

Cranial Electrical Stimulation is used to stimulate brain tissue to produce neurochemicals up to a level of prestress homeostasis. Research findings state that CES appears to stimulate the production of these beta endorphin levels (supporting the hypothesis that a mild effect is produced at the hypothalamic area of the brain) which, in turn, tend to "inhibit the increased levels of norepinephrine from unduly stimulated neuroreceptors on the locus ceruleus so that anxiety and associated panic states are effectively blocked." (Budzynski 1990).

The locus ceruleus is a cluster of neurons located in the dorsal brain stem, adjacent to the fourth ventricle. More than half of the noradrenergic neurons in the central nervous system are located within its boundaries. This relatively small collection of neurons has numerous and important projections to the cortex, the limbic system, the medullary and spinal centers affecting cardiovascular sympathetic activity, hypothalamus, and other important brain neurotransmitter systems.

A study by Gold (1979) has indicated that endorphins and exogenous opiates inhibit the activity of the locus ceruleus. Drugs (or CES) which inhibit the function of the locus ceruleus and block elicited behaviors and visceral phenomena, may be hypothesized to be useful in the medical treatment of opiate withdrawal. This was Gold's hypothesis and he found that clonidine (a drug which inhibits the locus ceruleus and locus ceruleus mediated noradrenergic activation) is an efficacious nonopiate treatment for opiate withdrawal. This finding supports the data found with CES since it also inhibits the locus coreleus and produces the same effect as clonidine of blocking anxiety.

CES AND METHADONE

One of the most important findings resulting from CES studies is that CES is highly effective when used in conjunction with methadone withdrawal for heroin addicts. (Methadone is often used with heroin addicts - substituting one addicting drug for another.) A study by Gomez (1978) shows a major decrease in withdrawal time coupled with a significant reduction in anxiety.

CONCLUSION

A significant amount of research has been conducted in the field of CES. There have been other successful studies concluded in the areas of stress, anxiety, and reduction of pain (Smith 1985).

So far we have found that CES can be a valuable adjunct to existing therapy in the treatment of alcohol withdrawal. In substance abuse recovery programs CES stimulates brain tissue and produces an increase in beta-endorphin levels and also acetylcholine levels which block anxiety and improve cognitive functioning in alcoholics. Also, when used in conjunction with other modalities it results in quicker recovery in alcoholism, cocaine, heroin, and other drug abuse. New studies have shown CES benefits with opioid withdrawal (Westermeyer, 1990) and Kosten, et al., 1988).

CES has several advantages over many treatments of alcoholism in that it does not require the ingestion of another potentially addictive substance; once shown how to use the device it is easy to treat oneself. It appears to be effective in cases of chronic tension states, depression, and sleep disturbance. It reduces stress, and turning a switch on is much easier than learning a method of relaxation (e. g., Zen). Finally, there are no side effects when properly used. As stated by Ostrander, there is no other treatment modality designed to help the brain bring its neurochemistry back to pretrauma levels of homeostasis; or to allow cognitive functioning to return to normal patterns within weeks instead of the usual months or, in some cases, years, which is often the case with substance abuse situations.

CES is becoming more widely used in the United States, but for some reason it is not widely known. We are currently researching the effect that different frequencies and milliamps have on results. Most drug users can tolerate and enjoy higher milliamps than patients with anxiety, depression, and insomnia. Already, different frequencies have FDA "approval" for chronic pain and PMS, and the age of electromedicine seems to be dawning. Stress reduction and relaxation seem to be important benefits of CES even in normal people. Drug addiction appears to occur commonly in people with significant depression, anxiety, and insomnia. CES may be both a treatment and prophylactic device. Braverman, et al., (1990) have shown through brain mapping that many serious disorders of the brain have electrical rhythm disturbances. CES may normalize a variety of these rhythm disturbances in diverse psychiatric conditions. The brain wave, P300, is significantly improved by CES. This wave is associated with drug craving and is probably a marker for decreased attention span. Braverman, *et. al.*, have provided other data for the mechanism by which CES corrects abnormal electrophysiology of the brain.

PROPOSAL FOR PROMISING NEW AREAS OF RESEARCH

Electrical stimulation is a growing field. There are many

questions that are still unanswered, confirming the need for continued research. Few experiments have been performed on young children in general and especially on young children with learning disabilities. If CES were used at an early age maybe we could help decrease the number of individuals turning to drugs and alcohol as a way to reduce stress or forget about the responsibilities of life. If CES can help an alcoholic recover some short term memory and cognitive brain dysfunction maybe it could help with learning disabilities and stimulate the brain to possibly change processes at an early age, thus eliminating or reducing problems later in life. These are two areas requiring consideration due to the increasing problems as we see the younger generations more readily turn to drugs and alcohol.

CES CASE HISTORIES: TREATMENT-RESISTANT DEPRESSION

R. C. is a 64-year-old man who had been suffering from severe depression for 40 years. He is diagnosed as having Organic Affective Syndrome (293.83). He described the following symptoms: being full of regrets, depression, memory problems, dizziness, stomach trouble, fatigue, sexual problems, concentration difficulty, anxiety, no appetite, tremors, paranoia, abnormal fears, obsessive thoughts, mind racing, insomnia, fear of people, antisocial feelings, and feelings of being looked at. He had tried Prozac, Elavil, Thorazine, Valium, Triavil, Depakote, Tegretol, Dilantin, Wellbutrin, Xanax, and clozapine. He was addicted to Valium, and underwent over 100 ECT's. He is normal height and weight and had a normal physical exam. He has an (full scale) IQ of 115, Verbal IQ at 113 and less Verbal at 116. He has elevated cholesterol and hypoglycemia. Neurotransmitter profiles showed low platelets, epinephrine, norepinephrine, metanephrine, dopamine. An MHPG level was low at 0.4. A low level of tryptophan at 5, and of cystine at 0 was noted. Trace metals studies were normal, EKG was normal, and a stress test was normal. R. C. had a biochemical imbalance, and no neurotransmitter treatment or biochemical use of amino acids could completely restore him. He did no better on Amino Stim, a mixture of methionine phenylalanine, and tyrosine; multivitamin; an antioxidant; garlic; magnesium; calcium; and fish oil.

A Brain Electrical Activity Mapping (BEAM) study was performed and an abnormal BEAM was obtained. The EEG was moderately and diffusely slow with an excess theta anteriorly. On the auditory evoked response (AER) he had delayed first component, and on the visual evoked response (VER), an early and aberrant second component. At this point he began cranial electrical stimulation (CES). He utilized the device for a period of one year, 1-2 hours nightly, and had a remarkable result in the first few months. He remained only on Pamelor and was able to reduce his Pamelor dosage from 150 to 100 mg.

His repeat BEAM test one year later had shown a normal EEG and normal theta waves. The VER and AER were also normal. It was noted, though, that his P300 was slightly delayed at 380 milliseconds and the voltage was slow at 4.28 microvolts. These were not measured in the previous BEAM, but indicated some of the biochemical and cognitive bases for his current depression. There was a borderline excess central positivity on the AER to 2.49 standard deviations. It must be noted that he was on Pamelor during both brain mapping tests and one could not determine what his brain map would be without it. Nonetheless, this is a remarkable improvement in an individual who clearly had a brain rhythm disorder that could not be corrected by ECTs/anticonvulsants or antidepressants but was corrected by CES.

CASE HISTORIES IN CES: TREATMENT-RESISTANT HEADACHES

I. F. is a 56-year-old woman who had migraine headaches which began about 13 years ago and used to occur about twice a month, but had become more frequent over the last 4 years. She was treated by a neurologist over the last 4 years with feverfew, Elavil, Cafergot, Reglan, Meclomen, Corgard, Calan, Blocadren, Vistaril, Norgesic, Periactin, Anaprox, vanquish, with only Blocadren giving some mild relief, but primarily no great change. She had an inability to concentrate, but otherwise was in good health and felt very good about her overall life. She had normal blood testing, except for a low iron level of 20 and a decreased copper level, which was thought to be due to polyps and hemorrhoids. Strikingly, on a brain mapping test she had a normal EEG but an abnormal auditory evoked response with aberrant localization of latency with negativity in the left central parietal region instead of at the vertex. There was also excess positive activation in the right posterior temporal region. On the visual evoked response there was aberrant localization of the midlatency positivity in the right central parietal region instead of at the vertex, and excessive positive activation in the left midtemporal region. There was also excessive negative activation in the right temporal region. In March 1990, the patient started taking Depakote, 500 mg t.i.d., and received 90% relief. In July 1990, she started using the CES device, and was able to reduce the Depakote to 500 mg twice a day in the first month. After using the CES device for about 2 months, she began to lower the Depakote to 750 mg a day. In March of 1991, we repeated the BEAM and it was drama-tically improved. Instead of an extremely abnormal auditory evoked response, it was now normal, and the visual evoked response only showed a right central excess negative to 2.67 standard deviations. We cannot say with certainty that this individual's lowering of the anticonvulsant dose over a period of a year for treatment of migraine headaches was due to nightly use of CES. The objective and subjective improvement suggest that CES may be a technique to change abnormal brain maps and lower medication dosages.

Positive Effects of CES

- enhanced cognition
- reduced anxiety
- reduced depression
- reduced insomnia
- reduced withdrawal symptoms
- improved P300
- improved brain wave disturbances
- enhanced neurotransmitter functions
- relapse prevention
- prevention of substance abuse in high risk individuals

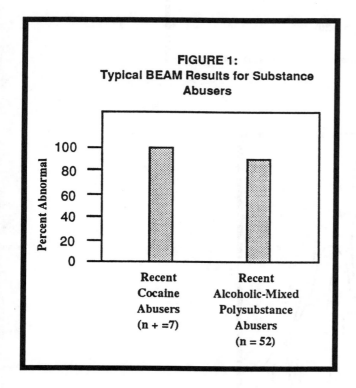

FIGURE 1:
Typical BEAM Results for Substance Abusers

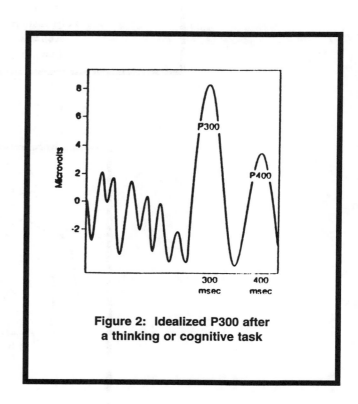

Figure 2: Idealized P300 after a thinking or cognitive task

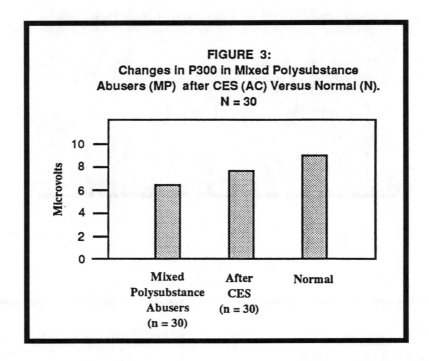

FIGURE 3:
Changes in P300 in Mixed Polysubstance
Abusers (MP) after CES (AC) Versus Normal (N).
N = 30

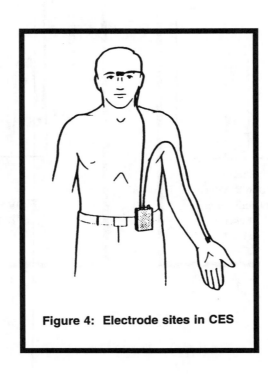

Figure 4: Electrode sites in CES

REFERENCES

Bobblit, W. E. (1969) Electrosleep as a Sleep Induction Method. *Psych Forum.* p. 9.

Braverman, E., et al., (1990) A Commentary on Brain Mapping in 60 Substance Abusers: Can the Potential for Drug Abuse be Predicted and Prevented by Treatment? *Current Therapeutic Research*, 48(4):569-585, 1990.

Braverman, et al., (1990) Modification of P300 Amplitude and Other Electrophysiological Parameters of Drug Abuse by Cranial Electrical Stimulation. *Current Therapeutic Research*, 48(4):586-596, 1990.

Budzynski, T. (1989) Cranial Electric Stimulation and the Practitioner. *CES Labs.* pp. 1-51.

Foote, S. (1987) Locus Ceruleus, George Adleman (editor) *Encycl. of Neuroscience.* pp. 596-597 (Boston, Birkhouser Inc.).

Gold, M. S. (1979) Endorphin-Locus Ceruleus Connection Mediates Opiate Action and Withdrawal. *Biomedicine* p. 1.

Gold, M. S. (1980) Clonidine in Acute Opiate Withdrawal. *NEJM.* pp. 1421-1422.

Gomez, Evaristo. (1978) Treatment of Methadone Withdrawal with Cerebral Electrotherapy (Electrosleep). *Brit J of Psych* pp. 111-113.

Krupitsky E. M, Buralov, A. M., Karandashova G. F., Katsnelson J., Lebedev, V. P., Grinenko A. J., Borodkin Jus, (1991) The Administration of Transcranial Electric Treatment for Affective Disturbances Therapy in Alcoholic Patients. *Drug and Alcohol Dependence* 27:1-6.

Philip P., Demotes-Mainard J., Bourgeois M., Vincent, J. D. (1991) Efficiency of Transcranial Electrostimulation on Anxiety and Insomnia Symptoms During a Washout Period in Depressed Patients: a Double-blind Study. *Biol Psych* 29:451-456.

Grinenko A., Drupitskiy, E. M., Lebedev V. P., (1988). Metabolism of Biogenic Amines During Treatment of Alcohol Withdrawal Syndrome by Transcranial Electric Treatment. *Biogenic Amines.* 5(6): 527-536.

Jarzembski, W. B. (1985) Electrical Stimulation and Substance Abuse Treatment. *Neurobehavioral Toxicology and Teratology.* pp. 119-123.

Kosten, Vinning E. (1988) Clinical Utility of Rapid Clonidine-Naltrexone Detoxification for Opioid Abusers. *Br J Addict.* pp. 567-577.

Kotter, GS, et al., (1975) Inhibition of Gastric Acid Secretion In Men by the Transcranial Application of Low Intensity Pulsed Current. *Gastroenterology.* pp. 359-363.

Ostrander, D. R. (1989) *CES: An Overview of the Effectiveness as a Treatment Modality.*

Schmitt, R. (1984) Cranial Electrotherapy Stimulation Treatment or Cognitive Brain Dysfunction in Chemical Dependence. *J Clin Psych.* pp. 60-63.

Smith, Ray (1975) Electrosleep in the Management of Alcoholism. *Biol Psych.* pp. 67-68.

Smith, Ray (1977) The Effects of Cerebral Electrotherapy on Short Term Memory Impairment in Alcoholic Patients. *The Intern J of Addictions.* pp. 575-582.

Smith, Ray, Cranial Electrotherapy Stimulation. Joel Myklebust (editor), *Neural Stimulation* (chapter 15, pp. 1-45). Florida: A Uniscience Publication, CRC Press, Inc.

Smith, Ray (1982) Confirming Evidence of an Effective Treatment for Brain Dysfunction in Alcoholic Patients. *J of Nervous and Mental Disease.* pp. 275-277.

Westermeyer, Joseph (1990) Rapid Opioid Detoxification with Electrosleep and Naloxone. *Amer J Psych* p. 7.

Wilson, L. F. (1988) Cranial Electrotherapy Stimulation for Attention to Task Deficit: A Case Study. *Am J Electromed.* pp. 93-99.

CES Placement Important to Health

New studies by Dr. Antonio Demazio, neurologist, University of Iowa Hospital and Clinics, showed that individuals with frontal lobe damage can no longer make ethical decisions. This fits with Dr. Henri Begleiter's original documentation that the right frontal lobe was particularly involved in drug use.

The battle for the forehead is on and we believe that the CES device can help modify the electrical activity of the frontal lobes when being worn on the main frontal spot. This can help the brain and individuals make more moral and helpful decisions. For placement see Figure 4 on p. 176.

Use of 3M Corporation CES/TENS Device

As described, the 3M CompTenz (TENS) device is a very useful electrical device currently available on the market and has the greatest health benefits for treating anxiety, depression, insomnia, drug abuse, and other organic brain diseases. The usual position when wearing the CES on the head is the left wrist and the forehead. One should note, though, that there are two channels on this device, allowing one to use the device, for example, over the abdomen for dysmenorrhea and on a muscle (e.g., for back pain) simultaneously. One channel should be selected for use as a CES (Cranial Electrical Stimulator), with electrodes placed on the forehead and left wrist over the radial pulse. The letter R stands for rate, and 100 Hz is the appropriate rate to be set for CES devices. Other rates that have been thought to be helpful are 80 Hz for drug addiction, 0.5 Hz for chronic pain, 5 to 10 and even 50 Hz for muscular pain, 15,000 (another alternative setting) for chronic pain, and even 280 for cocaine addiction. But most of the studies suggest that 100 Hz is the best frequency for anxiety, depression, insomnia, drug abuse, and organic brain disease.

Most CES devices have one to 2 millisecond pulse duration. This device will provide .25 milliseconds wavelength, which is a much shorter pulse duration. Therefore, it might be more comfortable on the head than are other devices. Shorter pulse widths for CES have no known problems but also no known benefits.

Setting the pulse width (W) at 25 (.25 milliseconds) is usually the most comfortable. Other patients find that they like it as high as 250. At a width (W) of 250 the device can be painful and frequently individuals can only tolerate it at 1/10 strength. Drug abusers and other individuals with severe organic brain diseases will be able to tolerate much higher amounts of electricity without side effects. My general recommendation is to set the width at 25 and to move gradually up the dial if this width is uncomfortable. Otherwise, the dial should be permanently set at 25. Somewhere between 15 and 35 on the intensity dial (W=25, R=100) will be tolerated by most individuals with garden variety anxiety and depression. It is important to be very cautious when handling the device because you can give yourself a shock (this is not dangerous and is very temporary) if you are not careful.

INSTRUCTIONS REVIEW

1. Electrodes -- left wrist, over radial pulse; forehead, between and slightly above eyes.
2. R -- set at 100.
3. W -- set at 25, to be moved up if no effect.
4. Amplitude or Intensity Dial - set at maximum comfort level.

TENS Settings

TENS, or Transcutaneous Electrical Nerve Stimulation, is extremely useful for a variety of pain syndromes. A complete review of this subject can be found in *Clinical Transcutaneous Nerve Stimulation* by Jeffrey S. Manheimer, M.A. and Gerald N. Lampe, B.S., published by F. A. Davis Company, 1984. They point out that there are many different parameters, such as strong, low rate acupuncture-like TENS, which is 1 to 4 hertz with a pulse width of 150 to 250 microseconds; and brief, intense TENS, which is 100 hertz with a pulse width of 150 to 250 microseconds. There are numerous rotations and placements, and there is virtually no part of the body where one cannot place the TENS unit. For temporoman-

dibular joint dysfunction and tension headache, TENS is frequently put on the temporomandibular joint and over the left hand or wrist. For cervical pain, one can put the electrodes directly on the spine or where the temporomandibular joint meets. Four electrodes can be used for certain TENS placements. One can place two electrodes on the back of the head, and both hands and the shoulders can be encapsulated by four different electrodes. TENS electrodes can be placed on the lower back region and along the back of the leg. Smaller TENS electrodes can result in greater pain relief, according to a recent study in the *Journal of Psychosomatic Research* by M. I. Johnson, et. al.

Electrical Parameters of CES Devices

UNIT	3M	SRS	HPAX
Rate (pulses/sec.)	100	100	100
Pulse Width (millisec.)	.25 ms	2 ms	2 ms
Duty Cycle	20%	20%	20%
Milliamperes	0 - 60 ma	0 - 15 ma	0 - 1.5 ma
Wave Form	Square	Sinusoidal	Square
Power Skc.	9 v.d.c.	9 v.d.c	9 v.d.c
Peak Voltage	40 - 80 v.	40 - 80 v.	40 - 80 v.

CODE:

3M = A TENS machine of 3M company

SRS = Self-Regulatory Systems CES device

HPAX = Health Pax - Health Directions Inc. CES device

Precautions

Many users report a feeling of induced relaxation while using CES. Though this relaxation response does not in any way impair reaction time, it is recommended that CES not be used while operating dangerous equipment, while driving, or in any other situation where mental alertness is required. Patients should be alerted to a possible increase in the incidence of vivid dreaming. This may be a sign of normalized or improved neurological functioning. Side effects are rare. Perhaps three persons out of one hundred have reported a slight headache when using CES. This is usually alleviated by simply turning the current down. If the headache should recur during regular use, the attending physician should be consulted.

Isolated cases of skin irritation may occur at the side of electrode placement, but this is very rare.

The physician/licensed practitioner should be informed of any changes in the medical condition of the patient while using the unit, such as pregnancy or negative changes in the patient's psychological or mental state.

A way to keep CES electrodes from drying out is to use a little bit of moisturizer on them. People have used water, but a dab of hand lotion also works.

Although the CES device can be used while watching T.V., reading, and relaxing, there may be additional benefit to using it while praying, meditating, and keeping absolutely still.

Electromedicine:
Some Frequencies of Reported Benefits

CES	MILLIAMPS 0.5-1	VOLTS 40-80	HERTZ 100	WAVE square	DUTY CYCLE 20
Seizure: Grand Mal	1.0	55	40 pps	sinusoidal	
Dental Pain	4	27	15000	square sinusoidal	50%
TENS - for muscle pain	50-100		10-200	square and more	.05-100%
Bladder	7.5			150 millisec. pulse	20 pps
Gastric Acid	0.1-1.5	57	100	sinusoidal	20%
Alcohol	0.5-1	40-57	100 110	sinusoidal square	100 pulse 20%
Hearing loss	2		7-55		
Pain	low frequency pain 1-200		1, 5, 10 Hz pulse width 200-500 millisec	sinusoidal square	4-50 pulses 90-160 width 9-350 10 pps
Alcohol withdrawal	1.5 0.5		370 80	square sinusoidal	3.5-4.0 millisec
Spinal injury	TENS				
Learning	0.15 0.25 0.6		5 pps slow theta 5 pps	square sinusoidal	100% 0.5 pps 20%
PMS	1.5	40-57	100	sinusoidal	20%
Skin healing	40		64 or 128		140 millisec
Stroke	0.25-2.3		15-50		4 sec steps 0.4-2.0 adj

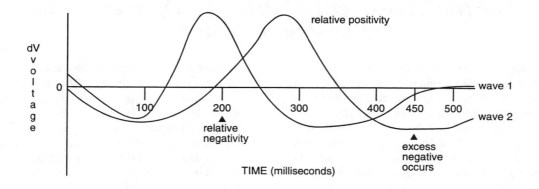

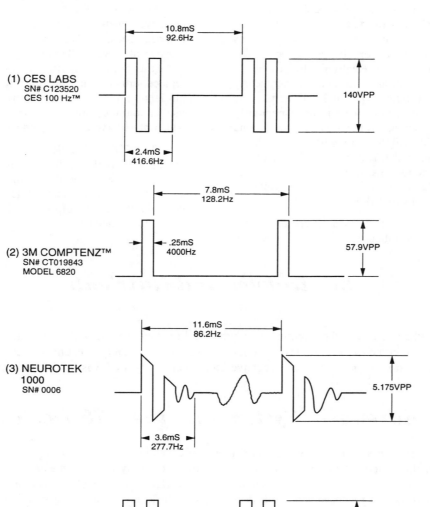

(1) CES LABS
SN# C123520
CES 100 Hz™

140VPP

(2) 3M COMPTENZ™
SN# CT019843
MODEL 6820

57.9VPP

(3) NEUROTEK
1000
SN# 0006

5.175VPP

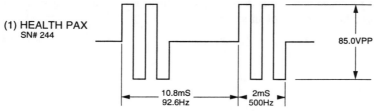

(1) HEALTH PAX
SN# 244

85.0VPP

Transcutaneous Electrical Nerve Stimulation (TENS)
For the Treatment of Primary Dysmenorrhea
(Menstrual Cramps)

Traditionally, we have been treating dysmenorrhea, or menstrual cramps, with nonsteroidal drugs such as Motrin or Ponstel. For some women it is so severe that they need to be placed on natural progesterone or birth control pills. For the women who do not obtain complete relief from pills, who have contraindications or side effects from using the nonsteroidal anti-inflammatory drugs, or who do not wish to use a medication, TENS is a new, non-drug method for relieving the pain of dysmenorrhea. A study was done using TENS for dysmenorrhea at the Department of Obstetrics and Gynecology at the University of Illinois College of Medicine. The TENS has 3 electrodes that are placed on each side of the umbilicus (belly button) and one right over the pubic area. The patient adjusts the amount of electricity to produce a comfortable tingling sensation or to achieve satisfactory pain relief. There are different types of TENS units. One unit is small enough that one can wear it inconspicuously while working or exercising. In the study that was done at Illinois, therapy with TENS also significantly reduced diarrhea, fatigue, menstrual flow, and clot formation, as compared with these conditions in women who were not using TENS. The TENS was safe and did not affect the length or amount of menstrual flow.

The reason why TENS is postulated to reduce dysmenorrhea involves two theories. One is called the gate control theory and the other is called the endorphin-mediated pain relief theory. The gate control theory is that one stimulates the sensory nerve fibers affecting the uterus, and this blocks the transmission of the pain related impulses. The second theory is the release of our natural endogenous endorphins. These endorphins are natural potent analgesics, and it has been demonstrated that these endorphins can be released with low frequency electrical stimulation. This effect may be potentiated by adding nutrients and/or medicine thought to potentiate endorphins, e.g., D-phenylalanine, Trexan. In summary, TENS is an effective method for some women in relieving dysmenorrhea. TENS also, obviously, can be used with nonsteroidal, anti-inflammatory drugs like Motrin. The nutrients, borage oil, fish oil, B-6, and magnesium, can replace drugs. In fact, the two together (TENS and nutrients) are even more effective. The TENS is a non-medication alternative that can be used for some women who want to avoid using medication.

The 3M TENS device has the dual advantage of having two outlets, allowing it to be used as a CES device. Interestingly, the setting for CES and TENS for dysmenorrhea is the same 100 Hz, 25 (.25 msec.) width or pulse duration. Therefore, this device can be used in two ways simultaneously.

Electrolytes and Nutrients

Without electrolytes and nutrients and the electricity they produce, life would be impossible. Electrolytes are compounds that, when dissolved, dissociate into charged particles called ions. These act as a battery, creating an electrical charge. The human body is like a machine that runs on positive and negative ions. Your body's CES is by the intercompartmental movement of electrolytes.

Adrenalin System and the CES Device

Children who watch television are exposed to approximately 70,000 violent murder scenes per year. This overstimulation "burns out" their adrenalin system. Neurotransmitters in the central nervous system become depleted and a craving for drugs which provide quick relief occurs. Drugs like alcohol, nicotine, caffeine and the like are commonly abused to help this "burned out" state. A substitute for these dangerous drugs is the CES device. Our next generation of children will depend on our guidance in a mega information, mega violent society.

11. Endocrinology

Aging Reversal Services

The PATH to wellness also has a PATH to longevity. Research has shown that male menopause can be treated with natural hormones, natural estrogens and natural progesterones, leading to increased longevity.

We now know that both males and females have adrenopause. When the adrenal gland falls asleep it can be awakened with natural adrenal DHEA and revitalization will follow.

Aging will never be the same again. People will have more active and abundant lives with greater strength, lower cholesterol, reduced heart disease, and improved sex lives from these natural hormone therapies. In addition, PATH Medical uses only natural thyroid therapies to help in maintaining body hemostasis.

Adrenal Gland Stress Tests

As we are able to stress the pancreas with a glucose tolerance test, the thyroid with a thyroid-stimulating test, the brain with a brain map, the heart with a stress thallium, we are also able to detect subtle abnormalities in the adrenal gland through the adrenal stress test. This ACTH rapid stimulation test requires 250 mg. of I. M. ACTH or adrenal corticotrophic hormone. Initially we draw a baseline cortisol, then inject ACTH. Then we draw another 30-minute baseline cortisol and then a baseline cortisol at 60 minutes.

It is probably also useful to do this test in conjunction with a urinary free cortisol test, but at a different time, in which you collect a 24-hour urine in a plastic bottle containing boric acid preservative. We need a 100 mg aliquot of a 24-hour urine sample and the total volume of the 24 hours.

These are both excellent tests of the functioning of the adrenal gland. Some individuals with treatment-resistant depressions or anxiety may need to be treated with Cortef (hydroxycortisone 5 mg, 4 times per day, which may be a safer form of steroid than prednisone).

New Testing for Blood Sugar Tolerance

There are numerous new tests to identify blood sugar besides the glucose tolerance test which is very difficult to take. Hemoglobin A1C evaluates blood sugar over three months, fructosamine levels evaluate blood sugar over one month, fasting blood sugar evaluates blood sugar over a given day and glucose tolerance test reveals the pancreas's ability to manage sugar stress. Hence, it is a pancreas stress test. Other ways to identify abnormalities in blood sugar relate to measuring insulin, protein bound glucose, and C peptides. Blood sugar abnormalities, particularly hypoglycemia and diabetes, impact brain mapping. Hypo-glycemic individuals will have lower P300 waves on a BEAM test and can look like alcoholics, schizophrenics, or attention deficit individuals during low blood sugar attacks on their health. Diabetics develop microvascular disease and can have brain maps like individuals with Alzheimer's, especially when they are poorly controlled diabetics and develop advanced blood vessel disease. Abnormal blood sugar affects the brain and the brain impacts blood sugar regulation through the control of the brain catecholamine synthesis.

Natural Steroid Therapy

Natural steroid therapy for aging glands is now available because of three independent research discoveries. One form of therapy is the use of hydrocortisone, rather than prednisone, in divided dosages up to 20 mg., which has been shown to have no side effects. The second is dehydroepiandrosterone (DHEA), a natural micronized therapy; and the third is injectable natural testosterone that stays in the system for two to three weeks. Along with Armour thyroid and natural estrogen and progesterone, these represent a host of improvements in therapy.

What is Aging? -- The Signs of Aging

The rate of aging varies enormously among individuals and even among different organs in the same individual. Nevertheless, some changes predictably occur in most humans.

1. **Memory** -- Often fades slightly in normal people in midlife, P300 test voltage goes down, time slows.

2. **Personality** -- No changes after 30 except through psychotherapy or dementing illness. Personality disorders worsen.

3. **Sense of smell** -- Declines slowly at age 45 and faster after 65. Vitamins like choline may help.

4. **Thymus** -- Begins to shrink at puberty. Immune response declines slowly. Antioxidants may help.

5. **Lungs** -- 40 percent drop in maximum breathing capacity between age 20 and 70. Aerobic exercises help. Pulmonary function tests predict longevity.

6. **Muscles** -- 20 percent to 40 percent of mass may be lost between 20 and 90 with lack of exercise; exercise prevents most loss. Growth hormone and amino acids may help.

7. **Ovaries** -- Dramatically slow production of estrogen, progesterone, and testosterone after 50.

8. **Blood vessels** -- Diameter of vessels narrows, arterial walls stiffen, 20-25 percent increase in systolic blood pressure. This can be tested by Doppler and treated with chelation and nutrients.

9. **Pituitary gland and hypothalamus** -- Secretion of growth hormone declines at 50, causing muscles to shrink and fat to increase. Nutrients and CES may help.

10. **Sight** -- Increased difficulty seeing nearby objects begins in the 40's. Ability to see fine detail does not deteriorate until the 70's.

11. **Hearing** -- Begins to decline about 20, and worsens faster in men than women.

12. **Bones** -- Begin to weaken after 40 through osteoporosis, especially in women. Hormones, calcium and other nutrients may help.

13. **Heart** -- No decline in resting output. Twenty percent decline in maximum rate during exercise after age 40 because the heart becomes less responsive to stimulation from the nervous system. Exercise and nutrients help.

14. **Adrenal glands** -- After 30, secretion of DHEA, which slows cancer and boosts immunity, declines; and after 70, production of the stress hormone cortisol soars. Supplementation of hormones and nutrients and even hydroxycortisone may help.

15. **Skin** -- Changes in collagen, a connective tissue, cause skin to lose elasticity in later years. Retin A and nutrients help.

16. **Nerves** -- Speed of messages along nerves drops 10 percent between age 40 and 80. CES and nutrients may help.

Breaking the Aging Barrier

Our quest to contribute to breaking the aging barrier continues at PATH as part of the long-standing biblical dream. As was written in the book of Isaiah, men will live to 100, and he who dies before 100 will be considered cursed (Isaiah 65). It now appears that the pausing of the various hormone systems in the body can be stopped so individuals can essentially stay at 50 years of age hormonally with natural adrenal hormone substitution DHEA, natural sex steroid hormone, testosterone with or without estrogens and progesterones, growth hormone which is now available in Mexico, and of course thyroid hormone which has long been available. It would appear that these hormonal manipulations will greatly slow down and retard the aging process while improving quality of life.

In addition, it is being studied why at puberty the thymus gland begins to diminish in function and whether or not thymus extract can be another intervention to slow the aging process.

We look forward to genetic repair as a way of reversing the aging process, and we hope that PATH Medical will continue to be on the forefront of slowing down the dying process. We will keep you posted as these things develop and hope you benefit from the natural hormone supplementation program at PATH which is being realized by patients all across New Jersey and the tri-state area.

Eldepryl and Brain Aging

Eldepryl is a new anti-aging of the brain breakthrough. Eldepryl has been used to slow down the development of Parkinson's. It's a powerful selective inhibitor of monoamine oxidase enzyme, MAO-B inhibitor enzyme which breaks down dopamine compounds when they are excreted. As we age, there is a rise in this MAO level which results in increasing depression, Parkinson's, Alzheimer's, and other aging of the brain. Dopamine producing neurons may be destroyed or made dysfunctional as a result of the side effects of the dopamine metabolism. Eldepryl inhibits the activity of one of the prime breakdown enzymes.

Eldepryl also protects dopaminergic neurons from toxicity caused by certain pesticides in chemicals, notably MPTP, and street drugs. Therefore, indirectly, Eldepryl may slow down the entire aging process.

Not until 80 percent of the brain cells are destroyed do we even begin to see the symptoms of Parkinson's disease. Basically most brain diseases don't show up until very, very late. The idea is prevention.

Eldepryl is a mild antidepressant, mild sexual stimulant, a prevention for Parkinson's, Alzheimer's and probably a total anti-brain aging therapy.

Tofranil Protocol

Dr Braverman's Tofranil protocol is Klonopin, one pill QHS 0.5 mg with Tofranil 25 mg. Add one pill of Tofranil every week until 100 mg. QHS is reached. If any symptom occurs, e.g., an increase in anxiety or any unusual feeling at all, go to Klonopin two with a Tofranil

dose. If symptoms are present, you can increase the dosage to three Klonopin. If there are any problems that are not included in this protocol, please call the office immediately.

DHEA Deficiency is also a Factor in Control of Blood Pressure and Heart Disease

New Studies show that the higher the concentration of DHEA, the less likely the man will have impotence. A study by Robert F. McGivern of Harbor UCLA Medical Center in the January 1990 issue of Teratology suggested that post-magnetic fields, low frequency, might result in demasculinization and that EMF may be another environmental feminizer which can be estrogenically producing cancer for women and affecting male health.

A new study reviewed in the January 8, 1994 issue of Science News that 39% of men with heart disease and 15% of men with hypertension had impotence. The most significant factor was not testosterone but DHEA. We are one of the first clinics to do DHEA blood testing on all men between 50 and 70, and we have been able to identify that low levels of this natural adrenal hormone result in a variety of problems, such as sexual dysfunction, premature aging, inability to handle stress. Essentially this is a state called adrenopause.

Male Menopause (Andropause)

Male menopause occurs in men over time. It probably begins anywhere from age 30 to 50, when men start losing DHEA (dehydroepoendostrione, pronounced dee-hi-dro-ep-ee-an-dro-ster-own) as well as levels of testosterone, free and total, and growth hormone diminishes and insulin increases. This is similar to what happens with women where their ovaries and adrenal glands start to deteriorate and get fewer signals from the hypothalamus and the aging/dying cycle begins. Both men and women can start replacing DHEA at early stages in their lives and may eventually be able to do low dose growth hormone replacement. Such replacements will result in a slowing of the aging process.

Male Menopause

New studies again highlight how common male menopause is. Men over 50 can have tremendous improvement with injections of male hormone. They may experience improvement in strength, balance, red blood cell count, lowering cholesterol, and reduction of angina, according to a study by Dr. Shi of St. Louis University School of Medicine, presented at the American Geriatric Society.

One of the main reasons for male menopause may be the estrogen producing and/or imitating pesticides.

Weekly testosterone shots are extremely successful. Men on these hormone shots, natural testosterone injection, also available in pill form, have significantly larger muscles, better strength and are significantly stronger than those individuals given placebo, as well as having lower cholesterol.

A similar study done by Dr. Phillips at Roosevelt St. Luke's Hospital in Manhattan showed that men have reduced heart attack risk when taking testosterone. He also confirms safety and effectiveness. There was no increase in prostate problems identified.

The amount of testosterone correlated with high density lipoproteins which protect against arteriosclerosis. It has been suggested that taking saw palmetto herb or zinc with testosterone will diminish the potential risk, if any, of prostate enlargement.

Patients are less likely to develop angina when taking the testosterone. Incidents of heart attacks increases as testosterone goes down. Better regulation of blood sugar may occur with men who take testosterone supplements. Men with angina have lower levels of testosterone.

These articles appeared in a scientific journal published by the American Heart Association (*Arteriosclerosis and Thrombosis*).

Several other studies have also shown that the administration of testosterone results in decreased risks of heart attacks. The correlation of low testosterone and coronary artery disease is now highly significant and relatively well established.

Adrenopause

More research has been done on adrenopause as we now start to better understand what dying is. Dying is the death of various glands, particularly those that are distant from the brain which are the source of life such as the testicles, ovaries, adrenal gland, thyroid and the pancreas, which produces growth hormone.

A paper presented at the American Psychiatric Association (subdivision Biological Psychiatry) submitted by Dr. Russe at the University of California at San Francisco showed that DHEA is low in people with declining memory and aging. Preliminary data has shown that cognitively impaired individuals have lower levels of this hormone and that therapeutic trials were recommended. These substances, DHEA and DHEAS (the sulphated form), are both low in individuals with aging memory problems as well as in individuals with depression.

DHEA -- Adrenopause:
Protecting Your Brain

At the American Psychiatric Association, Biological Psychiatry Division, a new study was presented showing that low levels of DHEA are associated with memory loss and cognitive deficits. 50 mg per day in individuals over 50 has remarkable effects on well being. [1] Low DHEA, like low thyroid hormone, is a marker of aging and dying.

DHEA and Adrenopause:
A New Sign of Aging and a New Treatment

We have all heard for a long time about menopause, where the ovary goes to sleep and no longer makes the hormones estrogen, progesterone, or testosterone. We can now raise this gland from the dead, so to speak, with natural estrogens, progesterones, and testosterones. In the case of the thyroid gland, many people go into thyropause, where natural hormone replacement is necessary for thyroid, T3 and T4. Male menopause is now also thought to be common, where men lose their sexual hormone functioning because they do not have adequate sex hormones. Without the natural testosterone, men can develop intellectual slowing and abdominal obesity associated with heart disease, as well as decreased sexual function.

Soon, growth hormone given for pancreopause, reviving a sleeping pancreas, should be more readily available.

There is now a condition known as adrenopause, where the adrenal glands seem to become depleted. This eventually occurs in autoimmune diseases of all types, such as multiple sclerosis, lupus, psoriasis, eczema, arthritis, and allergy conditions.

Probably some safe use of steroids, such as low dosages (5 mg, 4 times/day) of hydroxy cortisone can help the ailing adrenal gland. Adrenal stress tests may help identify the gland's reserve capacity and health.

A common phenomenon associated with aging, arthritis, cancer, obesity, diabetes, lowered immune system, susceptibility to infection, estrogen deficiency, prevention of Alzheimer's disease, and osteoporosis is the loss of the adrenal hormone called DHEA (dehydroepiandrosterone). DHEA is deficient in people as they age, and right before dying fails to remarkably low levels and is really in some ways an indication of overall bodily health. We believe that this new condition of adrenopause (where at least DHEA is deficient) must be treated when it usually occurs between the ages of 60 and 70.

---

1. Arlene J. Morales, et al., Effects of Replacement Dose of Dehydroepiandrosterone in Men and Women of Advancing Age, *Journal of Clinical Endocrinology and Metabolism*, vol. 78, #6, 1994.

DHEA is a steroid hormone produced by the adrenal glands. It is the most abundant steroid in the human bloodstream. Research has suggested that it may have significant antiobesity, anti-cancer, and anti-aging effects. DHEA blood levels drop naturally as people age. Additionally, DHEA, like the hormones estrogen and progesterone, may have an important role in cognitive enhancement.

DHEA protects brain cells from Alzheimer's disease and many other degenerative conditions. Nerve degeneration may occur readily under low DHEA conditions. Brain tissue naturally contains 6.5 times more DHEA than is found in other tissues. By adding low concentrations of DHEA to nerve cell tissue cultures, we can increase the number of neurons, their ability to establish contacts, and their differentiation. DHEA may also enhance long-term memory in mice. Perhaps it plays a similar role in human brain function.

Low levels in obesity are common as are high insulin levels and low growth hormone levels. DHEA may be an alternative for estrogen-intolerant individuals.

DHEA is now being administered to Alzheimer's patients in scientific studies. People with Alzheimer's may have 48 percent less DHEA than matched controls of the same age. DHEA may be low in other degenerative diseases, e.g., diabetes, Parkinson's, etc. DHEA deficiency probably should be treated in most cases.

In conclusion, today's medicine is slowly attempting to revive worn out body parts starting with dead glands like testicles, ovaries, thyroids, adrenal glands, and even the pancreas.

Reprinted from *Total Health*, February, 1994.

DHEA -- Treatment for Obesity and Adrenopause

DHEA or dehydroepiandrosterone (pronounced dee-hi-dro-ep-ee-an-dro-ster-own) is a steroid hormone produced by the adrenal glands. DHEA is the most abundant steroid in the human bloodstream. Research has suggested that it may have significant antiobesity, anti-cancer, and anti-aging effects. DHEA blood levels drop naturally as people age. Additionally, DHEA, like estrogen and progesterone, may have an important role in cognitive enhancement. Deficiency in various adrenal hormones, including DHEA, is probably linked to depression.

DHEA protects brain cells from Alzheimer's disease and other degenerative conditions. Nerve degeneration may occur readily under low DHEA conditions. Brain tissues naturally contains 6.5 times more DHEA than is found in other tissues. By adding low concentrations of DHEA to nerve cell tissue cultures we can increase the number of neurons, their ability to establish contacts and their differentiation. DHEA may also enhance long term memory in mice. Perhaps it plays a similar role in human brain function. Low levels in obesity are common as are high insulin levels and low growth hormone levels. DHEA may be an alternative for estrogen intolerant individuals.

DHEA is now being administered to Alzheimer's patients in scientific studies. People with Alzheimer's may have 48% less DHEA than matched controls of the same age. DHEA may be low in other degenerative diseases, e. g., diabetes, Parkinson's, etc. DHEA deficiency probably should be treated in most cases.

Update on DHEA

New studies on DHEA show that women with Lupus may experience relief of rashes, joint pain, headaches, and fatigue taking 50 to 200 mg of DHEA. The only side effect is that sometimes there is some mild acne.

DHEA has also been thought to limit burn damage. Aging mice and animals of all types do better with DHEA, which seems to help the immune system.

The *Harvard Health Letter* of July, 1994 says much work has been done with DHEA; Too much to ignore it as a major therapy for all sorts of illnesses and chronic diseases.

DHEA Supplements

The Department of Psychiatry, University of California is now recommending DHEA supplements upon failure of memory test or memory loss with depression (*Biol Psychiatry*, pp. 615-747, 1994).

DHEA and Other Hormones:
Availability

A prescription is required. In order to obtain DHEA and other hormones, a written prescription from an M.D. or D.O. is required.

Sources:

Medical Center Pharmacy
10721 Main Street
Fairfax VA 22030

1-800-723-7455 or 1-703-273-7311; FAX 1-703-591-3604

Hopewell Pharmacy	**Warren County Pharmacy**
1 West Broad Street	13 E. Washington Ave.
Hopewell NJ 08525	Washington NJ 07882
(609) 466-1960	(908) 689-0036
FAX (609) 466-8222	FAX (908) 835-0633

The charts on the next page list hormonal preparations available from the above three pharmacies, with approximate prices. Prices are listed here for your convenience, but are subject to change without notice. Shipping charges are additional.

An additional source of DHEA is:

College Pharmacy
833 North Tejon Street
Colorado Springs CO 80903

(800) 888-9358

The most common strengths, with prices subject to change without notice, in quantities of 100, are:

25 mg $77.50
50 mg $90.00
100 mg $145.00

Shipping charges are additional. Also, COD is available for a charge. For orders over $100.00 a small insurance charge is made.

PRODUCT	STRENGTH	FAIRFAX	HOPEWELL	WARREN
DHEA	10 mg	$34.00	$32.00	$32.00
	25 mg	$44.00	$40.00	$40.00
	50 mg	$58.50	$55.00	$55.00
	100 mg	$99.00	$95.00	$95.00
Progesterone	100 mg	$49.00	$49.00	$49.00
	200 mg	$59.00	$59.00	$59.00
	300 mg	$69.00	$69.00	$69.00
	400 mg	$79.00	$79.00	$79.00
Testosterone	2.5 mg	$23.50		
	5 mg	$25.50	$23.50	$23.50
	10 mg	$26.50	$25.00	$25.00
	25 mg	$29.50	$27.50	$27.50
	50 mg	$49.00	$45.00	$45.00
	75 mg	$69.00	$65.00	$65.00
	100 mg	$79.00	$75.00	$75.00
Estradiol	0.5 mg	$29.50	$25.50	$25.50

PRODUCT	STRENGTH	FAIRFAX	HOPEWELL	WARREN
Estradiol/ Estriol	0.5 mg 0.1 mg	$49.50	$47.00	$47.00
Estradiol/ Progesterone	0.5 mg 100 mg	$59.00	$57.00	$57.00
Estrone/ Progesterone	0.1 mg 100 mg	$79.00	$76.00	$76.00
Progesterone/ Estradiol/ Testosterone	100 mg 0.5 mg 25 mg	$89.00	$85.00	$85.00
Progesterone/ Estradiol/ Testosterone	100 mg 0.5 mg 5 mg	$69.00	$65.00	$65.00
Progesterone/ Estradiol/ Testosterone	100 mg 0.5 mg 2.5 mg	$59.00	$55.00	$55.00

DHEA References

GENERAL REFERENCES

Orentreich, N., et al., Age changes and sex differences in serum dehydroepiandrosterone sulfate concentrations throughout adulthood. *J. Clin. Endocrinology Metab.*, 1984; 59:551-555.

Kent, S., DHEA: "Miracle" drug? *Geriatrics,* 1982; 37:157-161.

Schwartz, A. G., Dehydroepiandrosterone: an anti-cancer and possible anti-aging substance, in *Intervention in the Aging Process: Part A.* (W. Regelson and M. Sinex, eds.), 1983; Alan R. Liss: New York, pp. 266-278.

Barrett-Connor, E., et al., A prospective study of dehydroepiandrosterone sulfate, mortality, and cardiovascular disease. *New Engl. J. Med.,* 1986; 315:1519-1524.

Nestler, J. E., Dehydroepiandrosterone reduces serum low density lipoprotein levels and body fat but does not alter insulin sensitivity in normal men. *J. Clin. Endocrinology and Metab.,* 1988; 66:57-61.

ARTHRITIS

Cutolo, M., et al., Androgen replacement therapy in male patients with rheumatoid arthritis. *Arthritis and Rheumatism,* 1991; 34:1-5.

Sambrook, J. A., et al., Sex hormone status and osteoporosis in postmenopausal women with rheumatoid arthritis. *Arthritis and Rheumatism,* 1988; 31:973-8.

Cutolo, M., et al., Sex hormone status of male patients with rheumatoid arthritis: evidence of low serum concentrations of testosterone at baseline and after human chorionic gonadotropin stimulation. *Arthritis and Rheumatism,* 1988; 31:1314-7.

CANCER

Bulbrook, R. D., et al., Relation between urinary androgen and corticoid excretion and subsequent breast cancer. *Lancet,* 1971; 2:395-398.

Schwartz, A. G., Dehydroepiandrosterone and structural analogs: a new class of cancer chemopreventive agents. *Advances in Cancer Research,* 1988; 51:391-424.

Pashdo, L. L., et al., Inhibition of DNA synthesis in mouse epidermis and breast epithelium by dehydroepiandrosterone and related steroids. *Carcinogenesis,* 1981; 2:717-21.

Nyce, J. W., et al., Inhibition of 1,2 dimethylhydrazine-induced colon tumorigenesis in Balb/c mice by dehydroepiandrosterone. *Carcinogenesis,* 1984; 5:57-62.

Schwartz, A. G., et al., Inhibition of 7,12-dimethyl-benz (a) anthracene and urethane-induced lung tumor formation in A/J mice by long-term treatment with dehydroepiandrosterone. *Carcinogenesis,* 1981; 2:1335-1337.

DIABETES

Coleman, D. L., et al., Therapeutic effects of dehydroepiandrosterone (DHEA) in diabetic mice. *Diabetes,* 1982; 31:830-833.

Coleman, D. L., et al., Effect of genetic background on the therapeutic effects of dehydroepiandrosterone (DHEA) in diabetes-obesity mutants in aged normal mice. *Diabetes,* 1984; 33:26.

Coleman, D. L., et al., Antiobesity effects of etiocholanolones in diabetes (db), viable yellow (A) and normal mice. *Endocrinology,* 1985; 117:2279-2283.

Coleman, D. L., et al., Therapeutic effects of dehydroepiandrosterone metabolites in diabetes mutant mice (C57BL/KaJ-db/db). *Endocrinology,* 1984; 115:239-243.

IMMUNE SYSTEM ENHANCEMENT

Loria, R. M., et al., Protection against acute lethal viral infections with the native steroid dehydroepiandrosterone (DHEA). *J. Medical Virology,* 1988; 26:301-314.

Lucas, J. A., et al., Prevention of autoantibody formation and prolonged survival in New Zealand Black/New Zealand White

F1 Mice fed dehydroepiandrosterone. *J. Clinical Invest.* 1985; 75:2091.

Henderson, E., *et al.,* Dehydroepiandrosterone and 16α-bromo-epiandrosterone: inhibitors of Epstein-Barr virus-induced transformation of human lymphocytes. *Carcinogenesis,* 1981; 2:683-686.

IMPROVED BRAIN FUNCTION

Flood, J. F., *et al.,* Dehydroepiandrosterone and its sulfate enhance memory retention in mice. *Brain Research,* 1988; 447:269-278.

Rudman, D., *et al.,* Plasma dehydroepiandrosterone sulfate in nursing home men. *J. Am. Geriatrics Soc.,* 1990; 38:421-427.

Bologa, L., *et al.,* Dehydroepiandrosterone and its sulfated derivative reduce neuronal death and enhance astrocytic differentiation in brain cell cultures. *J. Neuroscience Res.,* 1987; 17:225-234.

Roberts, E., *et al.,* Effects of dehydroepiandrosterone and its sulfate on brain tissue in culture and on memory in mice. *Brain Research,* 1987; 406:357-362.

INFECTION

Ben-Nathan, D., *et al.,* Protection by dehydroepiandrosterone in mice infected with viral encephalitis. *Arch. Virol.,* 1991; 120:263-271.

Moore, M. A., *et al.,* Early lesions induced by DHPN in Syrian golden hamsters: influence of concomitant Opisthorchis infestation, dehydroepiandrosterone or butylated hydroxyanisole administration. *Carcinogenesis,* 1988; 9:1185-1189.

OBESITY

Tagliaferro, A. A., *et al.,* The effect of dehydroepiandrosterone (DHEA) on calorie intake, body weight, and resting metabolism. *Federation Proc.* (abstract 201), 1983; 42:326.

Yen, T. T., *et al.,* Prevention of obesity in A vy/a mice by dehydroepiandrosterone. *Lipids,* 1977; 12:409-413.

Yoshimoto, D., *et al.,* Reciprocal effects of epidermal growth factor on key lipogenic enzymes in primary cultures of adult cat hepatocytes. Induction of glucose-6-phosphate dehydrogenase and suppression of malic enzyme and lipogenesis. *J. Biol. Chem.,* 1983; 258:12355-12360.

OSTEOPOROSIS

Buchanan, J. R., *et al.,* Effect of excess endogenous androgens on bone density in young women. *J. Clin. Endocrin. Metab.,* 1988; 67:937-943.

Drucker, W. D., Biological activity and metabolism of androgenic hormones: the role of the adrenal androgens. *Bull. N. Y. Acad. Med.,* 1977; 53:347-358.

ALZHEIMER'S/PARKINSON'S DISEASE

Nasman, R., *et al.,* Serum dehydroepiandrosterone sulfate in Alzheimer's disease and in multi-infarct dementia. *Biol. Psychiatry,* 1991; 30:684-690.

Regelson, W., *et al.,* Hormonal intervention: "buffer hormones" or "State dependency." The role of dehydroepiandrosterone (DHEA), thyroid hormone, estrogen and hypophysectomy in aging. *Ann. N. Y. Acad. Sci.,* 1988; 521:260-273.

Sunderland, T., *et al.,* Reduced plasma dehydroepiandrosterone concentrations in Alzheimer's disease. *The Lancet,* 1989; 2:570.

SUBSTITUTE FOR ESTROGEN REPLACEMENT

Cumming, D. C., *et al.,* Evidence for an influence of the ovary on circulating dehydroepiandrosterone sulfate levels. *J. Clin. Endocrin. Metab.,* 1982; 54:1069-1071.

Lebeau, M. C., *et al.,* On the significance of the metabolism of steroid hormone conjugates. In: *Metabolic Conjugation and Metabolic Hydrolysis* (W. H. Fishman, ed). 1973, Academic Press, NY; vol. 3, pp. 151-187.

Leifer, E. H., *et al.,* Androgenic and estrogenic metabolites in serum of mice fed dehydroepiandrosterone: relationship to antihyperglycemic effects. *Metabolism,* 1987; 36:863-869.

Melatonin: A Modified Amino Acid

Melatonin is a hormone produced by the brain's pineal gland, a light-sensitive gland that is sometimes referred to as our third eye. Melatonin is relatively benign in nature and low in toxicity. Some people think it shrinks tumors when taken in high doses. Unfortunately it is very difficult to obtain. Twenty and 30 mg pills are available by prescription; in some cases as much as 80 to 250 mg have been used to help individuals sleep and to regulate the hormonal cycle. Melatonin is now available in pure form and should not be purchased in any other form. It may help lower blood pressure in that it can relax, calm, reduce stress, and help improve sleep. It also may relieve heart cancer and decrease other cancer risks and development.

Melatonin is derived from the amino acid tryptophan by the action of two enzymes in the pineal gland. Dietary tryptophan is converted in the body to serotonin. Serotonin is then converted to melatonin by the enzymes N-aceytl-transferase (NAT) and Hydroxy-indol-o-methyl transferase (HIOMT). In essence, melatonin is a modified amino acid whose rate limiting step is NAT.

Human production of melatonin was thought to be independent of external light because melatonin levels did not increase in response to room light.

By 1980, it was shown that substantially brighter light, 2,500 lux or five times the usual intensity of room light was necessary to inhibit human melatonin production. Subsequent studies show that daily melatonin production could be shifted by timing bright light stimulus. Bright light scheduled in the morning advanced the melatonin rhythm, shifted the onset to an earlier time (wake up early, go to bed early). Bright light scheduled in the evening delayed it, so people stayed up later. We believe that the melatonin cycle best reflects the phase of internal circadian pacemaker. No surprise, the pineal gland was thought to be the seat of the soul (by Rene Descartes) at least it's the seat of the circadian rhythms!

Production of melatonin from the pineal glands stimulated by sympathetic neuro output from the super chiasmatic nuclei. Melatonin production begins in the evening, sometimes after dusk, somewhere around 8:00 pm and it peaks at about 12:00 and has another peak at about 4 am, and finally should be gone by 6 am. Morning melatonin levels are low daytime concentrations, although people differ at onset. Each individual variability is minimal.

Melatonin production is a useful marker for understanding the entire circadian rhythm pacemaking. If subjects are kept in dim light 30 to 50 lux, they avoid suppression of melatonin production. And bright white light can be used to shift cycles. If you take the melatonin around 8:00 at night you are getting a boost to your melatonin production. You are more likely to fall asleep and get into a deeper sleep. If you take it too late, you might find yourself waking up in the morning as if you are sleeping (the sleep hormone effect) but feeling as if it was four in the morning physically. So you must be careful with melatonin so that you don't get yourself into too deep a sleep because what it does is it puts your whole body to sleep. It can shift your entire sleep phase. So if you arrive on a jet lag and it's 2 am and you want to get to your destination time (say, California time, if you live in New York) you can start taking it right away at 8 pm at your destination time, or you can take it earlier on your plane ride and put yourself to sleep. Ten milligrams is frequently enough, others need 10 to 80 milligrams.

Light suppresses melatonin production in human beings, and therefore melatonin production seems to go up in the winter leading to some people having depression. On the other hand, if you take the melatonin earlier and get people sleeping better, sometimes you can avoid the winter depression. Early morning light, 2500 to 10,000 lux maybe is another way to get people out of the winter blues, gently nudging the sleep cycle. During this winter depression cycle, patients may appear to be bipolar type II, temporal lobe disorder or atypical depression. This of course, represents brain chemical imbalance which also occurs in the aged with low urinary melatonin metabolite secretion.

Melatonin Deficiency

A recent article (July, 1994) in the British Medical Journal, concluded that melatonin deficiency appeared to be a key factor in the incidence of sleep disorders among the elderly. It was further concluded that melatonin replacement therapy may in fact prove beneficial.

This article refers to a study in which patients with insomnia were found to have significantly lower peak levels of 6-Sulphatoxy-melatonin secretion, with delayed onset and peak times. Furthermore, elderly patients without sleep disorders were found to have no significant difference in melatonin secretion. This fact, once again, indicates that melatonin is strongly related to sleep disorders.

In addition, it was hypothesized that the lack of bright light in institutions may lead to a decrease in secretion of 6-Sulphatoxy-melatonin during one's elderly years.

Biological Rhythms

Plants can tell time and they are very sensitive to how long a day is. Leaves fall when the days shorten, and flowers usually bloom when the days lengthen. A plant in shade will grow spindly and tall, while one in full sunlight will grow more robust and shorter. Plants like humans tell time by distinguishing between light and dark. Light is perceived by pigments that plants have which are very similar to our hemoglobin pigments. Our body also tells time and is reactive to light through which it is mediated by our pigment center such as the chemical hormone melatonin, a derivative melanin from the pineal gland which is associated with biological rhythms. Many individuals experience seasonal affective disorder, which can be a neurobiochemical imbalance associated with imbalances of tryptophan, melatonin, phenylalanine, and tyrosine. Some renowned researchers suggest that white light can be useful in seasonal disorders. Others are even looking at different colored lights such as green, blue, and red to modify mood swings. Green and blue lights are supposed to be relaxing, while red light may be stimulating (adequate documentation of these effects is not available yet). We do know that fluorescent lighting can cause fatigue and hyperactivity and full spectrum lighting can affect our moods positively. Electromagnetic pollution varies throughout our society in the forms of video screens, electric blankets, power lines, etc., which are affecting behavior and causing anxiety associated with depression, etc. Like air and electromagnetic fields, light is another "nutrient" which affects our total health. Those who are affected by changes in light should put full spectrum lighting in their homes and evaluate the nutrients which may be beneficial to modify mood swings associated with changes in light, such as melatonin (chronoset). The benefits of chronoset may be further than just biological rhythms associated with changes in light and darkness because chronoset also may benefit the individual who suffers from Jet lag and PMS. Some people with fluctuating biological rhythms have neurological conditions on BEAM which respond to anticonvulsants and even medicines for manic depressive illness. Offer natural agents which may help with rhythm problems in the brain are GABA, taurine, melatonin, manganese, and possibly adenosine.

Hypothyroidism: Notes on Iodine and Thyroid

Hypothyroidism is the most common biochemical imbalance of the body that affects behavior and brain chemistry. Hypothyroidism commonly results in fatigue, depression, anxiety, mood swings, constipation, and irritability. Hypothyroidism can even present itself to the doctor's office as a pseudodementia. (Hyperthyroidism, although frequently marked by weight loss, can also be marked by the same symptoms of depression and anxiety.) Other symptoms of hypothyroidism may be heart disease, elevated cholesterol, lowered HDL, lowered triglycerides, and poor focus. Hypothyroidism is a very common illness. It can be identified by a thyroid stress test which is often called the Thyroid Stimulation Test. The Thyroid Stimulation Test is to the thyroid as a stress test is to the heart.

Hypothyroidism is probably common in our society because of excess iodine in our foods (especially fast foods) and as a result of soy milk infant formulas and lack of breast milk feeding. Hypothyroidism has also been linked to autoimmune disorders and may be a symptom of immune imbalance. Thyroid disorders are extremely commonplace and all patients need thyroid screening at least once a year.

Other causes of thyroid disorders include radiation exposure. Frequently patients who had cancer (e. g., Hodgkins) for which they were radiated later developed hypothyroidism. Toxins (e. g., lead, cadmium, aluminum) in our environment may be linked more and more to hypothyroidism. Certainly goitrogen foods such as cabbage, spinach, and kale can lower the thyroid function but have not frequently been implicated in hypothyroid disease. Fish is certainly beneficial. Kelp may be beneficial. Excessive dosage of iodine supplement is certainly harmful. Normal iodine supplements and low dose thyroid replacement in normal individuals probably reduces cancer risk (particularly breast). Although iodine supplements have beneficial effects in some individuals they can worsen acne.

Thyroid Hormones and Iodine

Abnormalities in thyroid hormones are the most common endocrinological problems that affect behavior. The thyroid hormone gets its instructions from the brain's hypothalamus (lower brain) which instructs the thyroid in how much thyroid hormones to make. Many patients with hyper- or hypothyroids have anxiety, irritability, fatigue, euphoria, and depression. Proper evaluation of thyroid function includes T4, T3, TSH, T3 uptake, T4 index, and in some cases, autoantibodies to the thyroid (indicative of the immune system attaching the thyroid) need to be measured.

Autoantibodies to the thyroid are often directed against thyroglobulin, mitochondria, and microsomes. Elevations in sedimentation rate can help predict thyroid inflammation and testing T-cells can help decide whether or not cancer is present, e. g., by observing whether a low T-helper/T-suppressor ratio occurs. Lithium will lower the thyroid hormone, while the addition of T3 Cytomel may be beneficial when added to any antidepressant, antipsychotic, or anticonvulsant regimen as an augmenter of improved mood. In individuals where thyroid abnormalities are not clear, a thyroid stress test or a TRH (Thyroid Releasing Hormone) stimulation test is indicated. TRH may have transient mood-elevating properties. Individuals who have thyroid problems should be evaluated for iodine deficiency. Iodine is an essential part of thyroid hormones. Individuals that are iodine deficient can be born with abnormal brain development or cretinism. Certain foods will lower thyroid levels, such as cabbage, broccoli, cauliflower, kale, and all cruciferous vegetables. These vegetables are also thought to have anti-cancer properties. Some people feel that low thyroid levels lead to lower cancer rates, while others feel that thyroid supplementation leads to lower cancer rates. I prefer the latter view about higher thyroid levels leading to protection against cancer and thyroid supplementation reducing cancer rate. There may be some positive effects of tyrosine, carnitine, and manganese on increasing thyroid function, although probably minimal. Thyroid supplementation may lower cholesterol levels to some degree especially in thyroid deficient patients. Extreme hypothyroidism is marked by elevated cholesterol. Thyroid deficiency is common in people with depression and anxiety, and should be evaluated in every patient. Estrogens, birth control pills, and Premarin falsely elevate thyroid, as can many medications.

The Thyroid Stress Test or TRH Screen

The purpose of this test is to determine if your thyroid is functioning properly. There is no more sensitive test to identify subtle thyroid deficiency. You will be injected intravenously with Protirelin, a synthetic Thyrotropin Releasing Hormone (TRH) which will cause release of the Thyroid Stimulating Hormone (TSH) from the anterior pituitary. TSH blood levels will be taken before and after injection of TRH, and by comparison of these serum levels, thyroid function can be determined. You will need to remain lying flat for the duration of the test. Please answer the following questions:

Do you have a history of?:

____ Heart Disease
____ Murmur
____ Mitral Valve Prolapse
____ Angina
____ Irregular Heart Beat
____ Low or High Blood Pressure
____ Bleeding Disorder
____ Asthma
____ Emphysema
____ Pulmonary Disease

Most common side effects are:

Nausea
Flushing
Urinary Urgency
Light-headedness
Headache
Dry Mouth
Abdominal Discomfort

I have answered the above questions truthfully. The procedure and possible side effects have been explained to me by the reviewer, and I hereby with my signature give consent for performance for the TRH test.

Signature of Patient _____   Date _____

Psychiatric Diagnostic Lab of America [1]

Name: _____ **Age:** _____ **Date:** _____

Fast Morning of Test. Patient must remain in supine position for test duration.

Baseline EKG   BP   P   Thyroid Prof. Fast

Hang normal saline solution and inject TRH IV push.   Keep normal saline solution KVO rate.

Any patient with hypertension will have D5W IV instead of normal saline solution.

15 min. BP   P   TSH

30 min. BP   P   TSH

60 min. BP   P   TSH

90 min. BP   P   TSH

Hydroxycortisone:

For Allergies, Depression, and Chronic Fatigue Disorder

The medication hydroxycortisone is a normal adrenal hormone. It is not prescribed in excess of the hormone in your body. Taken on an empty stomach it may cause some stomach discomfort and indigestion, and the tablets may taste bitter. If this is the case, they can be taken with milk or an antacid, preferably a sugarless form of Tums, Titralac, for example. Most medication is more effective if it is spread out throughout the day. A typical dose of hydroxycortisone is five milligrams, four times per day. It is not harmful to double the dose if a dose is forgotten. Because it is a normal hormone, hydroxycortisone will not interfere with other medications you may be taking. If you develop a cold or flu, double each dose and give me a call.

The scare of steroids does not necessarily apply to hydroxycortisone, which is different from the glucocorticoid, prednisone, which affects your blood sugar and can cause cataracts, ulcers, psychiatric problems, etc. Hydroxycortisone has been successfully and safely used for a variety of problems, including autoimmune disorders, diabetes, thyroid conditions, chronic fatigue, respiratory infections, and allergic disorders.

Reference:

Williams Jefferies, *Safe Uses of Cortisone,* Charles C. Thomas Publishers: Springfield, Illinois, 1981.

---

1. South Plainfield, NJ (1-800-237-PDLA)

Nutrition and Endocrinology

Dietary factors can impact on endocrinology through a variety of hormonal systems. Certain foods contain estrogen, such as black cohosh and yams. A fat-containing meal reduces testosterone concentrations without affecting the luteinizing hormone. Fatty acids modulate testosterone production by the testes. Other studies suggest that high fat diets (saturated fats) raise testosterone. After low fat, high fiber diets, 16 or 17 premenopausal women had lower levels of estrogen than while on the standard western diet. Elevated estrogen is a risk factor for breast cancer and again fiber and low fat diets can impact it. Large meals can result in a decrease in progesterone and cortisone levels. Progesterone peaks are low for vegetarian amenorrheic women. In contrast, peak estradiol level is high for vegetarian amenorrheic women.

Certain fibers can inhibit steroids such as estrogen and testosterone, which also may be a mechanism by which fiber reduces the risk of prostrate cancer by modulating hormones. Steroids will lower the levels of various amino acids such as tryptophan and tyrosine in a similar way that branch chain amino acids affect them. Amino acids such as tryptophan, phenylalanine, tyrosine, methionine, histidine, leucine, isoleucine, and valine may actually stimulate growth hormone release. But it is unclear benefit is obtained by growth hormone elevation since its activity must be mediated by other hormones. Girls with fat localized predominantly in the hips have the highest level of sex steroids and gonadotrophins. Fat distribution may affect ovarian activity.

Girls with predominantly abdominal fat were more obese and had increased plasma levels of total E2 (estrogen) and a lower androgen estrogen ratio in plasma. Brain injury, or encephalopathy, will result in precocious puberty. Most notable is the fact that fish oil and polyunsaturated oils will increase prostacyclines made by the uterus. The removal of the uterus may have damaging endocrine effects in that the body cannot make various prostacyclines that it did previously, hence causing the post-hysterectomy syndrome. These are just some of the basic influences which nutrition and diet have on hormones.

Estrogen:
Natural Hormones for Lowering
Blood Pressure
and Stabilizing Heart Disease

PATH Medical continues to do its natural hormone treatments. These treatments are beneficial for male menopause and women who are looking for a non-period, low side effect natural estrogen. Evidence is not suggesting that Estriol, another form of natural estrogen which is high during pregnancy, will actually prevent breast cancer and may need to replace Estradiol and Estrone. Articles by Dr. Follingstad in 1978 and Dr. Lemon in 1966 were generally ignored, but new suggestions by Dr. Julian Whitaker and Dr. Jonathan Wright suggest that this might be an alternative way of supplementing estrogen. We are looking into it and trying to evaluate the data, but it certainly may be worth a try in many women. The ideal hormone replacement would be a combination of Estriol, Estradiol, progesterone, and natural testosterone. This can lower blood pressure, reverse or stabilize heart disease. All natural hormone therapies have been shown to positively impact heart disease, the degree of reversal and stabilization depends on each patient. It depends on each patient's deficiencies, supplement level, and biochemical individuality.

Rosacea

In rosacea, the cheeks, nose, and the chin are red, thickened, oily, and the site of itching and stinging. Blood vessels in affected skin are often noticeably enlarged and there may be raised lesions similar to those of acne. The redness and discomfort are often made worse by spicy food, alcohol, sweating, or exposure to hot sunlight or cold winds. The nasal skin may get so thick that the nose becomes greatly enlarged and bulbous, and plastic surgery may be needed to restore its shape and size to normal. No one cause adequately explains all cases of rosacea, but its onset often coincides with use of hydrocortisone cream on the face, excessive sunburn, and exposure to other irritants. In such cases, the doctor may prescribe applications of metronidazole gel (trade-name MetroGel),

doxycycline, erythromycin, oral Flagyl, or antifungal cream. *In menopausal women, estrogen deficiency has been recognized as a common cause of rosacea. These cases often respond to estrogen replacement* (possibly worsened by DHEA), a regimen that also strengthens the bones and helps to prevent coronary heart attacks and strokes. If, after the redness and thickening subside, unsightly enlarged blood vessels remain, a dermatologist can get rid of them with laser therapy.

Sources: *Current Medical Diagnosis and Treatment* 1993 (Lange) p. 93, and *Rosacea Review*, (Winter 1994, p. 3), a newsletter for rosacea victims published by the National Rosacea Society, 220 Cook St., Suite 201, Barrington, IL 60010.

Pharmaceutical Purchases

Some pharmaceuticals can be purchased for less from various mail order specialty pharmacies that deal in bulk. Examples of these are:

Mail Order Pharmacy
P.O. Box 787
Watersville, Maine 04903
(800) 452-1976
(207) 873-6226

Family Pharmaceuticals
P.O. Box 1288
Mt. Pleasant SC 29465-1288
(800) 922-3444

12. Environment and Toxins

Air Pollutants

We have all been exposed to numerous air pollutants, acid rain, etc. In addition, many buildings have sick building syndrome, with enormous accumulation of indoor air pollutants. The concept of electronic ionizers is an interesting one, particularly in that it may impact seroton-in levels and other brain neurotransmitters. More research needs to be done in this area, but it is a new and exciting area, modifying our environment so that we might have total health. This modification also includes aroma therapy which can even impact cognitive function.

Toxic Metals

Toxic metals still remain a very serious problem in our society. (See *Zinc and Other Micronutrients*, in which my contributions were acknowledged by Dr. Carl Pfeiffer, its author.) When writing that book, we reviewed the number of ways in which lead poisoning, elevated copper levels, cadmium poisoning, arsenic poisoning, and mercury poisoning exists in our society. We still often see individuals with elevated lead levels. Since the writing of this book in 1976-77, recommended safe blood lead levels have fallen from 80 to 20 and lead has been removed from gasoline; still lead pollution exists. Elevated lead levels are present particularly with abnormal psychiatric syndromes such as bulimia, psychosis, depression, and lupus. Elevated cadmium level is usually common in smokers or people who live around smokers, and cadmium contributes to high blood pressure. Elevated copper levels contribute to depression. Elevated mercury levels may occur in some individuals who have problems with dental fillings. An analysis of toxic minerals is a worthwhile test for many individuals. We have extensive information on all of these toxins, including aluminum, which has been implicated recently in memory loss. Probably the best way to measure lead is through erythrocyte and zinc protoporphyrin in blood even if the blood lead test is not positive. Blood testing can be very accurate in regard to the other toxic metals, but hair tests may be the most sensitive general screening procedure for toxic metal poisoning. Although hair tests (pubic hair may be best used due to its longer life and less exposure to elements) reveal a low yield, they should be part of a total health screening.

Chelation: Heavy Metal Toxicity

In the first studies done to determine lead toxicity, 80 parts per million was thought to be toxic. Then it was lowered to 60, then 40, then 20, and now there is no threshold. Lead toxicity is quite common. In fact, all people, as they get older, accumulate heavy metals and probably should have some chelation to cleanse out these metals. Simple tests can identify the severity of this heavy metal burden. Hair tests or pubic hair tests will identify those individuals with the highest burdens.

Dimethyl Succimer, DMSA, is a very benign chelating agent which is safer than the previous ones used, such as D-penicillamine, EDTA and DMPA. DMSA at 250 mg, two tablets q.i.d. for three days with a 24-hour urine test on the second day for heavy metals, collected for doctor's data, will identify severity of heavy metal burden. EDTA chelation drugs can help cleanse the body of toxins in virtually all people. See Chelation Therapy, pp. 234, 235.

Chelation: Side Effect

Chelation can have an effect similar to a diuretic where good nutrients are pulled out resulting in fatigue. Fortunately, with high dosages of a multi-vitamin and zinc, this effect is usually completely negated.

Mercury Toxicity

Recent concern over mercury toxicity has increased with the discovery that mercury gas is released from dental fillings. A mercury vapor test shows that intraoral mercury (in the mouth) is significantly proportional to the number of fillings, and is a reliable indicator of mercury poisoning. Mercury from fillings is the major contributing factor to total daily mercury dose. Furthermore, subacute levels of mercury toxicity may have subtle effects. The symptoms of chronic mercury poisoning are below.

EXTENT OF THE PROBLEM

Swollen gland and tongue
Ulceration of oral mucosa; gingivitis
Dark pigmentation of marginal gingiva; gingival recession
Metallic taste; foul breath
Excess salivation
Nephritis
Pneumonia
Birth defects in offspring

SYMPTOMATOLOGY OF CHRONIC MERCURIALISM

Symptoms of chronic mercurialism include the following:

Muscular tremors (first observable sign) starting with handwriting and progressing to convulsions
Loss of appetite; nausea; diarrhea
Nervous excitability; insomnia
Headache; mental depression
Edema of face and legs
Speech disorders
Anxiety
Depression

Our testing suggests very few patients (about 1%) with multiple dental fillings may have any effect from mercury fillings. Affected patients will show an elevated level of mercury in the blood and/or hair. However, following chelation more of the mercury can be found elevated in the urine relative to the normal population. Despite this observation, it appears that most if not all filling-related mercury toxicity is treatable by vitamin E, cysteine, selenium, and other antioxidants.

The dental profession is at high risk. Probably as much as 1% of all dentists have mercury toxicity. The level of mercury in dentists has been shown to be proportional to the amount of work on fillings and other mercury-related work. It has been proposed that other natural substances, e. g., zinc, be used in amalgams. The subchronic nature of mercury exposure in dentists may be a factor related to the high rate of suicide and job stress in this profession.

Cigarette Smoking

There are numerous techniques for stopping smoking. Dietary factors include: high bicarbonate intake, e. g., seltzer, alkaline vegetables (spinach, cabbage, brussels sprouts, etc.). Elimination of sugar, alcohol, and white flour, etc., is also important. Nutrients such as methionine, tyrosine, and phenylalanine can help by their stimulant properties. Psychological factors are also involved. Antidepressants, e. g., doxepin and Prozac are helpful, as can be clonidine and Xanax. Depression has been found to contribute to patients resuming cigarette smoking. Hypnosis, psychotherapy, biofeedback, etc., may help as well. Nicorette can be another useful method. Nicotine patches now are the newest and most effective way to quit smoking. Anyone who wants to stop smoking can receive medical help to do it.

Environmental Sensitivities

In this day and age we are constantly being exposed to new and undefined chemicals throughout our entire environment. It is very important when a person suffers from allergy-like symptoms (stuffy nose, asthma, headache, rash, moodiness, fatigue, and irrational fears) to look at our entire environment to search out potential causes.

For instance, we must look at installation methods of, and materials used, in heating, wiring, floor tile and rugs, walls and ceilings, furniture, window coverings, light fixtures, appliances, ornaments and decorations, all of which could contain synthetics and give off ozone, gases, and dust. Many parts of our homes can grow different types of mold. Varnishes, waxes, bleaches, and fumes can also be a problem. There are numerous odors (tobacco smoke, auto exhaust, glue, cooking odors) which can also be harmful. It's important to always keep our houses clean, using water and air purifiers, and to search for gas leaks, etc., when treating allergies and environmental sensitivities. Allergies usually increase the risk of environmental sensitivities. Antihistamines or natural antihistamine vitamins (methionine, quercetin, calcium, and vitamin C) may be helpful.

Radiation

Radiation is likely to become an increased hazard. Fortunately, a possible solution exists. Certain radioactive chemicals such as radioactive iodides, radioactive cesium, radioactive strontium, and radioactive barium are *not* toxic even in high doses in their non-radioactive form. Hence it may be possible to eliminate radioactive elements, for example, when they have invaded the water supply, by flooding the system with large amounts of non-radioactive salts like cesium, potassium iodide, strontium, etc. or precipitating out radioactive elements present in the water supply. Further research is necessary to explore this possibility in the event of a radioactive accident.

Household Appliances

Cleaner Cleaners

Once you've emptied your shelves of hazardous waste, the best way to keep safe is to avoid bringing further polishes, drain openers, and other toxic products into your home. But does that mean you have to be unarmed in the "war against waxy yellow buildup"? Hardly. Here are some environmentally safe alternatives that will accomplish the same chores.

HAZARDOUS	NONHAZARDOUS
Furniture Polish	Two parts olive or vegetable oil, one part lemon juice.
Floor Wax Stripper	Pour club soda on the floor. Allow it to soak for several minutes and then scrub.
Floor Wax	Rub floors with a mixture of one part thick boiled laundry starch with one part liquid soap.
Air Fresheners/Deodorizers	An open box of baking soda; cinnamon and cloves boiled in water.
Drain Cleaner	Try a plunger first. If still clogged, mix one cup each of baking soda and salt. Pour it down the drain along with one cup of white vinegar. Wait 15 minutes. Flush the drain with boiling water.
Window Cleaner	Equal parts vinegar and water.
Silver Cleaner	Soak silver for five to ten minutes in warm water with one teaspoon baking soda, one teaspoon salt, and a small piece of aluminum foil; wipe with soft cloth.
Oven Cleaner	Apply a paste of baking soda and water, then loosen grime with a scrubber.
Mothballs	Cedar chips; dried lavender; peppercorns.
Bug Spray	Avon Skin So Soft -- oil based perfume.
Toothpaste Whitener	Baking soda and peroxide.

Chlorine

Chlorine has become a serious toxin in our environment. It is used in the manufacture of pulp and paper. Chlorine is shown to cause cancer and birth defects. Waste water discharges seem to affect the food chain through fish and other animals. Our country needs to reduce the use of chlorine.

Those who swim in chlorine frequently have chronic bronchitis and various health problems. Chlorinated water and our drinking water may be a problem as well.

As our society seeks total health, try to avoid chlorine. New ways to deal with pools may be to ozonate them, rather than chlorinate them. Chlorine in the pool can worsen cough, asthma, etc.

Indoor Air Pollutants and Sources

Indoor air pollution is very common. It occurs from:

- Radon
- Car exhaust
- Humidifiers
- Air conditioners
- Paneling
- Aerosol propellants
- Unvented gas stoves
- Drapes
- Curtains
- Moisture off propellants
- Pressed wood furniture and cabinets
- Stored hobby products
- Wood stoves and fireplaces
- Unvented clothes dryer

- Tobacco smoke
- Mites
- Household chemicals
- Asbestos pipe wrap
- Asbestos floor tiles
- Air fresheners
- Car exhaust
- Carpets
- Paint and painting supplies
- Moth repellents
- Pesticides
- Stored fuels
- Pressed wood subflooring
- House dust

With the use of air cleaners you should notice a decrease in coughing, sneezing or wheezing, reduction of dust which settles in a room, smoke clears out faster and odors do not linger as long. Trapped pollutants should be observable in air cleaner filters after a period of use. Place an air filter near an inlet or outlet.

Bacteria and viruses need moisture. They die when they are filtered out.

The types of filters to choose are generally mechanical filters, electrostatic filters, (precipitators and ionizers). Ionizers may produce ozone and should be avoided until they are better perfected. The plates in electrostatic filters can reduce their efficiency.

13. Food

Biologic Classification of Foods: Establishing a Food Rotation Diet

Animal Foods

Mollusks:	Abalone	Mussels	Scallops	Clams	
Crustaceans:	Crayfish	Lobster	Shrimp	Squid	Octopus
Amphibians:	Frog				
Fish:	Flounder	Sole	Chub	Perch	Harvestfish
	Salmon	Trout	Mackerel	Haddock	Swordfish
	Pollack	Sturgeon	Tuna	Pompano	Codfish
	Bluefish	Sardine	Smelt	Butterfish	Scrod
	Carp	Sunfish	Bass	Whitefish	Snapper
Dairy:	Butter	Cheese	Goat's milk	Cow's milk	
Meat:	Lamb	Venison	Mutton	Rabbit	Beef
Reptiles:	Turtle				
Mammals:	Beef	Veal			
Birds:	Chicken	Duck	Goose	Turkey	
	Chicken Eggs	Duck Eggs	Goose Eggs	Guinea Hen	
	Squab	Pheasant	Partridge	Grouse	

Plants

Grains:	Wheat	Oats	Rice	Wild Rice
	Gluten Flour	Graham Flour	Sorghum	Cane
	Bran	Rye	Barley	Cane Sugar
	Wheat Germ	Malt		Molasses
	Corn	Corn Starch	Corn Oil	Corn Sugar
	Corn Syrup	Cerulose	Dextrose	Glucose
Buckwheat Family:	Buckwheat	Rhubarb		
Spurge Family:	Tapioca			
Potato Family:	Potato	Tomato	Eggplant	Red Pepper
	Cayenne	Green Pepper		
Arrowroot Family:	Arrowroot	Psyllium		
Arum Family:	Taro	Pol		
Composite Family:	Leaf Lettuce	Head Lettuce	Endive	Escarole
	Artichoke	Dandelion	Oyster Plant	Chicory
Morning Glory Family:	Sweet Potato	Yam		
Gourd Family:	Pumpkin	Squash	Cucumber	Cantaloupe
	Honey Dew	Persian Melon	Casaba	Watermelon
Legumes:	Navy Bean	Kidney Bean	Lima Bean	String Bean
	Soybean	Soybean Oil	Lentil	Black Eyed Peas
	Pea	Peanut	Peanut Oil	
	Acacia	Senna		
Sunflower Family:	Sunflower Seed	Sunflower Seed Oil		Jerusalem Artichoke
Pomegranate Family:	Pomegranate			
Lily Family:	Asparagus	Onion	Garlic	Leek
	Chive	Aloes		
Ebony Family:	Persimmon			
Rose Family:	Raspberry	Blackberry	Loganberry	Youngberry
	Dewberry	Strawberry		

Mustard Family:	Mustard	Cabbage	Cauliflower	Broccoli
	Brussels			
	Sprouts	Turnip	Rutabaga	Kale
	Collard	Celery Cabbage	Kohlrabi	Radish
	Horseradish	Watercress		
Goosefood Family:	Beet	Beet Sugar	Spinach	Swiss Chard
Banana Family:	Banana			
Laurel Family:	Avocado	Cinnamon	Bay Leaves	
Parsley Family:	Parsley	Parsnip	Carrot	Celery
	Celeriac	Caraway	Anise	Dill
	Coriander	Fennel		
Apple Family:	Apple	Cider	Vinegar	Apple Pectin
	Pear	Quince	Quince Seed	
Olive Family:	Green Olive	Ripe Olive	Olive Oil	
Citrus Family:	Orange	Grapefruit	Lemon	Lime
	Tangerine	Kumquat	Tangelo	
Plum Family:	Plum	Prune	Apricot	Nectarine
	Almond			
Heath Family:	Cranberry	Blueberry		
Pineapple Family:	Pineapple			
Myrtle Family:	Allspice	Clover	Pimento	Paprika
	Guava			
Gooseberry Family:	Gooseberry	Currant		
Papaya Family:	Papaya			
Honeysuckle Family:	Elderberry			
Grape Family:	Grape	Raisin	Cream of tartar	Kiwi
Mint Family:	Mint	Peppermint	Spearmint	Thyme
	Sage	Marjoram	Savory	

Foods with Monamine Oxidase Inhibitors to be Avoided

(See Section 9, p. 116.)

Corn

Sensitivity to corn is one of the most common causes of food allergy (milk, dairy, and wheat are the most common) and, in general, corn is the most difficult food in the diet to avoid.

I. Mode of Exposure

Corn may be a cause of allergic symptoms as the result of ingestion, inhalation, or contact. The most common inhalant sources are the fumes of popping corn and the steam of boiling corn on the cob. The other exposures of this nature include body powders, bath powders and while ironing starched clothes. Occasionally corn is a cause of troubles as an inhalant when all other sources of corn are tolerated. More rarely, contact exposure to starched clothing or shoes containing corn adhesives will result in symptoms in the highly sensitive individual. In general, the ingestion of corn and corn-containing products represent by far the greatest corn exposure.

II. Forms of Corn

In some instances there is a difference in the effect of exposure to the different forms of corn. Sometimes one is able to eat unripe corn without having symptoms but will have a reaction if he uses any of the ripe forms or products containing ripe corn fractions such as sugar, starch or oil.

The various edible forms of unripe and ripe corn are listed herewith and in a subsequent listing all foods containing corn or made of corn are given in alphabetical order.

Ripe Forms of Corn

- Corn flakes
- Corn flour
- Corn meal
- Corn Oil "Mazola"
- Cornstarch
- "Kremel"
- "Linit" (often used as food)

- Corn Sugar
- "Cerelose"
- Dextrose
- "Dyno"
- Corn syrups
- "Cartose"
- Glucose

- "Karo"
- "Puretose"
- "Sweetose"
- Grits
- Hominy
- Parched corn
- Popped corn

Unripe Forms of Corn

- Fresh
- Canned

- Frozen
- Roasting ears

- Fritters
- Succotash

Food Groups: Guide to Labels

One must be extremely careful when reading labels since modern food labels are filled with deceptions. Numerous foods attempt to prove themselves to be low in cholesterol but are actually high in the more dangerous saturated fat. Numerous foods that claim to be low sugar are actually high in different forms of other toxic sugars. Foods that claim they have no saturated fat, often have modified hydrogenated toxic products. Foods that claim to be natural often have very few natural ingredients. It is best to bring labels in to your doctor. Eventually, PATH hopes to develop a PATH seal that will be put on foods to make it easier for patients to identify appropriate health foods.

Yeast: A Brief Description of Common Sources of Contacts

THE FOLLOWING FOODS CONTAIN YEAST AS AN ADDITIVE INGREDIENT IN PREPARATION (OFTEN CALLED LEAVENING):

Breads: Crackers   Hamburger buns   Hot dog buns   Rolls, homemade or canned
Canned ice box biscuits: Borden, Pillsbury, and General Mills

Cookies: Pastries   Cake & cake mix

Pretzels: Flour enriched with vitamins from yeast:
General Mills, Inc., Flour Corporation
    flour and enrichment wafers, Pfizer lab. enrichment products

Milk: Fortified with vitamins from yeast

Meat: Fried in cracker crumbs

THE FOLLOWING SUBSTANCES CONTAIN YEAST OR YEASTLIKE SUBSTANCES, BECAUSE OF THEIR NATURE OR NATURE OF THEIR MANUFACTURE OR PREPARATION.

Mushroom: Truffles

Cheeses: All kinds, including buttermilk   Cottage cheese

Vinegars: Apple, Pear, Grape, and distilled. These may be used as such, or they will be used in these foods:

Catsup	Mayonnaise	Olives	Pickles
Sauerkraut	Condiments	Horseradish	French Dressing
Salad dressing	Bar-B-Q sauce	Tomato sauce	Chili peppers
etcetera	Mince pie	Gerber's oatmeal and barley cereal	

Fermented Beverages:

Whisky	Wine	Brandy
Gin	Rum	Vodka
Root beer	etcetera	

Malted products: Cereals   Candy and milk drinks which have been malted

Citrus fruit juices: Either frozen or canned. Only home made are yeast free.

Dormison rest capsules

THE FOLLOWING CONTAIN SUBSTANCES THAT ARE DERIVED FROM YEAST OR HAVE THEIR SOURCE FROM YEAST.

Vitamin B capsules or any other tablets if made from yeast.

Multiple vitamins, capsules or tablets with Vitamin B made from yeast.

Zylax, Zymalose, Zymanol, Lilly's vitamin products which contain B-12.

U. S. Vitamin products: Laxo-Funk, Phoscaron-D, VI-LitronDrops, Mead Johnson's vitamins which contain B-12.

Squibb's vitamins products if indicated on the label.

Parke Davis's vitamin products: VIBEX.

Merck, Sharpe & Dohme vitamin products which contain B-12, Lederle's vitamin products, Endo's vitamin products and Massengill vitamins.

THE FOLLOWING PRODUCTS ARE THOUGHT TO BE FREE OF YEAST:

Pioneer Flour Mills, Gladiola Flour Mills International.

Abbot's vitamins: Dayalets, Vi-Daylin, etc.

Robins' vitamins: Aloe with C.

U. S. Vitamin products, except Laxo-Funk, Phoscaron-D and Vi-Litron.

Mead Johnson's vitamins if free of B-12.

Tips for Cooking

The freshest, most natural, least processed foods are best and have the most vitamins. Frozen foods are quite acceptable if not kept in the freezer more than three months or so. Canned foods (except fish packed in water) are not for everyday use as they have been cooked longer which destroys vitamins. (They also tend to be salty or have other additives.)

Fish can be broiled fairly quickly, generally requiring a few minutes per side. Both chicken and eggs can carry salmonella, so cook chicken well, bake 45 minutes at 350 and cook eggs over low medium heat. Remove the skin from poultry before cooking, otherwise the fat under the skin will soak through the meat and this is not a healthful fat.

Do not cook with oils often, even with healthful oils, (e. g., safflower, olive). Whenever possible use a nonstick pan. Saute or stir fry vegetables in water. Add a tablespoon of oil to a cooked dish just before eating, if desired. Healthful oils can be transformed by heat into oxidized oils which may clog the arteries. For this reason choose raw sunflower seeds over roasted.

Most vegetables can be steamed in 5 to 8 minutes though some of the more fibrous ones (e. g., carrots, beets, potatoes, collards) may require 12 to 18 minutes. Raw vegetables are higher in vitamins but light steaming may help break down the cell walls, permitting the body access to more vitamins. So eat some of both (raw and steamed) each day unless otherwise directed by your doctor. You can get a steaming basket which holds the vegetables above the water in the pan at most supermarkets.

Baking powder should not contain aluminum. Rumford's is a good brand, available at your health food store. Also, do not use aluminum pans. Food flavoring (e. g., vanilla extract) can usually be obtained at your health food store. Mrs. Dash is a good herbal substitute for salt. No Salt has potassium in place of sodium and is generally acceptable for people on sodium-restricted diets, though you should check with your doctor. Experiment with herbs. Garlic is actually beneficial for both cholesterol and blood pressure. A little parsley can mitigate garlic's strong odor.

Always read labels. You will be amazed at the number of crackers still made with lard, or at best, hydrogenated palm oil (a very saturated fat likely to clog arteries). Many products contain sugar disguised by chemical names (e. g., dextrose, maltodextrin, fructose, sucrose). Especially avoid sucrose and even dextrose, while fructose is okay. It is probably best to avoid syrup and honey, but small amounts of molasses, rice syrup, or barley malt (less sweet and richer in minerals) are acceptable when used infrequently. Diabetics should avoid all of these and perhaps consider a high protein, low carbohydrate, high fiber diet under the direction of their doctor.

Some of these menus may seem strange to you. Another important aspect of good nutrition is variety. A repetitious diet containing 3-4 foods will lack certain nutrients. Our culture emphasizes sweets, fats, and salt. All of these have negative health implications, so, broaden your diet, experiment, learn to appreciate new tastes.

Microwave Radiation

Beside the fact that a microwave oven puts out large amounts of milligauss toxic energies, it will probably turn out that the preparation of radiated foods makes certain toxic amino acids that increase our requirements for anti-oxidants. It should be noted that other forms of cooking, including grilling and oven-baking (especially if burning occurs) may also do similar destruction to a variety of amino acids, as frying hydrogenates fat. It is unclear at this point what the least toxic way is to prepare food, although *microwaving may be one of the most toxic techniques.* Its one benefit may be in complete sterilization. Possibly this may be sufficient to cancel out other side effects.

14. Gastroenterology --
Stomach, Colon, and Intestine

Constipation: Some Causes

Metabolic:
Amyloidosis
Diabetic neuropathies
Porphyria
Uremia

Endocrinal:
Hypothyroidism
Hyperparathyroidism
Panhypopituitarism
Pheochromocytoma

Electrolyte:
Hypercalcemia
Hypokalemia

Neurogenic:
Brain tumors
Cerebrovascular disorders
Multiple sclerosis
Paraplegia
Parkinson's disease
Pseudo-bowel obstruction
Tabes dorsalis

Psychiatric:
Psychosis
Depression
Anxiety

Other:
Diverticulitis
Drugs
Hernias
Irritable bowel syndrome
Pregnancy
Stress/anxiety
Strictures
Tumors

Cystic Fibrosis and Nutrition

The lack of nutrition, that is, malnutrition due to improper digestion and absorption of nutrients, is a primary manifestation of this disease, which is the most common lethal genetic disease among children. Because pancreatic enzymes are deficient in patients with cystic fibrosis (CF), they are unable to digest food adequately. As a result, they suffer from poor weight gain, ravenous appetite, distended abdomen, thin extremities, and sallow skin with poor turgor (normal rigidity).

Vitamin supplementation is very important to patients with CF, as they are deficient in the fat soluble vitamins A, D, E, and K, as well as the trace elements selenium and zinc. Two grams a day of taurine may improve fat absorption.

As there is currently no cure for CF, the main concern of the physician is to make the patient as comfortable as possible. Nutritional therapy can help do this, as well as help prolong life. Many patients with CF, as in any chronic disease, suffer from depression and emotional upset. BEAM testing can help determine the diagnosis of and therapy for this problem. A new DNA therapy may be available for this disease in the near future.

Dry Mouth

Dry mouth can be an uncomfortable side effect from a variety of medications. It may contribute to cavities. And it can cause difficulty speaking.

Many people seek relief from hard candy and throat lozenges, which further damages the enamel of the teeth. Possible substitutes are choline which can sometimes induce an increased moisturizing effect.

Other causes are pregnancy, smoking, snoring, radiation, stress, aging, diabetes, and hypertension.

A new substitute is Salix (215-453-2505), which has been studied in Swedish medical journals as a potential effective agent.

Flatulence or Gas

Flatulence can be produced by different types of foods: excessive fruit ingestion (particularly dried fruit), beans (due to the high amounts of nitrogen which can be converted into gas), high lactose foods (particularly milk or aged cheeses), and junk foods (white flour because of the lack of nutrients and excess of yeast).

Various medical conditions can also lead to gas, e. g., diverticulosis, colon disease, or aging with the weakening colon. Many nutrients can also lead to gas formation: magnesium, vitamin C, N-acetyl-cysteine, methionine, garlic, excess calcium carbonate or Tums. Eating too quickly (swallowing air with too many vitamins

at one time) also promotes gas formation.

Treatment for flatulence or gas can be the elimination of harmful foods that cause the condition as well as dealing with the underlying ailment itself. Simethicone is a natural "gas" reliever available in many forms (e. g., Mylicon 80). Flatulex, a combination of simethicone and charcoal, is probably the most effective combination. Tums, or if need be, Zantac or Tagamet (which can be prescribed) are all helpful antacids. Antianxiety medication can also help with gas problems, e. g., Librax.

Heartburn

Heartburn is a burning sensation behind the breast bone and can result in nausea, belching, bloated sensation, and sore throat from acid reflux. One afflicted with heartburn should avoid smoking, and alcohol, and exercise with moderation. Avoid deep-fried foods, spice, coffee, tea, and tomato products. Do not lie down or bend shortly after eating. Avoid tight belts or other restrictive clothing. CES device can cut acids, as can zinc or any of the antioxidants. Heartburn is primarily a stress reaction. Treat it before you end up with serious disease problems such as pre-ulcer symptoms. See the article about ulcers for more information.

Gastrointestinal Dysbiosis

In a healthy human being, certain parts of the body are in interaction with microorganisms (bacteria). Gastrointestinal dysbiosis occurs when the normal balance of good bacteria and yeast is changed to a more toxic state. There is a delicate balance between these potential vehicles of disease and the body. The bacteria are attacking living things, and living things respond by hiring them to do jobs, i.e., a symbiotic relationship develops in which these microorganisms are channelled to serve the human being. In some cases, and possibly in all diseases, the immune system, chemistry, and rhythm of the body

change and there is an overgrowth of either yeast or bacteria. It is important to view this problem as only a symptom of a primary disease -- similar to finding water on the floor in a house that has a bad roof: the roof is leaking; the floor is not sweating.

It is probably not of great value to do stool testing, where one sees decreases in the healthy bacteria such as lactobacilli, E-coli, and strep faecium, and increases in the disease-producing bacteria such as hemolytic or mucoid E-coli, Klebsiella, and hemolytic streptococci, etc. Individuals with this overgrowth condition can have arthritis, fibromyalgia, autoimmune disorders, chronic fatigue syndrome, anxiety, or depression. It is no surprise that in some cases individuals can take an antibiotic and end up treating their arthritis or other atypical syndromes successfully. In some cases there may be a bacterial overgrowth or disease-producing agent such as Mycoplasma or chlamydia. Some individuals, as a result of excess intake of simple sugars, and pervasive, repetitive use of antibiotics, may have a problem in slowing of bowel transport. Correction of this overgrowth of yeast and bacteria, or what is called dysbiotic syndrome, requires the same total health approach as delivering health care, e. g., dealing with brain rhythm, changing diet from simple sugars to complex carbohydrates, adding fluid and fiber, recolonizing the intestinal tract with good bacteria and adequate nutritional supplements, etc.

Lactose Intolerance

Lactose intolerance is very common in our society and is easily determined.

FREQUENCY OF LACTOSE
INTOLERANCE IN ADULTS

Ethnic Group	% Intolerant
African Blacks	97-100
Dravidian Indians	95-100
Orientals	90-100
North Amer. Indians	80-90
South Amer. Indians	70-90
Mediterraneans	60-90
Jewish descent	60-90
North Amer. Blacks	70-75
North/Central Indians	25-65
Middle Europeans	10-20
North Amer. Caucasians	7-15
Northwestern Indians	3-15
North Europeans	1-5

The actual numbers quoted on the table for North American Caucasians is probably much higher, as it is for North Europeans.

Milk intolerance is easily identified by RAST IGG blood testing. It can also be identified by the breath test for lactose malabsorption. Symptoms of lactose malabsorption are diarrhea, mild to explosive bloating, abdominal cramps, discomfort, flatulence, and even depression and mood swings.

Millions of Americans cannot digest lactose and other sugars and frequently don't know it. Most people, as they become adults, cannot tolerate lactose.

Reference: Courtesy of Great Smokies Diagnostic Laboratory.

Inflammatory Bowel Disease

Recent studies suggest that anxiety is significantly associated with increased disease activity and discomfort. Such anxiety should be appropriately evaluated and treated in patients with inflammatory bowel diseases. Decreased anxiety will result in less severe exacerbation and will increase one's quality of life.

Nutrition and Gastrointestinal Diseases

There are numerous roles for nutrients in various gastrointestinal diseases.

A. Bowel Motility

Calcium carbonate, niacin, B vitamins, and possibly vitamin A, reduce the frequency of bowel movements while magnesium oxide, safflower oil, vitamin C, and lecithin increase bowel frequency. Diets high in non-pectin containing fruit, bran, and vegetables increase bowel frequency, while diets high in protein, cheese, and sugar reduce bowel frequency. Other alterations in treatment include the mildly toxic atropine drugs (Lomotil, Imodium) and Pepto Bismol. Kaopectate, or pectin found in fruits, is probably the best treatment of diarrhea besides vitamins. Fiber is the most important treatment of irritable bowel syndrome (diarrhea and constipation) and has the additional effect of protection for the heart and cardiovascular disease by reducing cholesterol. Calcium carbonate is very constipating and turns stool to stone. Magnesium is the antidote.

B. Gall Bladder

Gall stones are a common occurrence in fat, forty year-old women. This predisposition is due to high estrogens in the diet, e. g., dairy and meat (due to hormone injections). A diet high in vegetables may reduce gall bladder disease. Furthermore, patients with cholestasis (bile duct blockage) need more fat soluble vitamins, e. g., vitamins E, A, D, and K. Methionine has been a useful therapy for cholestasis in some patients. Taurine, which conjugates bile, may also have a role. Most large stones do not pass spontaneously, yet even large stones often remain asymptomatic for a long time. There are new techniques to dissolve them (chemical and ultrasound) to avoid surgery. Actigall is particularly promising for radiolucent stones.

C. Crohn's Disease

This disease is an inflammation of the small intestine (ileum) and is marked by potassium, magnesium, zinc, vitamin A, and thiamine deficiency. Crohn's may be marked by such severe malnutrition that parenteral feeding may be necessary. Antioxidants and the anti-inflammatory fish oil (EPA) may be other useful therapies for Crohn's disease. Primrose oil and saturated fat may increase inflammation. Vegetarian or oligoantigenic diets can be helpful.

D. Ulcerative Colitis

This inflammatory disease of the large bowel is treated like Crohn's. Yet, fish oil may increase bleeding, and copper may be useful for its anti-inflammatory effect. Antioxidants are extremely important for protection against the increased risk of cancer associated with ulcerative colitis. Under medical guidance calcium and fiber can be used to reduce frequency of bowel movements. Certain drugs like Asendin can also be helpful; they stop frequent bowel movements as well as reduce depression and anxiety.

E. Appendicitis

High vegetables diets reduce the risk of appendicitis. Vitamin C and other antioxidants in vegetables are probably responsible for the reduced risk.

F. Motion Sickness and Nausea

Ginger is helpful for motion sickness. Scopolamine (Transderm) may also be helpful. The niacin flush (atropine-scopolamine-like effect) eventually produces nausea. Vitamin B-6 has been used in certain preparations for treating nausea of pregnancy and may be deficient in patients with frequent nausea. Zinc supplements can produce nausea.

G. Gilbert's Syndrome

These patients have a mild, nonhemolytic, unconjugated hyperbilirubinemia. They may be more sensitive to the toxicity of a high dose (3 grams) of niacin.

H. Chronic Hepatitis

This is due to the after effects of hepatitis B- or C-virus or a drug toxicity. Methionine and other antioxidants especially N-acetyl-cysteine may be helpful in addition to conventional treatments.

I. Gastrointestinal Cancer

Salt and butyric acid (from ginkgo tree) promote cancer in the gastrointestinal tract. Nitrates also can contribute to cancer. A possible prevention for stomach cancer is the use of antioxidants and zinc.

J. Pancreatic Diseases

Zinc is highly concentrated in the pancreas where it is depleted by alcoholism or any pancreatic disease. Low plasma zinc is the hallmark for pancreatic disease. Folic acid also may be an important nutrient in healing the pancreas.

K. Diverticulosis

Both diarrhea and constipation must be regulated in this disease. Bran and other fiber sources, antioxidants, calcium, garlic (tetracycline effect), and avoidance of seeds, nuts, and corn are critical.

L. Familial Polyposis

This disease of the colon leads to an increased risk of cancer which may be reduced by antioxidants.

Gallstones

There are many types of gallstones: cholesterol gallstones, calcified gallstones, and pigment gallstones. There are many ways to image gallstones. The easiest is through the ultrasound. X-ray and CT scanning can also be very helpful. The gall bladder is also very easily imaged with an oral cholecystogram, or Hida scan. It is estimated that 30-50 percent of the patients in the United States with gallstones are asymptomatic, with 1.5 percent of these patients undergoing cholecystectomy each year. Risk factors for gallstones include being fat, female, forty, and fertile. Many individuals have chronic cholecystitis from gallstones.

There is a new treatment for the prevention of gallstones in high risk individuals and individuals who are dieting and may be at risk for gallstones. This new drug also may be used as treatment of certain individuals already suffering from gallstones. This is Actigall (ursodiol -- a natural bile acid) which is a natural treatment. It is found in small quantities in the normal human gall bladder, and the gall bladder of certain species of bears, where it was originally derived by the Greeks and dried for the treatment of gall stones. Numerous studies suggest that Actigall can result in dissolution of stones. Ninety percent is absorbed in the small bowel after administration. Actigall is indicated for patients with radiolucent, non-calcified, gall bladder stones, less than 20 millimeters in diameter, in whom elective cholecystectomy would not be undertaken because of increased surgical risk. It is probably useful in any individual at high risk for gallstones and those who have chronic dyspepsia.

Actigall will not dissolve calcified cholesterol stones, radiopaque stones, or radiolucent pigment stones. Patients with such stones are not candidates. Also, unremitting acute cholecystitis, cholangitis, biliary obstruction, gallstone pancreatitis, and biliary gastrointestinal fistula are thought not to be candidates for Actigall. It is now thought that chronic hepatitis may also benefit from Actigall. A typical dose of Actigall is 300 milligrams, twice to three times daily depending on the individual. Side effects are relatively limited and include allergy, rash, sweating, hair thinning, cholecystitis, flatulence, headache, fatigue, back pain, and rhinitis. Ultrasound images of the gall bladder should be taken at six month intervals during the first year of therapy.

In the future we hope to be able to identify early thickening of bile so the therapy can be used earlier for prevention. Gallstone dissolution with Actigall treatment generally requires 6 to 24 months of therapy. Dissolution progression may be confirmed by sonography in as early as six months. Complete dissolution does occur in many patients and recurrence of stones within 5 years has been observed in up to 50% of patients who dissolve their stones using bile acid therapy.

Motion Sickness

There are a number of ways to avoid motion sickness:

1. Eat a small, low fat, low protein, starchy meal before travelling.

2. While driving on winding roads, watch the curves out the window.

3. On a boat, use the horizon as a reference to remind yourself that you are indeed rocking.

4. Minimize body movements, especially head movements. Astronauts in the early space vehicles with virtually no room for head movements experienced very little nausea.

5. Stay busy with other thoughts. People involved with mental problems and tasks get sick less frequently.

6. Don't worry. Anxiety can stimulate some of the hormonal reactions that precipitate nausea.

7. Use either ginger or daily dosages of 200-500 milligrams of B-6, and/or magnesium.

8. Drugs like Dramamine, scopolamine, and Promethazine have side effects but can be useful.

9. Keep in mind pregnancy is like motion sickness.

Ulcers

Causes of Ulcers

Anyone who is a Type A personality -- always working hard -- is prone to ulcers. Cigarettes, caffeine, spicy foods, and aspirin abuse may contribute to their development. Of these three, smoking is probably the greatest risk factor for ulcer disease. Nicotine affects acid secretion in the stomach by indirect mechanisms and leads to the high, intense type of Type A life-style. Stopping smoking often heals ulcers better than the use of medication.

Caffeine drinkers should also be aware that they are at a high risk for ulcers. Caffeine increases acid secretion. This includes both coffee and tea. Males in their forties are more prone to ulcers than any other group of people. This is due to the large amount of stress and responsibility that surrounds their lives. They work as if they are young, but their bodies cannot take the pace any more. Less caffeine and less smoking is the needed response to this stress.

Spicy foods also contribute to ulcer formation, e. g.,

pepper, salt, chili powder, etc. Garlic, on the other hand, protects against ulcers. Foods that may prevent ulcers are: alkaline foods (asparagus, beans, cabbage, cauliflower, and celery). Acid foods (orange or tomato juice) are very bad for ulcer patients, whereas bananas (especially plantains) are very beneficial.

The biggest cause of ulcers is the overuse of aspirin. Fish oil can replace most aspirin therapy. Nonsteroidal drugs (Advil, Motrin) are extremely ulcer causing. Fish oil (5-15 grams) replaces much of the need for these medications. Cytotec protects against side effects of drugs like Motrin.

Zinc, beta carotene, vitamin E, and especially cysteine, are antioxidants which may be important in the preventive treatment of ulcers. Antioxidants are anti-cancer vitamins, and it is not surprising that bleeding ulcers can often become cancerous.

Conventional Treatment of Ulcers

Antacids can be used for treatment. Tagamet and Zantac (antihistamine, antiacid secreting drugs) are beneficial when frequent antacids upset the stomach or are inconvenient. These drugs also can help regulate the immune system and correct autoimmune diseases. The disadvantage of drugs is their side effects, which can be infertility, enlarged breasts, and more. Taking antacids alone is not any less effective than taking drugs. Any antacid that contains aluminum must be discouraged, even though its toxic effect does not show up for years. There are studies that say that gradual accumulation of aluminum

can be a contributing factor in Alzheimer's disease and memory loss. The best antacids are Riopan, which has the advantage of being low in sodium; milk of magnesia or magnesium carbonate, which is a laxative; or Tums (calcium carbonate), which is constipating. Ask your pharmacist for the equivalent of Tums with nutrasweet.

Most ulcers can be prevented through a wise diet and the use of nutrients, e. g., calcium or magnesium carbonate. Always consult a physician before medicating yourself with vitamins or antacids.

Heidelberg Test

The Heidelberg test is used for assessing gastrointestinal function. The doctor may order this test if you have reported gastrointestinal symptoms (bloating, gas, irritable bowel, or stool abnormalities), or if your blood tests or stool analysis indicate a problem absorbing nutrients (vitamin, mineral, or protein deficiencies).

The test involves swallowing a capsule containing a miniature high-frequency transmitter which is encapsulated for swallowing and which transmits Ph values from the gastrointestinal tract. The frequencies transmitted are picked up by a belt antenna system (worn by the patient). The receiver then displays the values on a meter and simultaneously records them on the machine's graph (pH gastrogram). The capsule will be eliminated without complication in a bowel movement.

Some problems that are commonly diagnosed with this test are:

hypochlorhydria (too little stomach acid) which may worsen an ulcer or gastritis.

hyperchlorhydria (too much stomach acid) which may worsen an ulcer or gastritis.

stomach empties too quickly indicating that foods are not properly digested when reaching the small intestine, and often results in allergies or frequent loose bowel movements.

stomach empties too slowly indicating that foods remain in the stomach too long. Often this is associated with feelings of "fullness" or constipation.

Based on the findings of the Heidelberg test the physician will design an appropriate program of supplements and/or dietary modifications. It is desirable to repeat the test three months after the initiation of your program to monitor your progress and make adjustments if necessary.

Flexible Sigmoidoscopy:
Patient Preparation Instructions

Please follow these directions carefully in order to achieve the best results possible during your screening examination. Everyone over 50 should have this test.

4 Days Before the Procedure:

Stop all vitamin C, red meat, iron supplements, aspirin or aspirin-like products (unless used by prescription). You may resume all of these after the screening.

Take two Fiber Con tablets every 8 hours.

3 Days Before the Procedure:

Continue to take two Fiber Con tablets every 8 hours.

2 Days Before the Procedure:

Eat a very light breakfast and an equally light lunch. For dinner, eat only clear soup, jello, clear fruit juice, and clear liquids. Tea and coffee are allowed.

1 Day Before the Procedure:

Purchase four Fleet or similar enemas. The price range should be from $.59 to $.99 each. If you are used to another form of enema, you may use that enema instead.

The Evening Before the Procedure: Eat a light dinner. After dinner, ingest only clear liquids and avoid any liquids with caffeine or stimulants. No laxative is necessary.

The Morning of the Procedure:

Drink only clear liquids for any meals before the procedure. About two hours prior to your office appointment (depending on how far you are from the office) begin giving yourself the enemas. You should repeat the enemas until the returns are clear. It is very important to completely clear the colon of brown stool so that I may see the inside of the bowel. The enemas must be repeated until no more solid or colored material comes out, only water and the enema solution. This usually takes two enemas, but sometimes takes three or four.

By the same token, do not continue to give yourself enemas if the returns are *clear* after one or two. You may dehydrate yourself or you may stimulate stool from higher up to come down.

Most local pharmacies will take back unopened enemas if you so wish. Or, you may choose to save them for future use (hopefully only for this procedure).

Then, come to the office as relaxed as possible. Please let us know of any questions or concerns you may have. If you wish to see what we have seen through the scope, please ask.

After the Procedure:

Treat yourself to a wonderful meal and be reassured that you have taken a major step toward preventing colon cancer. Remember also, if a polyp is found, it can often be cut out as an outpatient-type procedure, without major surgery.

Guaiac Card or Hemoccult: Stool Blood Test

This is a test for microscopic bleeding in the gastrointestinal tract. The most common etiologies of the bleeding would be hemorrhoids, peptic ulcers, inflammatory bowel disease, and - rarely - carcinomas. This test should be done at least yearly.

False positive tests can occur, and therefore there are some special diet instructions. This guaiac card diet should be started two days prior to and during the test period.

You May Consume:

Generous amounts of cooked and uncooked vegetables such as lettuce, corn, and spinach.

Plenty of fruits such as plums, grapes, and apples.

Moderate amounts of bran cereal, peanuts, and popcorn.

Tuna fish, roasted chicken, and turkey.

Do Not Consume:

Rare and lightly cooked meats.

Cauliflower, horseradish, red radishes, turnips, broccoli, and cantaloupe.

Aspirin and medications which may cause gastrointestinal irritation. For patients on prescribed medications in this category, ask your care coordinator for specific instructions.

If any of the above dietary items are known to cause discomfort, please advise your physician.

Directions for doing the test

1. Answer the three questions listed below.

2. Fill out the required information on the front flap of all three slides.

3. Upon completing the first bowel movement, open the first slide's front flap and follow the printed directions. Use one applicator to obtain two stool samples from the toilet bowl. Apply a thin stool smear to each window, then close the flap.

4. Repeat this procedure for the next two bowel movements using the second and third slides and applicators.

5. Place all three slides in the envelope and return to the address designated by your examining physician.

Specimen collection should not be attempted during menstrual or hemorrhoidal bleeding.

Question 1: Special diet followed: Yes ____ No ___

Question 2: I am on medication: Yes ____ No ____

Question 3: This medication is: _____

15. *Heart Disease, Cardiovascular and Peripheral Vascular Health*

Cardiac Disease Reversal Program

The PATH wellness organization has a very successful cardiac reversal program. This program utilizes both techniques of Nathan Pritikin and Bob Atkins in dietary reversal.

After we have had success with various diets for cardiac reversal, we use medications to lower cholesterol, as well as combinations of nutrients such as Mevacor and niacin. We have successfully achieved cholesterol levels lower than 100. Our techniques have resulted in PET scan and SPECT scan documented cardiac reversal.

In addition to the above, we can use stress reduction techniques such as biofeedback and in some cases, dietary and nutrient therapy to reduce the necessary drugs like Lasix. We have found lower morbidity when we switch from Coumadin to Ecotrin, and attempt to do so when plausible.

In conjunction, we use the BETH Israel cardiac PET scanning unit, as well as the University of Pennsylvania PET scanning unit to document pre and post changes.

Out of hundreds of patients with advanced cardiac disease we have yet to lose a patient to coronary artery bypass, angioplasty, or transplant. Many have been recommended for bypass by their doctors and have been told that they couldn't avoid it, yet with our program, patients are successfully avoiding it.

We are constantly consulting with Lance Gould, who is the world's leader in cardiac reversal at the University of Texas Medical Center at Houston.

As an adjunct to this program, we use chelation.

Doppler Test

The Doppler test is a scientific way of determining how well your arteries and veins are circulating blood throughout your body. Arteriosclerosis is a disease in which plaques and clots build up in blood vessels and block blood flow to vital organs such as the heart and brain. This process can eventually result in heart attacks or strokes if it goes untreated for too long. Fortunately, now with the Doppler test, blood supply to your brain, legs, and arms can be accurately measured without side effects. Segmental blood pressures can also assist identification of blood vessel blockages.

Procedure: There is no special preparation needed for this test. You may be asked to change into a loose-fitting gown in order to make it easier to perform the required measurements. First, blood pressures will be taken in your arms. Then you will lie down and four different pressures will be taken in each leg. An advanced computerized instrument will then accurately measure a

tracing of your blood flow in your arteries and veins of the legs, arms, and neck. The entire test may take about an hour since such extensive and thorough readings are needed. There are absolutely no needles used and the procedure is completely painless. In the best quality machines a color picture will be available for your review.

Purpose: Heart disease, strokes, kidney failure, high blood pressure, leg gangrene, venous phlebitis, varicose veins, leg edema (or swelling), cold hands or feet are just some of the conditions caused by circulation troubles. Hardening of the arteries, or atherosclerosis, is a gradual process of starving the body of oxygen since red blood cells carry cholesterol within the blood stream. Sometimes symptoms such as chest pain or leg cramps (especially in the cold or after walking) can be symptoms of this process. Most of the time, however, there is no way to detect the process until it is so advanced that a serious medical problem results. The Doppler test is one of the few ways to detect any early signs of blood vessel disease even before it causes any damage. If discovered early, it is possible to reverse the process (with diet, nutrients, drugs, and chelation) before it is too late.

Even the slightest blockages suggest a high risk of stroke. Forty percent of the people die from stroke. Half a million Americans sustain a stroke each year. The purpose for Doppler carotid testing is to identify high-risk patients for stroke.

Doppler Testing -- Vascular Screening

New ultrasound machines are able to search virtually the entire arterial and vena system in the hands, feet, legs, arms, and neck for blockages. Individuals who are at risk for blockages are people with leg pains, cramps, non-healing ulcers, leg swelling, varicosities, numbness, impotence, and change of skin color. Particularly at risk are hypertensive patients, diabetics, smokers, victims of stroke, T. I. A.'s (small reversible strokes), geriatric patients, overweight patients, and pregnant women. The exam is very safe and painless. The duplex color flow doppler procedure is done with photo cells, infrared light waves, and high frequency sound waves (ultrasound) which record light reflections and sound waves in the arteries and veins. Sound waves and reflected light patterns are converted to signals which appear on a strip chart or television-like screen. From these wave forms it is possible to determine if blockages or clots are present.

During the exam, the patient should lie quietly and refrain from talking. Blood pressure cuffs can be placed and small probes can be taped to the fingers and toes during the exam. The blood pressure cuff will be inflated on a rotation basis and gives the physician information on the blood supply to the extremities.

Symptoms for arterial studies include absent or diminished pulses, claudication, wrist pain, vasospastic disease, ulcers, pre- and postoperative surgical evaluations. Venous studies can help give information on acute deep vein thrombosis, edema, pain, postphlebitic ulcers, high risk for pulmonary embolism, valvular incompetency, both deep and superficial systems, carotid cerebral studies, transient ischemic attacks (T. I. A.'s), asymptomatic carotid bruits, branchial blood pressure differences, diminished pulses, post-endarterectomy follow-up.

Many diseases require this type of peripheral vascular study, including peripheral arteriosclerosis and arterial-sclerosis of any type, high cholesterol, Raynaud's syndrome, Berger's disease, thoracic outlet syndrome, venous insufficiency, vasculogenic impotence, carotid artery stenosis, long-standing diabetes, claudication, ischemic ulcers, subclavian steal syndrome, phlebitis or thrombophlebitis, cerebral thrombosis, etc.

Tobacco, caffeine and other vascular constrictors used shortly before testing can distort test results. Cold hands or feet can produce falsely abnormal digit wave forms. The patient must lie quietly and not talk during the exam, and must try to reduce test tension for more accurate results.

Indications for Non-Invasive Vascular Testing

ARTERIAL	CEREBROVASCULAR-CAROTID
Skin color changes or ulceration *	Cervical or carotid bruit *
Preoperative and postoperative evaluation *	Cluster-type headaches *
Diminishing / absent distal or pedal pulses *	Lapse of memory
Distal extremity hair loss (Trophic changes) *	Loss of balance
Intermittent claudication *	Loss of vision
Leg pain, rest pain, night cramps *	Visual disturbances
Medical-legal documentation *	Transient ischemic attack (T.I.A.; recovery within 24 hours) *
Gangrene *	Vertigo *
Extremity weakness or fatigue *	Increased vessel wall rigidity found during palpation *
Differentiation of various paresthesias	Unilateral paresthesias
Diabetic neuropathy	Aphasia
Numbness	Amaurosis fugax
Positive Allen's Test	Dizziness
Coldness in an extremity	Syncope
Raynaud's phenomenon	Dysarthria
Thoracic outlet syndrome	Fluctuating confusion
Subclavian steal syndrome	Loss of memory
Hypertension	Motor deterioration
Frostbite (cold injury)	Bruit
Skin or nail infections	RIND (recovery > 24 hours)
Lower extremity bone fractures	Stroke
Cigarette smoking	Ataxia
Heart disease	Drop attacks (sudden muscular weakness)

VENOUS
Monitoring patients with high risk of venous thrombosis *
Presence of pitting edema *
Varicose veins with symptoms *
Venous thrombosis and postphlebitic syndrome *
Skin color changes (Hemosiderin deposition) *
Extremity weakness or fatigue *
Pulmonary embolism
Oral contraceptive use
Ulcers
Cellulitis
* Most frequent indications

Vascular Patient History

Diagnosed conditions

Diabetes	_____ years
Hypertension	_____ years
Hyperlipidemia	_____ family history
Prev vasc surg	Syncope
Stroke/TIA	Varicose veins
Heart disease	Impotence
Angina	Bruit

Risk factors

Cigarette/tobacco use
    Years smoked: 0.0   PPD: 0.0   years quit: 0.0   pack years: 0
Sedentary
Oral contraceptives

Current symptoms

Gangrene	Rest pain
Limb hair loss	Paraesthesia\weakness
Skin color changes	Burning sensation
Stasis dermatitis	Ulcerations
Trophic nails	Cyanosis
Cellulitis	Rubor
Absent PT pulse	Headaches
Absent DP pulse	Vertigo
Pulse Grade PT	Edema
Pulse Grade DP	
Pulse Grade POP	
Pulse Grade FEM	
Claudication	

Pain at:
        thigh/buttock
        calf
        arch
        toe

Pain relief: rest
             exercise
             legs elevated
             legs down

Distance walked before pain (blocks)

Vascular and Venous Blood Testing

Vascular and venous. BF (blood flow) is evaluated by Doppler ultrasound, and Plethysmography, (Photoplethysmography, PPG and Pressure Cuff Recording(PCR))

Doppler Ultrasound

A probe is placed on the skin over blood vessels to capture the sound of blood coursing through them. The sound waves from the doppler strikes RBCs and bounce back to the sound head. The pitch indicates how fast the cells are moving, the higher the sound, the faster they are moving. Loudness determines the number of RBCs flowing through the vessel. The greater the number, the louder the sound.

Normal vessels: RBCs near the wall move slower and are lower in pitch. The loudness remains constant.

Obstructions: The number of RBCs decreases, so the sound is lower, but the pitch is high at the location where the RBC's break free. The sound is louder at the proximal end of the obstruction because it is here that the RBC's will have accumulated.

Plethysmography

Plethysmography is composed of:

1)   PPG photo plethysmography which measures BF

2)   PCR pressure cuff -- recording which measures changes in volume in a limb
Arterial System: with each heart beat, blood volume increases and then decreases as it empties. PPG and PCR measure changes in vascular volume over a short period of time.

Venous System: it is driven by respiration cycles. Oxygen-depleted blood flows back to the lungs and heart. Valves in vessels prevent blood from flowing back into the veins. As the venous system fills with blood, venous PCR measures the change in limb volume.

ABI (Ankle Brachial Index) Test

ABI (Ankle Brachial Index) test with Doppler to screen indication of patient for arterial disease in the lower extremities. The Doppler assesses the BF.

Method: A doppler probe and pressure cuff are used to obtain the right brachial pressure first. Then the right ankle at the site of the posterior tibial artery. The left side is then tested in the same manner. The pressure is increased in the upper extremity from 150-240 mm hg. In the lower extremity the cuff inflates to 60 mm hg. The wave form measured is the first wave form attained after the pressure cuff is released and the pulse becomes audible.

Results: The ABI is a ratio. Ankle systolic pressure/brachial systolic pressure. This ratio assesses the integrity of the vessels in the lower extremities.

Precautions: Increasing pressure in the upper extremities to the upper ranges if the patient has calcification of vessels restricting the BF as seen in insulin dependent patients.

Interpretation: Brachial pressures should be within 20 mm hg of each other.

Values: normal > 0.96

mild obstruction 0.71-0.96
moderate obstruction 0.31-0.70
severe obstruction .00-0.30

Indications of abnormality:

1)   Waveform differences side to side
2)   Loss of the dicrotic notch
3)   Drop in waveform amplitude

False Positives:

1) Patients with calcium deposits, partially occluded arteries
2) Room temperature must be 72-77^0. Patient must rest 10 min. after the cuffs are on.

Plan of Action:

1) If results are abnormal progress to the segmental test with Doppler
2) If results are normal, but the patient symptomatic, proceed to the hyperemia or post-exercise test

Segmental Testing

Indications: The patient has an abnormal ABI

Method: Similar to the ABI, but additional cuffs are put on the lower thigh and below the knee bilaterally.

Results: Pinpoints the location of the abnormality

Interpretation: The brachial pressures should be within 20 mm hg of each other. The lower extremity blood pressure should increase in value as you move proximally

1) The ABI less than 1 indicates an obstruction
2) The normal upper thigh pressure should be 10 mm hg > than the brachial pressure
3) Pressure difference between adjacent cuff sides should not exceed 20-30 mm hg of each other
4) A pressure difference of 30 mm hg over the entire leg may indicate an obstruction

False positives:

1) See ABI
2) Obese or muscular patients may show elevated pressures in the thigh

Plan of Action:

1) If the ST is normal, but the patient is symptomatic, you may want to perform the reactive hyperemia or post-exercise test.
2) Obtain toe pressure and PCR waveforms

Venous Reflux Test

Indication: To evaluate value competency of the patient's superficial and deep venous system in both legs. In normal patients the value in the venous system of the legs prevent reflux of the blood. In this test, photo plethysmography measures changes in the capillary BF. The PPG probe records instantaneous changes in the blood content of the skin that occur when there are changes in the venous pressure.

Method: A PPG probe (using the reflux disks) is placed 10 cm above the left at the malleolus. The patient is seated in a chair with the seat flat on the floor. The patient is asked not to talk during the test. The patient must be quiet and still for 2 minutes prior to exercising. The patient then flexes the ankle ten times. The motion must be maximum. A minimum of 5 heel raises are needed. If the patient cannot do this, the technician then manually squeezes the calf 10x. In this situation, each leg is done separately.

Results: The refill time represents the venous filling time; a time of over 29 sec. is normal. If the results are abnormal, the test must be repeated, or perform the test with a tourniquet below the knees or thighs.

Interpretation: *Venous test without tourniquet*

normal -- refill time is greater or equal to 20 sec indicating that the values are competent and that the arterial system begins to refill the venous system as blood is forced out of the leg.

abnormal -- refill time is less than 20 sec. meaning that the values are allowing blood to flow backwards in the legs during the resting phase.

Venous test with tourniquet

normal -- means the deep veins are competent but the superficial ones are not
abnormal -- the deep veins are incomplete and the superficial may or may not be competent.

False positives: Invalid studies can result from lack of venous emptying due to severe venous disease, venous thrombosis, or inability to dorsiflex adequately.

Plan of Action: A Doppler venous exam

Maximum Venous Outflow MVO for DVT (Deep Venous Thrombosis)

Indication: PCR is used to assess venous capacitance and max venous outflow. It is used to determine whether there is an acute and large deep vein thrombosis proximal to the calf.

Method: The leg veins are expanded to their maximum capacity using a special cuff on the thigh. The cuff inflates and hold a steady pressure of 60 mm hg for 1 minute to restrict venous outflow yet permit arterial blood to flow in. This is done 3x. Next a calf cuff inflates to measure the venous capacitance in that location, the MVO cuff is then deflated, and maximum venous outflow is measured 2 sec, at the calf site.

Results: Two parameters are measured to determine if the venous outflow is sufficient: (1) venous capacitance and (2) second venous outflow.

$$MVO = \frac{2 \text{ sec. venous outflow}}{\text{venous capacitance}}$$

Interpretation: An MVO ratio greater or equal to .61 is normal. A ratio less than or = to .5 is abnormal. An abnormal ratio means there may be an obstruction.

False+/-: Swelling or edema may limit calf expansion, as well as positioning, relaxation.

Plan of action: Further scanning or venography

Direct Doppler Carotid Test

Indication: The doppler is used to evaluate the patency of the common, internal, and external carotid arteries in patients with acute and severe disease.

Method: The doppler probe is placed on the artery sites, and the maximum waveform recorded of the clearest and loudest sound. The systolic and end diastolic points are measured.

Interpretation: Comparisons are made of waveforms at the same site. If both common carotid and brachial waveforms have been quantified, these indices are done.

Peak Systolic/Brachial Index (PS/Br)
Carotid Asymmetry index (CAI)

$$RPS/Br = \frac{Rt \text{ Peak Systolic}}{Brachial \text{ Peak Systolic}}$$

$$LPS/Br = \frac{Rt \text{ PS}}{BPS}$$

$$CAI = \frac{Rt \text{ Peak S}}{LPS} + \frac{Rt \text{ end Diastolic}}{Lt \text{ ED}}$$

Values: Normal flow

RPS > .9 and
LPS/Br > .9 and
CAI > 0.9 < 2.5

Plan of Action: Ultrasound imaging

Digital Test

Indication: To evaluate and characterize the arterial BF in the hands and feet using PCR and PPG

Method: Arterial waveforms and pressures are recorded from the digits bilaterally. Cuffs are inflated at the base of the toes or hands with 50 mm hg of pressure while PCR waveforms are recorded.

Precautions: If arterial flow is not occluded at 240 mm hg, there may be a medical reason for this.

Results: PPG waveforms that are rounded and low in amplitude may indicate an obstruction.

Interpretation:

$$\text{Finger/Brachial Index} = \frac{\text{FSP}}{\text{BP}}$$

$$\text{Toe/Brachial Index} = \frac{\text{TSP}}{\text{BP}}$$

Indications of Obstruction:

1) Bilateral distinguishable difference
2) Smoothing or loss of the dicrotic notch
3) Smoothing is the lack of 2 distinct peaks

False positives: Can be obtained if vasoconstricting or vasodilating agents are taken by the patients. Cigarettes, coffee, and cool room temperature can alter blood flow.

Plan of Action: If abnormal perform a Raynaud's test or thoracic Outlet syndrome test.

Reactive Hyperemia Test

Indication: To detect small changes in peripheral blood flow when the patient can not perform a treadmill test (e.g. patients with cardiopulmonary disease or severe claudication). It is used to simulate exercise and increase BF to the extremities.

Method: To increase blood flow, thigh cuffs are inflated above the systolic pressure and held at that pressure for a minimum of 3 min to completely shut down arterial flow to the lower legs. This stress on the arterial system creates the same effect as exercises. The pressure in the cuffs is released, and ankle pressures are taken every 30 sec. for the next 3-10 minutes. The test can be done with PPG, obtaining the waveforms at the ankle cuff or with doppler.

Results: Ankle pressure will drop following release of the upper thigh cuff, in patients without obstruction; ankle pressure will drop no more than 33% and return to baseline within one minute.

Interpretation: If the ankle pressure falls more than 33% below the resting value within 15 seconds after deflation of the cuff, and it takes longer to return to resting pressure, then arterial occlusive disease is indicated. A graph is displayed plotting systolic pressure to seconds after occlusion.

Precautions: It should not be done in limb with femoral or popliteal graphs. The test only tests the extremity distal to the occlusion cuff.

False positives: Can be obtained if the room temperature is cool.

Post-Exercise Test

Indication: Identifies borderline and symptomatic patients who have normal results in the ABI test.

Method: The ABI test is first done. Two methods can be used, the PPG test or the doppler. With the PPG test, cuffs are placed on the ankles, and then the patient exercised, (walking for 5 min, step ups for 3 min, or a treadmill -- 2 mph at 10% gradient -- for 5 min.). Immediately following the exercise, or if patient complains of pain, cuffs are placed on the ankle and great toe. The cuffs are inflated and waveforms recorded 5 times. The Doppler can be used to record waveforms at the post-tibial artery after cuff deflation.

Results: If the patient's arteries are unobstructed, BF will increase after exam or remain the same. If ankle pressures decrease, it is indicative of an occlusion.

Precautions: The patient must be monitored for signs of cardiac stress during examination.

Interpretation: The normal response to exercise is a rise in pressure when exercise is stopped, with a gradual decrease to resting pressure as the patient rests. If ankle pressure falls after exam and slowly rises to resting pressure, arterial occlusion disease may be indicated. A graph is displayed plotting resting systolic.

Impotence Test

Indications: Used to determine a vasculogenic cause of sexual dysfunction.

Method: Either PPG or PCR can be used. With PPG a cuff is inflated around the penis. A waveform is recorded, then the cuff is inflated to 200 mm hg. The waveform disappears, the cuff then bleeds down. When the pulse waveform returns, it is recorded with PCR. A cuff is used and inflated to 60 mm hg. The waveform is recorded at that time.

Results: PPG waveforms and pressure test

Interpretation: Penile brachial index = Penile pressure highest brachial pressure.
Normal values are > .75, if less than .60, arterial occlusive disease may be indicated prox. to the cuff. A ratio .6-.74, suggests further testing. Waveforms are examined for this amplitude and contour.

False positives: The penis must be placid and the cuff wrapped adequately and securely.

Chelation Therapy

The word chelation is derived from the Greek word, "chel," meaning "to claw." Chelation is a common reaction in both the biological and chemical world. The chelation reaction is used by both organic and inorganic chemists. EDTA, ethylene diamine tetra acetic acid (an amino acid), was first synthesized by Franz Munz, a German chemist, for use in textile and fabric production. Chelation therapy, in conjunction with sodium citrate, was first used in medicine for lead poisoning.

Over the last several decades, the medical application of chelation therapy has continued to grow, although some opposition has grown as well. Some of the early studies using EDTA have found it removes heavy metals from the body, especially calcium. This characteristic was severely criticized by orthodox medicine. Orthodox physicians pointed out that chelation robs the body of vitamins, mainly B-6, and may even chelate an abundance of calcium from the bones and teeth. Newer applications of this therapy have been accompanied by a vitamin regimen designed to replace whatever is lost. The decalcification of teeth or bones with chelation therapy cannot occur under these conditions. Protocols instituted by the new American Board of Chelation Therapy have reduced side effects to virtually zero.

Oral EDTA was used at first, but this actually increased lead and heavy metal absorption from the lower intestines. Today, this method of delivery is strongly discouraged. Early studies also tended to encourage the infusion of too high an EDTA concentration too quickly. This caused problems in patients, especially those on cardiac drugs. Now, over 3 million chelation treatments have been given to over 300,000 patients.

EDTA the chelating agent, donates an electron to the ligand, which is usually calcium or another metal. Once bound, this complex can be eliminated through the urine. Chelation therapy has been used for arteriosclerosis, lead or other heavy metal intoxification, memory loss, senility, Alzheimer's disease, diabetic gangrene, impaired vision,

kidney stones, high blood pressure, and a host of other maladies. In one case, a 54-year-old chiropractor had been saved from a leg amputation for diabetic gangrene by chelation therapy. Another doctor used chelation to lower his cholesterol (which it did), and noticed a great improvement in his memory. Certain eye diseases, for example, macular degeneration where circulation is diminished, are greatly helped by EDTA chelation therapy due to its cleansing effect on the blood vessels.

Although it has had numerous applications, perhaps the most widely used one is for treatment of cardiovascular disease, including high blood pressure and arteriosclerosis. EDTA is a non specific chelator, although it focuses on calcium since this is in abundance. By doing this, EDTA stabilizes intracellular membranes of the cells of the arteries. In addition, it helps to correct enzyme inhibition which is concomitant with the advancing of the disease. It also assists in stabilizing the electric charge of platelets, and thus reduces platelet leukocyte interaction leading to a reduction in unnecessary clotting. It can act as a calcium channel blocker and thus lower unnecessary arterial vasoconstrictions. The process of calcification is intimately associated with sclerotic hardening, and this can be reversed by EDTA chelation.

While the potential benefits of chelation therapy are currently unobtainable anywhere in orthodox medicine, it can save countless cardiovascular patients from the horrors of bypass surgery and other high risk, low success rate techniques. Chelation therapy is possibly a great, overall antioxidant technique. (See also Chelation: Heavy Metal Toxicity, Section 12, p. 157.)

The PATH cardiovascular reversal program continues to progress, with patients routinely showing cholesterol levels in the range of 90-111 while undergoing niacin medication therapy, vitamin therapy, and chelation. Apparently, chelation in and of itself has a great cholesterol lowering effect, which is worthwhile for patients with severe heart disease.

Chelation Therapy Facts [1]

Chelation therapy is a safe, effective treatment administered orally or intravenously, which has been used successfully to prevent and treat hardening of the arteries for over forty years in the United States. New evidence reveals that it may help to control, and in some cases reverse, the effects of arthritis, glaucoma, gangrene, cancer, stroke, osteoporosis, metal toxicity, irregular heartbeat, and senility as well as a host of other degenerative diseases.

The word "chelation" is derived from the Greek work "chel" meaning "to claw". EDTA, Ethylene Diamine-TetraAcetic Acid (an amino acid), was first synthesized by Frank Munz, a German chemist, in 1941 as a method for removing lead poisoning. EDTA is presently considered experimental under the Federal Drug Administration guidelines.

The research protocol was designed in consultation with the FDA. If final results prove the benefits of EDTA chelation therapy, the FDA will approve EDTA for treatment of many diseases.

The infusion solution consists of five hundred milliliters (500 cc's) of sterile water with the following additives (individualized for each patient):

- **EDTA:** Maximum 3 gm/20cc. The dosage is based upon an individual's age, body weight, height, and lab valves (creatinine clearance). It removes toxic metals, aluminum, lead etc.

- **Magnesium:** has two functions; (1) it prevents pain from the EDTA, and (2) it is therapeutic for many conditions treated with EDTA. Most patients are deficient in magnesium.

- **Sodium Bicarbonate:** to buffer the infusion solution to physiological pH.

- **Local Anesthetic:** to prevent pain at the infusion site.

- **Heparin:** to reduce the incidence of localized phlebitis proximal to the site of infusion. Heparin may be contraindicated for patients with bleeding tendencies and for patients who are already receiving full anticoagulating doses of warfarin. This small amount of heparin is not enough to cause systemic anticoagulation.

- **Ascorbate Vitamin C:** is synergistic with EDTA. Ascorbate enhances the ability of EDTA to remove lead from the central nervous system. Ascorbate is also an antioxidant and free radical scavenger.

- **Miscellaneous:** B-complex vitamins including B-1, B-6, and B-12, these vitamins are synergistic with antioxidant defenses (Crarton 94, 94, 96, 97).

EDTA is administered intravenously for not less than three hours. A 25 gauge butterfly needle is preferred by most physicians. This small needle serves two purposes: (1) it is easier and less painful to insert (2) the small lumen prevents an excessive rate of infusion.

Frequency of treatment depends on an individual patient's tolerance and convenience. Patients vary in their individual tolerance to EDTA. The treatment schedule for each patient will depend on clinical judgment and the results of a renal function test.

The American College of Advancement in Medicine is a nation wide, traditionally trained group of physicians who have formally adopted EDTA Chelation Therapy as their standard method of medical treatment for patients diagnosed with occlusive vascular disease and many other diseases. ACAM records indicate that about 500,000 Americans have taken chelation treatment. Members of the ACAM protocol have to follow the strictest standards for chelation therapy. The records show that with both long term and short term chelation therapy, 82% of chelated patients showed great improvement, both objectively and subjectively, as a result of their treatment program.

Chelation therapy provided by the ACAM protocol with proper application has been shown to be absolutely safe. Physician members of the ACAM including Dr. Eric Braverman, Medical Director of PATH, believe it is unfair to patients not to receive all alternatives of medicine. The American Medical Association, the American College of Chest Physicians, and other professional associations, along with other vested interest groups, will protect their own endeavors. In fact, these interest groups are competing with chelation therapists for patient dollars.

---

1. By Jan Lupa, R.N., with permission.

The physician members of the ACAM are board certified physicians. Some are cardiovascular surgeons, who could be performing bypass surgery and making a phenomenal amount of money, but these medical physicians choose alternative medicine for the best treatment possible for a patient.

Many medical physicians have become increasingly critical of bypass surgery. Bypass surgery does not cure patients; its overall effect on the patient is stressful and negative. A decade of scientific study has shown bypass surgery does not save lives or even prevent heart attacks. Regardless of the medical fees for bypass surgery, patients who suffer from coronary artery disease, and for those who are treated without surgery, enjoy the same survival rates as those who had open heart surgery. Yet many United States American Medical Doctors and Surgeons continue to prescribe surgery immediately upon the appearance of angina or chest pain.

Arteriograms are a major marketing tool for bypass surgery along with balloon (or now laser) angioplasty. Catheterization and arteriograms are too often used to frighten patients into accepting unnecessary "dangerous and expensive" surgery or angioplasty when nonsurgical treatment such as chelation would be equally effective, or more so, with less danger and expense. The risk of harm or death to the patient is high during heart surgery.

Another reason to delay surgery whenever possible has been touted by a recent report of accelerated atherosclerosis in coronary arteries after they have been subjected to bypass. Plaques grow faster after surgery.

When bypass is performed, an artery which is obstructed is often replaced by a vein turned inside out so the valves are located on the outside to prevent obstruction of blood flow. Thrombosis (an embolism) and total occlusion can easily occur, creating total dependence on a thin-walled and weaker vein graft. When that vein graft fails, the patient is much worse off than before surgery.

The American Medical Association has publicized in its *Journal of the American Medical Association* that forty-four percent of all bypass surgeries performed in the United States are done for inappropriate reasons.

Angioplasty often fails in less than a year, leading to repeated angioplasty or bypass surgery. Angioplasty can also damage an artery, exposing collagen to platelet aggregation and rapid clotting and emboli formation, making Chelation Therapy, and other nonsurgical treatments, less effective.

As discussed earlier, patients are rarely told about chelation therapy before bypass surgery or angioplasty, although chelation treatment is thousands of times safer at a smaller fraction of the cost. If asked, cardiologists and bypass surgeons will usually criticize chelation therapy and press for the much more profitable catheterization etc., etc., etc.

The American College of Advancement in Medicine maintains an extensive library of chelation therapy. A careful search of the scientific literature shows no data which refutes the usefulness of EDTA chelation therapy. Most criticisms of chelation therapy continue to originate from individuals with vested interest in competing therapies.

Politically powerful and traditional medical interest groups have a very large vested interest in catheterization studies and in arterial bypass surgery. This is a two billion dollar per year business in the United States. Many hospitals would be in financial difficulty and many cardiologists and surgeons would be forced to find other methods for their medical skills without these procedures. To get information from the medical society concerning EDTA chelation therapy, is comparable to asking "the fox to guard the henhouse."

While cardiologists and vascular surgeons enthusiastically promote the utilization of very expensive, highly invasive, and potentially dangerous catheterization followed by bypass surgery, there are estimated to be approximately one thousand physicians in the United States, and others overseas, who routinely and successfully treat occlusive arterial disease with intravenous EDTA. Medical insurance companies are repeatedly advised not to pay for chelation therapy but to pay instead for much more expensive cardiovascular surgery. This advice to medical insurance companies seems to be coming from consultants who are biased toward arteriography and bypass surgery.

History is replete with examples of innovators, initially labeled charlatans, only years later to be recognized as geniuses.

- Dr. Edward Jenner who was labeled as a quack, experienced his share of difficulties establishing a vaccine for small pox.

- Another famous physician, Ignaz Semmelweis, stated that handwashing would prevent infection from spreading (infection control). He proved himself right by minimizing obstetric ward mortality. His peers remained unimpressed and ultimately drove him out of the country.

Chelation physicians are routinely and maliciously attacked by organized medicine, licensing boards, governmental agencies, interest groups by organized medicine and health insurers. The tactics used against chelation physicians include smear campaigns, entrapment, illegal wiretaps, and politically inspired IRS audits. Some chelation physicians spend almost as much time defending their right to practice, as they do treating patients -- an obviously costly, time-consuming, and ego-bashing undertaking.

Presently, members of congress such as Senator Hatch (R. Utah), Senators Harry Reid (D. Nevada), and

Frank Murkowski (R. Alaska) have strong convictions for preventive health. Senator Hatch, a leader in the fight to oppose the Federal Drug Administration's battering of the natural food industries as well as the benefits of nutritional supplements, has been vocal on these issues.

Chelation: Side Effect

Chelation can have an effect similar to a diuretic where good nutrients are pulled out resulting in fatigue. Fortunately, with high doses of a multivitamin and zinc, this effect is usually completely negated.

Stroke

Every year over 500,000 strokes can occur. Nearly 150,000 people die of strokes per year and 300,000 are crippled. Only one third of people who have small strokes ever exhibit carotid bruits. Only 1 in 4 adult Americans can name a single risk factor concerning stroke, and only 1 in 5 know a single symptom of stroke. To get to know if someone is going to have a stroke, a physical exam is of minimal value. High cholesterol is somewhat predictive. An MRI tells you if someone is already having a small stroke, but the best stroke predictor is duplex and regular carotid artery scanning. This test has up to an 86% accuracy rate.

Symptoms of stroke are blocked blood vessels in the brain, blood clot or hemorrhagic stroke. Most are blocked blood vessels. Other symptoms are sudden weakness or numbness to the face, arm, or leg (usually one side of the body), loss of speech or trouble talking or understanding speech, dimness or loss of vision (particularly in only one eye), unexplained dizziness, unsteadiness or falls, or sudden severe headache.

In order to avoid stroke, lower blood pressure, lower cholesterol, eliminate fat, and eat a well balanced diet. If you have diabetes, keep it under control. Don't smoke, don't use alcohol, and consider all the antiplatelet nutrients, from herbal, willow bark, aspirin, vitamin E, garlic, onions, ginger, fish oil, etc.

From a nutritional point of view, the nutrient most associated with reducing the size of an infarct is carnitine, probably by its cholinergic action. My guess would be that it works by building up acetylcholine in the brain, which is the main memory compound, which would allow the brain to shift memories from damaged cells to other parts of the brain. The brain is extremely "plastic" or flexible. Let's say you added some memories and information stored in an area where the stroke was, if there is sufficient choline. Using an analogy with computers, what the brain will do is down load to another disk, so to speak, or it will shift off to a different directory. So the C directory can throw all its information into the D directory, but to do that it needs acetylcholine, and so acetyl-carnitine or carnitine are the most recognized to do this, and probably choline also.

The toxic effect of stroke occurs as a result of the release of calcium into the cells and the release of the neurotoxic amino acids glutamate and aspartate. GABA may be calming to a degree and can be tried in post-stroke patients up to 3 grams. Also, studies have definitely documented the benefit of vitamin A in reducing infarct size, as well as possibly the general category of antioxidants which include vitamin E, selenium, cysteine, vitamin C, and beta carotene. Dosages can range from 3 grams of cysteine, vitamin E 1600-1800 IU, selenium up to 400-500 micrograms, vitamin C to several grams, and beta carotene 25-100 mg. It may be possible, although I do not have much experience with it yet, that this should be included in some kind of TPN solution with high amounts of vitamin C and B-complex. There may be some additional benefit in giving low dosages of Dilantin post-stroke. With stroke, 5-15 percent of patients may have seizure. It is not that highly recognized at this point, but Dilantin has had some amazing benefits to patients over the years. There is no worsening of prognosis in patients who do seize following a stroke according to some studies. The Ginkgo Biloba in France has also been thought to be helpful in cerebral insufficiency. That is available as Cognitex or pure Ginkgo Biloba. Dosages are not exactly clear at this point. Long-term prevention of stroke and benefits to stroke prevention include the use of ginger, onion, garlic, even cayenne pepper, all (like fish oil, vitamin E, and aspirin) with natural antiplatelet activity. Basically, the people who use these things are using natural antiplatelet agents, which is the basis of most embolic strokes. We, of course, recommend to all patients and families who have embolic stroke histories that they get yearly carotid checks with our Doppler, just like we do cardiograms. Anger and frustration, anything from retirement to marital problems have been associated with high rates of stroke, even in nonhypertensive patients. Fish oil has been thought to increase infarct size so it should be used with caution in patients at risk for bleeding.

References

Vitamin A may mitigate stroke. Prevention October 1992:34.

Ebihara T, Sekizawa K, Nakazawa H, Sasake H. Capsiacin and swallowing reflex. Lancet 1993; 341:432.

Matsumoto Y, et al., Do anger and aggression affect carotid atherosclerosis? *Stroke* 24(7):983-986, 1993.

Steiner M, Vitamin E: More than an antioxidant. *Clin Cardiolo* 16(Suppl I):I-16 -- I-18, 1993.

Eldershaw T, et al., Pungent principles of ginger (Zingiber officinale) are thermogenic in the perfused rat hind limb. *International J Obesity* 16:755-763, 1992.

Kleijnen J, Knipschild P, Ginkgobiloba for cerebral insufficiency. *Br J Clin Pharmac* 34:352-358, 1992.

Wong M, Haley EC, Calcium antagonists: Stroke therapy coming of age. *Stroke* 21(3):494-501, 1990.

Rosadini G, et al., Acute effects of L-acetyl-carnitine on regional cerebral blood flow in patients with cerebrovascular disease. *Clin Trials J* 25(Suppl 1):35-46, 1988.

Dominkus M, Grisold W, Jelinek V, Transcranial electrical motor evoked potentials as a prognostic indicator for motor recovery in stroke patients. *J Neurology* 33:7-15--7-18, 1990.

Slivka A, Silbersweig D, Pulsinelli W, Carnitine treatment for stroke in rats. *Stroke* 21(5):808-811, 1990.

Fujimoto S, et al., The protective effect of vitamin E on cerebral ischemia. *Surg Neurol* 22:449-454, 1984.

Blood Clots

INTRODUCTION

Many diseases are marked by excessive clotting or increased viscosity of the blood. Many strokes are due to clots that form in the blood vessels. Clots occur when platelets (small cells of the blood) get too sticky and aggregate. These clots circulate in the blood as an emboli (traveling clots). Phlebitis is often caused by local clots in blood vessels and embolic clots. Most myocardial infarctions or heart attacks are caused by embolic clots. With advanced age, there occurs increased viscosity of blood that is secondary to an increased lipid or fat content. It is therefore, extremely important and beneficial to have the blood mildly anticoagulated or thinned.

Exciting research has been done in the field of nutrients and the prevention of clots. Until recently, physicians have only been able to prescribe an aspirin a day (or Persantine) for patients who feared heart attack, stroke or recurring stroke. Phlebitis patients were left on potentially hemorrhaging producing drugs such as Coumadin or Heparin. Today, we have more sophisticated nutritional forms of treatment.

MAX-EPA

The most exciting of nutrient blood thinning treatments are the fish body oils that contain eicosapentaenoic acid (EPA), which diminishes platelet aggregation and can actually prolong bleeding times in humans. The Eskimos on their oily, high fish diet, bruise very easily. Hence, do not take Max-EPA before surgery or with other anti-clotting drugs. Furthermore, the consumption of this nutrient in a fish diet has been associated with a decreased risk of heart disease. It also reduces the development of plaque in blood vessel walls by lowering both cholesterol and triglyceride levels of the blood.

The reason Max-EPA works is that it blocks the metabolism of arachidonic acid. Arachidonic acid in platelets is an important factor that makes them stick together. Arachidonic acid is made from linoleic acid and linoleic can encourage clotting if not combined with Max-EPA, although some studies suggest linoleic acid alone can decrease clotting. Studies have shown vitamin E is also an anti-clotting agent. (The Shute brothers used mega-dosages of E in heart disease.) Vitamin E's anticlotting ability in large doses is undoubtedly a factor in its beneficial role in heart disease.

Max-EPA is the most interesting nutrient anticoagulant and inhibits arachidonic acid incorporation into human platelet phospholipids, thereby diminishing platelet aggregation. Arachidonic acid is converted to prostaglandin E2, while Max-EPA will block that conversion and will eventually be converted to other forms of prostaglandins (prostaglandins 1 and 3). It is, therefore, not surprising that prostaglandins 1 and 3, which come from Max-EPA and dihomogamma linoleic acid (primrose oil) are anti-clotting. Prostaglandin El itself has been used as an anti-clotting substance. Hence, primrose oil unlike linoleic acid can be used in patients who need to have their blood thinned.

What dose of Max-EPA? In elderly people, 300 mg a day (one capsule) can have significant antiplatelet or anti-clotting effects. We frequently use as much as 1200 mg a day. Furthermore, Max-EPA has an anti-triglyceride and anti-cholesterol effect, but this may not be manifested until doses reach 5 grams or more daily. In addition, we have our patients use ginger, onion, and garlic as daily condiments.

VITAMIN E

The next most valuable nutrient in the treatment of clotting disorders is vitamin E, which prevents platelet abnormalities induced by estrogen. Estrogens are known to cause excessive clotting. Vitamin E -- 600 units a day -- has been found to be extremely effective in these thromboembolic diseases. Vitamin E also inhibits platelet aggregation. It can also inhibit the normal synthesis of several clotting factors. It is also not surprising that vitamin E can help intermittent claudication which may be secondary not only to impaired circulation but mild platelet aggregation. Vitamin E is also an antioxidant which can decrease the arachidonic-linoleic acid ratio. There is a higher proportion of linoleic acid in the membranes, which reduces the platelets from sticking. We have found that vitamin E is extremely helpful in clotting disorders.

TRACE METALS

Each year more material becomes available on the effects of trace metals and clotting. Zinc has a procoagulant effect on fibrin clot formation. Furthermore, there are new roles for copper in that blood-clotting factor 5 contains copper. Copper deficiency can also affect clotting. Excess copper probably increases clotting in human beings. Topical zinc heals ulcers and can prevent excessive clotting due to injuries. Yet, we are cautious with the use of zinc alone in patients who have a tendency for strokes or myocardial infarctions because of reported procoagulant effects.

Selenium has been shown to reduce the ability of platelets to aggregate. Platelets which tend to concentrate selenium have more difficulty forming collagen and thrombin. A high selenium diet or selenium supplements are extremely important because plasma selenium levels and platelet selenium levels are directly related. Hence, selenium is an extremely important anti-clotting nutrient.

Other nutrients that have a role in clotting are gold, which has an antithrombotic activity which may explain its antiarthritic effect. Folic acid is reduced in serum by aspirin. Hence, we think that folic acid has a pro-clotting effect and should be avoided by those patients who are prone to stroke or myocardial infarction. High elevation of tyrosine in blood in newborns (a congenital condition) can produce clotting defects. Vitamin K deficiency can induce bleeding disorders. Antioxidants, such as vitamin C and cysteine, may have mild anticoagulant effects. The antioxidant BHT can cause hemorrhagic death in high doses.

FOODS TO PREVENT CLOTTING, STROKES, HEART ATTACKS

The everyday diet can also be a factor in abnormal clotting. Onion, garlic, and ginger all inhibit platelet aggregation and are natural anti-clot materials. Ginger, used widely as a spice in India, is also used to relieve pain in the joints, like aspirin. Ginger can also correct the nausea and vomiting of early pregnancy.

OTHER HABITS

Exercise and alcohol habits should be considered. Alcohol increases the synthesis of arachidonic acid, while exercise may reduce it. Hence, alcohol should be avoided by those who are susceptible to clotting. Daily exercising to tolerance helps prevent heart attacks, clotting, etc.

CONCLUSION

In sum, vitamin E, Max-EPA, primrose oil, selenium, foods with onion, garlic, and ginger, are extremely important nutrients for the prevention of and treatment of clots, myocardial infarction, or other diseases. Folic acid, tyrosine, and copper may need to be used sparingly. Many nutrients have a significant role to play in prevention of stroke, phlebitis, and heart disease.

EKG and Echocardiogram (Echo)

Every adult over the age of thirty should have an electrocardiogram (EKG) once a year and adults at high risk, twice a year. An electrocardiogram is an electrical tracing of your heart activity. It measures whether or not the pumping function of your heart is working efficiently, or if there is an electrical conduction delay resulting in uneven heart muscle contraction. It can tell if the different chambers of your heart are working in rhythm with each other or if they are "out of step." All sorts of irregular beats and their causes can be detected. In addition, the EKG can often detect whether you have had a "silent" heart attack in the past and can show if there are signs of

an impending one. Finally, an enlarged or hypertrophied heart may show up as an abnormal tracing. A normal EKG can be a great reassurance that your heart is functioning well and working harmoniously with your body to contribute to your good health. This is especially true when the EKG has been analyzed by computer and/or accompanied by an echocardiogram. An echo is a safe ultrasound picture of the heart valves and functions and is a great predictor of heart size and pump efficiency. An ejection fraction of greater than 50% is a positive indication of heart function and well-being.

Exercise

There are so many benefits to exercise -- you can live longer, be healthier, and reduce triglyceride and cholesterol levels. There can be problems with long-term exercise, e.g., marathon running, in that it can decrease fertility and sex drive. Many studies have shown that exercise reduces hypertension, which is (next to obesity) the best predictor of reduced life span.

Sedentary people can have shriveled up hearts; they actually have a shrinking heart muscle. Inadequate exercise can indicate that a person will not live as long as the person that does exercise, because exercise can lower blood pressure from 10 to 15 points. Walking is an exceptionally good form of exercise, whereas long-distance running depletes zinc, chromium, and magnesium. Depletion of magnesium can cause instant death. Marathon running can reduce the male sex drive as well as cause anemia. Also common in marathon runners are tibial fractures and pelvis stress fractures.

Moderate exercise is a healthful activity in that it has many benefits. It can reduce the chance that a woman will develop osteoporosis. Weight-lifting and aerobic exercise seem to reduce triglycerides. Exercise lowers the fat in the blood, thus reducing the risk of heart disease. Exercise also increases metabolic rate, thus reducing weight. Exercise is particularly useful in high calorie diets.

An athlete in training will experience: a loss of choline, vitamin B-6, riboflavin, vitamin C (reduces lung

stress), as well as the loss in sweat of zinc and chromium. High complex carbohydrate diets are highly recommended for endurance training. Yet, sugar or refined carbohydrates can cause a loss of energy during an athletic performance.

Some preparation tips for exercise are: 1) eat at least 3-4 hours before a major athletic event; 2) eat complex carbohydrates (whole grains, brown rice, whole wheat toast); 3) limit protein intake (the more protein you eat, the more you urinate); 4) eliminate gassy foods and sugar (a quick sugar high stimulates insulin secretion which can result in hypoglycemic episodes, thus draining energy); 5) drink plenty of water; and 6) avoid caffeine and alcohol.

It's important to exercise consistently and moderately. The need for B vitamins, zinc, chromium, carotene, choline, potassium, and magnesium increases with strenuous exercise. Heavy sweating can result in depletion of potassium or magnesium levels and can create heart rhythm problems. Additionally, long distance runners may have less breast cancer because of a reduction in sex hormones, i.e. testosterone and estrogen.

Severe exercise can increase endorphins (natural pain killers). A runner's high comes from the release of natural pain relievers, endorphins. Marathon running is like a short-term antidepressant. Yet, the overall effects of extreme exercise (marathon training) are not beneficial. In contrast, swimming is excellent for osteoporosis and arthritis.

Exercise: A Summary

HOW MUCH EXERCISE SHOULD I DO?

The more active a person is the stronger his/her bones will be. Becoming more active is a gradual process. You can begin by working more physical activity into your everyday routine. Make a point to walk more during your day and to take the stairs instead of the elevator or escalator.

If you are presently engaging in aerobic, weight-bearing exercise which is of moderate intensity (e.g., aerobic dancing, slow jogging or brisk walking) you should aim to participate in this activity for a minimum of three days a week for at least 20-30 minutes. This level of activity is adequate for preventing the development of osteoporosis. You also may wish to increase the level of routine activity that you do by increasing the amount of walking you do. You may also wish to add some exercises to increase strength in your arms, shoulders, chest, and back.

If you are not presently exercising regularly consider beginning a program of regular walking. Walking is generally the recommended exercise for preventing and treating osteoporosis since it is a safe, effective exercise that everyone can endure.

HOW MUCH WALKING SHOULD I DO?

The amount of exercise you should do depends on several factors including your age, health, and physical condition. The intensity of the exercise will also affect how often you exercise. Mild exercise, such as walking at a comfortable pace, can be done daily. Thirty minutes of walking a day is believed to be enough exercise to stimulate bones and keep them strong and healthy. Moderate exercise, such as brisk walking, can be done 3-5 days a week, for 20-30 minutes. If you are not used to exercising regularly, or if you have any medical or orthopedic problems, you will need to gradually work up to this level of exercise. Begin slowly and progress gradually. Set small goals for exercise each week. For example, you may wish to begin with 10-15 minutes of walking, three days per week. As you feel stronger, gradually increase the amount of exercise you do. Listen to your body and don't push yourself.

EXERCISE BENEFITS

Exercise releases neuromuscular hormones into the brain, and this has a beneficial effect on depression, anxiety, insomnia, etc. Exercise may even improve nutrient absorption and utilization. Exercise has tremendous psychological and physical health benefits.

Leg Cramps

Leg cramps are usually of two types: 1) those that occur during the day due to exercise, and 2) those that occur at night. Daytime leg cramps due to strenuous exercise (or even walking) are usually a sign of vascular insufficiency. There are numerous nutrients that have been suggested to be helpful, e.g., fish oil (Mega-EPA), vitamin E, and garlic, which are antiplatelet, aspirin-like drugs that thin the blood. Niacin may also be useful because of its vasodilating effect (like the drug Vasodilan and others). Potassium must also be considered, because potassium deficiency can cause muscle spasm. Calcium and magnesium can also decrease daytime cramping. Tegretol, which reduces stickiness of red cells, can also be used.

Night cramps are often precipitated by stretching or extending legs during rest or light sleep. Walking sometimes brings relief. Others claim that raising the foot off the bed by nine inches is also helpful. Some drugs can cause nocturnal cramps, which disappear after drug withdrawal. Quinine, on the other hand, is sometimes helpful in low dosages because it is a mild muscle relaxant and blood thinner. Excessive use of quinine (an herbal) can cause tinnitus, nausea, and headache, and it should not be used during pregnancy. We try to stick to the use of vitamin E, calcium, magnesium, potassium, niacin, fish oil, and diet to treat both day and night cramps.

Diet and Anticoagulants

While you are on anticoagulant therapy you should eat less of the following foods (containing vitamin K):

Broccoli	Cabbage	Cauliflower	Kale	Kiwi fruit
Liver	Onions (fried or boiled)	Papaya (raw)	Pineapples (raw)	Salad greens
Soy meal, soybean oil	Spinach	Turnips	Green tea	

You should eat none of the following:

Caffeine (coffee, tea, cola, etc.)   Alcohol

Caution: Cooking oils that contain silicone additive will decrease absorption of your anticoagulant medication.

High Triglycerides and High Cholesterol

Nutritional treatment of high triglycerides is very successful. Seven capsules daily of EPA can lower triglycerides from 800 to 150 (normal) in just six months. EPA (fish oil) lowers almost all forms of triglycerides. Niacin is also effective in lowering triglycerides (type 4) but the flushing may be uncomfortable (Willner, Brason or other forms of time release may eliminate this problem but liver enzymes must be checked every 3 to 6 months). Diet is very important. Avoid sugar and alcohol, which frequently may do more to raise triglycerides than cholesterol levels. Saturated fat intake, e.g., cream, whole milk, frying or baking with oil, fatty meat, and butter, should be reduced or eliminated. Fish daily and two tablespoons daily of safflower or sunflower oil (possibly olive oil if there is no hypertension) are very helpful. Supporting nutrients (selenium, chromium, magnesium, pantothenic acid, and primrose oil) are helpful in the treatment of high triglycerides.

High cholesterol is more difficult to lower than high triglycerides. Most cholesterol levels go down with a reduction of refined carbohydrates. The same dietary approach as above is necessary. Sometimes red meat or even whole grains need to be reduced. Primrose oil or safflower oil (2-4 tbsp. per day) is helpful. Lecithin may be helpful (2-10 tbsp. per day). Olive oil may also be useful, especially in improving HDL ratios. Niacin and fish daily can also be helpful. Arginine and methionine are amino acids that can lower cholesterol slightly. HDL -- the good cholesterol -- is raised by exercise, EPA (fish oil), garlic, carnitine, pantetheine, vitamin C, and niacin daily. One drink per day (not more) may also raise HDL, but the bad side effects of alcohol outweigh this one possible good effect. Other supporting nutrients are the same as for treating high triglycerides. Zinc and vitamin E in very large doses raise LDL levels (the bad form of cholesterol). Overall, antioxidants probably protect against the side effects of high cholesterol.

Causes Of High Cholesterol Levels

1. Excess dietary sugar
2. Excess dietary starches, especially refined carbohydrates like flours and pasta
3. Excess hydrogenated or processed fats (lard, shortening, cottonseed oil, palm oil, margarine, etc.)
4. Liver dysfunction
5. Amino acid deficiency
6. Essential fatty acid deficiency
7. Deficiency of natural antioxidants such as vitamin E, selenium and beta carotene
8. Increased tissue damage due to infection, radiation, or oxidative activity (free radicals, etc.)
9. Fiber deficiency
10. Vitamin C deficiency
11. Carnitine deficiency
12. Biotin deficiency
13. Food allergies
14. Alcoholism

Causes of Low Cholesterol Levels

1. Immune decline
2. Chronic hepatitis
3. Cholesterol lowering drugs
4. Essential fatty acid deficiency
5. Liver infection or disease
6. Manganese deficiency
7. Adrenal stress
8. Street drugs (cocaine, marijuana, etc.)
9. Excessive exercise (especially in females)
10. Low fat diets
11. Psychological stress
12. Cancer

Cholesterol

Although, in general, cholesterol levels are predictive of who is at risk for heart attack, people die of heart attacks with cholesterol levels of 150-200 and even less. We do not understand why this is, but it shows the mystery of medicine and how important it is for us to realize that sudden death relates to so many factors. At PATH Medical, we think the factors that influence whether or not you are going to die are DHEA level, hormone levels, cardiac rhythm, carotid and leg circulation as per doppler testing, immune system, and brain rhythm. The fact that the brain controls the body is evidenced by the most recent study that the brain can stop the heart at any time, causing an immediate heart attack when the brain (insular cortex) is not functioning. Therefore, we recognize that all those who are looking at cholesterol are really only taking care of the tip of the iceberg of their total health when they need to take care of the entire picture which starts with the brain and includes the carotids, hormones, glands, etc.

Cholesterol Update

A new research study in the Post-Graduate Journal reports that a cholesterol lowering drug when combined with nicotinic acid, had more benefit than when the two were used separately. Significant changes were observed in the HDL ratio. It is thought that when the HDL/cholesterol ratio is 2.5 or less, cardiac reversal occurs. The report that a drug when combined with a vitamin had more significant effects than either one alone is very significant and further supports the PATH Medical life-style changes and nutrition along with the best of modern conventional medicine. This combinational benefit has also been demonstrated with the use of antidepressants or psychiatric medication in combination with vitamin therapy.

Pregnancy/Cholesterol

One of the proofs of the hypothesis that elevated sex hormones result in high cholesterol is pregnancy. Women routinely have cholesterol levels in the 300 range during pregnancy as their body revs up to make extra sex steroids to make the child. Elevated cholesterol is like pseudopregnancy in adults. What we need to do is provide adequate sexual hormones so that they don't need it.

Angina

Angina is chest muscle cramping. Its symptoms are typically chest pain behind the breast bone, pressure, tightness or burning in the chest; pain radiating to the arms, neck, jaw or back; chest pain that occurs during exercise after a heavy meal or on a cold windy day. It can also occur when under stress. It is easy to prevent in some ways by not smoking, keeping weight off, exercising, lowering cholesterol, eating less fat, dieting, doing the PATH cardiovascular program, reducing stress and staying inside on extremely cold days.

Heart Disease Prevention

The time to start preventing disease, of course, is early, not waiting until 50 years old for menopause symptoms and heart disease. After all, the risk for a woman dying of heart disease isn't one in ten, it's one in two. Therefore, a heart disease program and nutrients and hormones required for bone replacement should be started as early as possible.

The Physical Link
Between Stress and Heart Attacks

Again, the brain/body connection total health link shows that acute mental stress stimulates a chemical reaction that promotes blood clotting which can trigger heart attacks. In fact, most people forget that a significant percentage of patients who suffer from heart attacks do not have significant blockages in the vessels supplying the heart.

The central nervous system triggers arrhythmia, blood clotting and heart attack through this process. This should come as no surprise since the brain is the largest neurological organ and can actually shut off the heart under stress, possibly even related to issues of conscience in some cases. The fact that just massaging the carotid bodies in the neck sometimes can stop supraventricular tachycardia is evidence that the brain controls the heart and the entire body.

This concept was also further elucidated by the fact that the neuropeptide Y, occurring in the brain, has been genetically linked to hypertension. Again, the brain synth-esizes this neuropeptide which causes hypertension. A recent study has shown that Galamin, a peptide identified in the brain, affects fat craving. Again, the brain controls the body.

The main controller of the brain's stressed state is norepinephrine and tyrosine. According to a study in the *Aerospace Medical Association* in 1992, tyrosine can minimize and reverse stress induced performance losses. When tyrosine is deficient, some of these destructive peptides in the brain are made which raise blood pressure and increase fat craving. Therefore, so many of our patients are on Amino Stim.

So important is diet to the brain that a pregnant mother's diet has been shown to affect the child's risk of having a brain tumor. Mothers and their children who have had adequate amounts of vitamin C, vitamin A and folic acid did not develop brain tumors with nearly as much frequency as those with vitamin deficiency.

Sudden Death

All of us are interested now in who dies from sudden heart attacks. Increasing evidence in a recent study in the *British Heart Journal* has shown that the cardiogram and the echocardiogram are more than adequate to predict who will die. The most important predictor of all is an ejection fraction of less than 40 percent as proven by an echocardiogram. The second most important predictor are major ventricular conduction defects or ventricular tachycardia as proven by either EKG or 24-hour cardiogram. Other things that can be helpful in predicting heart attack are the use of diuretics, history of congestive heart failure, diabetes, atrial fibrillation, severe atrial arrhythmias, frequent PAC's, and use of antihypertensive medications. Beta blockers may actually reduce sudden cardiac death.

Fish Oil and Sudden Death

A recent study has shown that fish oil might ward off sudden death. About 250,000 people a year die of sudden cardiac death, where the heart's normal arrhythmic pulsing turns inexplicably chaotic, a condition known as ventricular fibrillation. The causes can be arterial sclerosis, heart attack, certain drugs, etc.

A new study with fish oil has shown that fish oil decreases the risk of sudden death by protecting the heart from going into a full ventricular fibrillation. Animals fed with fish oil, as opposed to other oils, such as sunflower oil, have much higher risk of ventricular fibrillation. Fish oil is by far the best oil for protecting the heart from going into a dangerous rhythm. Therefore, since all of us are under stress in this society, all of us are at increased risk of ventricular fibrillation. By taking fish oil on a frequent basis, we can reduce our chance of dying suddenly or of a slow protracted death.

Nutrients to Prevent Heart Attacks

Niacin reduces cholesterol and probably reduces the risk of heart attacks. At least one gram daily is needed to lower cholesterol and raise HDL. Because niacin in doses of that size opens (dilates) blood vessels, flushing occurs. Patients should start at doses of 100 mg twice a day with meals, doubling the dose every three days. If the flush is too great at any dose, the next dose should be cut by 1/2 or 1/4. The flush effect can be reduced by aspirin.

Hard water (high calcium and magnesium) protects against heart disease, while soft water with too much copper from the pipes promotes heart disease. Zinc and vitamin C can be used to reduce heavy metal levels, especially copper, lead, and cadmium. Magnesium is in hard water and is a useful therapy in various arrhythmias, and when deficient can produce arrhythmia and increase the size of the heart attack. Type A (overachiever) personalities more easily lose their magnesium. Twenty percent of patients admitted to Intensive Care units show decreases in magnesium. Magnesium is nature's physiologic calcium channel blocker, similar in its effects to the use of such drugs as verapamil and diltiazem. Magnesium, particularly as an oxide, is useful in the treatment of hypertension. Diuretics deplete potassium, magnesium, and zinc as well as other electrolytes significantly.

A recent study of fish consumption (in the *New England Journal of Medicine*) suggested that as little as one or two dishes per week may be of preventative value. Fish oil, like niacin and garlic, can raise HDL (the good cholesterol). Fish oil anticoagulates the blood as does aspirin.

Several other nutrients have been found to be deficient in patients with coronary artery disease. Low plasma chromium is found in coronary artery and other heart disease patients. Serum selenium has been found to be significantly reduced in patients with acute myocardial infarction. Cardiomyopathy has been associated with vitamin E deficiency. Decreases in serum linoleic acid (polyunsaturated oil) have been implemented in predisposing individuals to reinfarction. Antioxidants have a positive role in patients with coronary artery disease, probably reducing the risk of death. Vitamin B-6 has important diuretic properties and is essential to the lowering of blood pressure.

Other dietary suggestions are to follow a high vegetable, low fat, reduced meat diet, and to avoid all saturated fats and hydrogenated oils. It is advisable to eat large amounts of whole grains, use polyunsaturated oil (i.e. safflower or sunflower oil) liberally on salads, and consume high pectin fruits (apples, bananas).

Thrombosis

Measuring protein C and S low levels may indicate individuals at risk for stroke or blood clots.

PET Scanning at PATH

PET scan is another great innovation at PATH Medical, Positron Emission Tomography (PET) which can show the amazing breakthroughs in Cardiac reversal. We are able to get PET scanning which we believe replaces cardiac catheterization and stress Thallium testing completely. We have been able to demonstrate cardiac vascular reversal using this non-evasive, nontoxic technique. It also is capable of diagnosing cancer malignancies and may decrease the need for much of today's cancer biopsies. When having a PET scan performed, it is best to fast four hours prior to the test.

Another PATH innovation has been the use of Doppler, noninvasive, intravascular, ultrasound screening of blood vessels. Stroke is so common in our society: in people over 50 or 60, in smokers, in diabetics, in overweight patients, in those with high cholesterol and high blood pressure, in those who are inactive or bedridden, and in those who have a family history of heart attack or stroke. Deposits build up in the walls of our arteries and veins (arteriosclerosis) which causes narrowing and less blood flow to our toes, feet, fingers, head and brain. This can be picked up early. This probably occurs in at least one of four Americans, to a significant degree. Reversal can be achieved with a PATH program of exercise, diet, special shoes or stockings, medications, nutrients, ways to stop smoking, and chelation therapy.

It is very simple to test for both peripheral and carotid

vascular disease utilizing the new Doppler technique.

Get your pipes checked at PATH Medical and prevent the disease. Once you have a completed stroke, no one can adequately reverse it.

Whole Body PET Scan

Whole body Positive Emission Tomography (PET) scanning is a new breakthrough technique that finds cancers throughout the body better than any other technique currently established. Although there are certain areas where PET scanning may not be as good as other techniques, Pet scanning seems to be outstanding for ovarian cancer, colon cancer, lung cancer, musculoskeletal cancers, and staging of a wide variety of tumors.

Without invading the body and without any significant radiation, it can find all the hot spots in the body from bone to tissue. *One test* can tell whether or not you have a malignancy, where it is, and how much.

PET scanning is available from my colleague, D. Abass Alavi, Department of Radiology, Hospital of the University of Pennsylvania, 3400 Spruce Street, Philadelphia, PA, 19104.

All patients participating in the early research protocols will be required to pay only 20% co-pay to have this procedure done.

One of the great benefits is PET's ability to evaluate the internal mammary nodes. These are neglected by most surgeons. PET is accurate except for identifying cancer cells. Ninety five percent of the time it can be thrown off by fibrous tissue, inflammation or necrosis. Roughly, 3.5 times greater metabolism 2,3DPG indicates a cancer because there is such an increase in glucose transport with cancer. PET scanning can identify the cancerous stage and its malignancy status.

When preparing to have your PET scan, please have no oral intake (NPO) for four hours prior to the scan. Also, take no coffee, alcohol, nitrates, or nicotine for about 12 hours prior to the scan.

Pre-PET Scan Instructions

1. If your PET scan is scheduled before 1:00 p.m., do not eat or drink anything after the midnight prior to your test.

2. You may take medications with a small amount of water unless the medications are: Theophilline (Theodore, aminophylline, Slo-bid, etc.). Stop taking these medications 48 hours prior to your test -- **but do not discontinue any medications without first consulting your doctor!**

3. If you are currently taking dipyridamole (Persantine) do not take the morning dose on the day of the PET scan.

4. Cease smoking for six hours prior to the scan.

5. Please allow a minimum of three hours for the entire procedure.

6. If you are a diabetic, please consult with your physician for specific instructions.

7. Bring a signed and completed insurance form for your appointment.

8. If, for any reason, you are unable to follow the above instructions, you must inform the staff at the PET scan center, as well as your personal physician.

Body Composition Analysis

Body composition analysis is an important way of evaluating your muscle and body fitness. It will tell you the amount of body fat that you have, suggest a goal weight, and help you identify dietary ways in which you may improve your percentage of body muscle. It is also important for an individual to follow body composition while dieting to make sure that he does not lose muscle while dieting. Loss of muscle while dieting can be a very serious problem and affect your heart muscle.

Body components change throughout our life. For example, a fetus is 90% water, 0.6% fat, 6.3% protein while a premature child is typically anywhere between 82-86% water, 1-4% fat, 8-9% protein. Yet a full-term child is 71% water, 13.5% body fat and 12% protein.

Most adult males tend to be 60% water, 17% body fat, and 18% protein with the remaining fractions being minerals. As we age we all gain body fat. The ideal is probably 7 - 13% body fat.

If a person weighs 150 pounds and he has 20% body fat, then he has 30 pounds of fat and 120 pounds of what is referred to as lean mass. Muscle tissue increases or decreases depending on a person's diet, activities, exercise, and life style. While the average American typically loses muscle and gains fat steadily from age 20, this does not have to be so and weight training can actually benefit body components as well as total volume with age, and it can benefit overall health. The average American male has the following proportions of body fat:

Age	Percentage of body fat
20	10.3%
25	13.4%
30	16.2%
35	18.6%
40	21.0%
45	22.0%
50	24.0%
55	25.0%

Though a person may weigh the same at age 65 as he did at age 30, his body may have deteriorated substantially in terms of muscle mass. This can be responded to so that dieting and exercise can lead to the rebuilding of this muscle tissue. The body muscle can be continually built up at any age if proper exercise and diet are followed. Composition measures show what the scales won't show, whether, when a person goes off his diet and gains the weight back, he is gaining more fat and less muscle than he had originally.

Measuring body fat regularly will determine the effectiveness of an exercise/diet program being used. It is probably harmful for a man's body to be any lower than 6-7% fat because then there would be no reserve.

Body fat measurements can help direct a person how to diet and exercise -- how to recognize the need for better diet, calories, and nutrition. Individuals who are correct height and weight may actually have too much fat. Many individuals who appear to still be overweight while dieting will actually have added muscle and lost fat. The scale cannot give this type of information. For individuals who may be redistributing, the body composition device can help tell whether or not a person actually is redistributing, that is, adding muscle and losing fat. For some people who diet, this may be beneficial. Measuring body fat with skin fold calipers is very accurate.

The ideal amount of body fat in men as they get older is probably about 12%, and for women, 15-18%.

Body Composition -- Addendum

	Body Status	Percent Body Fat	Percent Lean Body Mass
Women	Very low fat	9-17	91-83
	Low fat	18-21	82-79
	Average	22-25	78-75
	Above average	26-29	74-71
	High fat	30-35	70-65
	Very high fat	35+	65-
Men	Very low fat	6-10	94-90
	Low fat	11-15	89-95
	Average	16-18	84-82
	Above average	19-20	81-80
	High fat	21-25	79-75
	Very high fat	25+	75-

Body fat is the reserve energy stored within body cells. This energy is measured in calories. For every 3500 calories consumed above the amount expended, the body creates one pound of fat. Serious health risks are associated with high body fat levels.

Lean body mass is fat-free weight composed of muscle, vital organs, body fluids, connective and other nonfat tissue. The greater the amount of muscle, the more efficiently the body metabolizes or "burns" fat. Dieting without exercise can result in a loss of 50% of fat content and 50% of muscle content, thus maintaining the same ratio of body fat to lean body mass. Exercise is therefore a necessity to the human body.

Body fat is probably a good correlation to coronary artery blockages and overall health.

Pretest Instructions for Body Composition Analysis

Your First Test Date: _____

First Retest Date: _____

Second Retest Date: _____

What is Body Composition Analysis?

Body composition Analysis (we call it BCA) is an extremely sensitive and accurate way to determine the ratio between body fat and lean body mass. It does this with a new technology called impedance plethysmography. Because this procedure takes into account the actual makeup of the body, it is far more useful than simple weighing when on a weight-loss or improved fitness program. The BCA computer not only calculates the mass ratios, but also predicts the risk of cardiovascular disease and supplies specific suggestions for exercise and weight reduction. When this test is repeated monthly (the second and subsequent tests are at a substantial discount from the first one), you get a "moving picture" of your progress. This method is gaining wide acceptance by sports trainers, exercise physiologists, and nutritionally-oriented physicians.

To monitor your progress, you should schedule another BCA one month after your first. Tests should be repeated at monthly intervals until you reach your weight/exercise goal.

How to Prepare for the Test

Although exceedingly accurate, certain factors *may* affect your results. Therefore, it important that you follow these directions in preparing for your BCA:

1. Minimize salt intake for at least 24 hours prior to the test.

2. Unless you regularly take diuretics (water pills or herbal preparations), do not take them.

3. No alcohol intake for at least 24 hours prior to the test.

4. Women should not schedule their test during the week before their periods. Follow-up tests should be scheduled at approximately the same time of the month as prior tests.

5. Do not eat for at least four hours prior to your test. You may, however, drink the normal amount of liquid customary for you.

6. Do not engage in strenuous aerobic exercise on the day of your test.

Twenty-Four Hour Blood Pressure Monitor

The twenty-four hour blood pressure monitor is an exciting new breakthrough in the management of high blood pressure. We all know that blood pressure varies greatly at different times of the day and under different stress conditions. Many individuals (especially those with generalized anxiety who come to the doctor) have falsely elevated blood pressure (white coat hypertension). Although this elevation may be an indication of a predisposition for high blood pressure, it frequently does not need to be treated. A twenty-four hour blood pressure monitor is very helpful in measuring average blood pressure and elevated blood pressures. Elevated twenty-four hour blood pressures are very predictive of risk for left ventricular hypertrophy (LVH). This means that as blood pressure increases the heart muscles have to work against more blood pressure and the heart increases in size. An enlarged heart muscle is not good. As the muscular wall thickens the inside volume is decreased. Furthermore, the blood supply to the ventricle does not increase in equal proportion to the muscle mass, and the risk of ischemia is increased. Therefore, you have to watch out for your heart becoming overly muscular as a result of high pressure. Fortunately, LVH is a reversible condition in many individuals.

The twenty-four hour blood pressure monitor is the ultimate in checking blood pressures; it measures a person's nighttime and daytime blood pressures and provides an average. In the future the established 140/90 goal as a standard upper ceiling of normal blood pressure may need to be lowered. It seems prudent to say that the blood pressure that is best for a person is that blood pressure which will not result in increased cardiovascular disease, e.g., increase in heart size, heart attack, or stroke. A lower blood pressure in age groups 40-70 (over 80 this may not be true), e.g., 120/80 or even 110/80 results in a reduction in total mortality. Yet, when individuals with high blood pressure have their blood pressure lowered to these values by drugs, it certainly results in more deaths.

See also material entitled *The Much Maligned Egg*, Section 9, p. 108.

Most drug treatments that lower pressure too much can be dangerous. If drugs are used, 140/90 is the goal pressure, without drugs 120/80 or 110/70. The blood pressure monitor can also be used to help the doctor understand if blood pressure has been satisfactorily corrected through treatment. So there are basically five main factors in the evaluation of hypertension:

1. Evaluate white coat hypertension

2. General blood pressure evaluation

3. Evaluation of the effect of drugs

4. Evaluation of left ventricular hypertrophy (may also require echocardiogram in addition to routine EKG)

5. Evaluation of the blood pressure lowering effects of a nutritional diet and healthful life style program

Holter Monitors

Holter monitors are very useful for measuring heart rhythms over a 24-hour period. They can detect subtle arrhythmias as well as life-threatening arrhythmias, thus helping a physician to decide which medication or even which nutritional approach might help in the treatment of cardiac arrhythmia. Holter monitors can also be utilized as event recorders. They frequently detect slow or sick sinus syndrome in adults who need pacemakers. Any patient with a potential cardiac arrhythmia history should utilize a Holter monitor.

16. Infectious Disease and the Immune System

Immunology

Immunology began in the laboratories of Pasteur and Koch, who sought to use the new science to solve the major health problems of their day -- acute infectious diseases. Their success lead to a period of intense concentration on the development of vaccines and sera, and justified the notion that the immune system existed for purposes of host defense. To this day, the prevailing explanation for the evolution and existence of the immune system is defense against invading microorganisms.

Immunological phenomena are regulated by physiological processes. The immune system has a dynamic interaction with cellular metabolism. The immune system proteins (autoantibodies, anti-idiotypes, and immunoglobulins) transport important nutrients, i.e., riboflavin, putrescine, and spermine, from the intestinal lumen to the cells for absorption. Immunoglobulins transport catabolic products of internal metabolism, i.e., denatured and degraded proteins, abnormal self or foreign cells to be lysed, excreted, or recycled.

Immunoglobulins (Ig's) regulate the response of target organs throughout the entire body to neurotransmitters and hormones. There are immunoglobulins which block and thereby regulate cell receptors for insulin, thyroid hormones, acetylcholine, parathyroid hormone, serotonin, and dopamine. B-endorphin may actually be an immunoglobulin fragment which regulates cell functions directly. (The immune system regulates metabolism by transport receptor blockade and controlling direct physiological functions.)

These autoantibodies (Ig's) are in all normal sera and normally regulate the above physiological processes. Antibodies occur in significant quantities in germ free environments in mice and man and thereby serve internal physiological functions. This explains why autoantibodies are present in virtually every known disease and are not necessarily indicative of pathology. Yet most diseases have abnormal autoantibody control because the disease process disrupts homeostasis.

The alteration of autoantibodies probably results from alteration in cell metabolism and products, i.e., homeostasis. Insulin, cholesterol, amyloid, and cortisol regulate the immune response, i.e., in disease condition autoantibodies clear more debris and transport more nutrients while other antibodies attack foreign agents. Autoimmune diseases such as Lupus, arthritis, and allergies are one form of abnormal regulation and the opposite are immune deficiency virus as seen with AIDS.

Because of the dynamic interaction between physiology and the immune system, principles from each can be applied analogously. Examples of *metabolic killing* of foreign or self products or cells via hyper or hypothermia, pH changes, and nutrient sequestering are host defense mechanisms. In addition, the concept of *immune* homeostasis explains alterations of immunoglobulins in disease as well as explaining why tonsillectomy and appendectomy can be harmful.

Finally, because the immune system is dynamically related to general metabolism, nutritional therapies can be designed to help treat "immune disorders." Nutritional deficiencies and imbalances are associated with increased allergy, i.e., food allergy. Megavitamin dosages of B-12 may continue to improve immune function above normal levels. Zinc is the key nutrient in thymus function; zinc deficiency can cause IgA deficiency.

Autoimmune Disorders

It is often more difficult to treat autoimmune disorders with nutrition, but Tagamet, aspirin derivatives, and nonsteroidal drugs can be helpful. Nutrients that may help the autoimmune disease are not yet well-studied since most individuals are working on building their immune system to fight off cancer and infection. It is probably true that most autoimmune diseases initially begin with infection. When the body fights off the infection, or the depletion of the immune system, it goes too far and begins to attack itself. Autoimmune diseases are frequently encountered in individuals who for a long time have depleted immune systems and tried to fight off the disease, stress, or infection, and now instead of fighting off the enemy are attacking themselves. It is very important to have your immune system studied through T-cell tests on a regular basis. There are both natural and atypical medication regimens as well as conventional medication regimens that can treat the immune system, whether it is depleted or overactive. We have not seen beneficial results from

thymus extracts. Immune suppressing drugs like Cyclophosphamide, Azathioprine, Hydrochloroprine, and steroids, except for the safe use of Cortef, are to be avoided in autoimmune disorders. Vaccination is another way of stimulating the immune system in some individuals. Flue shots, pneumonia shots, TB vaccinations, and other vaccinations can temporarily boost the weakened immune system.

An interesting study at Wayne State University in Detroit gave six zinc supplements, 30 mg a day, to 13 elderly zinc deficient men and women. After six months of extra zinc, they found improvements in immune function, increased blood levels of the thymus hormone thymosin, of which zinc is a key ingredient. You cannot make enough mature T-cells without zinc. The Wayne State study found that nearly 30% of a large group of healthy, affluent people over 50 were zinc deficient, according to their article in *Nutrition*, May/June 1993.

EMS (Eosinophilia Myalgia Syndrome)

EMS is caused by contaminated tryptophan. It works like an autoimmune disease similar to lupus. Treatment can be high doses of fish oil, antioxidants, and any anti-autoimmune disease agent whether it be Tagamet to chemotherapy, which of course we don't recommend, to drugs like Fastin, Ritalin, etc.

Other treatments might include DHEA, thyroid, etc., and of course steroids which again we usually do not recommend because of the side effects.

Middle Ear Infections

Make sure you take the full course of prescribed antibiotics. If infections reoccur, ask your doctor about permanent drainage tubes, although I prefer to avoid this. Allergies can be dealt with as a cause. Antihistamines, decongestants, and other medications improve the eustachian tube function. Avoid exposing susceptible children to colds, flu, and other viral illnesses.

Symptoms of middle ear infections include acute stabbing pain in the ear, prolonged crying, tugging or rubbing of the ear, pus discharge from the ear (discharge will most likely occur if eardrum ruptures to relieve pressure from fluid), fever and general fussiness (especially if child also has a cold), nausea and vomiting especially in young baby, and temporary hearing loss.

Infection: Modification by Food, Nutrients, and Behavior

INFECTION: CAUSE OF MANY DISEASES

Infection can begin with a cold and be as serious as AIDS. Some infections are in fact linked to cancer. Cryptocoides, a rare form of bacteria, can be a precursor to cancer. Viral infections may have a role in rheumatoid arthritis and schizophrenia can sometimes be caused by infection. Every single day we are fighting off an infection, either from being in contact with people who are sick or just normal bacteria exposure. This is why it's important to consider which nutrients can be beneficial. The Industrial Revolution has produced the Infection Revolution, and many believe that polio wasn't so much conquered by the vaccine as it was the changes in sanitation. Vaccinations were effective, but were not greatly effective until the control of hygiene and infection was prevalent.

NUTRIENTS AND INFECTION

Zinc is one of the main compounds that is found to be deficient in infectious individuals. It has been used to fight bacterial infections, because of stimulating interleukin and T-helper cells that fight infection. Studies on the common cold showed that zinc and zinc lozenges are effective in fighting the cold virus. Data does support that zinc does in fact help fight many viruses.

Too much iron can promote infection. Overnutritionizing yourself can have negative affects in fighting disease. Another vitamin, like zinc that raises the T-helper immune system, is B-12 in shot form (3-10 cc per week). It also raises energy levels. All the antioxidants are beneficial in infection. The key antioxidant, glutathione, decreases with infection. The use of vitamin C, cysteine, selenium, and vitamin E is important in fighting infection. Phenylalanine levels only increase with infection.

Branched chain amino acids (BCAA) -- leucine, isoleucine, and valine -- may have an important role in infection. Any individual who is deficient in nutrients should try this vitamin compound. When a person gets infected their muscles become drained and are sore. BCAA protect muscles. The role of lecithin in viral hepatitis is extremely important in its treatment. It may help to fight other virus infections.

MOOD AND INFECTION

Positive moods build immune functions to a degree. Joy, laughter, prayer, song, and all forms of love will benefit the infected person at appropriate times. Let us move toward health and holiness joyfully and nutritionally!

AIDS

Precautions that can be taken by the general public and by persons in special risk groups to eliminate or reduce the risk of contracting or spreading AIDS are:

- Do not have sexual contact with any person whose past history and current health status is not known.

- Do not have sexual contact with multiple partners or with persons who have had multiple partners.

- Do not have sexual contact with persons known or suspected of having AIDS.

- Do not abuse intravenous (IV) drugs.

- Do not share needles or syringes (boiling does not guarantee sterility).

- Do not have sexual contact with persons who abuse IV drugs.

- Use of a latex condom during sexual intercourse may decrease the risk of AIDS.

- Do not share toothbrushes, razors or other personal implements that could become contaminated with blood.

- Health workers, laboratory personnel, funeral directors, and others whose work may involve contact with body fluids should strictly follow recommended safety procedures to minimize exposure to AIDS, hepatitis B and other diseases.

■ Persons who are at increased risk for AIDS or who have positive HTLV-III, HIV antibody test, or hepatitis B test results should not donate blood, plasma, body organs, sperm, or other tissue.

■ Persons with positive HTLV-III antibody test results should have regular medical checkups and take special precautions against exchanging body fluids during sexual activity.

■ Women who have positive HTLV-III antibody test results should recognize that if they become pregnant their children are at increased risk for AIDS.

In sum, to be truly safe, have sex only with your spouse who was tested -- no extramarital sex; no premarital sexual relations.

Lyme Disease

Lyme disease, an infection similar to syphilis, is carried by deer ticks. Mankind is in a dynamic relationship with society and animals as disease spreads to human beings. When we are out of balance with nature, diseases get transmitted from us to animals and back to us (either through sex, ingestion, or through insect vectors). This is probably the case with Lyme disease, which is the transformation of a syphilis-like lifecycle with human beings in the chain. Lyme disease can be the great masquerader and affect the nervous system, the joints, etc. It can be treated effectively with antibiotics but can be a relapsing and recurring disease, somewhat similar to the way genital herpes acts and the way AIDS may eventually manifest itself. Techniques for testing lyme disease include various ELISA tests, western blot techniques, and consultation with an infectious disease specialist. The earlier Gunderson antibody test may be an even more accurate test.

Lyme disease is a nasty infection and rash at the site of a tick bite, usually with expanded rays with a circle and clear center. Flulike symptoms, headache, fever, fatigue, chills, sore throat, hoarseness, stiff neck, loss of appetite, nausea, vomiting, diarrhea, abdominal cramps may result. Other complications include hot, swollen, and painful joints.

Neurological complications include paralysis, often of the face, abnormal skin sensation sensitivity, irregular, rapid, or slow heart beat; chest pain, dizziness, or shortness of breath. Pregnant women can incur miscarriage or stillbirth.

Psychological complications include depression, dementia, and psychosis.

Avoid tick exposures, walk along clear and paved surfaces rather than walking in grass or in the woods. Wear long-sleeved shirts, buttoned at the wrist; long pants tucked into socks. Choose light colored fabric and use insect repellents containing deet or permethrin. Use flea and tick collars on your pets. Brush them carefully after they have been outdoors.

If you have been bitten by a tick, remove it immediately by grasping it with tweezers. Tape the tick to a 3x5 card and bring to a physician for identification.

Avoid areas where deer ticks are common, mow the weeds and grass around the house, and try to discourage birds that harbor ticks.

Warning: it is imperative that all women of child bearing age who are about to receive Lyme disease treatment (i.e., with Doxycycline) have a pregnancy test. Additionally, it is unwise to become pregnant within six months of this treatment.

Chronic Fatigue Syndrome

Chronic fatigue syndrome (CFS) is not really a disease but describes a symptom in which there are many possible causes. Some of these causes include abnormalities in brain chemistry, which are treated with tyrosine, phenylalanine, and sometimes antidepressants; or seizure disorders, which are treated with anticonvulsants; anxiety disorders, which are treated with CES devices and psychotherapy; immune disorders treated through the brain chemistry or allergy treatments; anemia; diabetes; thyroid and endocrinology conditions; abnormalities in the adrenal gland; infectious causes that need to be treated with antibiotics, such as Lyme disease; rare neurological causes such as M.S. and Alzheimer's disease; or enceph-alopathy treated with medications. Most chronic fatigue patients tend to have a brain biochemical imbalance, which can be treated through a combination of natural and/or drug therapies. Chronic fatigue is a treatable condition, and in most individuals has primarily a biochemical basis. Counselling can be helpful in terms of support, but will not successfully treat the condition. What is CFS? CFS is defined by major, minor and physical criteria. The definition requires (1) both of two major criteria, signs of 11 minor criteria and two or three physical criteria or (2) two major criteria and eight minor criteria. Major criteria are:

1. New onset of persistent or relapsing fatigue, with no previous history, which does not resolve with bed rest and is severe enough to reduce or impair average daily activity to less than 50 percent for six months.
2. Exclusion of other clinical conditions that may produce similar symptoms by a thorough evaluation, including the history, physical examination and appropriate laboratory tests.

Minor criteria (symptoms) are:

1. Mild fever.
2. Sore throat.
3. Painful cervical or axillary lymph nodes.
4. Unexplained generalized muscle weakness.
5. Muscle discomfort or myalgia.
6. Prolonged (24 hours or longer) generalized fatigue after levels of exercise that previously would have been easily tolerated by the patient.
7. Generalized headaches different from those that previously may have occurred.
8. Migratory arthralgia without joint swelling or redness.
9. Neuropsychologic complaints which may include photophobia, visual scotoma, forgetfulness, irritability, confusion, difficulty in thinking, and depression.
10. Sleep disturbance (hypersomnia or insomnia).
11. Initial development of the main symptom complex over a few hours or a few days.

Physical criteria, which must be documented by a physician on at least two occasions that are at least one month apart, are:

1. Low-grade fever.
2. Nonexudative pharyngitis.
3. Palpable or tender cervical or axillary lymph nodes.

Important Information About Pneumococcal Disease and Pneumococcal Polysaccharide Vaccine [1]

WHAT IS PNEUMOCOCCAL DISEASE?

Streptococcus pneumoniae is a bacterium that causes much illness and death in the United States each year. This bacterium, also called the pneumococcus, can cause serious infections of the lungs (pneumonia), the bloodstream (bacteremia), and the covering of the brain (meningitis). About five persons out of every 100 who get pneumococcal pneumonia, about 20 out of every 100 who get bacteremia, and about 30 out of every 100 who get meningitis, die of these infections. Anyone can get pneumococcal disease; however, persons over 65 years of age, the very young, and persons of any age who have special types of health problems have the greatest risk.

People are more likely to die from pneumococcal disease if they have problems such as alcoholism, heart or lung diseases, kidney failure, diabetes, or certain types of cancer. Older persons as a group are more likely to die from pneumococcal disease. Forty out of every 100 persons who have these special health problems die when they develop pneumococcal bacteremia and 55 out of 100 with these special health problems die if they get pneumococcal meningitis. The high risk of death occurs in spite of treatment with drugs like penicillin. Because of the risk of serious complications from pneumococcal infection, vaccination is recommended for older persons and children, as well as for adults with special health problems.

PNEUMOCOCCAL POLYSACCHARIDE VACCINE:

The pneumococcal polysaccharide vaccine contains material from the 23 types of pneumococcal bacteria that cause 88 percent of pneumococcal bacteremias. Most healthy adults who receive the vaccine develop protection against most or all of these types of pneumococcal bacteria 2-3 weeks after vaccination. Older persons and those with some long-term illnesses may not respond as well or at all. Children under two years of age also are not protected by the vaccine. The vaccine probably provides long-term protection for most people. However, some people may lose protection about six years after vaccination and require revaccination. The vaccine is given by injection.

WHO SHOULD RECEIVE PNEUMOCOCCAL POLYSACCHARIDE VACCINE?

Vaccination is recommended for the following:

Adults

1. All adults aged 65 years and older and adults of all ages with long-term illnesses that are associated with a high risk of getting pneumococcal disease, including those with heart or lung diseases, diabetes, alcoholism, cirrhosis, or leaks of cerebrospinal fluid (CSF, the fluid surrounding the brain and spinal cord).

2. Adults with diseases that lower the body's resistance to infections or who are taking drugs that lower the body's resistance to infections, including those with abnormal function or removal of the spleen, Hodgkin's disease, lymphoma, multiple myeloma, kidney failure, nephrotic syndrome (a type of kidney disease), or conditions such as organ transplantation.

---

1. *Pneumococcal* 9/1/89.

Lupus

Systemic lupus erythematosus (SLE) is a chronic inflammatory disease of unknown origin which can affect virtually all organ systems. Common symptoms of the disease are marked by malar or discoid rash, arthritis, photosensitivity, serositis (pleuritis, pericarditis), kidney disease (proteinuria or casts), neurologic disorder (seizures or psychosis), hematologic disorder (hemolytic anemia, leukopenia, lymphopenia, thrombocytopenia), immunologic disorder (abnormal ANA, LE, anti-DNA, anti-Sm), cardiolipin antibodies, histone antibodies. The disease primarily affects white females. Many drugs, e.g., phenelzine, hydrazine derivatives (e.g., aniline, isoniazid, tartrazine, sulfonamide, etc.) can also cause lupus.

Ninety percent of patients with lupus have fatigue, arthritis, and arthralgia. Eighty percent have fever; 70% have anemia; 60% have butterfly rash, anorexia and weight loss; 50% have alopecia, serositis, lymphadenopathy, personality disorders, and purpura. Lupus can also be present with depression and psychosis.

Conventional therapy includes steroids (may worsen condition in long run), immune suppressing drugs (e.g., cyclophosphamide, azathioprine), hydroxychloroquine (for skin), and aspirin-like drugs for fever and inflammation.

Nutrient treatments which have been suggested to be helpful for lupus are: beta carotene, vitamin A, fish oil, vitamin E, calcium, magnesium, and potassium. The vitamin A drug, isotretinoin (Accutane), 80 mg/day, may be effective in both chronic or subacute cutaneous dentoid lupus erythmetosis. Vitamin E (800-2000 I.U.) has been effective in discoid lupus. Dr. Atkins has suggested that phosphetamin in combination with calcium, magnesium, and potassium may be helpful. An arginine derivative (L-canavanine) may worsen or induce lupus.

Immunosuppressive drugs that affect brain chemistry can benefit lupus, e.g., Wellbutrin, Nardil, Desipramine and possibly Parlodel.

Sporonox

Sporonox (itraconazole) is a new oral antifungal agent which is extremely useful in a variety of fungal infections such as histoplasmosis and blastomycosis. It remains in the tissues (nail fungus) up to 28 days after discontinuation of the therapy, and does not enter into the brain. It is demonstrated with an outstanding safety profile up to three years. Common side effects are nausea, rash, and vomiting, and the only serious side effects have been reported when taken with Seldane or terfenadine. Sporonox should not be used with hypoglycemic drugs (used for diabetes) or with alcohol. See the before and after treatment color pictures.

Rare Diseases Information

Assn. of Biotechnology Companies, 1666 Connecticut Ave. N. W., Suite 330, Washington, DC 20009; (202) 234-3330.

Alliance of Genetic Support Groups, 35 Wisconsin Circle, Suite 440, Chevy Chase, MD 20815; (800) 336-4363.

Coalition for Heritable Disorders of Connective Tissues, 382 Main St., Port Washington, NY 11050; (516) 883-8712.

Division of Research Grants, National Institutes of Health, Westwood Building, 533 Westbard Ave., Bethesda, MD 20892; (301) 496-7543.

General Clinical Research Centers, Rare Disease Network, AA 3223 MCN, Vanderbilt University Medical Center, Nashville, TN 37232-2195; (615) 343-0124 or (800) 428-6626.

March of Dimes, 1275 Mamaroneck Ave., White Plains, NY 10605; (914) 428-7100.

Industrial Biotechnology Assn. 1625 K St. N. W., Suite 1100, Washington, DC 20006; (202) 857-0244. (Inquiries from organizations only.)

Metabolic Information Network, PO Box 670847, Dallas TX 75367-0847; (214) 696-2188 or (800) 945-2188.

National Library of Medicine, 8600 Rockville Pike, Bldg 38, Bethesda MD 20894; (301) 496-6095 or (800) 272-4787.

National Center for Education in Maternal and Child Health, 38th and R Streets N.W., Washington, DC 20013-1133; (800) 456-3505.

National Information Center for Orphan Drugs and Rare Diseases, PO Box 1133, Washington, DC 20013-1133; (800) 456-3505.

National Institutes of Health, 9000 Rockville Pike, Bethesda, MD 20892; (301) 496-4000 (general information number).

National Organization of Rare Disorders, PO Box 8923, New Fairfield, CT 06812-1783; (203) 746-6518 or (800) 999-6673.

Office of Orphan Products Development, Food and Drug Administration, 5600 Fishers Lane (HF 35), Rockville, MD 20857; (301) 443-4903.

Pharmaceutical Manufacturers Assn., Commission on Drugs for Rare Diseases, 1100 15th St. N. W., Washington, DC 20005; (202) 835-3550.

World Life Foundation, PO Box 571, Bedford, TX 76095; (817) 282-1405 or (800) 289-5433.

The Immune System as Regulator of Homeostasis:

Implications for Nutritional Therapy

Through the serendipitous discovery of protective immunity during the last century, the conception of the origin and function of the immune system has been channeled in a single direction: the defense of the body against foreign agents. This postulate was partially based on the observation that organisms distinguish endogenous (self) from exogenous (nonself) antigenic substances (Ags). Furthermore, immunologic dogma originally postulated that the organism can react with "nonself" and not with "self" Ags as was expressed by the famous Ehrlich's phrase "horror autotoxicus." We now know that the body does attack itself by producing autoantibodies. The purpose of the immune system is to regulate internal physiological processes and protect the human body (self) from invaders (nonself). During the evolution of the immune system this dual role has led to a cross-reactivity resulting in the infamous antibody.

Immune system proteins (autoantibody immunoglobulins) transport important nutrients, i.e., riboflavin, putrescine, spermine, etc., from the intestinal lumen to the cells for absorption. Immunoglobulins transport catabolic products of internal metabolism, i.e., denatured and degraded proteins, abnormal self or foreign cells to be used, excreted, or recycled.

Immunoglobulins regulate the response of target organs throughout the entire body to neurotransmitters and hormones. There are immunoglobulins which block and thereby regulate cell receptors for insulin, thyroid hormones, acetylcholine, parathyroid hormones, serotonin, and dopamine. B-endorphin is actually an immunoglobulin fragment which regulates cell functions directly. The immune system regulates homeostatic metabolism by transport, receptor blockade, and direct physiological interactions.

The key principle to this physiological immune concept is understanding the nature of autoantibodies and autoimmune disease. From the point of view of the theory considering that immunological phenomena are "defense mechanisms," the appearance of autoantibodies represent a contradiction. Autoantibodies can exist in small amounts in normal organisms and appear in quantity after tissue destruction or alteration by exogenous agents. Assuming that the immunological phenomena originally are not a "defense mechanism" but rather a physiological system of handling metabolic and catabolic substances, the appearance of autoantibodies is a normal process. "Self" constituents are normally degraded by autolytic enzymes, but in cases of massive destruction of tissues, these enzymes can be inhibited by substrate excess. Cells capable of synthesizing autoantibodies which exist normally are then activated and autoantibodies appear; they facilitate phagocytosis. The same mechanism acts for "nonself" substances if undergraded by existing enzymes. Tolerogens, resulting from degradation, can block the receptors on immunocompetent cells. Possibly, they may differ from immunogens in possessing only one determinant group susceptible to it.

Immunoglobulins and Disease

The two immune defense mechanisms, immunoglobulins (antibodies) and lymphocytic system are primarily involved in the fighting of infection. Immunoglobulins are secreted by plasma cells. When cancerous, the plasma cell produces multiple myeloma wherein the Bence Jones proteins in the urine and blood can be any one of the various globulins, because the protein consists only of the common low molecular weight chains. Congenital deficiencies in immunoglobulin production are associated with poorly developed lymphoid germinal centers, which results in a decrease in the absolute number of plasma cells. Abnormal immunoglobulin levels are associated with various diseases.

The antibody molecule includes two equivalent high molecular weight polypeptide chains and two shorter light chains. Light chains contain one of two kinds of proteins - 1 or k, which can be distinguished immunologically. Heavy chains have five protein varieties, A, D, E, G, and M. Congenital or acquired deficiencies may occur in IgM, IgA, and IgG. The immunoglobulins occur in blood, muscle, intestinal mucosa, and skin.

FOOD INTOLERANCE AND THE IGE

The IgE is formerly known as the skin sensitizing antibody. The immunoglobulin combines with the allergen on the surface of tissue mast cells or circulating basophils and leads to the release of histamine and other biochemical mediators (SRS-A, bradykinin). Everyone produces IgE, but some patients have trouble turning off the manufacturing mechanism. An example is the body's response to attack by the parasite ascaris. The individuals with the highest and longest response have the greatest immunity.

Determination of serum IgE and specific IgE antibodies can be helpful in detecting obvious allergies. Slightly raised IgE levels in the first years of life indicate a tendency to acquire hay fever, asthma, and dermatitis. Even low RAST scores, early in life, for specific allergies, indicate a food allergy. The majority of food allergies appear to be IgE mediated. Later in childhood low levels of IgE antibodies in response to milk and eggs are common even when tolerance existed. IgG may have a blocking capacity for IgE but this is speculative. IgE levels usually don't change significantly in the first two years of life while IgG can increase.

CELIAC DISEASE AND IMMUNOGLOBULINS

Some studies have provided evidence that a deficiency of IgM or IgA is common in celiac patients. Others present evidence of an inexact correlation. Adult patients with hypogammaglobulinemia (congenital disorder symptomized by reduction and/or impairment of plasma cells) acquire sprue at a 20% rate. Sprue and celiac disease are basically identical and different from tropical sprue. Biopsy reveals that IgA, IgM, and IgG are often deficient in the intestinal mucosa of celiacs.

Antibodies for at least one cow's milk protein were identified in 91% of celiac patients. This IgE allergic response can often be avoided by heating milk, thereby denaturing the protein. (Celiac disease can be determined by a wheat gluten skin test or elimination diet.)

AUTOIMMUNE DISEASE -- characterized by production of abnormal globulins.

1. 27% of the patients with autoimmune disease were sensitized to horse IgG, while all other groups were less than 4%.

2. Autoimmune hemolytic anemia -- RBC's are coated with abnormal protein.

OTHER CONGENITAL DISORDERS BESIDES MULTIPLE MYELOMA

Ataxia telangiectasia -- a congenital disorder of low IgA. Victims show great susceptibility to pulmonary and sinus infections, and loss of muscular coordination as a result of cerebellar disease. In addition, telangiectasia of a mucous membrane covering the anterior surface of the eyeball (conjunctivitis) may occur.

THE LIFE OF AN IMMUNOGLOBULIN

No accurate half-life determination of any immunoglobulin has been made. In multiple myeloma the abnormal globulin (M-component) has been detected 20 years prior to development of the disease. In abnormal chain production (Franklin's disease), victims may survive from four months to four years. IgE changes are insignificant in the first two years, while IgG production begins earlier from changes in rival diseases. We can predict that different immunoglobulins will have different life spans which are dependent on the overall health status of the individual.

FOUR TYPES OF ALLERGIC REACTIONS

1. An immediate hypersensitivity, IgE mediated reaction with an inhaled or ingested antigen. The antigen-antibody reaction releases histamine and slow reacting substances, kinins, serotonin, and acetylcholine.

2. An antibody reacts with an antigen attached to a cell surface. The reaction (thermolabile substance in normal serum destructive to bacteria and other cells when brought into contact) produces an antigen-antibody complex which is toxic to the tissues.

3. These are reactions of the IgG and IgM groups. These circulating antibodies cause the patient to react by forming an immune complex which is a cause of allergic pulmonary alveolitis. The immune complex releases lysozymes, damages neutrophils, and produces edema, hemorrhage, and thrombosis.

4. Delayed hypersensitivity is caused by sensitized Undegraded, the kind of delayed reaction which occurs in tuberculosis and Candida testing.

References -- Immunoglobulin and Disease

Baker, P. G., and Read, A. E., Positive Skin Reactions in Coeliac Disease. *Quarterly J. of Med.* 45:603-610, 1976.

Beerthema, J. H., Diagnostic Significance of IgM Antibodies in Toxoplasmosis. *Lancet* 237:2135, 1977.

Ben-aryeh, H., *et al.*, Salivary IgA and Serum IgG and IgA in recurrent Aphthous Stomatitis, 42:746-752, 1976.

Berrens, L., *et al.*, Complement component profiles in urticaria dermatitis herpetiformis and alopecia areata, *Brit. J. of Dermatol* 95:145-152, 1976.

Brandtzaeg, P., and Baklien, K., Immunohistochemical Studies of the Formation and Epithelial Transport in Normal and Diseased Human Intestinal Mucosa, *Scandinavian J. of Gastroenterology*, Vol. 11, Supp. 36, 1976.

Casterline, C. C., Quantitative Levels of Immunoglobulin E in Advanced Tuberculosis, *JAMA* 236:2008, 1976.

Chua, Y. Y., *et. al.*, In vivo and in vitro correlates of allergy. *The J. of Allergy and Clinical Immunology*, 58:299-307, 1976.

Cooper, B. J., and Patterson, R., Elevated IgM Levels in Edema and Fatigue Syndrome, *Arch. Internat'l. Med.* 36:1366-1369, 1976.

Dannaeus, A., *et. al.*, Clinical and Immunological Aspects of Food Allergy in Childhood, *Acta Paediatrica* 66:31-37, 1977.

Gillespie, D. N., Detection to Nuts by the Radio Allergosorbent Test. *J. of Allergy and Clin. Immun.* 57:302-309, 1976.

Hamburger, R. N., Allergy and the Immune System. *Amer. Scient.* 64:157-164, 1976.

Hjalmarson, O., IgA Deficiency during D-Penicillamine Treatment, *JAMA* 238:172, 1977.

Husby, G., *et. al.*, Smooth Muscle Antibody in Heroin Addicts. *An. of Inter. Med.* 83:802-805, 1975.

Internal Medicine News. IgG Antibody Response to Sting Called Variable Among Patients. 10:25, 1977.

Jarnum, S., *et. al.*, Dysgammaglobulinemia in Tropical Sprue. *Brit. Med. Journal* 4:416-417.

Jones, S. E., Immunodeficiency in Patients with Non-Hodgkins Lymphomas, *JAMA* 238:172, 1977.

Kjellman, N., I. M. Predictive Value of High IgE Levels in Children. *Acta Paediatra Scand.* 65:465-471, 1976.

Atopic Allergy and Serum IgE in Randomly Selected Eight Year Old Children. *Acta Allergologica* 32:91-108, 1977.

Maccia, C. A., Platelet Thrombopathy in Asthmatic Patients with Elevated Immunoglobulin. *E. Journal of Allergy and Clinical Immunology* 59:101-108, 1977.

McBride, G., Antibodies Yield Their Secrets and Display Therapeutic Versatility. *JAMA* 235:583-595, 1976.

Medical World News. When Transplants Bring Cancer, 2 Nov. 1973.

Nahari, J., Effect of Malnutrition on Several Parameters of the Immune System of Children. *Nutrition and Metabolism* 20:302-306, 1976.

Nutritional Reviews. Call-Mediated Immune Response in Celiac Disease, 34:295-297, 1976.

D'Loughlin, S., *et. al.*, Serum IgE in Dermatitis and Dermatosis. *Dermatology* 113:309-315, 1977.

Proesmans, W., *et. al.*, D-penicillamine Induced IgA Deficiency in Wilson's Disease. *Lancet* 2:804-805, 1976.

Ring, J., High Incidence of Horse Serum Protein Allergy in Various Autoimmune Disorders. *JAMA* 238:82, 1977.

Ross, I. N., and Thompson, R. A., Severe Selective IgM Deficiency. *J. of Clin. Patho.* 29:773-777, 1976.

Sharma, D. P., Extrinsic Allergic Alveolitis: Easy to Miss Consultant, May 1976.

Strahilevitz, M., *et. al.*, Immunoglobulins in Psychiatric Patients, presented at the 1975 A. P. A. Annual Meeting, Anaheim, CA.

Weston, W. L., A Hyperimmunoglobulin E Syndrome with Normal Cherootaxis in Vitro and Defective Leukotaxis in Vivo, *J. of Allergy and Clin. Immunology* 59:115-119, 1977.

Wolff-Burgin, A., Immunofluorescent Antibodies Against Gliadin: A Screening Test for Coeliac Disease. *Helv. Paediat. Acta.* 31:375-380, 1976.

Building and Maintaining an Effective Immune System [1]

Before we decide how to build and maintain an effective immune system, we need a test to assess the immune system. Fortunately, there is now a very simple and cost-effective test called T-helper/T-suppressor ratios. By measuring these two cells and coming up with a ratio, a doctor gets a basic assessment of the overall immune state. When T-helper cells are equal to T-suppressor cells, there is a ratio of one. In AIDS patients, this ratio can be .4 or even .1, an almost complete loss of all T-helper cells. Cancer patients frequently have depletion of the immune system or the helper cells, with ratios of .6 or .8. Individuals with chronic colds and chronic infections can be .9 or 1.2. Virtually any infection and various cancers deplete this ratio. In contrast, individuals with arthritis, lupus, myasthenia gravis, multiple sclerosis, allergies, or who are in the acute phase of having an infection or a breakout of cancer can have T-helper/T-suppressor ratios of 2 or greater. A ratio of 1.8 is probably ideal.

Once the immune system is assessed, it can be augmented in the proper direction. Some immune regulation nutrients can be useful in both overactive and underactive immune systems. The immune regulating nutrients are zinc, typically 90 mg; beta carotene, 50-75 mg; vitamin E, 800 units; selenium, 400 mcg; cystine, 2 g; fish oil, 2 g; as well as B-complex and a multivitamin. In addition, nutrients such as vitamin D, even higher dosages of zinc, and the natural interferons which are now available may increase T-helper cells. Branched-chain amino acids also can be helpful in building the immune system. The brain appears to be the master regulator of the immune system, and Cranial Electrical Stimulation (CES) can be very helpful because of biochemical and stress regulation.

1 *Health News & Review* 2:2, 2nd Quarter, 1992.

Immunoglobulins

IMMUNO-GLOBULIN	IgA 134-297 mg%; 10% of Total Requires Zinc & B-6; Affords Protection Against Live Virus	IgE 10-50 u/l Trace Amounts Inhalant Allergens	IgG 770-1510 mg% 80% of Total Antibacterial, Antiviral, Antitoxic	IgM 67-208 mg% 10% of Total Heterophile, Anti-RF, Isohemagglutinin
LOW	1. Penicillamine (may reduce zinc) 2. Pyroluria (B-6, zinc deficiency 3. Possible celiac association 4. Congenital loss of muscular coordination, disease of cerebellum	No known deficiency	1. Serum of schizophrenics with severe hallucinations 2. Lymphoma 3. Tropical Sprue	1. Possible celiac disease 2. No immediate consequence in adults 3. Congenital in children (father inherited); infections and death result 4. In advanced TB
NORMAL	1. Allergic milk group 2. Hives & Alopecia Areata 3. Aphthous Stomatitis 4. Tropical Sprue	1. In some patients with multiple allergies 2. Levels higher in blacks than in whites 3. Higher in children than adults	1. Malnourished children 2. Hives and hay fever 3. Alopecia Areata 4. Needed for maintenance of normal intestinal mucosa 5. Antibodies to cow's milk, egg white common to many children, possible blocking capacity of IgE food antibodies	1. Malnourished children 2. Hives and hay fever 3. Alopecia Areata 4. Aphthous Stomatitis 5. Tropical Sprue

IMMUNO-GLOBULIN	IgA 134-297 mg%; 10% of Total Requires Zinc & B-6; Affords Protection Against Live Virus	IgE 10-50 u/l Trace Amounts Inhalant Allergens	IgG 770-1510 mg% 80% of Total Antibacterial, Antiviral, Antitoxic	IgM 67-208 mg% 10% of Total Heterophile, Anti-RF, Isohemagglutinin
HIGH	1. Severe malnutrition 2. White schizophrenic females 3. Black schizophrenics 4. Higher in black schizophrenics than in white schizophrenics 5. In serum of all psychiatric patients 6. Patients before a polyarthritic attack	1. Correlates to atopic disease, hay fever, urticaria eczema, etc. 2. Correlates to food allergies 3. Correlates to specific allergens of milk, soybean, egg, fish, nuts 4. Correlates to respiratory allergies, allergic rhinitis, bronchial asthma, etc. 5. Platelet Thrombopathy in asthmatic patients 6. Defective leukocyte migration 7. In response to worms (ascaris) and mosquitoes. The greater the level, the more protection	1. High levels following insect bites 2. Higher in schizophrenics whose urine was phenothiazine positive than schizophrenics who were negative 3. Relates to milder hallucinations in schizophrenics 4. In advanced TB	1. Toxicoplasmosis disease (positive) 2. Edema and fatigue patients 3. Heroin addicts

T-Cell or Immune System Ratios and Health

T-cells are immune cells derived from the thymus gland. Two of the most important thymus cells are the T-helper cells which help other cells (B-cells) make antibodies to fight disease and T-suppressor cells which suppress this and other processes. T-helper cells are elevated in autoimmune diseases in which our own antibodies attack our tissues and cells (see table p. 213). T-helper cells are depleted in cancer, AIDS, and various other immune-compromised patients. T-helper cells are also depleted for a short while during acute illness such as viral infections. Because of the AIDS epidemic, there has been much interest in pharmacologic elevation of T-helper cells. Accutane (vitamin A drug) and Motrin (a fish oil-like drug) have been suggested agents to elevate T-helper cells in the blood. T-helper cells are very dependent upon zinc. AIDS patients are low in zinc, and zinc deficiency depletes T-helper cells. Hence, it is not surprising we have seen elevations in T-helper cells with zinc therapy of 90-150 mg per day. Successful treatment of T-cell ratio abnormalities is possible with nutrients and drugs. Parlodel, Nardil, L-dopa, Wellbutrin and Cytotec are probably immune suppressive and helpful in autoimmune diseases. Deseryl and Prozac, on the other hand, most likely are immune-augmenting treatments. The brain controls the immune system and susceptibility to immune diseases begins in the brain.

Thymus Hormone and T-cell Life

We hope in the future to be measuring thymidine. Thymus pause may be the first step towards death.

Vaccines

Regarding vaccines, I recently wrote this letter:

Recently my child was offered hemophilus influenza B vaccine, which I refused. I also refused to let her have hepatitis vaccine as an infant. Regarding DPT, I put it off to four months of age. Regarding repeat pertussis, after a bad reaction, I will not give the third dose. I also refused the pertussis vaccine for my first child after the first dose caused serious side effects.

As a way of background, historically, George Bernard Shaw said, "Modern medicine has replaced both Judaism and Christianity, in essence, substituting vaccinations for universal baptisms and circumcision." Shots simply are not for everyone.

Enclosed is literature from *USA Today* documenting some of the brain damage associated with DPT. Also enclosed is a copy of my entire file (face sheets). These articles are available if you should want them. DPT vaccine is still associated with many problems. It would be perfectly reasonable for anyone to refuse (of course, depending on risk) DPT vaccination. There are whole textbooks devoted to the adverse effects of pertussis and rubella vaccines.

On the other hand, there seems to be quite a bit of high cost, and I have proceeded with hepatitis and measles vaccine. Nonetheless, multiple sclerosis and cancer associated with polio vaccines has more than made this a controversial issue. There is reason for parents to be very concerned and to reject certain types of vaccinations. Chicken pox is another example of a controversial vaccine. Possibly with pertussis vaccine there can be neurological diseases. Nonetheless, pertussis has made somewhat of a comeback in the United States. It made the comeback, ironically, in children who were properly vaccinated! Again, this raises the issues about the validity of vaccinations. Rene Dubois, Nobel Laureate, questioned various issues of vaccines (especially TB and polio vaccines.)

Obviously, it would not be reasonable for a health care worker working with blood and/or sick people to reject the hepatitis B vaccine. It depends on the situation, i.e., rejection of the vaccine.

References

1. Adult Immunization with Acellular Pertussis Vaccine, Edwards, Kathryn M., M.D., et. al., *JAMA* 269:1, 1993.

2. Adverse Effects of Pertussis and Rubella Vaccines, AMA Book Source, edited by Howson, Christopher P., et. al., *JAMA* 267:23, 1992.

3. Adverse Events Associated with Childhood Vaccines Other than Pertussis and Rubella, Stratton, Kathleen R., Ph.D., et. al., *JAMA* 271:20, 1994.

4. Adverse Events Following Pertussis and Rubella Vaccines, Howson, Christopher P., et. al., *JAMA* 267:3, 1992.

5. Chicken Pox Conundrum, Gorman, Christine, *Time*, 7/19/93.

6. Diphtheria, Tetanus, and Pertussis -- What You Need to Know, U. S. Dept. of Health & Human Services, 3/92.

7. Doctors Told to Boost Adult Immunizations, Jones, Laurie.

8. Efficacy of Whole-cell Pertussis Vaccine in Preschool Children in the United States, Onorato, Ida M., M.D., et. al., *JAMA* 267:20, 1992.

9. FDA Approval of Use of Diphtheria and Tetanus Toxoids and Acellular Pertussis Vaccine, *JAMA* 67:4, 1992.

10. Guide to Contraindications and Precautions to Vaccinations -- From Standards for Pediatric Immunization Practices, U. S. Dept. of Health & Human Services, MMWR 42:RR-5, 1993.

11. Healthy Youth 2000. The Challenge -- Advertisement.

12. Hepatitis B Virus: A Comprehensive Strategy for Eliminating Transmission in the United States Through Universal Childhood Vaccination, U.S. Dept. of Health & Human Services, MMWR 40:RR-13, 1991.

13. (The) Immunization Resource Guide -- Letter, Rozario, Diane, Patter Publications, 1993.

14. Impact of Haemophilus Influenzae Type B Polysaccharide-Tetanus Protein Conjugate Vaccine on Responses to Concurrently

Administered Diphtheria-Tetanus-Pertussis Vaccine, Clemens, John D., M.D., et. al., *JAMA* 267:5, 1992.

15. Low Vaccination Levels of U. S. Preschool and School-age Children, Zell, Elizabeth R, et. al., *JAMA* 271:11, 1994.

16. Malaria Vaccines: Scientific and Ethical Issues, Tosta, Carlos Eduardo, *Rev. Inst. Med. Trop.*, Sao Paulo, 1992.

17. Mass Voluntary Immunization Campaigns for Meningococcal Disease in Canada: Media Hysteria, Flanagin, Annette, RN, M.A. -- edited by, *JAMA* 267:13, 1992.

18. Measles, Mumps, and Rubella -- What You Need to Know, U. S. Dept. of Health & Human Services, 1992.

19. Monitoring Progress Toward U. S. Preschool Immunization Goals, Cutts, Felicity T., et. al., *JAMA* 267:14, 1992.

20. Nation Must Make Sure All Children Get Their Shots, Debate -- Opposing View by Fisher, Barbara Loe, *USA Today*, 12/11/91.

21. National Childhood Vaccine Injury Act -- Requirements for Permanent Vaccination Records, Reporting of Selected Events After Vaccination, and Distribution of Vaccine Information Pamphlets, Dunston, Frances JL, M.D., M.P.H., State Commissioner of Health, *Health Bulletin*, 4/15/92.

22. New Chicken Pox Shot: Worth the Cost? Katzenstein, Larry, *American Health*, 6/94.

23. Outfoxing the Pox, Curless, Maura Rhodes, *Redbook*, 5/92.

24. Pertussis Makes a Comeback in the U. S., Brett, A. S., *Journal Watch*, 8/1/94.

25. Polio -- What You Need to Know, U. S. Dept. of Health & Human Services, 3/92.

26. Protecting Physicians from Vaccine Liability, Mason, James O, M.D., DrPH, Asst. Sec. For health, Head of the Public Health Service, *JAMA* 266:21, 1991.

27. JAMA 100 Years Ago -- Protective Vaccination Against Cholera, Flanagin, Annette, RN, M.A., edited by, *JAMA* 268:15, 1992.

28. Public-sector Vaccination Efforts in Response to the Resurgence of Measles Among Preschool-aged Children United States, 1989-1991, *MMWR* 41:29, 1992.

29. (A) Renewed Push for Child Immunizations, Nachman, Barbara, *USA Today*.

30. Retrospective Assessment of Vaccination Coverage Among School-aged Children -- Selected U. S. Cities, 1991, *MMWR* 41:6, 1992.

31. Revaccinating Adults, Weinstock, Cheryl, *American Health*, Jan/Feb, 1992.

32. Risk of Seizures after Measles-Mumps-Rubella Immunization, *CP News -- A Monthly Health Letter*.

33. Risk of Serious Acute Neurological Illness after Immunization with Diphtheria-Tetanus-Pertussis Vaccine, Gale, James L., M.D., et. al., *JAMA* 271:1, 1994.

34. Severe Measles in Immunocompromised Patients, Kaplan, Leonard J., M.D., Ph.D., et. al., *JAMA* 267:9, 1992.

35. Status of Immunity to Tetanus, Measles, Rubella, and Polio Among U. S. Travelers, Eileen, M.D., et. al., *Annals of Internal Medicine* 115:1, 1991.

36. Update on Adult Immunization -- Recommendations of the Immunization Practices Advisory Committee (ACIP), U. S. Dept. of Health & Human Services, *MMWR* 40:RR-12, 1991.

37. Vacination Coverage of 2-year-old Children -- United States, 1991-1992, *JAMA* 271:4, 1994.

38. Vaccine Information Pamphlets Here, But Some Physicians React Strongly, *JAMA* 267:15, 1992.

39. Vaccines: Are They Really Safe and Effective? A Parent's Guide to Childhood Shots, Miller, Neil Z., Press Release/Order Form.

40. Vaccinia (Smallpox) Vaccine -- Recommendations of the Immunization Practices Advisory Committee (ACIP), U. S. Dept. of Health & Human Services, *MMWR* 40:RR-14, 1991.

41. When Should Parents Worry?, Aesoph, Lauri M., N.D., *New Hope Communications*, 9/92.

42. Youthful Immunity, *Prevention*, 10/92.

Ways to Improve the Immune System When You're Sick

There has been increasing discussion on ways to improve the immune system. A recent conference with Dr. Dowes of Germany and Dr. Kuperman of New York suggested the following standard approach to immune-depleted patients: 1) use of 800 mg Tagamet (bedtime); 2) 1000 mg vitamin D-3; 3) 90 mg zinc; 4) 75 mg beta carotene; 5) 800 units vitamin E; 6) 400 mcg selenium; 7) 2 gm cysteine; 8) 2 gm arginine and 9) 2 gm mega-EPA (fish oil). In addition, you may use 3 ampules of DHEA hormone, 3 times a week; and thymus injections, 2 times a week. When patients are on this regimen, they may require biweekly measurement of their fasting T-cell levels. If they have cancer they may require frequent measurements of T-cells, CEA, CA-125, 19-9, 15-3, PSA (Prostate Specific Antigen), LFT's, Total Protein, and other relevant antigens in their cancer. Tamoxifen and Accutane may also be immune adjunctive compounds. Interferon injections can also be helpful.

Balancing Your Immune System

It is a mistake to think that the immune system should be just built up. In reality, the immune system has to be balanced. The two most critical cells for the immune system are the T-helper and the T-suppressor cells. (The letter T stands for thymus.) Proper balance of these two groups of cells is approximately a ratio of 1.8 times as many helper cells as suppressor cells. Other important measurements of immune competence relate to the number of lymphocytes, neutrophils, macrophages, antibodies, and killer cell activity. Yet, the T-helper to T-suppressor ratio seems to be the most useful in identifying immune diseases. The T-helper and T-suppressor ratio is a good general marker for immune system functioning. Typically, in immune system diseases, you see low levels of T-helper cells in relationship to T-suppressor (Table 1):

Table I: Diseases of Immune Suppression

- mumps
- Epstein-Barr virus
- chlamydia
- Toxoplasma virus
- cancer
- herpes 1, 2, and 6
- hepatitis
- parasites
- cytomegalovirus
- common cold
- HIV

Also, various brain diseases result in immune suppression because the brain controls the immune system and impacts the T-helper/T-suppressor ratio. It is typical to see a relative loss of T-helper cells in depression, Parkinson's disease, drug abuse, or prison incarceration.

There are a number of diseases that cause an increase in T-helper cells and a relative decrease in T-suppressor cells such as:

Table II: Diseases of Immune Excess (autoimmunity)

- inflammatory disease
- stomatitis
- multiple sclerosis
- lupus
- organ transplantation
- rheumatoid and osteoarthritis
- bursitis
- myasthenia gravis
- leprosy
- allergies

Also, I believe some depressions as well will present autoimmune type reaction of unknown etiology.

Recent studies suggest that the brain can regulate the immune system. Norman Cousins, Bernie Siegal, Ken Pelletier and Norman Vincent Peale have all talked and written famous books about the affect of a positive attitude on the immune system. Similarly, not only can change in attitude affect the immune system, but a change in brain chemistry can affect the immune system. Some medications like Parlodel (used in heart transplant patients), which decrease prolactin (increase tyrosine and dopamine affects), have a very immune suppressive affect by acting on brain chemistry. Diets that eliminate the amino acids tyrosine and phenylalanine from the diet are also immune suppressants; this can be very helpful in autoimmune diseases. In contrast, medicines like tryptophan, Desyrel or Prozac tend to augment T-helper cell counts. There may be side effects resulting from modifying the immune system through brain chemistry.

Ratios of T-Helper to T-Suppressor Ratios in Various Diseases

Disease	T-Cell Ratios	T-Cell Defect [a]
Control	1.73 ± 0.83	
Rikers Island Inmates with leukopenic anergy	0.31	T-helper decrease
Aphthous Stomatitis -- ulcer (tissue site)	0.1	T-helper decrease
Sinus Histiocytosis X	0.9	T-helper decrease
2.4 Yrs. Post-Thymectomy (MG)	2.1 ± 0.4	T-helper decrease?
2-6 Yrs. Post-Thymectomy (MG)	2.1 ± 0.3	T-helper decrease?
6 Yrs. Post-Thymectomy (MG)	2.3 ± 0.4	T-helper decrease?
Post-Thymectomy-MG	2.0	T-helper decrease
Virus Infection -- CMV, Echovirus, Hepatitis, Mumps	0.5 - 1.0	T-helper decrease
Renal Transplant-Epstein-Barr Virus, Herpes Simplex Virus	1.0	T-helper decrease
AIDS	0.4 - 0.8	T-helper decrease
Drug Abusers	0.73 ± 0.36	T-helper decrease
Dioxin Exposure (severe 10%)	1.0	T-helper decrease
Pelvic Irradiation	0.5 - 1.0	T-suppressor decrease
Chronic Lymphocytic Leukemia	0.5 - 1.0	T-suppressor decrease
Rheumatoid Arthritis	2.36 ± 0.67	T-helper decrease
Systemic Lupus	2.41 ± 0.91	T-helper decrease
Myasthenia Gravis (MG)	2.2 + 0.2	T-helper decrease
Toxic Epidermal Necrolysis	2.0	T-helper decrease
Aphthous Stomatitis-healing ulcer (tissue site)	10.0	T-helper decrease
Erythremia Nodosum Leprosum (ENL) (skin)	2.1 ± 0.4	
Non-ENL Leprosy (skin)	0.6 ± 0.4	T-suppressor decrease
Tuberculosis	2.0	T-suppressor decrease
Hypergammaglobulinemia	2.9	T-suppressor decrease
Lupoid Hepatitis	2.0	T-suppressor decrease
Parasites	1.0 ± 1.5	T-suppressor decrease

a. The primary T-cell defect is listed although secondary defects are common, i.e., T-helper decrease can be accomplished by either relative excess or deficiency of T-suppressor cells.

The Immune System --
Imbalance of Autoimmune Disorders

Most autoimmune diseases may result from low grade infections. There is a changing of the immune system during acute infection; for example, the T-helper/T-suppressor ratio may drop as low as .4 from 1.8. On recovery there may actually be a rebound into an autoimmune sphere of 2.2-3.0. Thus we see that in many instances autoimmune disease may actually begin as low grade infections, but then the immune system overreacts and cannot get out of the overreactive pattern. Therefore, constant infection is often a precursor to autoimmune disorders, allergies, arthritis, etc. The brain may cease to regulate excessive immune reactions when adrenaline is used up in stressful situations.

Serum IgE Levels in Disease

ELEVATED

Allergic/Atopic Disorders

- inhalant allergy
- atopic rhinitis and sinusitis
- atopic asthma
- atopic dermatitis and urticaria
- bronchopulmonary aspergillosis
- hypersensitivity pneumonitis
- drug and food allergies

Immunologic Disorders of Uncertain Pathogenesis

- hyper-IgE and recurrent pyoderma (Job-Buckley syndrome)
- thymic dysplasias and deficiencies
- Wisksott-Aldrich syndrome
- pemphigoid
- periarteritis nodosa

Neoplasms

- IgE myeloma
- advanced Hodgkin's disease

Parasitic Infestations

DECREASED

- congenital hypogammaglobulinemia
- sex-linked hypogammaglobulinemia
- ataxia-telangiectasia
- IgE deficiency

T-Cell Ratios:
Modulation by Nutrition:
Case Report

Interest in T-cell function has been stimulated by the immunological abnormalities in AIDS patients. These patients are marked by abnormalities in T-cell or thymus cell function, such as cutaneous anergy, lymphopenia, and a decrease in T-cell proliferative response to mitogens; but most strikingly, a decreased number in the percentage of T-helper cells (Cohen, et. al., 1986).

T-cells are particularly valuable in relationship to the control of viral and fungal infections. T-cells play a major role in direct and indirect control of bacterial infections (Blumberg and Schooley, 1985; Braverman and Pfeiffer, 1982). Severe defects in T-lymphocyte functions can lead to an increased susceptibility to viral, fungal, and bacterial infections and may also be an indicator of the degree of exposure to environmental carcinogens and toxins (Blumberg and Schooley, 1985). Most T-lymphocyte immunodeficiencies are due to intrinsic abnormalities in the lymphoid-stem cells (Blumberg and Schooley, 1985). The only curative therapy for T-lymphocyte defects and genetic diseases is the replacement of the normal lymphocyte stem cells. Bone-marrow transplantation is the primary therapy for T-lymphocyte defects. Bone-marrow therapy may have a future role for patients with AIDS and/or other T-helper cell deficiencies.

I began studying T-cell ratios (T-helper/T-suppressor) because of the increasing number of patients that I saw complaining of viral-like illness of unknown etiology, e.g., sore throats, low-grade fever, weakness, persistent fatigue, and swollen glands. About 50% of these patients have had T-cell abnormalities. Decreases in T-helper cells are found in viral illness and chronic disease. There may be a new syndrome, a pre-AIDS related complex (pre-ARC). Increases in T-helper cells occur in autoimmune diseases, healing ulcers, and forms of leprosy. T-helper cell deficiency is likely to be an increasing problem even in non-AIDS patients.

Case History: Intermittent Viral Illness

A thirteen-year-old, blond, blue-eyed, 5'9" male, 120 lbs., BP 80/50, P 60, presented to us, complaining of intermittent viral-like infections. He was unresponsive to antibiotics and had a marked low-grade temperature, upper respiratory symptoms, stomach pains, and drowsiness. He had a loss of appetite, craving for sweets, and allergies to dust. The child had missed 50% of the school year and had almost been left back.

His initial treatment (3/85) was 20 mg of zinc, elemental as the sulfate, 50 mg of vitamin B-6, 4000 mg of vitamin C, 400 micrograms of selenium, and a multivitamin (Willvite) daily. When he returned for his next visit one month later, he showed no improvement, weighing 121 pounds, with blood pressure 80/55. The following tests results were noted: plasma histamine of 52.6 mg/ml, copper 95 mcg % (normal 80-120 mcg %), zinc 78 mcg % (normal 100-120 mcg %), iron 58 mcg % (normal 40-120 mcg %), urinary cryptopyrrole (KP) 21 mcg %. He showed an IgG of 657 mg/dl, which was low (normal 750-2000), and IgA 42 mg/dl which was low (normal 80-441 mg/dl). IgM levels were normal. Zinc dosage was increased to 40 mg a day and vitamin B-6 was increased to 200 mg a day (4/85). He was started on deanol, 200 mg per day. Eicosapentaenoic Acid (EPA) was begun at 1000 mg per day but was not tolerated (nausea). He returned four months later with an overall improvement. He finished summer school successfully and had gone two months without an illness or relapse (9/85). A T-cell study was done (9/85) which showed a helper-suppressor ratio of 0.9. T-helper cells and B-cells were depleted. Zinc was increased to 100 mg and later increased to 120 mg per day.

The patient reported notable improvement (11/15/85) and was now six feet tall at 137 pounds with a blood pressure of 90/54. He missed only five days in the first 2 1/2 months of his school year. He had a T-cell ratio of 1:2, while his IgA was still low but increased to 60. He continued to do well and on his last visit (4/1/86) his T-suppressor ratio was 1.4 with a T-helper cell ratio of 48% (normal 32-50), and B-cells normal at 10%.

Case 2

A 24-year-old male on Accutane (.5 mg/kg day for 2 months) developed a flulike syndrome which occurred intermittently for several weeks. On recovery, we checked his T-cell levels. T-helper cells were 55% (32-50% normal) with a T-helper to T-suppressor ratio of 2.4.

Accutane has been helpful in a variety of illnesses including immunosuppressive diseases (Fontana, et al., 1986; Goldman, 1984; Katz, 1986; Meyskens, et al., 1985; Meyskens, 1983). Accutane (a vitamin-A derivative) may stimulate T-helper cells. In vitro, retinol suppresses T-lymphocyte functions. Yet, increased cancer risks, immunosuppressor effects and low vitamin A levels in serum have been noted by Watson, et al., (1985).

Discussion

As an approach to overcoming T-helper deficiency injections of gamma globulin (Gupta, et al., 1986) and thymus extract (De Martino, et al., 1985) (2 mg for 9 weeks did not help a similar patient) have been used. The benefit of Accutane may be due to some interaction with zinc metabolism, which is intimately linked; e.g., retinol-binding protein is zinc-dependent; hence, zinc deficiency can cause a relative vitamin A deficiency (Goodman, 1984; Cousins and Swerdel, 1985).

Fraker and colleagues in 1978 reported that a dietary deficiency of zinc can cause rapid atrophy of the thymus and impaired T-helper cell function. Their data and others (Baer, et al., 1985) have shown that zinc-deficient young animals can have T-helper cell functions restored upon nutritional repletion. Braverman and Pfeiffer (1982) reviewed the critical role of zinc in the immune system, particularly in thymus cell function. There is evidence that the offspring of zinc-deficient mice are also immunodeficient (Beach, et al., 1982). It has been suggested that transient hypogammaglobulinemia in infancy is a manifestation of maternal zinc deficiency (Lentz and Gershwin, 1984). This patient's initial low serum zinc and decreased IgA may be the cause of his T-helper cell abnormality (Lentz and Gershwin, 1984). Zinc deficiency in AIDS is not uncommon (Weiner, 1984). Clinicians that do find T-helper cell deficiencies in patients should consider megazinc therapy in combination with beta carotene.

References

Bach, M. A., Chatenoud L, and Wallach, D., *et. al.*, Studies on T-cell subsets and functions in leprosy. *Clin. Exp. Immunol.* 44:491-500, 1981.

Baer, M. T., *et. al.*, Nitrogen utilization, enzyme activity, glucose intolerance and leukocyte chemotaxis in human experimental zinc depletion. *Amer. J. Clin. Nutr.* 41:1220-1235, 1985.

Barr, R. D., Sauder, D. N., and Bienenstock, J., Interactions of stem cells and T lymphocytes contribute to the physiological control of cell proliferation in rapidly renewing tissues. *Med. Hypothesis*, 19:387-396, 1986.

Beach, R. S., Gershwin, M. E., and Hurley, L. S., Gestational zinc deprivation in mice: persistence of immunodeficiency for three generations. *Science* 218:469-471, 1982.

Berrih, S., Lebrigand, H., Levasseur. P., *et. al.* Depletion of helper/inducer T-cells after thymectomy in myasthenic patients. *Clin. Immunol. Immunopathol.* 28:272-281, 1983.

Berrih, S., Gaud, C., Bach, M. A., *et. al.* Evaluation of T-cell subsets in myasthenia gravis using anti-T-cell monoclonal antibodies. *Clin. Exp. Immunol.* 45:1-8,1981.

Blumberg, R. S., and Schooley, R. T., Lymphocyte markers and infectious diseases. *Seminars Hematol.* XXII(2):81-114, 1985.

Braverman, E. R., and Pfeiffer, C. C., Essential Trace Elements and Cancer. *J. Ortho. Psych.* 11(1):28-41, 1982.

Carbone, A., Manconi, R., Poletti, A., *et. al.* Lymph node immunohistology in intravenous drug abusers with persistent generalized lymphadenopathy. *Arch. Pathol. Lab. Med.* 109:1007-1012, 1985.

Cohen, R. L., Oliver, D., Pollard-Sigwanz, C., Leukopenia and anergy as predictors of AIDS. *J A M A* 255(10):1289, 1986.

Cousins, R. J., and Swerdel, M. R., Ceruloplasmin and metallothionein induction by zinc and 13-CIS-retinoic acid in rats with adjuvant inflammation. *Proc. Soc. Exper. Biol. Med.* 179:168-172, 1985.

Cox, A., Lisak, R. P., Skolnik, P., and Zweiman, B., Effect of thymectomy on blood T-cell subsets in myasthenia gravis. *An. Neurol.* 19(3):297-298, 1986.

De Martino, M., *et. al.*, Undegraded in children with recurrent respiratory infections: effect of the use of thymostimulin on the alterations of T-cell subsets. *Int. J. Tissue Reset.* 6(3):223-8, 1984.

Doherty, P. C., Zinkernagel, R. M., T-cell-mediated immunopathology in viral infections. *Transplant Rev.* 19:89-120, 1974.

Fontana, I. A., Rogers, I. S., and Durham, J., The role of 13-CIS-retinoic acid in the remission induction of a patient with acute promyelocytic leukemia. *Cancer* 57(2):209, 1986.

Fossaluzza, V., Tonutti, E., and Sala, P. G., T-cell subsets in the differential diagnosis of rheumatoid arthritis and systemic lupus erythematosus. *J. Rheumatol.* 12(6):1199, 1985.

Fraker, P. J., DePasquale-Jardieu, P., Zwicki, C. M., and Luecke, R. W., Regeneration of T-cell helper function in zinc-deficient adult mice. *Proc. Natl. Acad. Sci.* 75(11):5660-5664, 1978.

Goldman, R., Effect of retinoic acid on the proliferation and phagocytic capability of murine macrophage-like cell lines. *J. Cell. Physiol.* 120:91-102, 1984.

Goodman, D. S., Overview of current knowledge of metabolism of vitamin A and carotenoids. *JNCI* 73(6):1375-1379, 1984.

Gupta, A., Novick, B. E., and Rubinstein, A., Restoration of suppressor T-cell functions in children with AIDS following intravenous gamma globulin treatment. *AIDC* 140:143-146, 1986.

Hoffman, R., Stehr-Green, A., Webb, K. B., *et. al.*, Health effects of long-term exposure to 2, 3, 7, 8-Tetrachlorodibenzo-p-dioxin. *IAMA* 255(15): 2031-2038, 1986.

Iida, N., Takahashi, F., and Shiokawa, Y., T-cell subsets in rheumatic heart disease. *Japanese Circulation Journal* 49(12):1268-1269, 1985.

Katz, R. A., Isotretinoin treatment of recalcitrant warts in an immunosuppressed man. *Arch. Dermatol.* 122:19-20, 1986.

Lahat, N., Nir, E., Horenstien, L., and Colin, A. A., Effect of theophylline on the proportion and function of T-suppressor cells in asthmatic children. *Allergy* 40:453-457, 1983.

Lentz, D., and Gershwin, M. E., Is transient hypogammaglobulinemia of infancy a manifestation of zinc deficiency? *Dev. Comp. Immunol.* 8:1-5, 1984.

Levandowski, R. A., Ou, D. W., and Jackson, G. G., Acute-phase decrease of T lymphocyte subsets in rhinovirus infection. *J. Infect. Dis.* 153(4):743-, 1986.

Merot. Y., Gravallese, E., Guillen, F. J., and Murphy, G. F., Lymphocyte subsets and langerhans' cells in toxic epidermal necrolysis. *Arch. Dermatol.* 122:455-458, 1986.

Meyskens, F. L., Goodman, G. E., and Alberts, D. S., 13-ClS-retinoic acid: pharmacology, toxicology and clinical applications for the prevention and treatment of human cancer. *CRC Crit. Rev. Oncol./Hematol.* 3(1):75-101, 1985.

Meyskens, F. L., *Vitamin A and synthetic derivatives (retinoids) in the prevention and treatment of human cancer. Nutrition Factors in the Induction and Maintenance of Malignancy.* New York Academic Press, Inc. 206-215, 1983.

Modlin, R. L., Bakke, A. C., Vaccaro, S. A., *et. al.*, Tissue and blood T-lymphocyte subpopulations in erythema nodosum leprosum. *Arch. Dermatol.* 121:216-219, 1985.

Perri, R. T., and Kay, N. E., Abnormal T-cell function in early-state chronic lymphocytic leukemia (CLL) patients. *Amer. J. Hematol.* 22:55-61, 1986.

Petrini, B., Wasserman, J., and Blomgren, H., T-cell subsets in patients treated with pelvic irradiation for cancer. *J. Clin. Lab. Immunol.* 17:147-148, 1985.

Rohrbach, M. S., and Williams, D. E., Undegraded and pleural tuberculosis. *Chest* 89(4):473,474, 1986.

Savage, N. W., Seymour, G. J., Kruger, B. J., T-lymphocyte subset changes in recurrent aphthous stomatitis. *Oral. Surg. Oral Med. Oral Pathol.* 60(2):175-181, 1985.

Schuyler, M., Gerblich, A., and Urda, G., Atopic asthma T-lymphocyte subpopulations. *Clin. Allergy* 15:131-138, 1985.

Stevens, R. H., Cole, D. A., Lindhol, P. A., and Cheng, H. F., Identification of environmental carcinogens utilizing T-cell mediated immunity. *Med. Hypotheses* 19:267-285, 1980.

Watson, R. R., and Moriguchi, S., Cancer prevention by retinoids: role of immunological modification. *Nutr. Res.* 5:663-675, 1985.

Weiner, R. G., AIDS and zinc deficiency. *IAMA* (252)11:1409-1410, 1984.

17. Kidney Disease

Kidneys and Kidney Stones

The kidneys can be found on both sides of the lower thorax. They are filled with millions of cells that filter the ocean of life. Kidneys clean out our blood, getting rid of our waste products. Each person has an enormous amount of kidney nephrons which are made up of millions of tubules with filters over them. Kidneys don't fail until you lose about 98% of the functioning cells. There is a lot of surplus.

The most common ways that kidneys function improperly are through kidney stones (early in life) or renal failure (later in life). Kidney stones form like the shape and texture of rock candy. The stones grow on top of one another, on the inside of the kidney. They pass down through the tubule, which is the pain people feel when they have kidney stones. It's like a stone passing through a straw. It is one of the most painful diseases.

Kidney stones are primarily composed of calcium oxalate. Oxalate is a chemical found in foods that contain oxalic acid, e.g., spinach, rhubarb, nuts, coffee, tea, and cocoa. Vitamin B-6 and magnesium deficiency can also cause oxalate stones. If the stones block the kidneys, they can cause kidney failure or uremia, which fills the body with toxins. Kidney stones can also be made of uric acid, i.e., a gout-related stone. This stone is related to stress and a diet rich in asparagus, anchovies, protein, and mushrooms. Nutrition can prevent the formation of these stones. Triple phosphate crystals can sometimes appear in the urine. They can appear as magnesium ammonium phosphate. The treatment is hydration or magnesium to reduce the risk of formation of these types of stones.

Once you have had kidney stones, it's highly probably (about 70%) that they will occur again in the future. Once you're a stone-former, you will usually be a stone-former.

The use of magnesium is an excellent therapy for calcium oxalate type stones. The tendency to get stones with calcium in them occurs with magnesium deficiency. Magnesium raises the calcium/magnesium ratio, and it keeps calcium soluble in the urine, thus preventing stones. Magnesium (500-1000 mg), as well as vitamin B-6 (100 mg), and/or potassium citrate (75 mg daily), prevent oxalate stones in adults. The use of bran is important in binding calcium. Ten grams of bran (several tablespoons a day) is used to treat people with stones.

Calcium supplementation can reduce other nutrient absorption. Women who are now taking more and more calcium for osteoporosis should watch the dosage: 1000 mg is the recommended dosage for a woman who is premenopausal and 1500 mg the recommended dosage for a woman who is postmenopausal. If calcium is taken with magnesium, vitamin B-6, Vitamin D, and bran the risk for stone formation will be reduced.

Low sodium diets and low fat diets also protect against stone formation. Too much magnesium or cysteine can cause magnesium stones. Remember, the first sign of kidney failure can be discovered through a blood test, and the first sign of stones can often be detected through urinalysis.

Kidney Stones: Questions and Answers

The pain endured by people "passing" kidney stones is well-known. The kidneys are a matched set of fist-sized, bean-shaped organs located one on each side of the mid-thorax; they are the body's blood filters. Through them pass 2,500 pints of blood each day. Waste products are removed and excreted in the urine. A stone is formed when normally dissolved material, filtered from the blood, condenses into a solid. Stones have the shape and texture of rock candy and grow, one on top of the other, inside the kidney. They may remain in the kidney or they may enter the ureters, the tubes that carry waste to the bladder. It is when a stone passes through the ureter that the often severe pain is felt. It's like forcing a rough stone through a narrow straw.

Kidney stones are composed primarily of calcium oxalate. Oxalate is a chemical found in foods containing oxalic acid, such as spinach, rhubarb, celery, and nuts. Caffeinated beverages are probably the number one cause of kidney stones. Oxalate stones also can be caused by vitamin B-6 and magnesium deficiencies.

Gout-related stones are formed from uric acid. These stones are related to stress and a diet rich in asparagus, anchovies, sardines, meat and mushrooms. Proper nutrition can prevent the formation of this type of stone. Once you have had kidney stones, it's highly probable -- about 70% -- that they will occur again without nutritional intervention.

The use of magnesium is an excellent therapy for calcium oxalate-type stones. Stones with calcium usually form when there is a magnesium deficiency. A correct magnesium-to-calcium ratio keeps calcium dissolved in the urine, preventing it from forming stones.

Magnesium (500-1000 milligrams), vitamin B-6 (100 mg) and/or potassium citrate (75 milliequivalent daily available as urocyst) prevent oxalate stones from forming in adults. The use of bran is important in binding calcium. Ten grams of bran a day has been used to treat people with stones. Of utmost importance is high amounts of citrate, which helps the calcium oxalate, and large quantity of water.

Women who are taking calcium for the prevention of osteoporosis should watch the dosage, as calcium supplementation can reduce other nutrient absorption. If calcium is taken with magnesium, vitamin B-6, vitamin D and bran, the risk for stone formation will be reduced. Urinalysis should be done 1-2 times yearly in individuals taking calcium supplements. 24-hour urine studies may benefit those patients at risk for developing stones by following their urine chemistry and preventing stone formation by adjusting their nutrient intake. See Kidney Stone Diet, p. 142.

Creatinine Clearance
(For Kidney Function)

Creatinine clearance is a marker of how well the kidney is clearing toxins and proteins from the blood. Creatinine is just one item that the kidney clears, and is usually cleared at about 120 milligrams per millimeter, or 120 mg/ml. It is an excellent indicator of overall kidney function and is followed as a marker for the success and failure of patients as they approach or have dialysis. Patients who have total kidney failure have a creatinine clearance of about 1-2, as opposed to the normal of 120. It is not atypical with age to have creatinine clearances of 60-70 or lower. At a creatinine clearance of approximately 20, patients can start having symptoms. Naturally, the interpretation of this test, as with all other tests, must be taken in the context of the entire medical picture. Creatinine clearance can also be calculated from height, weight, and blood creatinine by a computer program.

Method: Drink at least 2-3 glasses of water before the test, then void and discard first void of day. No tea, coffee, or drugs are ingested on the day of the test. Save all urine for 24 hours and keep refrigerated. Large orange container will have 1 boric tablet placed on the bottom. At the end of 24 hours record the volume in milliliters on the label of the small white bottle. Invert the large orange bottle to mix all urine and pour into the small white bottle. Only bring the white bottle back to the office.

Monitoring Renal Function for Chelation Therapy Infusion

Creatinine Versus Creatinine Clearance

Serial measurements of serum creatinine and a routine urinalysis should be considered in the monitoring of chelation therapy. Intravenous EDTA chelation can cause renal impairment and occasionally patients may be unpredictably susceptible to trends in EDTA natural toxicity. Serum creatinine levels, if we monitor during chelation therapy, are adequate to protect renal function. The Cockcroft-Gault Equation can be utilized to extrapolate glomerular filtration rate in terms of ml/min using serum creatinine clearance.

The Cockcroft-Gault Equation will overestimate renal function in massively obese or edematous patients and patients with rapidly deteriorating functions. However, one can make allowances for this overestimation. Serum creatinine levels rise approximately 30% in response to dietary intake during the day, falling again at night.

Because there are rare, documented instances where a patient has suffered serious renal impairment as a result of intravenous EDTA, it is essential that careful monitoring of serum creatinine be maintained throughout the course of chelation therapy. If a longer time is allowed between infusions and if the dose rate of EDTA administered is reduced to a level compatible with renal function, most patients can benefit safely from a series of EDTA infusions, despite mild to moderate rates of renal impairment. Continued treatment in the presence of rising creatinine levels, however, can cause serious renal impairment and may lead to renal dialysis.

Calcium Oxalate Kidney Stones and the Breast

When we think of calcium oxalate we think of kidney stones. Patients with deficiencies of magnesium and B-6, and individuals who consume too many caffeinated beverages, chocolate, and all the kidney stone forming foods frequently have too much calcium oxalate in their urine and are at risk for kidney stones. Another area of calcium oxalate stone formation is in the breast. We don't often speak of calcification in breast tissue, which is frequently biopsied and almost always negative. PET scanning will help us determine which biopsies are necessary and which are not.

Cystitis

Cystitis is an inflammation of the urinary bladder. It can cause burning, difficulty in urination, blood in the urine, pain and fever. An urge to urinate when the bladder is empty, pain in the pubic area, occasional discharge, chills, fever and backache can suggest kidney involvement. It causes painful and frequent urination, pubic pain, sometimes urethra irritation, and sometimes malodorous, grossly cloudy urine with bacteria. It can be caused by Trichomonas, Candida, herpes, chlamydia, HPV. Some patients will have accompanying nausea, vomiting, and fever. Some will have a persistent cystitis, which can be the result of a brain imbalance treatable with antidepressants, anticonvulsants, and antianxiety agents. Urinary tract infections may be prevented to some degree by acidifying the urine with cranberry juice, methionine, and vitamin C.

Often cystitis is a stress condition. Like an irritable urinary tract, drink fluids. One must wipe themselves from front to back to avoid contamination from the bowels. Women with frequent cystitis should drink a glass of water before intercourse and urinate completely, immediately after intercourse. Avoid vaginal deodorants, bubble baths, and other irritating substances. Avoid sitting in a wet bathing suit.

Stress reduction techniques, treating underlying stress disorder, anxiety, or depression, may be helpful. Nutritional therapies include cranberry juice, vitamin C, etc. Methionine may also have benefits.

Dialysis and Transplantation

Kidney dialysis makes a unique nutritional demand on the body. It frequently renders patients deficient in carnitine, arginine, zinc, iron, and many other nutrients, as well as amino acids and trace elements. Kidney transplant pat-ients require immune suppression for which there are numerous agents, which in some cases may be augmented by brain medicines such as Parlodel, Wellbutrin, etc., as well as typical agents such as cyclosporin, etc.

Chronic Renal Failure

Chronic renal failure is marked by elevation of blood urea nitrogen, i.e., nitrogen waste products. Individuals will become uremic, i.e., itching of skin, tremors of hand, pericarditis (inflammation of heart lining), and pleuritis (inflammation of lung lining). There are a lot of ways that we can get kidney failure. Anyone with hypertension, antibiotic toxicity, mercury, lead, cadmium, or bismuth poisoning, pancreatitis, injury or trauma from a car accident, lupus, drug-related vasculitis, etc., are all prone to kidney failure.

Nutrition can help in the treatment of renal failure. Low protein diets are helpful. The secret is to eat the essential amino acids -- leucine, isoleucine, valine, methionine, tryptophan, phenylalanine, histidine, lysine, and arginine (Fast PATH). An excess of protein often backs up in the kidneys, so it's important to eliminate the nonessential protein sources in your diet. A diet high in zinc is also important. Zinc becomes deficient, particularly in renal failure patients, and can lead to edema (leg swelling), i.e., water retention. It's important not to indulge in too much salt because this can cause swelling.

Choline, lecithin, and olive oil, all of which reduce cholesterol, are also important. Vitamin D deficiency is also common in kidney patients and may be a factor in osteoporosis. Anemia can occur as well. Vitamin E can sometimes be beneficial, but most of the studies claim it is not helpful.

Carnitine deficiency is also common in chronic renal failure patients. Carnitine is an amino acid which is not easily metabolized. Signs of carnitine deficiency can include neurological problems or high triglycerides. Vitamin B-6 is also important, because it can return immune functions to normal. A high fat diet is shown to be poor for kidney failure patients, in that it increases urination and other kidney problems. Heavy metals like copper, cobalt, cadmium, and mercury, accumulate more commonly in kidney failure patients. Zinc can be used as an antidote. Copper can be toxic, and it must be avoided if possible.

Dialysis machines, used to clean failing kidneys, use a lot of water to filter the kidneys. The water, which is softened with aluminum, can result in dialysis dementia in many patients. This is a type of senility caused by aluminum intoxication. Various antacids and aluminum cookware contain small amounts of aluminum, which should be avoided by patients with or without kidney failure.

18. Neurology and Brain Disorders

Depression, Addiction, and Anticonvulsants

PATH has pioneered documentation of the information that most serious behavioral disorders can be correlated with brain electrical activity imbalances. We use Harvard Medical School's device, the Brain Electrical Activity Map (BEAM), to discover, diagnose, and study electrical imbalances associated with anxiety, depression, insomnia, and other types of brain disorders ranging from Schizophrenia to Alzheimer's. These conditions are often easily treatable with anticonvulsants (medicine which stabilize brain activity). We should not assume that just because a person has a brain arrhythmia, or a disorder often called cerebral dysrhythmia, that he or she is having psychological problems, any more than we assume that someone who has a heart arrhythmia is a heartless individual.

Physical disorders of the brain can occur independently or may exist in a mutual dependence with psychological factors. We have found, however, that the so-called anticonvulsants (Dilantin [phenytoin], Tegretol, Klonopin, Phenobarbital, Mysoline, Diamox, and Felbamate, among others) have had remarkable success in treating brain disorders of all types and are very safe medications when given with nutrients. Please read and enjoy the two books on Dilantin, keeping in mind that everything said about Dilantin, to a great degree, can apply to the rest of these anticonvulsants.

It is important to know that the brain rhythm approach to brain disorders is also successful using non-drug approaches. For example, Cranial Electrical Stimulation (CES), achieved with a small electrical device, can do what Dilantin does. Additional non-drug approaches are brain exercises, such as biofeedback, which often helps regulate brain rhythm, and nutrients that have mild brain regulating properties, such as GABA, inositol, melatonin, magnesium, B-6, and B-complex. In some cases, the miracle of Dilantin, in our understanding of it, can be duplicated with CES, biofeedback, and nutrients.

It should be noted, however, that some people respond to Dilantin while others respond to different medications; therefore, it is a very complex set of judgments that goes into choosing which medicine is best for you. If you are not on Dilantin, please keep in mind that it is because it was felt that there are other substances more appropriate for you that can help regulate your brain rhythm.

Temporal Lobe Abnormalities

Temporal lobe abnormalities are so common in our society, causing mood problems and neurological symptoms. Risk factors are described in "Characteristics of Medical Temporal Lobe Epilepsy: I. Results of History and Physical Examination" by French, et al., from *Annals of Neurology* 34(6):774-780 (1993) and include infections, birth events, etc. Very few have no identifiable risk factors. Furthermore, virtually all patients (96 percent) have some type of aura.

Felbamate: A New Anticonvulsant

Felbatol (Felbamate) is a new anticonvulsant. Starting dose is at 300 milligrams in the morning and at 2 p.m. Some people find it stimulating unlike Tegretol. Dosages can then be moved to 600 milligrams BID up to 3600 milligrams over a QUID dosing.

It is a unique medication. It is thought to work by stimulating the amino acid GABA in the brain, which is an inhibitory amino acid that helps us resist excitement. Maybe it will be augmented by the use of GABA supplements. It is thought to be the sole drug in the treatment of partial complex seizures with and without grand real. It is helpful in children's seizures called Lennox Gastaut Syndrome and in generalized seizures.

It should, at this time, be avoided in combination with other drugs, when possible. It also can decrease the serum levels of Tegretol and increase the concentrations of Valproate.

The major side effects appear to be fatigue, headache, sleepiness, dizziness, and insomnia. Nausea, anorexia, vomiting, upset stomach, constipation are other common problems. Rarely you will get fever in children and somnolence, anorexia, vomiting, and upper respiratory infection.

We'll see whether or not the increased energy persists in some patients or somnolence will be the end result at the higher dosages.

The Neuropsychological Examination

The purpose of the neuropsychological examination is to assess the integrity of the brain (or the developing brain, in children) through neurobehavioral tasks which reflect the functioning of specific brain regions. The comprehensive evaluation provides information regarding a wide range of functional abilities and identifies strengths and weaknesses. This information is used to diagnose a brain disorder and to formulate an individualized treatment approach.

There are many reasons why a neuropsychological examination may be recommended. Among these are, to: a) identify an organic component to a current psychiatric presentation; b) rule out Attention Deficit Disorder without hyperactivity; c) rule out learning disability; d) identify the nature and extent of neuropsychological sequelae due to polysubstance abuse, stroke, tumor, or traumatic brain injury; and e) evaluate the physical and physiological state of the brain.

The neuropsychological examination involves a detailed evaluation of the following neurobehavioral-neurocognitive functions:

- Sensory Perceptual Functions (various sensory responses)
- Attention and Concentration
- Academic Abilities (learning skills)
- Intellectual Functioning (thinking; problem solving)
- Motor/Visual-Motor Functions
- Language Functions (expressive/receptive speech)
- Spatial Abilities
- Memory Functions (verbal, visual, associative, etc.)
- Personality Functions

Typically, the comprehensive examination lasts approximately four to five hours (but can be less or more, depending on the situation), during which a wide variety of standardized tests are administered. Following the interpretation of examination results and report preparation, a post-test consultation will be scheduled to discuss evaluation findings. Please notify us of your insurance status so that we can provide assistance with the handling of your claims.

The One-Hour Test

The one-hour test can be used with PHT (Dilantin), Klonopin, Ritalin, CES, or other medicines to see if there is rapid response to treatment. It can help us to find the right medications.

Part 1: Somatic Conditions

These questions pertain to how you feel now. If you answer yes to any question, grade your symptoms on a scale of 1 - 10 (1 - minimal; 10 - most severe).

Symptom	Before therapy	After therapy
Do you have a headache of any sort?	_____	_____
Any pain or blurring in the eyes?	_____	_____
Any ache or pain in the neck?	_____	_____
Any ache in the shoulders, back, or chest?	_____	_____
Shortness of breath?	_____	_____
Aches or pains in your arms or hands?	_____	_____
Aches or pains in your legs or feet?	_____	_____
Are your hands or feet hot or cold?	_____	_____
Any tingling sensations?	_____	_____
Any "knots" or "butterflies" in your stomach?	_____	_____
Are you trembling now? Hold out your hands and observe?	_____	_____
Do you feel a pulse, or beat, or throbbing sensation inside you?	_____	_____
How is your energy now?	_____	_____
Do you have any pain or discomfort not asked about?	_____	_____

Part 2: Thoughts and Emotions

It is useful to begin by asking the patient what he had for breakfast. When he tells you, remind him that he got the answer from his memory; it was not "alive" in his brain. Explain that is not what you want. What you are looking for are thoughts that are going on right now, that are difficult to turn off.

If there are such thoughts, ask the patient to write them on the left side of a piece of paper, explaining that you do not need to see them since they might be personal. It is the emotions that come with the thoughts that you want. Then ask the patient to think each thought separately, and write opposite to it the emotions that accompany it. Do this for each thought.

An hour after drug treatment, repeat the same questions.

BEFORE DRUG

Thoughts   **Emotions**

_____   _____

_____   _____

_____   _____

_____   _____

_____   _____

AFTER DRUG

_____   _____

_____   _____

_____   _____

_____   _____

_____   _____

Psychoneuroimmunology [1]

Psychoneuroimmunology is the study of the connections between the mind, the immune system, and the nervous system. We know that reactions to events can affect the immune system, and autoimmune diseases such as arthritis can be exacerbated by emotional trauma.

Individuals who are emotionally traumatized have greater susceptibility to illness. People whose spouses die have a higher chance of developing cancer in the year following the loss than the general population. Individuals who are emotionally and mentally traumatized have certain abnormal T-cell functions.

We know that diseases that are primary immune system diseases such as lupus and AIDS are accompanied by psychological symptoms, even psychosis.

We know that the immune system can be conditioned. For example, a chemotherapeutic drug can condition the immune system to remain suppressed even after withdrawing the drug. The best known example of conditioned response involves Pavlov's dogs which salivated when a feeding bell rang, even when food was not offered. In experiments rats can suppress their immune systems in response to similar conditioning.

A variety of hormonal factors affect the immune system as well as the brain: endocrine hormones, steroids, interferon, growth receptors for hormones, neuroendocrine substances, hormone, and thyroid. All immunologically competent cells have neurotransmitters, and neuropeptides.

Behavioral interventions such as psychotherapy, relaxation techniques, imagery, and biofeedback can also affect the immune system and then the resultant biochemical interactions can extend the effect.

The placebo mechanism -- faith that one will heal -- does promote healing. Mood elevation should be obtainable by behavioral and spiritual techniques.

Psychoneuroimmunology is nothing more and nothing less than the recognition that the mind can affect bodily health (psychosomatic phenomena recast into more specific terms). The degree to which the mind controls health may depend on the individual. We all know the teaching of popular psychology, i.e., that loneliness is dangerous and bad thoughts lead to bad health. This has led to a proliferation of techniques of healing emphasizing positive and nurturing attitudes such as biofeedback, hypnosis, massage, psychotherapy, meditation, and the use of crystals. The question arises: which is the best? Which spiritual, physical, or mood elevation approach leads to the best

---

When medicine discusses the degree to which attitude affects illness, it is really exploring an aspect of religion.

---

long term health? Norman Cousins, Leo Buscaglia, Ken Pelletier, M.D., Joan Borysenko, Ph.D., Herbert Benson, M.D., and Bernie Siegel, M.D., to name a few, have joined with Reverend Norman Vincent Peale and Reverend Schuller in promoting healing through positive attitudes: laughter, prayer, meditation, and love. Two questions arise: (1) to what degree will the mind control the health; and, (2) what aspect of the mind will control the health? In these case studies we do not address these issues but show that the mood elevation of an antidepressant is effective in a variety of physical diseases. Yet, this "brave new world" chemical solution to the human condition is not a permanent or best solution, only a currently necessary one in medical practice.

Case 1: Arthritis

A sixty-year-old man with high blood pressure (HBP), high cholesterol, and bilateral degenerative arthritis on the left and right knees came to see me. He was treated through nutrition and diet for HBP and high cholesterol, yet he continued to complain excessively of knee pain. The knee pain was getting worse for the last two to three years since an injury. He had been a construction worker all of his life and had done a lot of bending and carrying. He had been treated with Indocin, Motrin, Feldene, Clinoril, and aspirin, all of which aggravated or irritated his stomach while producing only minimal relief. The patient's orthopedic physician wished to schedule him for surgery. Despite the confirmed X-ray diagnosis of arthritis in his knees, his sedimentation rate and C-reactive protein were unremarkable, leading me to consider psychosocial causes which could lead to internalized conflicts and physical pain. Rather than send this patient to surgery, I suspected that this patient had atypical

---

1. *Health and Nutrition*, vol. 6, no. 2, pp. 2-6 (1991).

depression although he denied depression symptomatology. He was living with a younger girlfriend, divorced from his wife. He also had relationship problems with his children. I confirmed the depression biochemically by measuring the amino acids in his serum. I treated him with antidepressants, initially desipramine and later Prozac, and he had virtually complete remission of his experience of pain. He was encouraged to examine the issues of guilt, anger, and forgiveness regarding his family relationships.

Case 2: Multiple Sclerosis (MS)

A forty-four-year-old woman with a fifteen year history of multiple sclerosis came to my office. She initially developed optic neuritis due to MS (confirmed by NMR), but now walked with a cane. She was also taking Ditropan to prevent urinary retention and had been treated with traditional drugs for MS such as Lioresal and steroids without success. She had some constipation and she was put on a diet high in polyunsaturated oils, low in saturated fats and high in complex carbohydrates. Her blood tests were essentially unremarkable except for a low level of GLA, an essential fatty acid. She was treated with primrose oil (a source of EPA-GLA), fish oil, antioxidant, multivitamin, an antidepressant, amino acids such as methionine, tyrosine, and phenylalanine which produced some improvement. She was also counselled that, although a dismal prognosis often accompanies a diagnosis of MS, she did not have to believe she would be disabled. She was invited to cultivate a hopeful outlook. Seeing some improvement, she was placed on two antidepressants, Pamelor and later Prozac (which causes less dry mouth). She markedly improved. She threw away her cane and her numbness subsided dramatically. Her ability to move and her energy level improved with a nearly complete remission of fatigue. She continues with 40 mg of Prozac and 100 mg of Pamelor, with more than a sixty percent remission of her symptoms of Multiple Sclerosis.

Case 3: Back Pain

A forty-one-year-old male with a Masters in Business Administration and a degree in Engineering, presented with chronic fatigue of several years duration. He had seen many nutritional physicians and had a diagnosis of candidiasis. He came in taking 120 vitamins which he claimed were keeping him functioning as a salesman. He described all sorts of symptoms of forgetfulness, confusion, irritable bowel syndrome, muscle aches, back problems, and skin rashes. He was treated with Prozac for depression and avoidant personality disorder. He had been married for seven years and had marital difficulties. His wife was past the practical age for having children and this childlessness was a factor in his somatization of unrecognized depression.

With treatment, he had complete remission of his fatigue, and back pain, and his irritable bowel syndrome improved greatly. He reduced his vitamins to proper levels, including amino acids for depression as well as the preventive supplements for heart disease and cancer.

Case 4: Chronic Headache Sufferer

A sixty-year-old man presented with a one year history of severe headaches, having been unsuccessfully treated with lithium, Inderal, verapamil, and ergot derivatives. He was a heavy smoker who consumed large amounts of coffee, white sugar, and flour. He was put on a diet which eliminated white flour and sugar. He was tapered off his coffee and cigarettes and was put on the amino acids methionine, tyrosine, and phenylalanine for his chronic fatigue, which improved greatly. Yet, some headaches still persisted, which were relieved only by Fiorinal. He was then placed on 50 mg of doxepin at night. Within two weeks he stopped smoking and using coffee, and had a reduction in headaches. Like so many patients, he could not tolerate more of the tricyclic antidepressants hence, I added Prozac. He now has been one year without headaches.

Case 5: Epstein-Barr Virus

A seventeen-year-old female with a two-year history of chronic fatigue, stomach pains, nausea after eating, and headaches, came to my office. She described an episode of fever and had a tentative diagnosis of Epstein-Barr virus. She had also sustained a neck injury in an automobile accident four years earlier. For the last two years she had lost weight and had not functioned well, and had quit her job because of poor concentration, and fatigue. On taking a social history, I discovered she had a problem relationship with her boyfriend that had started two years ago. Her father did not approve of the relationship and this had become a significant family conflict. Epstein-Barr virus antibody and other test results were all within normal range. She was placed on tyrosine, phenylalanine, and tryptophan therapy (based on her amino acid tests) and she showed some improvement. Later, because of her desire for more rapid improvement, desipramine was added. The antidepressant resulted in a virtual remission of her symptoms, and a desirable weight gain of eight and a half pounds in a period of six weeks (from 97 1/2 to 104 pounds).

Case 6: Asthma

An asthmatic sixty-five-year-old man with a four-year history of asthma presented to my office; he was being treated with Theo-Dur, Proventil, Vanceril, Brethine, and steroids. He had mixed results from these medications. In addition, he was waking up in the middle of the night with shortness of breath. He wanted to try a different nutrient regimen using N-acetyl-cysteine along with certain vitamin recommendations for asthmatics, which included: pyridoxal phosphate and magnesium. He was still suffering from severe shortness of breath at night. As I got to know him I learned that he was running his own business and was a workaholic. He also was extremely isolated from his family and had few social support mechanisms. He had fears of the prospect of no longer working up to his capacity. At that point, he asked me if there were any other medications he could try.

Based on one study of treating asthma with Dilantin, he was started on this medication with poor results. After this failure he gave in and tried Prozac (I had urged an antidepressant previously), a simple antidepressant with very limited anticholinergic side effects. He called me back a week later and said he could not believe how great he felt. He no longer woke up at night with shortness of breath, and during the day he was no longer short of breath, and he had discontinued his Proventil and Theo-Dur. Prozac was extremely effective at the higher dose of two pills (44 mg). He came completely off and remains off all asthma medication two months after beginning Prozac.

This is a very common example of asthma in our society due primarily to depression or psychological factors. Simple mood elevation can solve the problem short term. The problem, of course, is that one hates to rely strictly on antidepressants to raise mood and improve so many different types of chronic conditions. I hope that another approach to effect mood (e.g., Cranial Electrical Stimulation) can incorporate some of the new techniques in psychoneuroimmunology. Somatic symptoms for psychiatric disease is widespread and often missed as a diagnosis. A recent study by the American Medical Association actually showed that 80% of those patients coming in for chronic fatigue syndrome in general practice had anxiety and depression. Although the alternative medical press seems to diagnose these patients with candidiasis, hypoglycemia, and mercury toxicity, it would seem that the great majority are depressed and would be better treated through psychological and/or biochemical intervention. The answer of antidepressants gives dramatic results. Yet, one has to be suspect of offering the chemical Messiah to these patients. On the other hand, one has to protect these patients from somatization and somatic delusions that their whole problem is physical. (It is, but in the brain, not the body.)

In summary, these are classic examples of individuals whose emotional and/or spiritual issues resulted in somatization: experience of physical symptoms such as headache, back pain, chronic fatigue, and stomach pains which can completely remit with mood elevation. Ideally, mood elevation would be accomplished ultimately by nutritional, emotional, or spiritual means, providing, however, some initial and quick relief from fatigue and hopelessness is administered, until the person feels strong enough to function well. For this purpose, an antidepressant is sometimes beneficial.

Lithium

Lithium has been useful in a variety of diseases: manic-depression, post-traumatic stress disorder, schizo-affective disorder, anorexia, PMS, obsessive compulsive disorder, alcoholism, violent behavior, individuals with bipolar traits, hypomania, and mild depression. Individuals with impulse control can respond to lithium the way they do to beta blockers. Many patients who present with schizophrenia are reacting to Dilantin and would do well with lithium. Lithium may be an essential trace element to life, but no known enzyme using lithium has been identified. It is thought, but not yet proven, that low lithium levels in the hair or blood are indicative of a need for this trace element. Doctors used to feel that the only place to start lithium therapy was in the hospital, but now it is possible to start outside the hospital under proper medical supervision.

Less than 0.5 milli equivalence per liter is a well-accepted dosage, and lithium is best given at night. Lithium levels of 0.9 to 0.15 are usually produced with 5-7 capsules, and lithium levels of 0.5 to 0.8 with 3-4 capsules. One to two capsules rarely produce side effects and can really take the edge off some patients as a natural treatment. Three to four tablets at 300 milligrams can lead to nausea, diarrhea, increased thirst and urination, and decreased thyroid function. Five to seven capsules will lead to severe increase in urination, tremors, lethargy, and tiredness. Patients have trouble overdosing on lithium, since too many tablets will cause nausea and vomiting. For this reason lithium is a good choice in individuals at high risk for suicide. Lithium is best used as Eskalith, or time-release lithium. Lithium is available for children as lithium citrate.

Tegretol Protocol

Tegretol can be a life-transforming medicine when used properly and safely. It is used for anxiety, allergies, mood swings, depression, manic depression, psychosis, environmental sensitivities, epilepsy, temporal lobe disorders, etc. Generic tegretol can contain a dye. If you are sensitive to medication, you may only require about a half dose, and you should do everything at half speed. A world renowned expert on tegretol suggests using only carbamazepine by Warner Chalcott. Initial dose is 1/2 tablet of 200 mg, two times a day by mouth, 9 am and 9 pm for two days. Then one tablet by mouth two times a day for two days. Then one tablet three times a day at 9 am, 3 pm, and 9 pm for two days. Then seven days at one tablet three times a day with two tablets at 9 pm. Then do a blood level at 9 am before taking medication. Tegretol reactions include elevation of liver enzymes (like high dose niacin), rash, and swollen nodes. We will monitor the liver enzyme level. However, call your doctor if any of the other problems develop.

Tegretol Protocol -- Revised:
For the Individual Who is Extra-Sensitive to Medication

Carbamazepine is generic tegretol. The generic version should be white and without dye. The medication should be taken as follows:

1/2 tablet twice a day (at breakfast & bedtime) for four days,

then . . . .

1 tablet twice a day (at breakfast & bedtime) for four days,

then . . . .

1 tablet three times a day (at breakfast, dinner and bedtime) for four days,

then . . .

1 tablet twice a day (at breakfast & dinner) and 2 tablets at bedtime for seven days.

At the end of the 19th day, a blood level should be taken at 9:00 A. M. with no tegretol taken that day.

The most common side effects are rash and sedation. If any side effects or changes that are bothersome occur, call your doctor.

If sedation occurs during the day, the dosing can be shifted to larger ones at dinner and bedtime: no daytime dose is taken; as a more strenuous measure, all medicine can be taken at bed if sedation affects are considerable.

Magnetic Resonance Imaging (MRI)

MRI, Magnetic Resonance Imaging, is one of the great breakthroughs, even greater than the CT scan, for imaging soft tissues of the body. An MRI is done on a scanner table, and an open-air MRI is available in Newtown, New Jersey for those people who feel claustrophobic. For an MRI scan you will be asked to remove all jewelry, watches, hair clips, dentures, glasses, hearing aids, keys, and wallets so that none of these things can interact with the MRI scanner.

During the examination you will hear a tapping sound, and it is important for you to be perfectly still. MRI's usually should be done with an injection of contrast material so as not to miss a rare but potentially serious problem of meningioma, which can only be seen during gadolinium dye injection. Special equipment such as ear plugs and claustrophobic glasses are available to make the scan more comfortable. No preparation is needed for the examination. For very nervous individuals, sedation may be necessary. If you have had studies such as CT scans, X-rays, ultrasound, and bone scans done at other hospitals or private facilities, you should bring them to the MRI so the radiologist can review them.

The MRI frequently identifies subtle aging in the brain, such as UBO's (Unidentifiable Bright Objects). This is found in approximately 9% of aging brains, and although it has not been thought to be associated with Alzheimer's disease, it is probably a marker for organic injury to the brain due to cerebral vascular problems.

If you have any of the following conditions, they may either prevent you from having an MRI or you may need special procedures: if you have a cardiac pacemaker or a cerebral aneurysm clip; if you have metal plates, cardiac valves, or neuro implants; if you are possibly pregnant; if you have had brain, eye, ear, or any other surgery; if your weight exceeds 300 pounds; if you have been exposed to metal fragments at work while welding, binding, or drilling metal and do not routinely wear goggles.

The MRI uses a magnetic technique to see internal organs. It allows the doctor to see soft tissue such as muscle, fat, and internal organs without the use of an X-ray. It can be very helpful, particularly in detecting multiple sclerosis, small tumors, neurological disease, and organic brain diseases, and it is also used now as a new breakthrough technique in imaging the pancreas, the prostate, the heart, and many other organs. The MRI is a new and great breakthrough that allows the doctor to look into the body without opening the body. MRI also reflects the miracle of medicine in how we diagnose disease with magnets, and it reflects the continuous creative breakthroughs in human health symbolic of our time. At PATH we diagnose with magnets and heal with electricity!

Chiropractic

Increasing evidence suggests that chiropractic adjustments may be an important dimension of wellness. A recent double-blind review of spinal manipulation and mobilization for back and neck pain gave promising results in certain patients who have this type of problem. Coz, et al., Spinal Manipulation and Mobilization for Back and Neck Pain, *British Medical Journal*, Nov. 23, 1991, pp. 1298-1303. We look forward to chiropractic being included as an important part of neuromuscular tension relief and relaxation. Certainly, chiropractic may be a better approach to anxiety relief than drugs such as Xanax, Klonopin, and Valium. We look forward to the contribution that chiropractic will make in the coming years as osteopathic, chiropractic, and conventional medicine merge -- a true PATH to wellness.

Tourette's Syndrome

Gilles de la Tourette's Syndrome is a neurological disorder that has been widely misunderstood and misdiagnosed. The symptoms of Tourette's often mimic other movement and neurological disorders. Tourette's should be distinguished from habit spasms and transient, allergic tics of childhood. Often, patients are seen by allergists, psychiatrists, and ophthalmologists before a neurologist.

Tourette's is characterized by tics, involuntary movements of the face, arms, and legs, usually beginning in childhood or early adolescence. Frequently, facial tics include eye blinks and nose twitches. Most cases involve several body parts displaying involuntary movement. Repetitive touching, as well as obsessive and compulsive rituals can occur. Verbal tics also occur in Tourette's and may include shouting, barking, grunting, or throat clearing. Occasionally repeating one's own words or someone else's occurs; involuntary shouting of obscenities is also seen in some cases.

Tourette's is not a degenerative disease. However, symptoms come and go, and are sometimes triggered by stress. Intelligence and life span of these patients are not affected. Many patients show that tics can be less severe and more controllable with age. The less severe forms usually show complete or partial remission over time.

The etiology of Tourette's has not been definitively established. Research has shown biochemical abnormalities in the basal ganglia brain region. An overactivity in dopamine metabolism (and possibly other neurotransmitters as well) seems to be found in Tourette's patients. There may be subtle abnormalities in brain waves. Allergy has been implicated in Tourette's because of high IgE levels.

The decision to treat Tourette's is based upon many factors: negative social impact due to the tics, concentration obstructions, negative performance as to schoolwork, as well as other life factors. Most forms of nonpharmacological approaches have proved fruitless. There are several drugs such as Haldol and Orap (like Clozaril) which inhibit dopamine metabolism and help the disease. Clonidine, another drug, may be useful in the treatment of Tourette's Syndrome. These drug regimens are long term and have the possibility of numerous side effects.

Our Tourette's patients are put on a well-balanced diet with basic supplementation. In addition, Haldol, the drug of choice for Tourette's, is sometimes given before bedtime. Also, lecithin or an even better acetylcholine precursor (deanol or choline) can be administered. Increasing this neurotransmitter seems to be beneficial for Tourette's patients. Finally, helping patients reduce stress is of great use, since Tourette's is thought to be correlated to stress.

Neurological Obesity

Neurological obesity is a condition in which individuals are addicted to carbohydrates, fat, or foods as a result of irregular rhythms in the brain. They think they can beat their problem with only willpower, but they can not because it is as physical a problem as height and weight. It is a neurological deficit documented on BEAM (Brain Electrical Activity Map). These people commonly have a P300 wave of 5-8, often centrally or frontally displaced.

Instead of in the back of the head, the burst of activity is in the front of the head. This is what we call Cerebral Dysrhythmia or Generalized Encephalopathy. The treatment often requires very high doses of stimulants such as Fastin and Tenuate (and/or with Pondimin) to give energy and is usually very effective. Hopefully, in the long run, CES (Cranial Electrical Stimulation) and amino acids can correct most of the problem.

Multiple Sclerosis

Multiple sclerosis is a relatively common neurological disorder that is chronic and often attacks young people, frequently in the optic nerve, spinal cord, and brain, with multiple sclerosing plaques where the myelin sheath, or insulation, around the nerves in the brain begins to erode. Classically, there is weakness, numbness, impaired vision, double vision, trouble swallowing, intention tremor, trouble walking (such as ataxia), impairment of deep sensation, bladder dysfunction, and altered emotional responses.

There can be as many as 1 to 10 years between minor initial symptoms and full diagnosis. The MRI test is extremely useful (it shows demyelinating lesions); and Brain Electrical Activity Mapping (BEAM) frequently shows abnormal electrical activity. CT scans and brain stem evoked potentials are practically useless. Multiple sclerosis can occur between the ages of 20 and 40, and there is a higher incidence in women compared to men. There may be a susceptibility gene or an immune gene which is related to human leukocyte antigens, which is why one of the best tests for evaluating multiple sclerosis is to measure the immune system (T-helper/T-suppressor ratios). As the T-cell ratio increases, the disease worsens. There is a familial tendency for the disease, and it is commonly found in Northern European groups farther from the equator and will show up even when people move to warmer climates. There is an increase in multiple sclerosis in farmers, possibly due to exposure to pesticides and toxins. One can produce multiple sclerosis in animal experiments in any number of ways, such as viral exposure, Epstein-Barr, herpes, etc. Trauma, although no longer thought to be a factor, was once considered a significant factor and may still cause some multiple sclerosis. Allergic encephalomyelitis, which can be a model for creating multiple sclerosis, infection, trauma, and pregnancy, is also thought to be a precipitating factor. Flu frequently precedes multiple sclerosis. During pregnancy there are exacerbations, as well as during surgery.

About 25 percent of all patients have retrobulbar optoneuritis, with visual loss that can recur with partial or total loss of vision in one eye. On rare occasions it is progressive. MS can induce a tingling electrical feeling down the back and, less commonly, the interior thighs, as well as unsteadiness in walking. Brain stem symptoms are diplopia, double vision, vertigo, vomiting, increased urination and hemiplegia; facial paralysis and deafness can occur in a small proportion of cases. There are variants in multiple sclerosis, which are cerebellar in their nature. In some cases multiple sclerosis can present the semblance of confusional psychosis. Multiple sclerosis can require steroid treatment and can render patients stuporous, comatose, decerebrate, or even injure a cranial nerve. Amaurotic form of multiple sclerosis can also occur. Mimickers and other types of multiple sclerosis -- Guillain-Barre syndrome and other viral-like conditions -- exist. Cerebral proteins frequently show an oligoclonal band and high levels of myelin basic protein.

Forms of lupus and syphilis can imitate multiple sclerosis. Vitamin B-12 deficiencies can imitate MS, as can ALS and subacute combined degeneration. MS can be found in recovering alcoholics. MS unfortunately affects the brain. It can cause amnesia, forgetfulness, aphasia, apraxia, agnosia, visual-spatial disorder, trouble swallowing.

Depression is the most common psychological deficit of MS. In addition, there are frequently impairments in performance I.Q., memory, attention, conceptual reasoning, and even verbal I.Q. Use of strong antidepressants, such as Nardil and Eldepryl, might slow the progress of the disease. On rare occasions sodium valproate has been used to treat the problem. It is now known, as with so many diseases, that the chronic course can be reduced by dietary change; particularly, high intake of polyunsaturated oils (e.g., safflower oil) has frequently been demonstrated to slow the progression of MS over a period of 35 years.

According to certain studies there may be some benefit of borage oil (fish oil) supplements. You can't underestimate in some cases the response of patients with MS to drugs like Symmetrel, clonazepam and Lioresal. It is suggested that vitamin C and calcium may benefit, especially in experimental models of producing MS. Because MS has an autoimmune basis, autoimmune treatments can be tried, such as colchicine, Parlodel, Wellbutrin, etc. Other rare forms of MS can be mimicked by neurobrucellosis and other rare infections. Certainly MS will be exacerbated by the normal process of aging. Certain antioxidant enzymes may protect the blood brain barrier against MS progression and development.

At this point, the majority of evidence suggests that T-cell levels can be followed, and an increase in T-cell ratios from 2.6 to 3.6 is particularly indicative of progressive MS. Although a ratio over and above 2, rather than the normal 1.8, frequently indicates MS is there. Progression and the origin of the disease probably begins after puberty. We still can't underestimate the immunomodulating factors and even chemotherapy has been tried. Other drugs such as Plaquenil, Cytoxan, Clinoril, and Azulfidine have been used less commonly. Common presenting symptoms: numbness, gait difficulty, weakness, visual loss, double vision, urinary difficulty, trouble swallowing, trouble moving a part of the body, severe fatigue, vertigo, impotence, convulsion, severe emotionality, trouble holding one's bowel movement, hearing loss, and movement tremor. Fifty percent will have either numbness or gait difficulty. It is thought that certain solvents, welding, and exposure to animals (such as birds) may be factors, although not yet demonstrated.

Abnormalities on MRI are common in MS, inasmuch as 99 percent will have white matter lesions. Neuro-psychological tests are probably the best tests for evaluating the severity of MS and its effect on cognitive functioning. A drug called copolymer is being researched. Polyunsaturated oils may be useful as well as various trace elements. B-12 shots can be tried. In some cases digestive problems may be associated with MS. The immune modulating drug levamisole, which may increase the cyclic effect of guanosine and antioxidant enzymes, has been thought to also help. Further research will be needed on how to use this agent -- 150-200 mg once a week for a 4-year period may help. Trials of hyperbaric oxygen have been looked at. Increasing evidence suggests that HTLV viruses are associated with MS. Some cases of MS may even appear as a narcolepsy-like syndrome. Neuropsychological examinations and brain mapping can evaluate the severity of cognitive effects. Certainly, cognitive disorders occur very early in MS and should be picked up and treated with medicine, nutrients, or cognitive remediation.

Parkinson's Disease

Parkinson's is a clinical syndrome consisting of 4 major signs: tremor at rest, rigidity, bradykinesia or slow movement, and loss of postural reflexes. Not all patients have these signs. Patients frequently have reduction in spontaneous movements and difficulty in involuntary movements. Parkinson's patients often have masked facial expressions, general slowing down of movement, decreased frequency of blinking, a staring expression, decreased swallowing resulting in drooling, soft voice, loss of speech modulation, impaired handwriting, micrographia, decreased amplitude in performing rapid repetitive movements, difficulty rising from a chair, difficulty turning in bed, short shuffling steps, loss of spontaneous gesturing and speaking. It affects approximately one million Americans.

Risk factors for Parkinson's can include a history of encephalitis, influenza, exposure to drugs or toxins, surgical removal of parathyroid glands, and previous strokes. The main therapy for Parkinson's disease is the amino acid, dopa. But there are numerous other therapies such as Parlodel; the antiviral agent Symmetrel (or amantadine) as well as anticholinergic agents Artane and Benadryl and Cogentin; antipsychotic agents Parsidol (a new prevention medicine), Sergelide or Eldepryl, and pergolide -- another dopa receptor agonist. Other agents include Akineton, Hemadrin, Larodopa, and Levsin.

There have been numerous studies about nutrients helping Parkinson's, such as antioxidants, methionine, tyrosine, phenylalanine, tryptophan, and even electrical therapies such as ECT and possibly CES. Certain nutrients should be used as an adjunct, with or without medications, depending on the doctor. There are many subtleties in dosing, and improvements can occur with drug holidays, various manipulations in drug timing, etc., all of which require a physician's experience and certain trial and error prescribing medicines and vitamins.

Epilepsy

**TABLE 1: INTERNATIONAL CLASSIFICATION
OF EPILEPTIC SEIZURES***

Partial (Focal, Local) Seizures

Simple partial seizures (consciousness not impaired)

Motor signs
Somatosensory or special sensory symptoms
Autonomic symptoms or signs
Psychic symptoms

Complex partial seizures (consciousness impaired)

Simple partial onset followed by impaired consciousness
Consciousness impaired at onset

Partial seizures evolving to generalized seizures (tonic, clonic, or tonic-clonic)

Simple partial seizures evolving to generalized seizures
Complex partial seizures evolving to generalized seizures
Simple partial seizures evolving to complex partial seizures evolving to generalized seizures

Generalized Seizures (Convulsive or Nonconvulsive)

Absence seizures

Typical (brief stare, eye flickering, no motion)
Atypical (associated with movement)

Myoclonic seizures
Clonic seizures
Tonic seizures
Tonic-clonic seizures
Atonic seizures

Unclassified Epileptic Seizures

---

*From the Commission on Classification and Terminology of the International League Against Epilepsy.

TABLE 2: INTERNATIONAL CLASSIFICATION OF EPILEPSIES, EPILEPSY SYNDROMES, AND RELATED SEIZURE DISORDERS*

Localization-Related (Focal, Local, Partial) Epilepsies, Syndrome Defined by Seizure Type and Other Clinical Features, Including Artatomic Localization and Etiology

Idiopathic

    Benign childhood epilepsy with centrotemporal spikes
    Childhood epilepsy with occipital paroxysms
    Primary reading epilepsy

Symptomatic

    Temporal lobe epilepsy
    Frontal lobe epilepsy
    Parietal lobe epilepsy
    Occipital lobe epilepsy
    Chronic progressive epilepsia partialis continua

Cryptogenic (presumed to be symptomatic but cause is unknown)

    Temporal lobe epilepsy
    Frontal lobe epilepsy
    Parietal lobe epilepsy
    Occipital lobe epilepsy
    Chronic progressive epilepsia partialis continua

Generalized Epilepsies

Idiopathic

    Benign neonatal convulsions (familial and nonfamilial)
    Benign myoclonic epilepsy in infancy
    Childhood absence epilepsy
    Juvenile myoclonic epilepsy
    Epilepsy with generalized tonic-clonic seizures on awakening

Cryptogenic

    West's syndrome (infantile spasms)
    Lennox-Gastaut syndrome
    Epilepsy with myoclonic-astatic seizures
    Epilepsy with myoclonic absences

Symptomatic

    Nonspecific etiology

        Early myoclonic encephalopathy
        Early infantile epileptic encephalopathy with suppression burst
        Other symptomatic generalized epilepsies

    Specific syndromes (disease states in which seizures are a presenting or predominant feature)

Undetermined Epilepsies

Generalized and focal features

    Neonatal seizures
    Severe myoclonic epilepsy of childhood
    Epilepsy with continuous spike waves during slow-wave sleep
    Acquired epileptic aphasia (Landau-Kleffner syndrome)
    Other undetermined epilepsies

Without unequivocal generalized or focal features

Special Syndromes

Situation-related seizures

    Febrile convulsions
    Isolated seizures or status epilepticus
    Seizures caused by an acute or toxic event, such as alcohol or drug overdose, eclampsia, or hyperglycemia

*From the Commission on Classification and Terminology of the International League Against Epilepsy.

Kinds of Seizures

SEIZURES -- Typical, Atypical

- Partial or focal seizures
- Psychomotor seizures
- Tonic-clonic-grand mal seizures

SYMPTOMS

- Psychopathological difficulties
- Schizophreniform or depressive psychoses
- Sinking or rising feeling
- Outcry
- Urinary or fecal incontinence
- With or without tongue biting
- May have hand tremors a few minutes to an hour
- Preceded by prodromal mood and/or other symptoms
- Change followed by deep sleep -- headache, muscle soreness at times; focal motor or sensory phenomena (look for focal lesion)

Seizures - Nutritional Control

Seizures are extremely difficult to control nutritionally, although studies suggest that vitamin E may help anticonvulsant work better and that other nutrients such as B-6, magnesium and taurine may have some beneficial effects. Common nutrients, like calcium and magnesium, may help depending on your concept of seizures. Seizures are on a continuum between anxiety, depression, insomnia, and panic. The end stage of the conditions listed above may be seizures. In other cases, a seizure can be full-blown, like a heart attack, manifesting irregular brainbeats similar to irregular heartbeats. Some seizures are due to head trauma, some are idiopathic. Fifty percent of all seizure patients have normal EEG's. Seizures due to brain damage are hard to control without drugs. Some psychiatric patients have seizures which never manifest themselves on the EEG. Brain mapping can help identify where the seizures are occurring, probably better than any other technique. Because nutritional control of seizures is so difficult, the concept of using Cranial Electrical Stimulation (CES) worn on the head or implanted in the left vagus may also be beneficial. One should always try to control seizures with one medication if possible.

Dyslexia

Dyslexia is a problem associated with a reversing of letters. It is often called dyslexia, dysgraphia, or even dyscalculia or other learning disabilities. It affects mostly reading and writing. Some people are born with it, others may get it through a traumatic injury, genetic injury, or even a virus. The brain in dyslexics has different electrical imbalances. Dyslexia sometimes can be treated by stimulants or anticonvulsants or even antidepressant medication along with nutrition and diet. Cure is usually not possible, but significant reduction in symptoms usually is, with medication, e.g., antidepressants, anticonvulsants, or even electrical stimulation.

Tinnitus

Tinnitus is a disease in which a person is highly sensitive to noise, or there is a spontaneous ringing in one or both ears. The former condition may be classified as objective; that is, a person hears a sound that arises externally. Objective tinnitus is often caused by temporomandibular joint dysfunction and the opening of eustachian tubes. Indeed, intracranial pressure, caused by stroke or brain tumor, can be another cause of tinnitus (angiograms may be necessary).

Subjective tinnitus (the spontaneous condition indicated above) is more common and often entails metallic ringing, blowing, buzzing, clanging, popping, roaring, or non-rhythmic beatings in one or both ears. A slight degree of tinnitus can be observed by almost everyone, if they concentrate their attention on auditory events in a quiet room. Extremely loud tinnitus can be manifested due to salicylate, quinine or quinine toxicity, ingesting large amounts of caffeine, being exposed to loud noises, or using nicotine or salt excessively. These things need to be avoided. Tinnitus can also be treated with sodium fluoride and zinc.

Orthodox medical treatment of tinnitus can include the use of intravenous lidocaine and anticonvulsants, particularly carbamazepine, Dilantin, and valproic acid. I have noticed that some tinnitus patients can have biochemical depression that can be treated with antidepressants. Even psychosis can be a factor in tinnitus. Other patients have elevated copper levels that can be treated by zinc, manganese, and molybdenum. The use of zinc may be helpful in general for this problem, although not in all cases. Food allergy may also be a factor. The majority of stress conditions reduce plasma amino acids, particularly the antioxidant sulfur amino acids. Hence, this may be a useful therapy.

The use of amino oxyacetic acid (oxylated glycine) as a palliative in tinnitus has been proposed. This treatment has been reserved for unresponsive patients, and, as far as we know, is not FDA approved.

Sleeping Better

There are many general rules for good sleep, e.g., avoid sleeping pills, sleep at regular times, get physical exercise, avoid sleeping during the daytime, quit smoking, avoid coffee, tea, cola drinks, cocoa (all caffeine), TV watching and exciting reading before bedtime, take a warm bath or at least a footbath before going to bed, have a cup of soothing herb tea, keep your bedroom well ventilated with low temperature and rather high humidity, and don't take your problems to bed with you. If you couldn't solve them today, let them wait until tomorrow.

Yet, despite adhering to these rules, many people cannot sleep. Nutrients can help, and unlike most drugs, they do not result in exacerbation of daytime psychiatric problems, i.e. depression or psychosis. Tryptophan (typically 1 gram) at dinner and bedtime (up to a total of 15 grams) is effective in starting sleep, and, in some cases,

keeping a person asleep. Niacin (timed release) and niacinamide prolong the tryptophan effect. Melatonin (Chronoset) and GABA also can contribute to quality sleep.

Vitamin B-6, pantothenic acid, and other B-vitamins also increase dream recall and promote satisfying sleep. Inositol and vitamin C also can be helpful. If drugs are necessary, antianxiety drugs, antidepressants or anti-convulsants (e.g., Xanax, Klonopin, Tegretol or doxepin and/or antihistamines) are best. Occasionally, major tranquilizers, e.g., Haldol or Mellaril, are necessary. Barbiturates are too dangerous for regular use. The CES (Cranial Electrical Stimulation) may be the best treatment of insomnia developed to date. Sleep is a measure of overall health. Good sleep leads to good life and is a barometer of brain health.

19. *Nutrients and Drugs*

The Nutrient Beatitudes

Blessed are those who breathe clean air for their bodies will be free from lead.

Blessed are those who drink living spring water for they will not be polluted by copper.

Blessed are those who eat fresh fruit for they will receive minerals and manganese.

Blessed are those who exercise and play for they will tone and tune the temple of their body.

Blessed are those who eat bran for their bowels will be regular.

Blessed are those who eat fresh vegetables for they will protect themselves from heart disease.

Blessed are those who eat essential oils for these will lower cholesterol.

Blessed are those who eat food supplements for they will find what they seek.

Blessed are those who glow with nutrients for their minds will ever grow.

Blessed are those who seek wholeness of body, mind, and spirit, for they will nourish the world.

Elements of Good Nutrition and Malnutrition [1]

Essential Nutrients

Elements	macro	calcium, magnesium
	micro	phosphorus, sodium, potassium, chromium, copper, iodine, iron, manganese, selenium, zinc
Carbohydrates	water-soluble	B-1, B-2, B-6, B-12, biotin folic acid niacin, pantothenic acid vitamin C
Proteins	nitrogen-containing amino acids	histidine, isoleucine, lysine, methionine, phenylalanine, threonine, tyrosine, tryptophan, valine
Fats	fat-soluble	vitamins A, D, E, K

Essential Nutrients -- Conditionally Essential Nutrients

Elements	macro	silicon, bromide
	micro	rubidium, nickel, vanadium, tin, boron, fluoride, cesium
Carbohydrates	water-soluble	inositol, bioflavonoids, glucose, PABA
Proteins	nitrogen-containing amino acids	deanol, para-aminobenzoic acid, nicotinic acid, alanine, arginine, aspartic acid, carnitine, cysteine, dimethyl glycine (DMG-B15), glutamic acid, glutathione, glutaurine, glycine, histidine, hydroxyproline, norleucine, ornithine, orotic acid, proline, serine, taurine, tyrosine.
Fats	fat-soluble	beta carotene, vitamin D, octacosanol, omega 3, 6, 9 and 12 fatty acids, cholesterol.

Marginal Nutrition/Malnutrition: Basic Causes -- Past and Present

A. Medical

1. Malabsorption -- diarrhea, parasites, IGA deficiency, celiac disease, (gluten enteropathy) sprue, lactose intolerance, intrinsic factor deficiency, pancreatic insufficiency, obstructive jaundice, operations, i.e., Billroth I or II, fistulas, etc.

2. Chronic disease -- infections, critical illness, cancer, hyperthyroidism.

3. Poor nutritional intake -- chronic emesis, hypogeusia, anorexia nervosa, alcoholism, dieting, bulimia, vitamin deficiency, myasthenia gravis, esophageal structure, oropharyngeal disease.

4. Increased metabolic requirements -- pregnancy, lactation, childhood puberty, rapid growth.

5. Inborn errors -- homocystinuria, porphyria, pyroluria, etc.

---

1. Source: Eric R. Braverman, Medical History and the Holistic Perspective, *The Journal of Orthomolecular Medicine*, vol. 3, # 4, pp. 195-196, 1988.

6. Excessive excretion -- protein losing enteropathy, Addison's disease, primary aldosteronism.

7. Faulty transport -- carnitine deficiency, abetalipoproteinemia, deficiency or retinol binding protein hyperproteinemia.

8. Medications -- antimetabolite, antivitamin, antimineralites (methotrexate, hydralazine, Dilantin, BCP, penicillamine, cholestyramine, phenobarbital, diuretics).

B. Food Acquisitions.

1. Quality of land fertilization, too limited using only nitrogen, potassium, phosphate, fertilization with too much copper phosphate nitrate or alkali. Soil deficiency in trace metals, i.e., molybdenum, selenium. Soil contaminated with pesticides, chemicals, poisoned water. Acid rain, natural catastrophes, etc.

2. Contaminated fish -- swordfish with mercury, seed grain with organic mercury, pigs with methyl mercury, rice with cadmium -- Ginger Jake paralysis -- triorthicresylators multiple neuritis milk with tremetol -- milk root poisoning.

3. Food Processing -- milling of grain that removes vitamins and trace elements, bleaching of grain, freezing with chelators which may reduce availability of nutrients, canning adds tin, may add some lead and cadmium. Addition of chemicals -- dyes, BHT, sulfur dioxide, nitrates, etc.

4. Food storage -- bacterial growth peanut fungus, aflatoxin, potato, carcinogen.

C. Social.

1. Poverty -- overpopulation, inadequate protein, poor economy, farming, ignorance, contaminated water.

2. Familial -- neglect of children, current diet habits, dietary foods.

3. Household -- aluminum cookware utensils, excess copper, lead with acid well water, copper plumbing, no hard water.

4. Cooking -- burnt food, nitrosamines, overcooked.

D. Environmental -- allergic etiology, ultimately nutritional depletion?

1. Air pollution, fluorescent light, fossil fuels, plastics, perfumes, rubber, hair sprays, tar-containing adhesives, bleaches, ammonia, mothballs, pine, tobacco smoke.

2. Geopathic zone, radio waves.

Essential Amino Acids:
The Protein You Need to Live

The human body has protein requirements which are satisfied by the essential amino acids. (See the Fast Path amino acid formula.)

ESSENTIAL AMINO ACIDS REQUIREMENTS

Amino Acid	Infant (4-6 mo)	Child (10-12 yr)	Adult	Amino Acid Pattern for High Quality Proteins, mg/g of protein
Histidine	33			17
Isoleucine	83	28	12	42
Leucine	135	42	16	70
Lysine	99	44	12	51
Total S-containing amino acids (includes methionine and cystine)	49	22	10	26
Total aromatic amino acids (includes phenylalanine and tyrosine)	141	22	16	73
Threonine	68	28	8	35
Tryptophan	21	4	3	11
Valine	92	25	14	48

Source: National Academy of Sciences, *Recommended Dietary Allowances*, 9th Edition, 1980, p.43.

We do not have a requirement for the nonessential amino acids because we can make them in our cells. The essential amino acids are the ones missing, and when present in only a low amount, the protein synthesis of the body will fall to a very low level or stop completely. In most foods containing protein, all the essential amino acids are present. In some foods, one or more of the essential amino acids may be present in significantly lower amounts than others, making it an incomplete protein. Animal foods have more complete protein sources. In addition, many foods have a limited number of essential amino acids in proportion, as opposed to other amino acids. For example, foods with low methionine are not well utilized by the body, and commercially available protein powders may be 60 or 70 percent nonessential amino acids, which means they give excess nitrogen and protein, which strain the kidneys without providing the essential amino acids required by the body to make muscle. Therefore, ironically, protein shakes are not likely to add to the muscle-making capacity of individuals.

It is also important to have an adequate amino acid balance. For example, food containing 100 percent of a person's lysine requirement but only 20 percent of his methionine requirement, results in only 20 percent of the protein in that food being used as protein in the body. When taking an amino acid supplement, it is important to complement it by adding all the essential amino acids. This is very difficult with tryptophan being unavailable on the market; it is, therefore, the essential amino acid lacking in most supplements. The importance of balancing the essential amino acids by obtaining the best possible protein in our foods cannot be overstressed.

FAST PATH INGREDIENTS

L-Isoleucine	73.64 mg
L-Leucine	98.21 mg
L-Lysine HCL	73.64 mg
Methionine	61.39 mg
L-Cysteine HCL	73.64 mg
L-Arginine HCL	86.03 mg
L-Phenylalanine	49.14 mg
L-Tyrosine	49.14 mg
L-Valine	86.03 mg
L-Threonine	49.15 mg

(temporarily missing L-tryptophan)

The supplement Fast Path best imitates this essential amino acid requirement because it contains only essential amino acids, and is therefore the only pure, essential amino acid supplement available.

The Amino Acid Blood Test

The amino acid (AA) profile is a test of your AA levels in blood plasma (a liquid part of blood). This test measures over 30-40 AA's. Amino acids are important to health because they are the building blocks of protein, hormones, brain neurotransmitters, muscles, immunoglobulins, etc. Your amino acid test can give us important clues about your health.

There are a number of diseases in which amino acids are completely reduced in plasma. Low plasma amino acids occur in patients who have anorexia, cancer, folliculitis, alcohol abuse, pregnancy, arthritis, or glucagonoma. Low plasma amino acids can occur during any severe stress (such as minor and major depressions). Fever and infectious diseases reduce most amino acids in serum, yet there is an increase in phenylalanine. Patients with hypoglycemia can have low alanine levels. In kidney failure, plasma tyrosine is often low as are threonine, valine, isoleucine, leucine, lysine, and histidine.

Allergy patients are frequently low in cysteine. Depressed patients may be deficient in taurine, phenalal-anine, tyrosine, methionine, glycine, and tryptophan. Psychotic patients can be deficient in tryptophan, histidine, and glycine. Serine, tyrosine, and phenylalanine can be elevated in psychotic patients.

Elevations in plasma amino acids are found with vitamin D deficiency, heavy metal poisoning, liver disease, pancreatitis, magnesium deficiency, vitamin C deficiency, Wilson's disease (high copper), and skin diseases. High copper can reduce histidine and tryptophan, as well as elevate other less valuable amino acids. Alanine is elevated in Cushing's disease and gout patients. Leucine, isoleucine, and valine are elevated in diabetics and dieters. Migraine patients have elevated tryptophan and GABA. Phenylalanine and tyrosine are elevated in hyperactive children, schizophrenics, and migraine patients.

All these possible abnormalities in amino acid levels make this blood test an important diagnostic tool for your health. Information concerning amino acid levels can be used by your doctor to predict which antidepressants can be most helpful.

Acute and Chronic
Supplementation of Amino Acids

iron and

INTRODUCTION

Of the four essential nutrient groups, amino acids may be the most fundamental to brain chemistry. The dietary dependence of the neurotransmitters dopamine, serotonin, and histamine upon their amino acid precursors, is now well established (Wurtman, et al., 1980). Many other neurotransmitters, which are either made from amino acid precursors or are amino acids, are likely to be dietary dependent. Plasma amino acid levels have been demonstrated to be directly proportional to brain neurotransmitter levels (Wurtman, R. J., 1980; De Montis, M. G., et al., 1977). Therefore, neurotransmitters can be influenced to a great degree by the amino acids in the diet or by supplementation (Benedict, et al., 1983).

Interest in amino acids in therapeutics is growing. Tryptophan (Trp) has been utilized in insomnia, depression, pain relief, and mania. Methionine (M) has been utilized in depression (Muscettola, G., et al., 1984), gall bladder diseases (Frezza, M., et al., 1984), and other medical conditions (Braverman, E. R., and Pfeiffer, C. C., 1984-85). Taurine (T) is a common therapeutic in Japan, where it is used as an inotrope (Azuma, J., et al., 1983) and anticonvulsant (Muscettola, G., et al., 1984). Hence, we studied the effects of acute and chronic supplementation of amino acids on plasma amino acid levels. This is because plasma amino acids are directly correlated to neurotransmitter content in the brain.

METHODS AND RESULTS: ACUTE LOADING OF TRYPTOPHAN AND OTHER AMINO ACIDS

Five fasted normal subjects were loaded with five grams (per 70 kg) of Trp; plasma amino acids, trace metals, polyamines, growth hormone, and Metpath Lab Flex profile were measured. Trp levels in plasma were 7.8 ± 1.6 uM/DL at 0 hour (before load) 39 ± 10 uM/DL at two hours and 31 ± 8 uM/DL at four hours. Changes in Trp were significant at the less than .001 level (Figure 1). Trp will return to normal in about six to eight hours (Zarcone, V., et al., 1973). A downward trend of valine, leucine, glycine, threonine, asparagine, proline, lysine, and histidine (Table 1) was noted, but was not significant when compared to a fasted control group that had blood drawn at 0.2 and 4 hours. Fasting alone decreases plasma amino acids. There were upward trends in serum

growth hormone. All differences in biological variables but tryptophan were N. S.

Similar studies were done for 22 other amino acids (Table 3). Rates of absorption are shown in Table 4. The sulfur amino acids, taurine and methionine, are best absorbed. Munro (1972) and others have suggested that amino acids are better absorbed as peptides.

Table 1
Amino Acids as Precursors of Neurotransmitters

Amino Acid	Neurotransmitters
cysteine	cysteic acid
glutamine	GABA, glutamic acid
histidine	histamine
lysine	pipecolic acid
phenylalanine	phenylethylamine plus same as tyrosine
tyrosine	dopamine, norepinephrine, epinephrine, tyramine
tryptophan	serotonin, melatonin, tryptamines

Amino Acids as Neurotransmitters

Amino Acid	Function
alanine	inhibitory or calming
GABA	inhibitory or calming
glycine	inhibitory or calming
taurine	inhibitory or calming
glutamic acid	excitatory
aspartic acid	excitatory

Figure 1:
Effect of Acute Tryptophan Loading

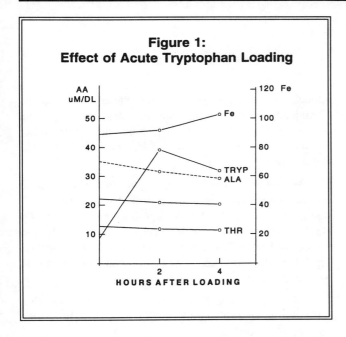

Table 2:
Absorption of Individual Amino Acids
1 gm/70 kg -- % increase VS controls

A.A.	hr 2	hr 4
TAUR	663.1	256.9
MET	291.7	172.3
HPRO	155.1	107.8
SER	135.5	62.5
PROL	121.1	54.2
ILE	116.4	121.8
PHE	101.8	52.6
ORN	100.6	42.2
TRP	77.5	57.9
GABA	64.0	.0
THR	62.2	52.3

Table 3:
Absorption of Individual Amino Acids
1 gm/70 kg -- % Increase VS Controls

A.A.	hr 2	hr 4
VAL	60.1	52.6
ASP	40.1	.0
ASN	31.7	14.6
HIS	30.4	12.2
LYS	26.3	8.5
LEU	18.5	5.5
ARG	15.0	18.8
TYR	14.3	21.4
ALA	7.1	1.5
GLN	2.2	.2
CYS	.0	11.7
GLY	-1.4	15.7

Table 4:
Absorption of Individual Amino Acids
g/70 KG - % increase VS controls

Average % increase for hours - 2 and 4

Tau	4600	....
Met	2320	....
Hpro	1314	....
Ile	1191	....
Ser	990	....
Pro	877	....
Phe	772	....
Orn	714	....
Trp	677	....
Thr	573	....
Val	563	....
GABA	245	...
Asn	231	...
His	213	..
Tyr	179	..
Lys	174	..
Arg	169	..
Asp	141	..
Lea	120	.
Gly	72	.
Cys	58	
Ala	43	
Gln	12	

METHODS AND RESULTS: CHRONIC SUPPLEMENTATION OF TRYPTOPHAN AND OTHER AMINO ACIDS

Data on four patients loaded with 2.5 grams (per 70 kg) of tryptophan (Trp) daily for an average of 6 weeks were analyzed retrospectively. The mean Trp level for these patients was 12.8 ± 3 uM/DL compared to 7.1 ± 2.2 uM/DL for a matched control group of 96 patients (Table 7). The difference was significant at the less than .001 level. There was a significant increase of asparagine, arginine, threonin,e and alanine (p less than .05) when compared to several matched control groups. Comparison of chronic loaded Trp patients showed significant elevations of these amino acids (p less than .02) and T (p less than .05) compared to the acute loaded group at the times determined. These data show that the downward trend in plasma amino acids observed with tryptophan loading is not seen in chronic loading. Furthermore, postulated decreases of amino acids that compete with Trp for absorption do not occur.

Twelve grams of Trp loaded daily to manic patients increased plasma levels to twice normal at two weeks due to homeostatic compensation (Chouinard and Colleagues, 1978). We have had children with plasma Trp twice normal without decreases in other plasma amino acids. Chronically loaded tryptophan increases other plasma amino acids. We have observed this with other chronically loaded amino acids, i.e., taurine and methionine.

We retrospectively analyzed plasma amino acids in patients loaded with M alone (N= 3, 1400 mg/70 kg-11 weeks), M ± T (N=4, M 1800 mg/70 kg-13 weeks, T 600 mg/70 kg-11 weeks), Trp alone (N = 4, 2500 mg/70 kg-6 weeks) and M ± Trp (N= 4, M 800 mg/70 kg-9 weeks, Trp 900 mg/kg-10 weeks). We compared these groups to two control groups.

M alone (Table 5) increased plasma M and other sulfur amino acids T and Cysteine (Cys), as well as Abu, Glycine (Gly) and Asn (P less than .01).

M + T (Table 6) increased the above amino acids plus Orn and Hpr (p less than .03). M compared to M + T showed only T to be significantly elevated.

Table 5

Significant Increases in Plasma Amino Acids with Chronic Methionine Therapy

Dose 1400 mg/70 kg for 11 Weeks

N = 3   CTRL = 16   P < .1

Methionine Only		Control		
MET	10 ± 3.6	3	±	0.9
CYS	4 ± 1.0	2.3	±	1.5
TAU	7 ± 2.6	5	±	1.3
ABU	3.7 ± 0.6	2	±	0.8
GLY	37 ± 13.9	23	±	5
ASN	14 ± 4.0	7.1	±	1.8

Table 6

Significant Increases in Plasma Amino Acids with Chronic Methionine Plus Taurine Therapy

MET (1800 mg/70 kg 10 Weeks		TAU (600 mg/70 kg 14 Weeks		
N = 4		CTRL = 16		
MET & TAU (P < 0.3)		Control		
MET	7.5 ± 2.1	3.0	±	0.9
TAU	15 ± 6.1	5	±	1.3
ABU	3 ± 0.8	2	±	0.8
GLY	31.8 ± 15	23	±	5
ASN	9.5 ± 2.3	7.1	±	1.7
HPR	4.3 ± 1.3	2.6	±	1.4
ORN	8.5 ± 3	5.8	±	5.8

Trp alone (Table 7) elevated Trp, Thr and Arg (p less than .03). M ± Trp (Table 8) elevated M, Thr, Arg, and T, Lue, Ile, Val, Phe, Tyr, Set, Hpr, and Lys (p less than .03).

The addition of a second amino acid again accentuated the increase in other plasma amino acids. All four groups combined (N = 15) compared to controls (N = 26) showed increases in 10 amino acids (p less than .05) and trends upward in all plasma amino acids. Chronic supplementation of M, T, or Trp leads to an elevation of many other plasma amino acids.

Table 7

Significant Increases in Plasma Amino Acids with Chronic Tryptophan Therapy

Dose 2.5 g/70 kg for 6 Weeks

N = 4   CTRL = 10   P < .3

	Tryptophan Only			Control		
ASN	9.8	±	1.9	7.5	±	1.7
ARG	11.8	±	0.9	9.1	±	1.6
THR	15	±	2.9	11.8	±	2.2
ALA	46.3	±	8.9	34	±	7.6
TRP	12.8	±	2.9	7.9	±	1.4

Table 8

Significant Increases in Plasma Amino Acids with Chronic Methionine Plus Tryptophan Therapy

MET (800 mg/70 kg 9 Weeks   TRP (900 mg/70 kg 10 Weeks

N = 4   CTRL = 16

	MET & TRP			Control			
LEU	19.5	±	4.8	12.3	±	2.7	
ILE	11.0	±	3.4	6.2	±	1.4	
VAL	29.2	±	6.2	21.8	±	4.4	
MET	7.25	±	0.9	3.1	±	0.9	
TAU	14.1	±	9.0	5	±	0.94	
PHE	8.25	±	1.7	5.6	±	1.2	
TYR	8.8	±	1.7	6.3	±	1.0	
SER	13.5	±	2.4	9.9	±	2.5	
HPR	9	±	8	2.6	±	1.5	
ARG	12.3	±	1.3	9.1	±	1.7	
LYS	26	±	4.7	18	±	2.5	
TRP	8.3	±	0.9	7.9	±	1	N.S.

DISCUSSION

Conditions of stress, pregnancy, zinc deficiency (Mora, R. J., and Lyefly, A., 1985), infection, surgery, and cancer consistently lower many plasma amino acids. Hypo-aminoacidemia occurs in anorexia, cancer, alcoholism (Ericksson, T., et al., 1983), pregnancy (Gard, P. R., and Handley, S. L.), stress (Milakofsky, I., et al., 1984), chronic hospitalization, hypothermia, fever and infection, (phenylalanine is elevated), and renal failure (except tyrosine). Pellagra is marked by decreases in tryptophan and branched chain amino acids. Rheumatoid arthritis has decreased histidine as do allergy patients who have low plasma histamine. Allergy patients can also have decreases in plasma ornithine (unpublished results). Gout patients are marked by decreased glycine. Scurvy is marked by a decrease in threonine, glycine, lysine, leucine and arginine. Elevated serum copper in females decreases plasma tryptophan and histidine (unpublished results). Decreases in tryptophan, methionine, taurine, tyrosine and/or glycine have been reported in depression (Braverman, E. R., et al., 1984).

Aging is marked by deficiency of glutathione due to failure to meet increased need for sulfur amino acids with age. Hence, aging is marked by a relative deficiency of sulfur amino acids and aromatic amino acids.

For example, elevated plasma amino acids have been found to improve recovery from surgery and therapeutic drug responses to antidepressants and penicillamine have been correlated to elevations in plasma amino acids. Hence, elevation of plasma amino acids may be used in the treatment of a variety of disorders. The most recent example has been the use of BCAA (branched chain amino acid) solutions (intravenous, preoperatively) and essential amino acid solutions (Moss, G., 1984) to reduce trauma (Adibi, S. A., et al., 1984) from surgery and sepsis. See also for BCAA solutions, Mizock, A., 1985. Interestingly, the 'Atkins Ketogenic Diet' raises BCAA by 30%, (unpublished results).

We studied chronic supplementation of amino acids over several weeks and found that combinations of individual supplementation lead to increases in several plasma amino acids. Elevation of plasma amino acids with dietary supplement of essential amino acid has also been found by Rosell and Zimmerman, 1985. These increases include amino acids other than the supplemented ones.

This effect is probably related to nitrogen sparing and has many interesting applications to medical therapeutics. Already mega amino acid therapy is commonly recommended in the scientific literature: tryptophan -- 3 g for pain, 6 g for obsessive compulsive, 2-6 g for depression and 2 g for migraine, tyrosine 6 g for depression and cocaine abuse, etc. The use of mega amino acids in the doses described is probably not hazardous and may have additional therapeutic benefits not previously suspected.

ACKNOWLEDGMENTS

Special thanks to Monroe Laboratories for their expert technical assistance in plasma amino acid determinations.

REFERENCES

Adibi, S. A, Fermi, W., Langenbeck, U., and Schaer, P. ed.: *Branched chain amino and keto acids in health and disease.* p. 1-14, Larger, Base, 1984.

Azuma, J., Saw, A., Await, N, Hasenpfeffer, H., Ogura, K., Harada, H., Ohta, H., Yamauchi, K., and Kishimoto, S.: Double blind randomized crossover trial of taurine in congestive heart failure, *Cur. Thera. Res.* 34, 4: 543-557, 1983.

Benedict, C. R., Anderson, G. H., and Sole, M. J.: The influence of oral tyrosine and tryptophan feeding on plasma catecholamines in man, *Amer. J. Clin. Nutr.* 38: 429-435, September, 1983.

Braverman, E. R., LaMola, S., Solder, A, Pfeiffer, C., Low plasma tryptophan in depressed outpatients. Abstracts of IVth World Congress of Biological Psychology, Philadelphia, PA, September, 1983.

Braverman, E. R, and Pfeiffer, C. C.: *Healing Nutrients Within: Amino Acids,* New Canaan, CT, Keats Publishing, Inc., 1986.

Chouinard, G., Young, S. N., Annable, L. Sourkes, T. L., and Kiriakos, R. Z.: Tryptophan nicotinamide combination in the treatment of newly admitted depressed patients. *Commun. Psychopharmacol.* 2:311-318, 1978.

DeMontis, M. G., Olianas, M. D., Mulas, C., and Tagliamonte, A.: Evidence that only free serum tryptophan exchanges with the brain. *Pharm. Res. Commun.* 9:2, 1977.

Egberts, E. H., Schomerus, H., Hamster, W. and Jurgens, P.: Branched chain amino acids in the treatment of latent portosystemic encephalopathy. *Gastroenterology* 88:887-895, 1985.

Eriksson, T., Magnusson, T., Carlsson, A., Hagman, M., and Jagenburg, R.: Amino acid balances and its relationship to requirements. *Journal of Studies on Alcohol* 44,3:215-221, March, 1983.

Fisher, H.: Essential and nonessential amino acids. *Biomed. Infor. Corp.,* New York, NY, 1984.

Frezza, M., Pozzato, G., Chiesa, L., Stramentinoli, G., and DiPadova, C.: Reversal of intrahepatic cholestasis of pregnancy in women after high dose S-adenosyl-L-methionine administration. *Hepatology* 4,2:274-278, 1984.

Gard, P. R. and Handley, S. L.: Human plasma amino acid changes at parturition. *Horm. Metabol. Res.* 17:112, 1985.

Mantovani, J., et al.: Effects of taurine on seizures and growth hormone release in epileptic patients. *Arch. Neur.* 36:672-674, 1979.

Milakofsy, L., Hare, T. A., Miller, J. M., and Vogel, W. H.: Rat plasma levels of amino acids and related compounds during stress. *Life Sciences* 36:753-761, 1984.

Mizock, B. A.: Branched-chain amino acids in sepsis and hepatic failure. *Arch. Inter. Med.* 145:1284-1288, July, 1985.

Mora, R. J. and Lyerly, A.: Amino acid loss of jejunum and colon during perfusion with isotonic and hypertonic solutions. *Life Sciences* 36:2515-2531, 1985.

Moss, G.: Elevation of plasma amino acid level correlated with enhanced wound healing, host sepsis resistance, and shortened hospitalization. *ACN* 3:335-342, 1984.

Munro, H. N.: Basic concepts in the use of amino acids and protein hydrolysates for parenteral nutrition. Symposium on total parenteral nutrition. Nashville, TN, Jan. 17-19, 1972.

Muscettola, G., Galzenati, M., Balbi, A.: Same versus placebo: a double-blind comparison in major depressive disorders. *The Lancet,* p.

198, July, 1984.

Rosell, V. L. and Zimmerman, D. R.: Threonine requirement of pigs weighing 5 to 15 kg and the effect of excess methionine in diets marginal in threonine. *J. Animal Sci.* 60:2, 1985.

Wurtman, R. J., et al.: Composition and method for suppressing appetite for calories as carbohydrates. *United States Patent*, 4:210,637, July, 1980.

Zarcone, V., Kales, A., Scharf, M., Tan, T. L., Simmons, J. Q., and Dement, W. C.: Repeated oral ingestion of 5-hydroxytryptophan. *Arch. Gen Psychiatr.* 28:843-846, June 1973.

Branched Chain Amino Acid (BCAA), Anabolic Properties and Future First Thought for I. V. Feeding

BCAA, as an abbreviation, refers to the branched chain amino acids valine, isoleucine, and leucine which are structurally similar essential amino acids, because they have a branched carbon chain. All three are essential to man. Despite the structural similarities, the branched amino acids have different metabolic routes with valine going solely to carbohydrates and leucine solely to fats and isoleucine to both. The different metabolism accounts for different requirements for these essential amino acids in man -- 12 mg/kg, 16 mg/kg, and 14 mg/kg of valine, leucine and isoleucine, respectively. Furthermore, these amino acids have different deficiency symptoms. Valine deficiency is marked by neurological defects in the brain, while isoleucine is marked by muscle tremors.

Many types of inborn errors of BCAA metabolism exist, and are marked by various abnormalities. The most common form is the maple syrup urine disease marked by an unusual urine smell. Other abnormalities are associated with a wide range of symptoms, such as mental retardation, ataxia, hypoglycemia, spinal muscle atrophy, rash, vomiting, and excess movements. Most forms of BCAA metabolism errors are corrected by dietary restriction of BCAA and at least one form is correctable by the supplementation of 10 mg of biotin daily. Many people may suffer minor inborn errors of metabolism which may account for increase in vitamin needs for biotin and other nutrients.

BCAA are useful because they are metabolized primarily by muscle. Stress states, surgery, trauma, cirrhosis, infections, fever, and starvation require proportionally more BCAA than other amino acids and probably proportionally more leucine than either valine or isoleucine.

BCAA and other amino acids are frequently fed intravenously by Total Parenteral Nutrition (TPN) in malnourished surgical patients and in some cases of severe trauma, gall bladder, sepsis, liver failure, etc.

BCAA, particularly leucine, stimulate protein synthesis, increase reutilization of amino acids in many organs, and reduce protein breakdown. Furthermore, leucine can be an important source of calories, and is a fuel superior to glucose (dextrose).

Leucine also stimulates insulin release, which stimulates protein synthesis and inhibits protein breakdown. These effects are particularly useful in athletic training. BCAA may also reduce the need for steroids, the use of which is common among weight lifters. Individuals with Huntington's chorea, tardive dyslexia, amyotrophic lateral sclerosis, and probably other muscular degenerative disorders have low serum BCAA. BCAA, particularly leucine, are among the most essential amino acids in muscle building.

Cysteine - Glutathione: The Body's Strongest Antioxidant

Cysteine is important in energy metabolism and, like cystine, it is a structural component of many tissues and hormones.

But what makes cysteine and all the chemical variants of it that are used in modern medicine -- N-acetylcysteine, D-penicillamine (dimethylcysteine), gamma glutamyl cystine, and cysteamine -- so active pharmacologically is that cysteine is a precursor of the ubiquitous tripeptide glutathione.

Glutathione has many roles, in none of which does it act alone. It is a coenzyme in various enzymatic reactions. The most important of these are redox reactions, in which the thiol grouping on the cysteine portion of cell membranes prevents peroxidation and conjugation reactions, in which glutathione (especially in the liver) binds with toxic chemicals in order to detoxify them. Glutathione (GSH) is also important in red and white blood cell formation and protection, and in the immune system.

Through these basic functions, glutathione is important in all of our lives. We are all likely to be exposed to many of the pollutants GSH detoxifies. These include lead, mercury, radiation, pesticides, herbicides, fungicides, plastics, nitrates, cigarette smoke, birth control pills and other drugs, etc. At the same time, cysteine, by its rapid conversion to GSH, protects against these problems.

Glutathione's clinical uses include the prevention of oxygen toxicity in hyperbaric oxygen therapy, treatment of lead and other heavy metal poisoning, lowering of the toxicity of chemotherapy and radiation in cancer treatments, and prevention of cataracts. In one study, oral glutathione was able to reverse advanced liver cancer in rats. Other potential uses may be in increasing the recovery chances of stroke victims, preventing or even reversing liver cirrhosis, and alleviating arthritis, psychosis, and allergy.

Cysteine itself, in addition to the detoxifying function that results from its ability to increase glutathione levels, has clinical uses ranging from the treatment of baldness to psoriasis to preventing smoker's hack. N-acetylcysteine is available in liquid or aerosol form and is useful for mucus-burdened bronchial passages. Oral cysteine therapy has been used for treatment of asthmatics, enabling them to reduce theophylline and other drugs.

In the future, cysteine may play a role in the treatment of hair loss, cobalt toxicity, diabetes, sclerosis, and seizures. Cysteine also enhances the effect of topically applied silver, tin, and zinc salts in preventing dental cavities.

At PATH our "standard dose" of L-cysteine is 500 mg/day, often given with selenium. Plasma sulfur amino acids are often a useful guide to therapy. Jean Carper says in *Food Your Miracle Medicine* how food can prevent and cure over 100 symptoms and problems. She also coauthored the best selling *Food Pharmacy*. She claims, although I don't know the documentation, that the acetylcysteine in chicken soup, which builds the glutothine in the brain and it works as the best antioxidant that we described in *Healing Nutrients Within*, is the basis for success.

5-Hydroxytryptophan

5-Hydroxytryptophan is a metabolite of tryptophan and, in low doses, is thought to have benefits for attention deficit, sleep disorder, and concentration. Unfortunately it is very expensive and there have not been enough studies done on the right dose. 5-Hydroxytryptophan is also thought to augment the benefits of antidepressants, and it may also cut the carbohydrate appetite. Because it has a paradoxical stimulating effect in some patients, it should be taken in the morning. For those on whom it does not have a stimulating effect, it should be taken at night to build the serotonin level.

Histidine:
Vasodilator and Antirheumatism

Histidine is an essential amino acid for infants but not adults. Infants from 4-6 months old require 33 mg/kg of histidine. Adults make histidine. Dietary sources probably account for most of the histidine in the body. Inborn errors of histidine metabolism exist and are marked by increased histidine levels in the blood. Elevated blood histidine is reflected in a wide range of symptoms from mental and physical retardation to poor brain development, emotional instability, tremor, ataxia, and even psychosis.

Histidine in medical therapies has its most promising trials in rheumatoid arthritis (RA) where up to 4.5 grams daily have been used effectively. RA patients have been found to have low serum histidine levels. RA patients remove histidine rapidly from their blood. Histidine and other imidazole compounds (levamisole) have anti-inflammatory and anticancer properties. Histidine may accomplish this function through a complex interaction with threonine or cysteine and possibly copper. Yet copper is usually elevated in RA patients.

Histidine may have many other possible functions, because it is the precursor of the ubiquitous neuro-hormone-neurotransmitter-histamine. Histidine increases histamine in the blood and probably in the brain. Low blood histamine with low serum histidine occurs in RA patients. Low blood histamine also occurs in some manic, schizophrenic, high copper, depressed, and hyperactive groups of patients. Histidine is clinically proven to be a useful therapy in all low histamine patients. The only other patients besides RA patients that have been found to be low in serum histidine are patients with chronic renal failure.

Histidine as therapy has been claimed to have been useful in hypertension because of its vasodilatory effects. Claims of its use in connection with the libido and allergies are without proof at present.

Histidine is abundant in body proteins and foods. One gram of histidine can be found in a cup of wheat germ. About 200-300 mg of histidine are found in a cup of oat flakes, an ounce of most cheeses, an egg, a cup of whole milk, a cup of chocolate and a cup of yogurt. Beef, pork, poultry and wild game contain the largest amounts of histidine.

The combination of high dose histidine with use of the CES device requires further research. Drugs like peracitin, which have an antihistamine effect, increase appetite. Many antidepressants have an antihistamine effect and can increase appetite as well, e.g., Doxepin, Elavil, etc.

L-Carnitine:
An Oxidizer of Fat

L-carnitine is an important amino acid which the body makes from lysine. Although it is not a vitamin, it has a role in nutrition and in general medicine. Its most important known metabolic function is to transport fat into the mitochondria of muscle cells -- including the heart -- for oxidation. Inborn errors of carnitine metabolism can lead to brain deterioration like that of Reye's syndrome, gradually worsening muscle weakness, Duchenne-like muscular dystrophy and extreme muscle weakness with fat accumulation in muscles. Carnitine is an essential nutrient for preterm babies, certain types (nonketotic) of hypoglycemia, kidney dialysis patients, cirrhosis, kwashiorkor (protein calorie malnutrition), type IV hyperlipidemia, heart muscle disease (cardiomyopathy), and propionic or organic aciduria (acid urine resulting from genetic or other anomalies). In all these conditions, and the inborn errors of carnitine metabolism, carnitine is essential to life and carnitine supplements are useful.

Carnitine therapy may also be useful in a wide variety of clinical conditions. Carnitine supplementation has improved some patients who have angina secondary to coronary artery disease. Carnitine supplementation may be worth a trial in any form of hyperlipidemia or muscle weakness. Carnitine supplements may be useful in many forms of toxic (Valproate) or metabolic liver disease and in cases of heart muscle disease. Carnitine may augment the beneficial effects of Depakote and other anticonvulsants. Hearts undergoing severe arrhythmia quickly deplete their stores of carnitine. Carnitine supplements may be useful in arrhythmia-prone hearts.

Athletes, particularly in Europe, have used carnitine supplements for improved endurance. Carnitine may improve muscle building by improved fat utilization and may even be useful in obesity. Carnitine joins a long list of nutrients which may be useful in male infertility due to impaired motility of sperm. Pregnant women and hypothyroid individuals also join the long list of clinical conditions where deficient serum carnitine levels have been identified. Carnitine may be a useful adjunct therapy in these conditions as well.

Carnitine is available in health food stores or from pharmacists by prescription. *The Physicians' Desk Reference* recommends 1-2 tablets of 600 mg three times a day.

Deanol

Deanol, a choline substitute which may have adrenergic properties, as well as cholinergic properties, invented by my mentor, Dr. Carl Pfeiffer, has been used for hyperactivity, concentration with modest benefits over the years. Until further research documents whether or not it is good, time will tell whether or not choline or phosphatidyl choline are better. At this point I recommend Phospholine over deanol.

Methionine:
for Arthritis, Parkinson's, and Depression

Methionine is one of the essential amino acids for humans. Bacteria can make it from aspartic acid. Some methionine may be absorbed from the bacteria flora of the gut under starvation conditions. The average human needs 10 mg/kg of methionine and cysteine or as much as 700 mg a day of methionine. Homocysteine plus extra B-6 in the diet can obviate most of the need for methionine.

Methionine-deficient diets in experimental animals result in impaired growth and elevated blood spermidine (a cancer maker). Normal methionine metabolism depends on the utilization of folic acid which can be elevated in the serum of methionine-deficient patients. Some foods are rich in methionine. A cup of low fat cottage cheese can contain up to a gram of methionine. Most cheeses contain 100-200 mg per ounce of methionine. Methionine supplements lower blood histamine by increasing the breakdown of histamine. Methionine is also a useful treatment for copper, lead, and heavy metal poisoning and lowers serum copper.

Methionine supplementation is usually in the D, L form, which is more effective than just the L form. This is probably due to D-L salt formation. Methionine is well absorbed in the brain where it is converted into S-adenosylmethionine, which may increase catecholamines in the brain. Methionine, a methyl donor, may produce active brain stimulants and may lower blood histamine. Methionine supplementation has been particularly useful in depression of the high histamine or allergy type. For these patients, methionine is almost as effective as MAO inhibitors (antidepressants). Methionine may be useful in the type of schizophrenia that has a strong component of depression.

Methionine is also a useful adjunct therapy in Parkinson's disease, because it stimulates the production of L-dopa. By lowering copper, methionine is also of value in acrodermatitis enteropathica, a rare disease of zinc deficiency. Two to seven grams of methionine may be effective in the treatment of osteoarthritis.

Methionine supplementation may help patients with heroin addiction. These patients are unusually high in histamine and have a low pain threshold. (Tolerance to the CES device reveals pain threshold). Methionine may be useful for patients with chronic pain and is thought to be a lipophilic agent which lowers blood cholesterol.

At present, we use methionine in patients with depression, high copper, high cholesterol, chronic pain, allergies, and asthma.

Pain and Nutritional Supplements

One in three Americans suffers some kind of chronic or recurring pain. Seventy-six million have back pain, thirty-six million endure the pain of arthritis, twenty million have migraine headaches and 800,000 have cancer-related pain. Having so much company is very little comfort if you are one of them.

Pain is a symptom, and its causes are multiple. The direct and indirect costs of combating pain each year total billions of dollars. Physiologic manifestations of pain are treated with sedative painkillers (opiates) and anti-depressants. Five (5)-hydroxytryptophan, which has some documentation as a painkiller, works in similar fashion. D-L phenylalanine (DLPA) also may have opiate agonist qualities to reduce pain. Methionine can help reduce pain in the manner of antihistamines, and fish oil (EPA) is similar in action to the typical anti-inflammatory treatment provided by medications such as Motrin.

Three to ten grams of EPA is particularly effective in arthritis and migraine and two to seven grams of methionine may be effective in osteoarthritis. Methionine is not as well studied as another form of methionine -- which is S-adenosylmethionine -- for osteoarthritis. One to three grams of 5-hydroxytryptophan may be useful in almost all pain disorders. Other nutrients such as vitamin B-6, zinc, and manganese are essential to deal with the stress caused by pain. Mega doses of B-vitamins may be beneficial in some pain disorder. Chronic pain can be treated by devices of very high or very low frequency electrical stimulations worn on the earlobes, mastoids, wrist, or forehead position. The FDA has permitted two such devices to be used in this manner, the alpha-stim and the Liss device.

Phenylalanine: Fatigue and Pain Relief

Phenylalanine is an essential amino acid and precursor of the neurotransmitters called catecholamines; these are Adrenalin-like substances. Normal metabolism of phenylalanine requires biopterin, iron, niacin, vitamin B-6, copper and vitamin C. Phenylalanine is highly concentrated in the human brain and plasma. An average adult ingests five grams of phenylalanine per day and may optimally need up to eight grams daily.

Phenylalanine is highly concentrated in high protein foods, such as meat, cottage cheese, wheat germ, etc. A new dietary source of phenylalanine is Nutrasweet. Nutrasweet is safe and nutritious except in hot beverages. However, to be totally safe it should be avoided entirely by phenylketonurics and pregnant women. Phenylketonurics have a genetic error of phenylalanine metabolism causing elevated serum plasma levels up to 400 times the normal. Mild phenylketonuria can be an unsuspected cause of developmental problems in children.

We have found that about 10-50% of depressed patients have low plasma phenylalanine, and phenylalanine is an effective treatment. Elevated phenylalanine levels occur during infection. Phenylalanine levels are lowered by caffeine ingestion as the brain takes up more phenylalanine. Phenylalanine probably is most effective in treating mild depressions, particularly in countering the symptom of fatigue.

DL-Phenylalanine can be an effective pain reliever. Its use in premenstrual syndrome and Parkinson's enhances the effects of acupuncture and electric transcutaneous nerve stimulation (TENS). Phenylalanine and tyrosine, like L-dopa, produce a catecholamine effect. Phenylalanine is better absorbed than tyrosine and may cause less headaches. Low phenylalanine diets have been prescribed for certain cancers with mixed results. Some skin tumors (primarily melanomas) can have increased phenylalanine requirements. The approach most likely to succeed is not dietary restriction, but medication to reduce the absorption of phenylalanine.

In sum, phenylalanine is an antidepressant and pain reliever with many potential therapeutic roles. L or DL phenylalanine supplements are widely available and have an important role in general medicine and health.

Taurine:
for High Blood Pressure,
Seizures, and Depression

Taurine is a sulfur amino acid like methionine, cystine, cysteine and homocysteine. It is a lesser known amino acid because it is not incorporated into the structural building blocks of protein. Yet, taurine is an essential amino acid in preterm and newborns of humans and many other species. Adults can synthesize their own taurine, yet are probably dependent in part on dietary taurine. Taurine is abundant in the brain, heart, breast, gall bladder, and kidney and has important roles in health and disease in these organs.

Taurine has many diverse biological functions: a neurotransmitter in the brain, a stabilizer of cell membranes, a facilitator in the transport of ions such as sodium, potassium, calcium, and magnesium. Taurine is highly concentrated in animal and fish protein, which are good sources of dietary taurine. Taurine is synthesized from cysteine. Deficiency of taurine occurs in premature infants, neonates fed formula milk, and in various disease states.

Inborn errors of taurine have been described, with low blood taurine resulting in early signs of depression, lethargy, fatigability, sleep disturbances, progressive weight loss, and depth perception impairment. Later, a Parkinson's syndrome may develop, progress to coma and then death.

Another inborn error of taurine metabolism has been described with mitral valve prolapse associated with a rapidly progressive form of congestive cardiomyopathy. These patients have elevated urinary taurine levels and depressed levels of myocardial (heart muscle) taurine. There may be a subcategory of taurine responsive mitral valve prolapse.

Taurine, after GABA, is the second most important inhibitory neurotransmitter in the brain. This effect is one source of taurine's anticonvulsant and antianxiety properties. Taurine also lowers glutamic acid in the brain. Preliminary clinical trials of taurine suggest it may be useful in some forms of epilepsy. Taurine in the brain is usually associated with zinc or manganese. The amino acids alanine and glutamic acid as well as pantothenic acid inhibit taurine metabolism, while vitamins A and B-6, zinc and manganese help build taurine. Cysteine and B-6 are the nutrients most directly involved in taurine synthesis. Taurine levels have been found to be significantly decreased in many patients with depression. The reasons for the findings are not entirely clear because taurine is often elevated in blood of epileptics. It is often difficult to distinguish compensatory changes in human biochemistry from true deficiency disease.

Low levels of taurine are found in retinitis pigmentosa. Taurine deficiency in experimental animals produces degeneration of light sensitive cells. Therapeutic applications of taurine therapy to eye disease are likely to be forthcoming.

Taurine has many important metabolic roles. Taurine supplements can stimulate prolactin and insulin release. The parathyroid gland makes a peptide hormone glutaurine (glutamic acid-taurine). We need further understanding of taurine's role in endocrinology. Taurine increases bilirubin and cholesterol excretion in bile, critical to normal gall bladder function. Taurine seems to inhibit the effect of morphine and potentiate the effects of opiate antagonists.

Mega-taurine therapy has been proven to be useful in many patient groups, e.g., those with postmyocardial infarction, congestive heart failure, elevated cholesterol or preventricular arrhythmias. The dying heart muscle quickly becomes depleted of taurine. Taurine levels are low in high blood pressure and supplementation with 3 grams of taurine is mildly effective and very low in side effects. It may prove to be useful in patients with epilepsy, gall stones, mitral valve prolapse, hypertension, hyperbilirubinemia, retinitis pigmentitis, photosensitivity, and diabetes. Effective supplements range from 500 mg to 5 g orally. Therapy can be guided by a plasma amino acid determination. Taurine is very low in toxicity.

Tryptophan:
A Sleep and Anti-Aggression Nutrient

Tryptophan is an essential amino acid, one of the key nutrients the body needs to maintain health. Tryptophan is the precursor of serotonin, which is a brain neurotransmitter, a platelet clotting factor and neurohormone found in organs throughout the body. Metabolism of tryptophan to serotonin requires nutrients such as B-6, niacin, and glutathione. A metabolite of tryptophan, called picolinic acid, may increase zinc absorption. Niacin is an important metabolite of tryptophan. High corn or tryptophan deficient diets can cause pellagra, which is a niacin-tryptophan deficiency disease, associated with dermatitis, diarrhea, and dementia.

Inborn errors of tryptophan metabolism exist where a tumor (carcinoid) makes excess serotonin. Hartnups's disease is a disease in which tryptophan and other amino acids are not absorbed properly. Tryptophan supplements may be useful in each condition -- in the carcinoid, by replacing the over-metabolized nutrient; and in Hartnup's, by supplementing a malabsorbed nutrient. Some disorders of excess tryptophan in the blood may contribute to mental retardation.

Assessment of tryptophan deficiency is done through studying excretion of tryptophan metabolites in the urine or blood levels. Blood may be the more sensitive test because this amino acid is transported in a unique way. Increased urination of tryptophan fragments correlates with increased tryptophan degradation, which occurs with oral contraception, depression, mental retardation, hypertension, and anxiety states.

The requirement for tryptophan and protein decreases with age. Adults' minimum daily requirement is three mg/kg daily or about 200 mg a day. This may be an underestimate for there are 400 mg of tryptophan in just a cup of wheat germ. A cup of low fat cottage cheese contains 300 mg of tryptophan and a pound of chicken and turkey contain up to 600 mg per pound.

Tryptophan supplements up to three grams a day have been used in various intractable pain conditions.

Furthermore, tryptophan supplements decrease aggressive behavior. Abnormalities in tryptophan metabolism occur in aggressive mentally retarded patients. There are increased violent crimes where corn is a major dietary staple. B-6 and tryptophan supplements can correct some of the biochemical disorders related to aggression. Drugs (e.g., Nardil or bromocriptine) which increase the opposite neurotransmitter -- dopamine -- can produce rage reactions as do drugs which can inhibit B-6 (e.g., isoniazid, which inhibits metabolism of tryptophan to niacin). The tryptophan effect may be augmented by melatonin (Chronoset), which may be substituted for hydroxytryptophan.

Tryptophan is also a useful treatment for insomnia, reducing significantly the time taken to fall asleep. Effective dosage ranges from 500 to 2000 milligrams. Disorders of REM sleep may require doses of three to five grams.

Suicidal patients have a significant decrease in serotonin levels. These patients, as well as agitated, depressed patients, do well with tryptophan supplements. Most antidepressants prolong the effects of serotonin by preventing reuptake of this neurotransmitter and catecholamines. Tryptophan at night and tyrosine in the morning can probably mimic the effects of most antidepressants. Levels of the neurotransmitters are directly dependent on dietary tryptophan and other amino acids.

Tryptophan has many other reported desirable effects. Appetite for carbohydrates is decreased and blood sugar is raised by tryptophan supplements. Tryptophan is a growth hormone and prolactin stimulant. Tryptophan is also beneficial in some forms of schizophrenia, probably by balancing dopamine excess, and in Parkinson's by inhibiting tremor, and possibly in progressive myoclonic epilepsy. Patients with kidney failure, on birth control pills, or with Down's syndrome, may need more tryptophan. Hydroxytryptophan may be substituted in some cases, yielding a more stimulating action.

Tyrosine:
Anti-Fatigue Adrenalin Builder

Tyrosine is an essential amino acid that readily passes the blood brain barrier. Once in the brain, it is a precursor for the neurotransmitters dopamine, norepinephrine and epinephrine, better known as adrenalin. These neurotransmitters are also an important part of the body's sympathetic nervous system. Tyrosine is not found in large concentrations throughout the body, because it is rapidly converted to active amine. Folic acid, copper, and vitamin C are cofactor nutrients for these reactions. Tyrosine is also the precursor for thyroid, estrogens and the major human pigment, melanin. Tyrosine is an important amino acid in many proteins, peptide and even enkephalins, the body's natural pain relievers. Branched amino acids, tryptophan and possibly methionine, may reduce tyrosine absorption.

A number of genetic errors of tyrosine metabolism can occur, most commonly in the form of increased tyrosine in the blood of premature infants. The increase is marked by decreased motor activity, lethargy, and poor feeding. Infection and intellectual deficits may occur. Vitamin C supplements reverse the disease. Some adults also develop elevated tyrosine in their blood, possibly indicating the need for more vitamin C.

Tyrosine therapy is very useful in a variety of clinical situations. An average human equivalent dose of two to six grams intravenously can raise the blood pressure in blood loss shock in experimental animals. An average human dose equivalent of 500 mg tyrosine intravenously reduces susceptibility of life-threatening ventricular fibrillation in experimental animals.

More tyrosine is needed under stress, and tyrosine supplements prevent the stress-induced depletion of norepinephrine and biochemical depression. One stress that tyrosine may not be good for is psychosis. Many antipsychotic medications inhibit tyrosine metabolism which is the most publicized hypothesis for their function.

L-dopa, which is directly used in Parkinson's, is made from tyrosine. Tyrosine, the nutrient, can be used as an adjunct or sole treatment of very early Parkinson's. Peripheral metabolism of tyrosine necessitates large doses of tyrosine, as contrasted with L-dopa, which goes directly to the brain.

Drugs which prolong the effects of tyrosine fragments have been used as an aphrodisiac. Tyrosine supplements may stimulate sex drive in large doses (and may raise blood pressure) by elevating the level of catecholamines.

Tyrosine, like amphetamines in extremely large doses (i.e., greater than 20 grams daily), paradoxically, reduces appetite; but low doses have a less consistent effect on appetite. Tyrosine therapy increases resistance to stress and is the body's natural adrenalin builder.

Physicians at Harvard Medical School have pioneered the use of one to six grams of tyrosine for the effective treatment of medication-resistant depression with good results. Metabolism of tyrosine and its metabolites is decreased in some forms of depression. Many antidepressants work by prolonging the action of tyrosine metabolites. Plasma tyrosine levels can be used to help predict which antidepressant can be most helpful. Use of tyrosine is safer, although the results may be less dramatic in the short term than the antidepressants. Lower doses have been found to be effective clinically as well in experimental animals; e.g., as little as 500-1000 mg. The minimum daily requirement for adults of tyrosine and its precursor, phenylalanine, is 16 mg/kg a day or about 1000 mg total. Hence, six grams is six times the minimum daily requirement.

Tyrosine therapy may be useful in treating drug addiction, temporarily replacing cocaine and amphetamines as methadone did for heroin addicts. Tyrosine can be used as a safe and lasting therapy, useful in a variety of clinical situations: hypotension, ventricular fibrillation, Parkinson's disease, low sex drive, and appetite suppression. N-acetyl-tyrosine may be the better absorbed form of supplemental tyrosine.

Proline

Proline and hydroxyproline are nonessential amino acids and are highly concentrated throughout the body, except in the cerebrospinal fluid. Collagen is an important protein, which is the major source for the amino acids. Proline can be synthesized in the body from amino acids, either ornithine or glutamic acid. Proline can be broken down into ornithine and thereby reduce the requirements of ornithine and arginine.

Excess proline, due to genetic errors, can lead to convulsions, elevated blood calcium and osteoporosis. Dietary restriction is a useful treatment, probably because we depend on dietary proline to meet some of our proline needs. Hence, proline deficiency probably can occur under some conditions. At least one patient with Parkinson's disease has been identified with low proline in blood.

Elevated proline levels can occur in alcoholics with cirrhosis and probably in depression, severe allergy and even learning disability. We have observed elevated hydroxyproline levels in several cases of acute psychotic depression. These patients also may require extra vitamin C.

Proline is modified in smokers and becomes a carcinogen. Drugs which inhibit proline metabolism have anticancer properties. Low proline diets may be useful in some forms of cancer treatment. Proline may be useful in wound healing. Proline peptides are involved in important neurological proteins. Knowledge of proline supplementation is limited.

Proline is concentrated in high protein foods like meat, cottage cheese, and wheat germ. There is more proline in dairy protein relative to meat protein; whereas, most of the other amino acids are found in higher concentrations in meat protein than in dairy protein.

Threonine

Threonine is an essential amino acid thought to be beneficial for treatment of immune deficiency, specicity, and possibly weed allergy. It may help build GABA and serine in the brain.

Arginine

A useful amino acid in kidney failure and possibly cancer, cholesterol lowering, and body building. It is also converted to ornithine. For more information on amino acids, see Dr. Braverman's book, *The Healing Nutrients Within: Facts, Findings and New Research on Amino Acids*, New Canaan, CT: Keats Publishing, 1987.

N-Acetylcysteine

N-Acetylcysteine has been used for chronic bronchitis (600 mg, 3-4 times a day); for otitis media (200 mg, twice a day); for heavy metal detoxification; as an anticarcinogen (up to 7 g daily); for HIV patients to convert to glutathione; for cardiovascular protection, raising lipoprotein A, for angina, and helps Nitro work better. It has been used for gastric damage and alcohol gastritis, and it is a type of "universal antidote" (see *Healing Nutrients Within*).

Amino Acids Build Neurotransmitters
That Initiate Behavioral Response(s)

Effect of Amino Acids:

Phenylalanine, Glutamine, Tyrosine and Tryptophan

On Neurotransmitters:

Serotonin, GABA, Dopamine, Norepinephrine, Epinephrine, Endorphins and Cholecystokinin

Agrawal, H. C., Bone, A. H., Davison, A. N., Effect of phenylalanine on protein synthesis in the developing rat brain. *Biochem J*, 1970, Apr: 117(2):325-31.

Algeri, S. C., Cerletti, Effects of L-dopa administration on the serotonergic system in rat brain: correlation between levels of L-dopa accumulated in the brain and depletion of serotonin and tryptophan. *Eur J Pharmacol*, 1974, July, 27(2):191-7.

Bell, C., Dopamine as a postganglionic neurotransmitter. *Neuroscience*, 1982, Jan; 7(1):l-8.

Blundell, J. E., Hill, A. J., Nutrition, serotonin and appetite: case study in the evolution of a scientific idea. *Appetite*, 1987, Jun; 8(3):183-94.

Burns, D. D., Mendels, J., Serotonin and affective disorders. *Curt Dev Psychopharmacol*, 1979, 5:293-359.

Deakin, J. F., Owen, F., Cross, A. J., Dashwood, M. J., Studies on possible mechanisms of action of electroconvulsive therapy; effects of repeated electrically induced seizures on rat brain receptors for monoamines and other neurotransmitters. *Psychopharmacology* (Berl), 1981, 73(4):345-9.

Dunner, D. L., Goodwin, F. K., Effect of L-tryptophan on brain serotonin metabolism in depressed patients. *Arch Gen Psychiatry*, 1972, Apr. 26(4):364-6.

Edwards D. J., Rizk, M., Effects of amino catecholamine synthesis in the brain. *Prog Neuropsychopharmacol*, 1981, 5(5-6):569-72.

Eichelman, B., Catecolamines and aggressive behavior, pp. 146-50. In: Usdin, E., et al., ed., *Neuroregulators and Psychiatric Disorders*. New York Oxford Univ Press 1977. WM 100 N494 1976.

Feltkamp, H., Meurer, K. A., Godehardt, E., Tryptophan-induced lowering of blood pressure and changes of serotonin uptake by platelets in patients with essential hypertension. *Kiln Wochenschr*, 1984, Dec. 3;62(23):1115-9.

Green, A. R., Grahame-Smith, D. G., Processes regulating the functional activity of brain 5-hydroxytryptamine: results of animal experimentation and their relevance to the understanding and treatment of depression. *Pharmakopsychiatr Neuropsychophalmakol*, 1978, Jan. 11(1):3-16.

Hartmann E., Chung, R., Sleep-inducing effects of L-tryptophan. *J Pharm Pharmacol*, 1972, Mar. 24(3) :252-3.

Kahn, R. S., Van Praag, H. M., Wetzler, S., Asnis, G. M., Barr, G., Serotonin and anxiety revisited. *Biol Psychiatry*, 1988, Jan. 15; 23(2):189-208.

Kapatos, G., Ziqrmond, M., Dopamine biosynthesis from L-tyrosine and L-phenylalanine in rat brain synaptosomes: preferential use of newly accumulated precursors. *J Neurochem*, 1977, May 28(5):1109-19.

Kkarobath, M., Diaz, J. L., Huttunen, M. O., The effect of L-dopa on the concentrations of tryptophan, tyrosine and serotonin in rat brain. *Eur J Pharmacol*, 1971, May 14(4):393-6.

McBride, W. J., Hyde, T. P., Smith, J. D., Aprison, M. H., Lane, J. D., Effects of tryptophan on serotonin in nerve endings. *J Neurochem*, 1976, Jan. 26(1):175-8.

McEwan, M., Parsons, P. G., Inhibition of melanization in human melanoma cells by a serotonin uptake inhibitor. *J Invest Dermatol*, 1987, July 89(1):82-86

Moir, A. T., Eccleston, D., The effects of precursor loading in the cerebral metabolism of 5-hydroxyindoles. *J Neurochem*, 1968, Oct 15(10:1093-108.

Nicklas, W. J., Berl, S., Clarke, D. D., Interaction of catecholamine and amino acid metabolism in brain: effect of pargyline and L-dopa. *J Neurochem*, 1974, July 23(1):149-57.

Pickar D., Cohen, M. R., Naber, D., Cohen, R. M., Clinical studies of the endogenous opioid system. *Biol Psychiatry*, 1982, Nov. 17(11):1243-76.

Pratt, O. E., Kinetics of tryptophan transport across the blood-brain barrier. *J Neural Trans Suppl*, 1979, (15):29-42.

Schaechter, J. D., Wurtman, R. J., Serotonin release varies with brain tryptophan levels. *Brain Res*, 1990, Nov 5;532(1-2):203-10.

Smith, R. J., Wilmore, D. W., Glutamine nutrition and requirements. *JPEN J Parenter Enteral Nutr*, 1990, July-Aug. 14(4 Suppl):94S-99S.

Vinnars, E., Hammarqvist, F., Von der Decken, A., Wernerman, J., Role of glutamine and its analogs in posttraumatic muscle protein and amino acid metabolism. *JPEN J Parenter Enteral Nutr*, 1990, July-Aug. 14(4 Suppl):125S-129S.

Wurtman, R. J., Dietary treatments that affect brain neurotransmitters. Effects on calorie and nutrient intake. *Ann N Y Acad Sci*, 1987, 499:179-90.

Wurtman, R. J., Growdon, J. H., Dietary enhancement of CNS neurotransmitters. *Hosp Pract*, 1978, May 13(3):71-7.

Yehuda, S., Mostofsky, D. I., Bracha, T., Increased serotonin level via augmented tryptophan diet and its effect on escape learning. *Int J Neurosci*, 1981, 15(4):193-6.

Stress Causes Imbalances of Neurotransmitters Therapy Impairing Brain Functions

Effect of Stress on the Biosynthesis or Metabolism of:

Serotonin, GABA, Dopamine, Norepinephrine, Epinephrine, Endorphins, Dynorphins and Cholecystokinin.

Anisman, H., Pizzino, A., and Sklar, L. S., Coping with stress, norepinephrine depletion and escape performance. *Brain Res*, 1980, June 9,1991(2) :583-8.

Bliss, E. L., Ailion, J., and Zwanziger, J., Metabolism of norepinephrine, serotonin and dopamine in rat brain with stress. *J Pharmacol Exp Ther*, 1968, Nov. 164(1):122-34.

Blizard, D. A., Freedman, L. S. and B. Liang, Genetic variation, chronic stress, and the central and peripheral noradrenergic systems. *Am J Physiol*, 1983, Oct. 245(4):R600-5.

Boranio, M., Perlcic, D., Poljak-Blazi, M., Sverko, V., and Marotti, T., Suppression of immune response in rats by stress and drugs interfering with metabolism of serotonin. *Ann N Y Acad Sci*, 1987, 496:485-91.

Curzon, G., Effect of adrenal hormones and stress on brain serotonin. *Am J Clin Nutr* 1971 July 241(7):830-4.

Emrich, H. M., and Millan, M. J., Stress reactions and endorphinergic systems. *J Psychosom Res*, 1982, 26(2):101-4.

Glavin, G. B., Stress and brain noradrenaline: a review. *Neurosci Biobehav Rev*, 1985, Summary 9(2); 233-243.

Hendley, E. D., Burrows, G. H., Robinson, E. S., Heidenreich, K. A. and C. A. Bulman, Acute stress and the brain norepinephrine uptake mechanism in the rat. *Pharmacol Biochem Behav*, 1977, Feb 6(2):197-202.

Matlina, E. S., Main phases of catecholamine metabolism under stress, pp. 353-65. In: Usdin, E, et al., ed. *Catecholamines and Stress*. Oxford: Pergamon Press, 1976. W3 IN916P 1975c.

McGivern, R. F., Mousa, S., Couri, D. and Berntson, G. G., Prolonged intermittent footshock stress decreases Met and Leu enkephalin levels in brain with concomitant decreases in pain threshold. *Life Sci*, 1983, July 4;33(1):47-54.

Millan, M. J., Stress and endogenous opioid peptides: a review. *Mod Probl Pharmacopsychiatry*, 1981, 17:49-67.

Palkovits, M., Brownstein, M., Kizer, J. S., Saavedra, J. M. and Kopin, I. J., Effect of stress on serotonin concentration and tryptophan hydroxylase activity of brain nuclei. *Neuroendocrinology*, 1976, 22(4):298-304.

Roth, K. A., Mefford I. M., and Barchas, J. D., Epinephrine, norepinephrine, dopamine and serotonin: differential effects of acute and chronic stress on regional brain amines. *Brain Res*, 1982, May 13;239(2):417-24.

Shisetomi, S., Buu N. T., and Kuchel, O., Dopaminergic abnormalities in borderline essential hypertensive patients. *Hypertension* 1991 June 17(6 Pt 2):997-1002.

Stone, E. A., Neurochemical and behavioral effects of severe stress. *Psychopharmacol Bull*, 1975, July 11(3):71-2.

Telegdy, G. and Vermes, I., Changes induced by stress in the activity of the serotoninergic system in limbic brain structures. pp. 145-56. In: Usdin, E, et al., ed., *Catecholamines and Stress*, Oxford: Pergamon Press, 1976. W3 IN916P 1975c.

Weick, B. G., Ritter, S., and Ritter, R. C., Plasma catecholamines exaggerated elevation is associated with stress susceptibility. *Physiol Behav*, 1980, May 24(5):869-74.

Uses of Fish Oil

Fish oil is usually a combination of eicosapentaenoic acid (EPA) and docosahexaenoic acid (DHA). Unlike cod liver oil, it does not include vitamin A. EPA is the primary active ingredient, and it can be measured in plasma when deficient. Effective therapeutic levels can also be measured in blood tests. EPA is easily converted into DHA and is most abundantly prevalent in salmon and mackerel, and less so in other fish like trout and bluefish. It is relatively low, though, in shellfish, which is high in cholesterol. EPA does occur naturally in vegetables but not in high quantities.

EPA is a natural enzyme inhibitor of the same enzyme, cyclooxygenase, that aspirin inhibits. Therefore its uses are very similar to those of aspirin in that it is an anti-inflammatory, mild antipyretic, and can thin the blood. It has additional benefits in that it raises HDL, a good form of cholesterol, and lowers total cholesterol and blood pressure, as do recent aspirin-like derivatives such as interleukin. Fish oil has also been thought to prevent various cancers (e.g., breast) and gallstones. Moreover, because it is a polyunsaturated oil, it is considered to be corrective of the excess saturated fat and all the diseases to which saturated fat contributes. The therapeutic uses of fish oil, particularly cod liver oil, date back even to the book of Tobit in the Apocrypha of the Bible, where Tobit's vision is restored with a type of fish oil.

Products for Achieving Total Health (PATH):

Supplements and Their Possible Benefits

1. **Heart Formula.** This formula is primarily garlic, magnesium, and taurine. These nutrients have been shown to be useful adjuncts in lowering blood pressure, thinning blood through an anti-platelet effect, and reduce or even possibly help reverse microcirculatory arteriosclerosis. This formula also contains other important nutrients as well, such as zinc, selenium, and potassium which are also believed to contribute to a reduction of blood pressure. Beta Carotene, which is thought to be associated with reduction of cardiac disease, and chromium, which has been found to be low in the plasma of heart attack victims, round out this formula.

2. **Antioxidant Formula for Detoxification.** This formula contains vitamin C, beta carotene, cysteine, vitamin E, and selenium. These nutrients are well-documented as treatments for individuals undergoing chemotherapy, individuals who are exposed to toxic chemicals from smoke to alcohol, and individuals who have liver damage or any chronic disease from heart disease to cancer. These nutrients protect the body from the toxic effects of oxygen waste products. There is a small amount of niacinamide in the formula to buffer the vitamin C. Cysteine is dominant because of its powerful antioxidant effect.

3. **The Calcium - Bone Formula** is used for treatment of osteoporosis, and calcium also plays an important role in the prevention of colon cancer. It is also found useful in the treatment of high blood pressure and is helpful with irritable bowel syndrome. The proper absorption of calcium requires adequate manganese, vitamin D-3, boron, and strontium. Boron is thought to have a natural estrogen effect, and strontium is an interesting trace element with antitoxin effects that may have other beneficial health effects on nails, skin, and hair. Manganese may be helpful for osteoarthritis and other illnesses.

4. **Magnesium Formula - Intestinal Health and PMS Formula.** This includes B-6 and zinc so that it has a natural diuretic effect, and magnesium and zinc are often used together, particularly for PMS, high blood pressure, toxemia in pregnancy, osteoporosis and constipation. This formula is a useful adjunct to other formulas. It is particularly an effective natural laxative and bowel cleaner.

5. **Multivitamin and Mineral Formula - An All-Purpose Stress Formula.** Here is a basic all purpose nutritional supplement. It does not contain high amounts of vitamins so it can be used during pregnancy when vitamin A might be toxic. Some individuals can take 4-6 pills a day under medical supervision.

6. **Amino Stim Formula -- the Energizer.** [1] Amino Stim contains the adrenaline producing amino acids phenylalanine, tyrosine, methionine, as well as the oil octacosanol, which is thought to be helpful in chronic fatigue and possibly Parkinson's. Multiple studies suggest that these nutrients can be helpful in osteoarthritis, chronic fatigue, treatment resistant depression, and can help augment the effects of many antidepressants.

7. **Branched Chain Amino Acid Complex - Muscle Building and Anabolic Formula.** This formula contains the amino acids most thought to have an anabolic steroid-like effect for muscle building without the associated risk. They can be used for a variety of diseases including liver trauma, tardive dyskinesia, olivopontocerebellar atrophy, and possibly even anorexia.

8. **Vitamin A Complex - the Antiviral Formula.** This contains nutrients that are thought to have anti-viral actions and it is even thought that vitamin A may have an action against measles. Vitamin C and garlic are thought to have a mild

---

1. This formula is a unique combination of the amino acids DL-phenylalanine, methionine, and tyrosine. Methionine has been shown to increase the absorption of phenylalanine and tyrosine. Numerous studies show that DL-phenylalanine reduces pain and can help with fatigue; that tyrosine helps with stress and helps people tolerate cold better; and both DL-phenylalanine and tyrosine have been shown to be antidepressants. They can help people quit smoking, reduce their coffee craving, and in some cases can even help reduce sugar craving.

tetracycline-like effect, and zinc has been thought to have antiherpes-like effects.

9. **Zinc Complex - the Trace Metal Formula**. This is used as a general trace element and includes rare trace elements such as iodine, vanadium, and rubidium. Iodine is thought to have a beneficial effect on cancer prevention and vanadium and rubidium are mood stabilizers. Zinc also helps to prevent toxic heavy metal buildup in the body by virtue of its chelating actions.

10. **Vitamin C Complex - the Allergy (Antihistamine) Formula**. This is useful as an antihistamine, as are methionine and quercetin, and it has antiallergy properties.

11. **Methionine Complex - the Arthritis Formula**. Methionine complex is thought to have an antiarthritic effect. Methionine has been compared to ibuprofen for treatment of osteoarthritis. A form of methionine (same as S-adenosyl-methionine) is useful in treating depression by methylating histamine. It also may acidify urine or may help beat urinary tract infections.

12. **Fast Path Formula - the Diet Formula**. Included are the fundamental, essential amino acids in proper dietary proportions so it can be used as a protein supplement by patients with kidney failure, a dieting supplement, and an amino acid supplement for the brain. A higher proportion of these amino acids is central to all weight loss programs and in maintaining balanced diets.

13. **Save** is a multivitamin, which also has the properties of Amino Stim for energy and treatment of chronic fatigue.

14. **Carnitine** is an amino acid thought to be helpful in lowering triglycerides, promoting weight loss, lessening side effects from anticonvulsant drugs, and building the brain chemical memory compound, acetylcholine.

15. **Choline - Triple Strength** is high potency choline used to build up brain acetylcholine, a neurotransmitter.

16. **CoQ10** is a vitamin E derivative that is useful in heart disease, low energy, and periodontal disease.

17. **Fiber Complex** is a type of rice bran and guar gum that lowers cholesterol and helps insulin regulation better than any other fibers.

18. **N-acetylcysteine** is an amino acid that helps detoxify many chemicals and is the strongest antioxidant.

19. **Pantetheine** is a nutrient thought to have mild triglyceride and cholesterol lowering effects.

20. **Fish oils** are used to help lower blood pressure, triglycerides, and cholesterol. They have an anti-inflammatory effect which treats arthritis, helps to thin the blood and prevent heart attacks.

21. **Borage Oil** is like primrose oil and gammalinoleic acid; it is useful as a diuretic and in the treatment of PMS and high blood pressure.

22. **Chronoset** contains melatonin, which helps with sleep and resets sleeping rhythms associated with jet lag and sleep disorders, and may also reduce carbohydrate craving.

23. **Hydroxytryptophan** is a tryptophan metabolite, as L-dopa is a tyrosine metabolite. It is a unique antidepressant and has an anticarbohydrate craving action, and is very useful in sleep, obsessive-compulsive disorder, depression, mood swings, and many other abnormal neurotransmitter conditions.

24. **Chromium** may help with muscle tone, carbohydrate craving, metabolism, regulation of blood sugar in diabetes, and hypertension.

25. **Guar Gum** is a fiber used for control of blood sugar, or control of the bowels, and as an appetite suppressant. It is a useful fiber but can produce gassiness.

26. **Cognitex**. Some studies suggest that it may raise the P300 wave of the brain. Unfortunately, the dosages currently available may not be high enough, but at the present time there are very few natural alternatives for the stimulation of brain function.

27. **Choline** is a precursor of acetylcholine that has been shown to have many different benefits, including cholesterol lowering, antimania, mood stabilization, and improved memory and concentration. It also antidotes the side effects of various antidepressant and antipsychotic medications. It may also increase the P300 wave of the brain.

28. **Coherin**. This may be useful as another technique for increasing cerebral vascular circulation and raising acetylcholine directly in the brain. It may also benefit the P300 brain wave as well as brain chemical imbalances.

29. **GABA and GABA Plus**. These are amino acids that are precursors for antianxiety compounds in the brain. Unfortunately they are not thought to be well absorbed, but may have benefits in high dosages in certain individuals. They are the body's own natural Valium, but are not addictive.

30. **Norival** is another version of tyrosine (acetyltyrosine) that is reportedly better absorbed.

31. **Niacin** is one of the great vitamins that is used not only for mood stabilization, treatment of depression, alcoholism, high cholesterol, and schizophrenia, but in high dosages can actually increase circulation to the heart. Niacin can have serious side effects, such as gout, fatigue, stomach upset, nausea, and vomiting, and should be administered only by a doctor. There are dozens of brands of niacin, and virtually anyone can find some brand that he can tolerate in a time-release form with relatively few side effects.

32. **Cayenne Pepper** is an herbal preparation that can reduce appetite, but may also upset the stomach.

33. **Slow Fe** is the best absorbed form of iron, although some debates about ferritin and other forms of iron are now coming into the medical literature. Slow Fe has been less constipating and very effective in our practice. Iron deficiency is still the most common deficiency in many conditions; however, it can exacerbate arthritis, heart disease, and other inflammatory conditions and should be given sparingly.

34. **Safflower Oil** is a polyunsaturated oil that can lower blood pressure and cholesterol level and works as a natural diuretic. Some people feel that too much safflower oil may contribute to cancer risk and acne.

35. **Ultra Fuel** is a unique glucose polymer combination used to improve glycogen levels. It is extremely beneficial in giving energy and helping individuals store weight or prepare for a carbohydrate challenge such as significant exercise, e.g., a marathon or other sport events.

36. **Linseed Oil** is a vegetarian version of fish oil and can be utilized in place of fish oil to help lower cholesterol and triglycerides. It is easily digested.

Formulas 1-12 are the unique Total Health Nutrients (**P**roducts for **A**chieving **T**otal **H**ealth).

Formula Contents

ITEM		UNIT SIZE

1- Heart Formula #1 ... **100**

Garlic Powder (Odorless)	200	mg.
Taurine	200	mg.
Magnesium (Oxide)	50	mg.
Potassium (Chloride)	7	mg.
Selenium (Sodium Selenite)	20	mcg.
Zinc (Chelate)	4	mg.
Chromium (Chloride)	26	mg.
Niacinamide	50	mg.
Vitamin C	40	mg.
Molybdenum (Chelate)	40	mcg.
Vitamin B-6	50	mg.
Beta Carotene	1222	IU

2- Antioxidant #2 ... **100**

Beta Carotene	8500	IU
Selenium (L-Selenomethionine)	50	mcg.
Vitamin E	100	IU
Vitamin C	10	mg.
Ascorbic Acid	250	mg.
L-Cysteine	250	mg.

3- Calcium #3 ... **100**

Calcium (Citrate)	270	mg.
Manganese Chelate	15	mg.
Vitamin D-3	135	IU
Boron (Calcium Borogluconate)	35	mg.
Strontium Chloride	.5	mg.

4- Magnesium #4 ... **100**

Vitamin B-6	65	mg.
Magnesium (Oxide)	470	mg.
Zinc (Chelate)	15	mg.

5- Multi Vitamin & Mineral #5 ... **100**

Vitamin B-1	5	mg.
Vitamin B-2	5	mg.
Vitamin B-6	5	mg.
Vitamin B-12	60	mcg.
Pantothenic Acid	6	mg.
Biotin	50	mcg.
Folate	125	mcg.
Vitamin C	200	mg.
Vitamin E	20	IU
Vitamin A	1000	IU
Vitamin D	200	IU
Niacin, Niacinamide	15	mg.
Calcium (Carbonate)	15	mg.
Magnesium (Oxide)	12	mg.
Molybdenum (Chelate)	12	mcg.
Manganese (Chelate)	1	mg.
Zinc (Chelate)	5	mg.
Iron (Chelate)	5	mg.
Iodine (Kelp)	100	mcg.
Copper (Chelate)	.25	mg.
G.T.F. Chromium	60	mcg.

6- Amino Stim #6 ... **100**

dl-Phenylalanine	225	mg.
L-Tyrosine	125	mg.
Methionine	60	mg.
Octacosanol	2000	mcg.

7- BCAA Complex #7 ... **100**

L-Leucine	200	mg.
L-Isoleucine	135	mg.
L-Valine	65	mg.
L-Ornithine	65	mg.
L-Arginine	65	mg.
B-6	15	mg.

8- Vitamin A Complex #8 ... **100**

Vitamin A	16000	IU
Zinc (Chelate)	20	mg.
Vitamin C	165	mg.
Garlic Powder(Odorless)	30	mg.

9- Zinc Complex #9 ... **100**

Zinc (Gluconate	20	mg.
Manganese (Chelate)	1	mg.
Iron (Chelate)	.5	mg.
Boron (Calcium Borogluconate)	130	mcg.
Molybdenum (Chelate)	130	mcg.
Iodine (Kelp)	30	mcg.
Vanadium (Chelate)	30	mcg.
Rubidium (Chloride)	30	mcg.

10- Vitamin C Complex #10   **100**
Vitamin C   160 mg.
Niacinamide   10 mg.
Quercetin   130 mg.
Bioflavonoids   65 mg.
DL-Methionine   65 mg.

11- Methionine Complex #11   **100**
Methionine   250 mg.
Niacinamide   150 mg.
Vitamin C   25 mg.
Pantothenic Acid   80 mg.
B-6   10 mg.
Vitamin E   30 mg.

12- FAST PATH #12   **100**
L-Isoleucine   75 mg.
L-Leucine   100 mg.
Lysine   75 mg.
Methionine   60 mg.
Cysteine HCL   75 mg.
Arginine   85 mg.
Phenylalanine   50 mg.
Tyrosine   50 mg.
Valine   85 mg.
Threonine   50 mg.

13- SAVE   **100**
dl-Phenylalanine   133 mg.
L-Tyrosine   133 mg.
Octacosanol   0.67 mg.
Zinc (Chelate)   3 mg.
Selenium (Sodium Selenite)   14 mcg.
Chromium (Chloride)   13 mcg.
Iron (Chelate)   3 mg.
B-6   7 mg.
B-1   1.3 mg.
B-2   1.3 mg.
Niacin   1.3 mg.
d-Cal Pantothenate   1.3 mg.
Beta Carotene   1110 IU
Vitamin E   6.7 IU
Manganese (Chelate)   133 mcg.
Folate   13 mcg.
B-12   2.7 mcg.
Magnesium (Chelate)   26.7 mg.
DL-Methionine   50 mg.
Molybdenum (Chelate)   33 mcg.
Biotin   20 mcg.

14- Carnitine   **100**
L-Carnitine   250 mg.

15- Choline Caps   **100**
Choline (from Choline Bitartrate)   350 mg.

16- CO-Q10   **100**
Co-Enzyme Q10   30 mg.

17- Fiber Complex   **200**
Defatted Rice Bran   266 mg.
Beet Fiber   200 mg.
Guar Gum   66 mg.

18- N-Acetyl L-Cysteine   **100**
N-Acetyl L-Cysteine   50 mg.

19- Pantethine   **60**
Pantethine   150 mg.
Pantothenic Acid as d-Cal Pantothenate   150 mg.

Treatment Sheet: Section of Vitamins

Vitamins are best taken 1/2 hour before meals but 5 minutes before or during meals is okay if necessary. KEY:
B=Breakfast, L=Lunch, D=Dinner, Bd=1 hr before bedtime, 1Tsp=1teaspoon. In the event of difficulty in taking the vitamins several
times a day it is permissible to take them at one time or more spread out. Refrigerate all oils.

FORMULAS	B	L	D	Bd	VITAMINS-CARBOHYDRATES	B	L	D	Bd
Heart #1					Children's Multi Vit.				
Anti-Oxidant #2					Choline				
Calcium #3					Co-Q10 (Ubiquinone)				
Magnesium #4					Hy-B Complex				
Multi-Vitamin #5					Juicy C				
Amino Stim #6					Niacin				
BCAA Complex #7					Niacin (Zero Flush)				
Vitamin A Complex #8					Pantethine				
Zinc #9					Phoschol				
Vitamin C #10					Vitamin A (Drops)				
Methionine # 11					Vitamin D				
Fast Path #12					Vitamin E (Liquid)				
Save					Vitamin E (Capsules)				
AMINO ACIDS-PROTEINS					**DIGESTIVE AIDS**				
Arginine					Medifast				
Cayenne-Capsaicin					Fiber Complex				
Coherin-Ginko-NAC					Ultra Fuel				
Cognitex					Papaya Enzyme				
Cysteine					Pancreatin				
GABA					Ephedra				
GABA Plus					Citronate				
Carnitine									
Threonine					**ESSENTIAL OIL-FATS**				
Lysine					Borage Seed Oil				
Melatonin					Emulsified Fish Oil				
N-Acetyl-Cysteine					Linseed Oil				
Norival-N-Ac-Tyrosine					Cod Liver Oil				
Phenylalanine					Safflower Oil				
Saw Palmetto					Twin EPA				
Taurine									
Tryptophan					**ELECTRICAL THERAPY**				
					CES TENS Device				
MINERALS & METALS					Electrodes				
Boron									
Chromic Fuel					**NATURAL ANTI-AGING-HORMONAL THERAPIES**				
Copper					DHEA				
Lithium Orotate					Testosterone				
Manganese					Estradiol/Progesterone				
Molybdenun									
Potassium					**PRESCRIPTION ITEMS**				
Selenium									
Silicon									
Time Release Iron									
Strontium									
Vanadium									
Special Instructions:									

Mineral Analysis

WHAT ARE MINERALS?

Like the liquid inside a battery or like the spark plugs in the engine of a car, minerals are the small but essential parts which make things work. Without zinc and other trace elements, our bodies can not function. We can not make these elements so we must obtain them from food. Modern food processing often strips away these minerals, as does our water supply. As many as 10-15 percent of all patients are deficient in magnesium, and about a third of all elderly patients may be deficient in at least one mineral. Toxic levels of bad minerals, such as lead and mercury, can replace the good nutrients, such as zinc and selenium, resulting in temporarily lowered I. Q. and impaired mental functioning.

Mineral levels can be measured in the blood plasma; in red blood cells, which may be the most sensitive test; in white blood cells, which may be the most short-term way of measuring minerals; and in hair, which can indicate toxins. On the next page is a table which describes symptoms associated with some specific mineral deficiency states.

COULD YOU BE MINERAL DEFICIENT?

Recent surveys by the Center for Disease Control has shown that surprisingly high numbers of people in the United States are deficient in essential minerals, such as magnesium, calcium, iron, and zinc.

Magnesium, a necessary element in 300 different enzyme reactions in the body, has been found to be low in half of the adults measured, and only 10 - 13% of patients deficient in this mineral were even recognized as being clinically deficient. This is very significant, given new evidence linking magnesium deficiency to heart attacks and hypertension, diseases that are often recognized too late.

CAN MINERAL DEFICIENCY AFFECT HEALTH?

Nutritional research is increasingly uncovering the intimate connection between trace element deficiencies or toxicities and many common health problems. Zinc is critically important to proper immune function. Low selenium levels have been associated with increased risk of cancer.

Chromium and manganese have been used effectively to treat adult-onset diabetes. Magnesium supplementation is proving to be a life saver in patients who suffer heart attacks and can significantly lower blood pressure. Subtle iron deficiency has been linked to learning disabilities in the young.

Toxic metal accumulation in the body is also being recognized as a growing health problem. Low level lead exposure has been associated with decreased IQ in children. Mercury accumulation was shown to cause immune suppression.

HOW TO TEST MINERAL LEVELS

Whether you have current or potential health problems due to inadequate mineral intake and assimilation depends on your environmental and health history. Your doctor can get clues to your needs from clinical signs, but generally a laboratory test is necessary to make an accurate determination of your needs.

Because there is so little of these elements in the tissues, determining whether you have enough or too much requires the most recent advances in laboratory technology.

Scientists have also found that it makes a difference which part of the body is used to measure mineral concentrations. Research has shown, for example, that the best measure of magnesium and zinc status are red blood cell levels.

Whether you have been exposed to toxic lead, cadmium or aluminum levels is best shown in your hair because such minerals are concentrated in the growing hair shaft.

A comprehensive mineral profile analyzes red blood cells, blood plasma, and hair for the five toxic heavy metals and most known essential nutrient minerals. By looking at these three different body tissues, one gets a more precise evaluation of your body's mineral requirements. An interpretive report is provided to aid in understanding the meaning of the data, and to suggest steps toward correcting any problems.

More Mineral Analysis

Symptoms Associated with Specific Mineral Deficiency States

Calcium: osteoporosis, high blood pressure, muscle cramping.

Magnesium: cardiovascular disease, high blood pressure, anxiety, irritability, fatigue.

Zinc: recurrent infection, slow healing, acne, irritable bowel syndrome, chemical intolerance, anorexia, immune suppression.

Chromium: diabetes, hypoglycemia, heart disease.

Manganese: bone fragility, glucose intolerance, connective tissue weakness.

Copper: heart disease, inflammation, immune dysfunction.

Selenium: heart disease, cancer, immune dysfunction.

Hair Testing

We sometimes underestimate the benefits of hair testing. It certainly is good for testing for toxic metals. We also know that magnesium, sulphur, calcium, copper, zinc, and chromium in the hair, in that order, have been linked to high risk of heart disease.

Some Guidelines [1] for Selecting a Specimen [2]

ELEMENT	RBC	PLASMA	BLOOD	URINE	HAIR
Sodium	40	100	40	80	10
Potassium	70	100	60	80	10
Sulphur	60	40	30	20	40
Phosphorous	50	100	30	60	40
Calcium	60	100	60	60	80
Iron	70	100	100	60	10
Magnesium	80	100	60	80	80
Silicon	40	30	30	60	90
Zinc	90	70	60	40	50
Selenium	90	70	80	80	90
Nickel	---	---	---	60	90
Manganese	80	---	70	40	50
Chromium	---	---	---	60	90
Copper	80	60	40	20	80
Molybdenum	---	---	---	40	60
Cobalt	---	---	---	50	90
Vanadium	---	---	---	60	90
Aluminum	100	40	60	50	90
Antimony	50	50	50	70	90
Arsenic	70	---	60	70	100
Barium	80	60	90	40	60
Bismuth	60	50	40	20	90
Boron	70	60	80	80	40
Cadmium	70	---	60	70	100
Germanium	40	40	60	70	70
Lead	90	---	80	70	100
Lithium	50	100	40	40	40
Mercury	70	---	60	70	100
Palladium	---	---	---	10	90
Platinum	---	---	---	10	90
Ruthenium	---	---	---	10	90
Silver	60	40	50	10	90
Strontium	60	70	50	10	90
Thallium	60	40	50	80	90

A total of 100 points or more will indicate clinical significance. For many elements, more than one specimen is required. 2/1/90

1. Based upon clinical significance, not on total body stores.

2. Chart reproduced with permission of BALCO (Bay Area Laboratory Co-Operative), 1520 Gilbreth Road, Burlingame, CA 94010, 1-800-777-7122.

Magnesium

Magnesium is one of the most critical elements and is involved in over 300 enzymes in the body. Magnesium is needed for growth, pregnancy, sleep, wound healing, cardiac function, muscle function. Magnesium deficiency has been associated with seizures, psychosis, delirium, tremors, heart attacks, heart arrhythmia, premenstrual tension, osteoporosis, abnormal calcium deposits, poor wound healing, hypertension of pregnancy, difficult pregnancy, difficulty swallowing, etc. Magnesium has some natural tranquilizing abilities and has been used as a natural anticonvulsant and a natural antiarrhythmic. Its deficiency is associated with brittleness of bones and teeth because it is so important for calcium absorption. Magnesium deficiency can be associated with hypoglycemia. Loss of magnesium occurs with trauma, surgery, and extreme athletic competition. Alcoholics frequently are deficient in magnesium. The best way to measure magnesium is probably red blood cell and white blood cell magnesium levels. Even when these are normal, magnesium as a supplement or therapeutic agent above and beyond normal levels can be useful, particularly in hypertension, PMS, seizure disorders, depression, constipation, chronic fatigue, and cardiac arrhythmia.

Many forms of magnesium, such as magnesium citrate, are used to clean out the bowels before sigmoidoscopy or barium enema. Magnesium oxide is a good supplement while milk of magnesia or magnesium hydroxide is a good antacid as well as laxative but not the best as a nutritional supplement. Chelated magnesium is expensive and probably no better than other forms of magnesium for absorption. Dolomite, which includes magnesium carbonate and calcium carbonate, may have toxins and does not have vitamin D, B-6, or other nutrients which help in absorption. Magnesium silicate may result in silicate kidney stones. Magnesium orotate and gluconate have hardly any magnesium, and the former is not valuable except for its orotate content. The best forms of magnesium are probably oxide from the hydroxide or chelated magnesium. Magnesium's uses have become so critical and better understood that it is now frequently used in emergency rooms around the country and in the intensive care and coronary care units because it is recognized that magnesium deficiency occurs commonly in patients on Digoxin, with heart attacks, and with rare arrhythmia such as torsade de points. Magnesium is a therapeutic agent that is becoming more and more widespread in medicine. Eventually, a new table salt using magnesium and other trace elements will probably be developed so that we get adequate magnesium from our environment, rather than too much sodium. Magnesium supplements help maintain adequate potassium supplementation in diuretic therapy and Bartter's syndrome. The diuretic Lozol may be somewhat magnesium sparing although most diuretics result in increased magnesium loss.

Magnesium Found To Aid Bypass Patients [1]

An inexpensive injection of a magnesium solution after bypass surgery reduced heart-rhythm problems by 50 percent and speeded recovery of patients, with virtually no side effects, a new study says. Magnesium, a mineral found in foods, is believed to relax blood vessel walls and improve blood flow.

The six-month study in the United States involved 100 patients randomly selected when they entered the New England Medical Center in Boston for bypass surgery. Biochemical studies were performed at Sinai Hospital of Baltimore. Fifty patients received an injection of magnesium chloride solution. The rest received a placebo.

Eight of the 50 treated with magnesium, or 16 percent, suffered heart-rhythm problems, while 17 of the placebo patients, or 34 percent, had erratic heartbeats, or dysrhythmia, following surgery. The magnesium, which costs around $1.50 for each dose, is about 10 times less expensive than other drugs used to treat irregular heartbeats. Chelation injections include large amounts of magnesium.

Results of the study were published in the November 4, 1992 issue of the *Journal of the American Medical Association*.

---

1. *New York Times*, Nov. 6, 1992.

Manganese

Although often ignored by nutrition-conscious individuals, manganese is an essential trace metal frequently deficient in our diet. A component of at least six known enzymes, manganese is required for efficient sugar metabolism and for the production of cartilage -- a vital structural component of our bodies.

We know that manganese deficient animals suffer impaired growth, reproductive problems, and a shortened life span. With a severe deficiency, animals cannot stand up because of defective cartilage formation. Humans with low manganese levels can suffer chronic joint pains, particularly around the knees and back. "Growing pains" can disappear when our young patients take adequate manganese with zinc along with their vitamins. And, since the discs between the vertebrae consist largely of cartilage, widespread manganese deficiency may contribute to the epidemic of back problems in this country.

In addition, scientists have long associated low manganese levels with epilepsy and schizophrenia. Studies dating back to 1929 indicate that schizophrenics can improve with supplementary manganese. Manganese-deficient patients may suffer depression which clears up when manganese is included in the treatment program. Seizure patients theoretically may respond to manganese.

Patients with either hypoglycemia or diabetes may need extra manganese to help normalize blood sugar levels. This isn't surprising, since scientists report that in manganese-deficient animals, the insulin secreting cells of the pancreas deteriorate -- and insulin is the body's crucial regulator of sugar metabolism. Interestingly, low levels of this trace metal during early development may lead to malformation of the ear's vestibular system, which is the body's machinery for maintaining balance. Young children who are slow to walk may require extra manganese.

Unfortunately, most diets, even the best planned, tend to be deficient in this important trace metal. Our manganese deficient farmlands often produce fruits and vegetables lacking adequate levels of this element. And, many of our frequently eaten foods fail to concentrate manganese even under the best conditions; for example, meat, even liver, provides little manganese. Foods rich in manganese include nuts, whole grains, spices, legumes, and tea leaves. Tropical fruits such as banana, papaya, and mango are particularly good sources of manganese.

However, patients with low manganese levels will probably need supplementary manganese in addition to a good diet. Fortunately, manganese is nontoxic, even at our high doses (up to 300 mg per day). However, occasionally in patients over forty, manganese can raise blood pressure and produce tension headaches. If this occurs, the manganese dose should be reduced until the blood pressure normalizes and the headaches disappear.

Zinc

Zinc was discovered in 1928, and is an essential nutrient. It is involved with as many as 70 or 80 enzymes in the body, unlike iron, which is only involved with about eight enzymes. Zinc is the most commonly used trace element in the body for biological functions. Zinc is removed from our foods, like so many other things, through the use of depleted soils and through food processing. Because zinc is involved with so many different enzymes, zinc deficiency has been found in individuals with retarded wound healing, joint pain, skin disorders, acne, endocrine problems, dwarfism, hypogonadism, loss of taste and smell, among other conditions. Zinc deficiency has been associated with lead poisoning and cadmium poisoning and has been used as an antidote for low toxic levels of both these metals. Zinc deficiency also may be involved to some degree in epilepsy, diabetes, and enlarged prostate. Zinc deficiency aggravates the side effects of oral contraceptives. Zinc is beneficial for treating sickle cell disease and Wilson's disease. Zinc deficiency has been thought to be a factor in impotency, retinal detachment, Reye's syndrome, breath odor, and coarse body hair. High copper in plumbing has been implicated as causing depression, and zinc is the antidote for the excess copper in the American water supply which affects so many.

A number of different studies also suggest that older people have an impaired immune function that relates to zinc deficiency; and if identified early, and treated, some of the immune function could be preserved.

Studies also demonstrate that alcohol and fiber

interfere with the body's ability to absorb zinc; therefore, people should drink in moderation and time their zinc intake differently from consumption of high-fiber breads and cereals.

Supplementation is a growing field of study, and zinc as a therapy has been helpful in increasing appetite and has been useful in treating the behavioral disorders of many children. Zinc is a great healing nutrient.

Selenium

In regions of the world where the people live on grains grown locally, the nutritional deficiency of the soil produces a corresponding deficiency in people. This has happened in the Keshan province of China where soil is deficient in selenium -- so much so that children of 10 and 11 years of age can die of congestive heart failure because of lack of glutathione peroxidase, an enzyme which contains four selenium atoms per enzyme. This peroxidase enzyme not only helps the heart but also prevents cancer.

The term 'dismembered' should be used for the processing of foods, such as wheat, where 25 nutrients are removed but only four are returned. Thus, the resultant white flour, with its "added" nutrients, can be called enriched rather than what it is -- dismembered and unfit to eat. Important minerals lost are selenium, sulfur, manganese, zinc and molybdenum.

We know that adequate selenium in the diet prevents cancer, and areas of the world where the soil is deficient in selenium have a higher incidence of cancer. Patients with cancer have a lower level of selenium in their blood than do normal controls. The degree of benefit from selenium supplements given after a heart attack is not clear.

With all this knowledge on the importance of selenium in nutrition the Federal authorities now allow 250 ppb of selenium to be added to animal feed. Both a 50 and 100 mcg selenium tablet are allowed to be sold by health food stores and pharmacies. Sodium selenite (in a form not derived from brewers yeast) is probably the best form. Doses of 100 mcg taken twice daily are usually without any toxic effect. Patients with cancer have gradually increased the dose of selenium under medical supervision. Some patients have gotten as high as 1 mg without any toxic signs or symptoms or changes in the laboratory tests. A single dose of 1 mg of selenium as the selenite may produce, however, all the symptoms of stomach flu including nausea and vomiting, diarrhea, fever, and even hematuria.

Your Trace Element Study

Today you will have a trace element study which includes over 30 trace elements relevant to your health -- calcium, magnesium, zinc, copper, chromium, selenium, vanadium, lithium, lead, mercury, cadmium, phosphorus, potassium, sodium, sulfur, and many others. These are extremely relevant to your health. There are many ways that you can be sick from some of them, i. e., lead toxicity from water and air pollution, mercury from fillings, cadmium from smoking and paints, copper toxicity from plumbing or birth control pills, deficiency of calcium from steroids or aging, or deficiency of magnesium from hypertension or constipation. This is the best study available today for accessing mineral and trace element nutrition. It may be necessary to do it in both plasma, red blood cells and whole blood. This is because some components of blood are not as valuable as others in measuring nutrients. We do feel that this study is very important in understanding and treating your health needs.

Vitamins Boost the Immune System

New studies by Dr. Ranjit Chandra reported in *The New York Times*, Nov. 6, 1992, suggest that various nutrients benefit the immune system. Vitamin A, beta carotene, thiamin, riboflavin, niacin, folate, as well as vitamins B-6, B-12, C, D, E, calcium, copper, iodine, iron magnesium, selenium, and zinc, given in about the daily allowances recommended by American officials, can boost the immune system in the elderly. About 30 percent of elderly patients will have a deficiency in one or more vitamins. The studies showed that the immune system, natural killer cells, CD-4 cells, production of interleukin 2, and antibody response to influenza vaccine can be boosted; that supplements can restore immune function in six months, and sometimes less than three months. In Dr. Chandra's study, other individuals took placebo capsules, which were not as effective. Those who took the nutrients had 23 days of infection-related illness as opposed to 48 days. There are a number of studies documenting that widespread nutritional supplementation in the elderly will boost their immune system and the ability to fight off infection.

Taking Your Vitamins

Some scientists feel that vitamin B-6 and amino acids should be taken before meals and all other vitamins after meals. We find this a cumbersome suggestion for most patients, and recommend all vitamins taken before or after meals. Most individuals digest their vitamins best when they are taken with meals or after meals. Certain vitamins, like fish oil, can repeat in patients, so many choose to take them before meals. Niacin can also cause flushing, so many choose to take it before or with meals. Many individuals find taking vitamins unpleasant, so it is suggested that they grind them in a blender or coffee grinder. Then put the powder into juice. The same can be done with open capsules. Vitamins, like tryptophan, niacinamide, etc., that are taken at bedtime, need to be taken one hour before going to bed for the best effect.

Niacin Therapy

Niacin is a great nutrient that can do so many important things, like lowering cholesterol, improving circulation, helping with heart disease, etc. In addition, it can help patients with Raynaud's syndrome and arthritis. Studies have shown that collateral circulation can increase in a patient taking one gram of niacin a day. Collaterals are extra blood vessels which form around the heart and can prevent people from dying from a heart attack.

Niacin therapy is best given in a time-released form, yet even then it can affect the liver enzymes. Fortunately, there are many different brands of niacin; so, a patient can find the brand that is right for him or her. We use Bronson niacin and Willner niacin, which sometimes cause flushing, and Natrol, which is a no-flush niacin. A baby aspirin taken at bedtime will frequently stop the flushing. Niacin may cause fatigue in some cases, which can be antidoted by Amino Stim or a low dose of tyrosine. We also use a new brand of niacin called Enduracin, which people claim has the best long-term absorption but is extremely expensive. Patients can pay up to 60 dollars for a bottle of niacin called Nicolar. Nicolar requires a prescription, or for $5 to $15 one can purchase a bottle of niacin here or at a local health food store.

The Wonders of Niacin

Niacin is a B-vitamin which can cause a severe flushing reaction. Some individuals turn bright red and itch all over. Others actually have an anxiety attack from the niacin. These symptoms are usually relieved quickly by aspirin. The next time, take less niacin on a full stomach; this will minimize the flush. Then, build up as tolerated. The flush is not dangerous; if you can tolerate it then take the full dose. Niacin in large dosages raises the HDL cholesterol, lowers blood pressure, reduces cravings for alcohol, and relieves anxiety. The warmth effect helps people with cold hands and feet and may be useful in arthritis. If you are taking niacin you need your liver enzymes checked regularly. A new brand of no-flush niacin seems to have much less side effects.

Vitamin Testing

In today's world of poor nutrition and environmentally-caused illness, more and more people are suffering from conditions which are caused directly or indirectly by vitamin deficiencies. In an attempt to replace missing essential vitamins, more and more people on their own are initiating self-styled vitamin regimens, often with little or no professional guidance. Some people take vitamins irregularly and still others are taking doses which are biologically ineffective for their particular personal biochemistry. As a result, millions of dollars nationwide and much personal effort are being wasted due to lack of knowledge. Fortunately, a test has been developed which clarifies much of this confusion. PATH offers a specific vitamin blood test. This measures the levels of specific vitamins in the blood, for example vitamin C and vitamin E as well as many others. This information provides a rational approach to adjusting vitamin supplementation as well as offering a means for detecting suspected deficiencies. Debate still exists over what should be considered the optional -- and optimal -- levels of vitamins.

The vitamin diagnostic test offers specific functional measurement for many of the B-vitamins. This means that this test can detect, e.g., whether B-2 or B-6 are enzymatically correct. This is the best test known for vitamin adequacy since your particular body might not be average. For example, your body may require twice the "normal" level of vitamin B-2, let's say; so that this "normal" level for your body would really represent a significant deficiency in vitamin B-2. Recently, conventional medicine recognized the value of the indirect approach to determine optimum vitamin levels. For example, measurement of methyl malonic acid, or homocysteine, was approved as an accurate gage of proper B-12 levels.

Despite the fact that human life cannot go on without vitamins, traditional physicians do not yet use vitamin measurements in the therapy of diseases. This is a great shame, since shortage of the antioxidant vitamins such as vitamin C and vitamin E may lead to conditions like degenerative arthritis, cataracts, and increased susceptibility to viral infections; while shortages of vitamin D can lead to osteoporosis (softening of the bones), and deficiencies of the B-vitamins can result in fatigue, depression, etc. The blood level of still other nutrients can be tested, e.g., fatty acids, carnitine, CoQ10 and trace metals. Traditional medicine has become so "disease oriented" that it has forgotten the best way to prevent disease -- by encouraging health!

Benefits of Nutritional Testing for Vitamins

Marginal vitamin deficiencies do occur, and they can affect the body's resistance to disease and infection. As much as 70 percent of the American population is deficient in vitamins. RDA's are not relevant because nutritional needs vary so much in each individual.

Urinary Methylmalonic Acid: To Detect B-12

This simple urine test can detect the presence of subtle vitamin B-12 deficiency, a condition which may result in anemia (low blood counts) and severe nerve damage. All patients over the age of 50 should be tested for this condition as well as any patient who has had stomach or intestinal surgery, anemia, depression, confusion or forgetfulness, or difficulty walking. In addition, any patient who has thyroid disease may be at increased risk. Once detected, vitamin B-12 deficiency is easily treated with monthly injections. If it goes undetected, this severe condition may progress to cause irreversible damage. Although many other ways to detect vitamin B-12 deficiency (e.g., homocysteine) exist, measurement of urinary methylmalonic acid is the most accurate. That is because this particular test adjusts for your own personal need for vitamin B-12. Other tests, such as a simple vitamin B-12 level, could be normal while your body still may require additional vitamin B-12 to function properly.

Nutrition:
Glaucoma And Other Eye Diseases

There are very few studies that suggest that individuals with glaucoma may have vitamin deficiencies. Some studies suggest that low levels of vitamin C deficiency may be associated with higher intraocular pressure and that higher dosages of vitamin C may reduce intraocular pressure. The same has also been said of rutin. Possibly other bioflavonoids and, on rare occasions, food allergies have been associated with glaucoma.

At present there is no strong evidence at this time for a relationship between nutrition and glaucoma. Other eye diseases may respond to a variety of natural approaches. For example, abnormalities in taurine metabolism result in an increase in the cataract crystals in lenses and an increase of the incidence of retinitis pigmentosa. Glaucoma may begin with different losses of chromatic color vision. GPC, giant papillary conjunctivitis, which occurs with contact lenses, and probably many other irritants, can be treated with vitamin A drops. Vitamin E may be helpful in the treatment of retinitis pigmentosa. N-acetyl-cysteine may be helpful with chronic macular edema in retinitis pigmentosa. Antioxidants can protect the brain against optic neuritis. Eye drops may help superior limbic keratocon junctivitis. Recent studies have shown that eye exercise and long-term physical training can help reduce the risk of glaucoma. Myopia can predispose an individual to glaucoma. Eyebright may help glaucoma.

Glaucoma is high pressure in the eye that leads to death of optic nerve cells. Death of cells leads to a loss of vision. Peripheral vision is lost first. Central vision can remain until the late stage, when 90 percent of the optic nerve is already destroyed. Glaucoma usually has no symptoms aside from silent painless loss of vision beginning peripherally. Glaucoma is the second leading cause of blindness in the United States and the leading cause in virtually every other country in the world. Over 70,000 people in the U.S. are blind from glaucoma -- 200,000 are blind in one eye, 2 million or more have some degree of visual damage and 8 million more are susceptible. Glaucoma is more common than diabetes and hyper- tension, probably because of abnormalities in blood sugar and blood pressure. Therefore it is extremely important to control these abnormalities. Risk factors are being black, myopia, diabetes, family history, hypertension, smoking, alcohol and other drugs, thyroid disease, arteriosclerosis, steroids and eye drops. Glaucoma is very often missed. Routine eye examinations are extremely important. Sometimes, glaucoma may occur with a low intraocular tension. Diurnal variations may be a factor, and therefore pressure must be checked extremely carefully.

Glaucoma is not one disease but a number of different diseases affecting the conditions of the eye and producing high pressure. There are two types of glaucoma -- angle closure and open glaucoma. Angle closure glaucoma is most common in Asians, least common in blacks and affects farsighted people. With an acute attack there is pain, red eye, blurred vision, and nausea. It is a medical emergency and can be cured with laser treatment, which is the primary definitive treatment. Open angle glaucoma is most common in blacks, least common in Asians. Exfoliation syndrome occurs in 20 percent of all glaucoma. The drain of the eye gets clogged by pigment, much like coffee grounds clogging a kitchen drain.

Pigmentary glaucoma may be more common than we realize, affecting maybe 250,000 people. Hereditary glaucoma affects young people 20-30 years old. It is, therefore, important to check family members. Over 1,000 patients currently at New York Eye and Ear who have glaucoma are under age 35. There is congenital glaucoma and infectious glaucoma. The goal of therapy is to minimize side effects of medication, lower the pressure, turn the so-called faucet down, and open the angle up and let things drain. Miotic drops such as pilocarpine and carbachol can be used. But side effects are very prominent in younger patients, including possible retinal detachment. Beta blockers, Timoptic, Betoptic and Betagan have few local side effects but could lower your pressure and cause other problems which might affect exercise tolerance, exacerbate asthma, congestive heart failure, memory loss, insomnia, depression and hallucinations. Carbonic anhydrase inhibitors or pills (e.g., Diamox or Neptazane) turn the faucet down. There are many new medications being tested. Nonsteroidal drugs may be helpful. Laser, surgical treatment, ultrasound and cyclodestructive procedures, e.g., laser sclerostomy, are being developed.

Drugs that worsen glaucoma are numerous, e.g., antipsychotics, antidepressants, inhibitors, antihistamines, anti-Parkinson's agents, anti-spasmolytic agents, and a variety of other agents that can cause idiopathic lens swelling, as well as sympathomimetic agents. As a rule, these are not prominent problems. Antioxidants are most useful in the prevention of cataracts, maybe they will someday be shown to benefit glaucoma. Antioxidants work to prevent cataracts probably by preventing damage by UV light. They also protect the aging macula.

Glaucoma also occurs frequently with increased sympathetic tone. It is possible that the CES device can reduce vagal tone. Forced unilateral nostril breathing induces selective contralateral hemispheric stimulation as measured by relative increases in EEG amplitude and the contralateral hemispheres alternating lateralization of plasma catecholamines. Forced right nostril breathing produces a functional vagotomy which lead to a bilateral decrease in intraocular pressure.

Light as a Nutrient

Light is an essential nutrient like air, food and water. Many people are daylight deprived. Daylight deprivation is common in individuals who 1) live in northern latitudes where daylight hours are shorter; 2) live in cloudy, overcast areas where dark days are common; 3) do not go outdoors without difficulty; 4) are homebound; 5) are sick, and 6) work regular hours or shift schedules, especially those who work at night.

The Impact of Daylight Deprivation

Daylight-deprived individuals can experience one of the following problems:

1. Moodiness, listlessness, low energy level, and doldrums.

2. Trouble falling asleep, waking up at bizarre times, and drowsiness during the day.

3. Trouble adjusting to an irregular work and travel schedule.

4. Decreased alertness and performance.

5. Carbohydrate craving.

Typically, individuals who are indoors at home or at the office have extremely low levels of light, where they are exposed to only 400-700 lux, while individuals who have a chance to get outside at 12:00 noon may be exposed to 92,500 lux. Possibly this makes a good case for everyone taking a short walk at lunchtime.

Light Levels in Our Environment

Condition	Light Level (lux)
Twilight	Below 750
Indoors At Home	200-500
Indoors At Office	400-700
Drafting Room	500-1000
Springtime Sunrise	
6:10 AM	750
6:20 AM	2,500
6:30 AM	5,000
6:45 AM	10,000
12:00 Noon	92,500
5:30 PM	10,000
5:45 PM	5,000
5:55 PM	2,500
Sunset 6:10 PM	750

These light levels represent the approximate illumination level, or lux, for clear sky conditions at the spring equinox for the middle of the United States. Sunrise and sunset are defined as half the sun's disk above the horizon. The indoor light levels represent typical light levels for all geographic areas.

Ultrabright light systems can be used to help set the body clock. The majority of photobiological researchers feel there is a body clock in the hypothalamic center of the brain. When light hits the retina, the retina transmits impulses to the body clock which helps to regulate the entire body and its metabolism. Ultrabright light systems of 10,000+ lux can be used for 20-30 minutes with success. Ultrabright mini-systems at 5500 lux will require 55-60 minutes for successful treatment. The purpose of these systems is to maximize light intensity, optimize visual comfort, and minimize glare. These particular systems tend to have more yellow and green light but do contain the full spectrum of bright light and contains less blue light proportionately. This can affect brain chemistry, brain rhythm, even brain metabolism, possibly by reducing porphyrins and bilirubin derivatives. It may be possible to measure reduction in porphyrins in the urine through various light treatments. Porphyrins will increase in the urine in a variety of conditions, such as PMS, anxiety, depression, stress, etc. (See Seasonal Affective Disorder, Section 22, p. 302.) The number to call to obtain a sunbox or white light device is 1-301-762-1786.

Prescribing Nutrients and Drugs

Both nutrients and drugs prescribed by the physician are to be used by the patient in given amounts for certain presenting symptoms to achieve set goals. Patients should adhere strictly to the physician's prescription in order to avoid the aberrant consequences of self-dosing.

Your Pharmacist and This Office

Frequently, pharmacists, meaning well, give patients advice, and can even frighten patients about medications. Pharmacists are used to dealing with medications and their typical prescribed route. Here at Path we have many creative uses of medications, as do other physicians. In fact, 70 percent of all medications are prescribed for reasons other than those of which the pharmacist will be aware. In addition, there is much information going around which is frequently inaccurate. For example, 40 years ago it was thought that smoking was not dangerous to your health and white bread was good for your bowels. Medicine is a constantly changing profession. Please use our office as your primary resource. We will be glad to answer any questions that you or your pharmacist may have.

Drugs for Many Purposes

Doctors use medications in many different ways. For example, aspirin, which is listed as an antipyretic (pyretic means fever), is a fever drug, yet we use it for thinning the blood for heart disease, for headache (ordinary), migraine, arthritis, pain, etc. Advil, while originally designed for fever, can be used for dysmenorrhea or even PMS. Antiseizure drugs, like Tegretol can be used not only for seizure, but also for brain dysrhythmia, manic-depression, depression, anxiety, and biochemical imbalance. Mellaril, which is listed as an antipsychotic, can be used for depression, melancholia, biochemical imbalance, and dopamine metabolic control. Antidepressants such as Prozac can be used for weight loss, appetite reduction, treatment of lower back pain, peptic ulcer disease, fibrositis, headache, peripheral neuropathy, rheumatoid disease, and irritable colon. All so-called antidepressants can be used for medical problems. In fact, 25 percent or more of all prescriptions of antidepressants are for nonpsychiatric disorders. Benzodiazapines, like Lonopin, can be used for anxiety but also seizure disorder, temporal lobe disorder, and biochemical imbalance.

Most brain chemical treatments have multiple uses, and no patient should be confused by the class of the drug, because its classification does not tell its multiple uses. The antianginal drug Procardia is used for hypertension and the antihypertensive drug clonidine is used for appetite suppression, mania and drug withdrawal from cigarettes, methadone and heroin. As much as 30-70 percent of all prescribing of drugs by physicians is for something outside the original purpose for which the drug was designed. This is also true of nutrients -- many nutrients have multiple purposes. Magnesium can help with angina and hypertension and also work as a laxative. Methionine can work for arthritis and allergies and work as an antihistamine. Other antihistamines like Benadryl can be used for insomnia or decongestion or even allergic reactions. In sum, most substances can't be classified as limited to treating just one or a limited number of diseases.

Reference

Broadhead, et al., Tricyclic antidepressant prescribing for nonpsychiatric disorders. *Journal of Family Practice.* Vol. 33, 1991.

Symptoms and Side Effects of Medications

- indigestion
- dizziness
- fatigue
- headache
- impotence
- depression

- palpitations
- constipation or diarrhea
- numbness or pain in the nerves
- breathing difficulty
- hair loss
- anxiety

Beta Carotene

Regarding the concept that beta carotene may promote cancer in smokers who take large amounts of beta carotene (50 milligrams), this is absurd and another example of the biased attack of the pharmaceutical industry against the benefits of anti-oxidants. Indeed, anti-oxidants may lack some benefits in certain situations such as smoking, but literature still supports the effective role of anti-oxidants against cancer.

Choline

Choline is the precursor to the neurotransmitter acetylcholine, which is found in the human brain and hippocampus. A choline precursor is deanol. The best absorbed choline (phosphatidyl) is present in many supplements as well as lecithin. There have been studies reporting the value of choline in tardive dyskinesia, Huntington's chorea, Alzheimer's disease, psychiatric disorders (particularly paranoia), Tourette's syndrome, and ataxia.

There have been reports of choline leading to improvements in tardive dyskinesia. This is unusual in that drugs that are anti-choline can also be useful in this condition. Some think that choline may even be a preventive of tardive dyskinesia. There is no question that tardive dyskinesia has Parkinson's-like attributes. Parkinson's disease is a result of dopamine deficiency due to prolonged therapy with neuroleptic drugs. It seems unlikely that choline-like drugs can treat tardive dyskinesia, but they may prevent it.

Huntington's chorea may be a disease with a true choline deficiency. This is clearly a movement disorder with an imbalance in dopamine and cholinergic function. Yet, anticholinergic drugs may be helpful.

Use of choline in Alzheimer's disease is more promising because it can help to restore memory. Phoschol, a highly purified form of lecithin (phosphatidyl choline) (7 times more pure than lecithin) is a good treatment (10 capsules a day). Phoschol should be combined with Prostigmin, an acetycholinergic. Psychiatric disorders may also respond to lecithin, particularly paranoia (up to 20 g/day). Ataxia patients have also tried 4-5 grams of choline, but have found no significant effect. Anticholinergics seem to be the more beneficial medication.

Tourette's syndrome may respond to Haldol, an anti-dopamine substance, and to choline which also is anti-dopamine. Myasthenia syndrome, an acetylcholine deficiency, is best treated by anti-acetylcholinergics which keep the acetylcholine alive the longest. Hence, it may be possible to supplement this disease with additional choline in the form of Phoschol.

The illnesses which may respond to choline supplementation are tardive dyskinesia, Huntington's, Alzheimer's, psychiatric disorders, ataxia, Tourette's syndrome and myasthenia. Alzheimer's, paranoia, Tourette's and myasthenia gravis are the most promising.

Quercetin

Recently much has been made of several forms vitamin C, e.g., cal-ascorbate and ester-C, that might be improved. Literature is still documenting the benefit of different super forms of vitamin C has been sorely lacking. Nonetheless there is a form of vitamin C in combination with a particular bioflavonoid called Quercetin that may be the most effective of all. Quercetin has already been shown to be the most powerful antihistamine and apparently anticancer agent of all the bioflavonoids and when combined with vitamin C may have additional properties.

In a recent study in cancer research, May 1, 1994, Quercetin was shown to down-regulate the P53 in the human breast cancer line. In particular P53 is the protein associated with genetic predisposition towards cancer.

Quercetin has been shown in other studies to have anticancer properties. Obviously at this point far better research literature supports a benefit of vitamin C in combination with quercetin and possibly thiamine which is the Total Health Nutrients' form of vitamin C that we recommend.

Dandruff

Dandruff can be a very stubborn condition. People should avoid white flour, sugar, and refined carbohydrates. Stress can make it worse. Zinc and vitamin A can help it significantly. If it becomes treatment-resistant, shampoos like Head and Shoulders, Selsun, and Nizoral, which is the strongest, can be used.

Nicotine

A recent study in the *New England Journal of Medicine*, 330:811-856 (1994), showed that nicotine cigarettes can help suppress the immune system. This suppression of the immune system may be of benefit for people with certain medical diseases. We now know it's clear that smoking is a self-medicating drug treatment, similar to taking Motrin. We know that the complex elimination of smoking requires replacement of what nicotine does for the human being. New studies will show us that we can replace nicotine addiction with the use of antidepressant, possibly nonsteroidal and the CES device. We now know that people are self-medicating their problems with cigarettes and the doctor has to find new ways of treating them.

Diet Pills and Obesity

There has been much written about diet pills lately: Are they dangerous? First of all, diet pills are misnomered. Diet pills are not diet pills. They are brain augmenting pills which increase Adrenalin in the brain so that individuals stop using food as a stimulant to their brain. By giving the brain more stimulation it cuts the appetite, thereby replacing food.

These drugs have been known to decrease levels of serotonin and increase Adrenalin, particularly Tenuate and Fastin. These drugs have been thought to injure the brain and are associated with stroke, etc. This information is contrary to the information in a consensus study of the National Institute of Health that says people take these medicines virtually for years without side effects.

We believe that if you take these medicines with a high protein diet; nutrients, B-complex, melatonin, and antioxidants, that there is no potential risk because you are supplementing what the drugs deplete.

The risk of obesity is, of course, enormous. For every ten pounds the cancer risk, stroke risk, and heart attack risk increase.

Obesity is still the number one predictor of who will live long and who will not, and who is going to live well and who will not. Medications are not the number one predictor. It is your weight which tells the doctor and life insurance companies what your prognosis for health and longevity is.

Reference: Miller M., "Fat Pharm," *Wall Street Journal*, 7/20/94.

20. Obstetrics, Gynecology and Women's Health

Estrogen and Testosterone Therapy at the Menopause

The adrenal and sex hormones make both sexes feel better. At puberty testosterone hardens the muscles of the teenager and estrogens give added energy to teenage girls. The rhythm of the hormones in the girl may produce menstrual letdowns which can cause depression, headaches, acne, and even seizures. Even the fetal and placental hormones may give relief to the pregnant woman from such illnesses as arthritis, asthma, migraines, and allergies. Some asthmatic women feel so much better that they try to stay pregnant year after year! The corticoid steroids are truly addicting in that they produce increased appetite, euphoria, need for less sleep, and relief of pain. Rheumatoid arthritic patients have a difficult time getting to a lower dose of prednisone, the commonly used corticosteroid.

The large-breasted woman is apt to have rheumatoid arthritis and depression at the menopause as she gets a letdown from the high estrogen dose that has produced and maintained the large breasts. This natural decrease in estrogens can be effectively treated with natural micronized estrogen which is the superior and best form of taking estrogen. This form has much less side effects and usually relieves both the depression and the arthritis.

In all species, testosterone excess tends to shorten life while estrogens prolong life, so testosterone therapy is used carefully in older males. Doctors know that testosterone can increase beta lipoprotein, cholesterol, and the low density lipids that increase heart attack risks. Testosterone injectables are mainly used in impotent males and have been shown to increase sexual libido, while decreasing nervousness, depression, and obesity. Testosterone may hold aplastic anemia, and other blood disorders, in check, and it increases sex drive in women who are deficient in it after menopause. Additionally, testosterone is used for the treatment of patients with breast cancer regardless of sex. On the other hand, estrogens have a wide use, and synthetic estrogens virtually have been replaced by the natural.

Research has shown that osteoporosis, often seen in elderly women, is directly related to the sharp decline in estrogen level following menopause. Much of the bone destruction occurs yearly with as much as fifty percent of the bone density being lost in the first seven years after menopause. Nevertheless, treatment is possible even late in menopause. Other factors which affect osteoporosis include aluminum intake, sedentary life, being of Caucasian or Oriental race, a slender body size, excessive alcohol consumption, low calcium intake, and smoking. Many believe that estrogens are indirectly linked to the parathyroid hormone, calcitonin, which promotes bone deposition and inhibits resorption. Estrogens stop the loss of calcium from bone in postmenopausal women, especially when accompanied by calcium, magnesium, and vitamin D supplements. Strontium, boron, fluoride and manganese are also important. Regular weight bearing exercise is also important in preventing bone loss, and should be started as soon as possible, even in adolescence. Since high continuous doses of estrogen have been linked to endometrial hyperplasia and cancer, progesterone needs to be taken along with estrogen. There are both synthetic and natural progesterone. Natural progesterone (from yams) appears to have less side effects. The doses used present negligible risk for cancer. Prevention of hot flashes (vitamin E doses of 400-800 IU daily may also be effective) and atrophic vaginitis also can be helped. Atherosclerotic disease is reduced as estrogen supplementation increases the levels of HDL's while depressing the levels of plaque forming LDL's and VLDL's (Progesterone may block this effect, however).

Estrogen treatment in males may be therapeutically useful in the case of recurrent prostate enlargement in the elderly. Although a male's sex life is usually absent after eighty, one must take care in explaining the impotency that will result from estrogen use. Impotency may be minor compared to the anticancer life benefits. Large dose estrogens should be used with caution if there is a clinical history of phlebitis or blood clotting disorders. High levels of estrogen have been tied to thromboembolic disease via an increase in clotting factors II, VII, X, fibrinogen, and copper. The incidence of gall bladder disorders such as cholelithiasis and cholecystitis have been slightly increased with the use of estrogens. These side effects can be prevented by the anticlotting effect of fish oil, vitamin E, and garlic, and anticholestosis nutrients of taurine, methionine, olive oil and niacin.

The more common, less serious side effects associated with the general use of female hormones include nausea, bloating, breakthrough bleeding, PMS-like symptoms, increases in the size of fibroids, breast tenderness or enlargement, and milk secretion. The related fluid retention may exacerbate such conditions as epilepsy, migraines, heart disease, or kidney disease. There may also be an increase in sexual libido. These effects do not seem to occur with natural estrogen plus progesterone.

Synthetic estrogens can be made very simply by the chemist, and since 1930 over 100 synthetic estrogens have been developed. Many are more potent than the natural estrogens (B-estradiol, estrone, estriol, and the conjugated estrogens). Being more potent, many of these synthetic estrogens are incorporated into the so-called "low dose" birth control pills. The estrogenic effect is equal to that of natural estrogens; however, the cancer-producing effect of these new compounds is not known in humans. Therefore, we believe only natural estrogen should be used therapeutically.

Although the cancer-producing effect of low doses of natural estrogens is minimal, the same is not true for progesterones. Progesterones were withdrawn in the sixties because of evidence linking hormones to malignant breast tumors in dogs. Synthetic progesterones, such as Provera, or the combination estrogen-progesterone drugs, have been connected to an increased risk for cervical cancer. Additionally, women taking progesterones are at greater risk for ectopic pregnancy and choriocarcinoma should conception occur. Synthetic progesterone therapy alone is usually not advisable due to these known cancer-producing effects. High dose progesterone can be helpful in breast cancer and weight loss. Insulin resistance precipitated by synthetic progesterone is also frequent. This possibility is of paramount importance when treating the elderly because maturity-onset diabetes mellitus may set in. Other common side effects of progesterone therapy include irregular bleeding, distended veins, irritability, weight gain, and depression. Many of these side effects can be attributed to the subsequent decrease in zinc levels resulting from estrogen/progesterone therapy. Women taking estrogen and/or progesterone, alone or in combination, should see their doctor at least once a year for a physical exam, pap smear, and mammogram.

Effects of Estrogen

To counteract the damaging effects of estrogen, eat phytoestrogens. Phytoestrogen foods are soy, legumes, peas, beans, and clovers. These prevent estrogen causing the terrible negative effects on growth and various organs.

Ways in which estrogen goes awry in our society is a result of detergents, DDT, and other estrogen like compounds.

Ways to see whether or not you have relative excess estrogen in women is elevated sex hormone binding globulin. Flax seed oil or borage oil may also help against bad estrogens to break them down properly. Oxines, of course, also protect against the side effects.

New Age in Natural Estrogen Hormone Therapy

PATH Medical continues to do its natural hormone treatments. These treatments are beneficial for male menopause and women who are looking for a non-period, low side effect natural estrogen. Evidence is now suggesting that Estriol, another form of natural estrogen which is high during pregnancy, will actually prevent breast cancer and may need to replace estradiol and Estrone. Articles by Dr. Foilingstad in 1978 and Dr. Lemon in 1966 were generally ignored, but new suggestions by Dr. Julian Whitaker and Dr. Jonathan Wright suggest that this might be an alternative way of supplementing estrogen. We are looking into it and trying to evaluate the data, but it certainly may be worth a try in many women. The ideal hormone replacement would be a combination of Estriol, Estradiol, progesterone, and natural testosterone.

The Hormone Diet:
Influencing Foods and Herbs

Since some mild natural estrogens and progesterones occur in foods, foods supplying (promoting) these hormones should be emphasized in the diet for the treatment of the following conditions:

- Symptoms of menopause
- Prostate problems
- Osteoporosis in menopausal women

Estrogen-promoting foods and herbs may need to be excluded (and estrogen-reducing ones emphasized) when treating:

- Breast cancer
- Premenstrual syndrome (PMS)
- Uterine fibroids
- Fibrocystic disease of the breast
- Ovarian cysts

Estrogen-Promoting Foods and Herbs

- Alfalfa, anise, garlic, licorice, parsley, sage
- Animal flesh, dairy foods, eggs
- Apples, cherries, olives
- Cereal grains, except rye, buckwheat, and white rice
- Yams, eggplant, tomatoes, potatoes, pepper

Estrogen-Reducing Foods and Herbs

- Any immature bean or pea such as string beans
- Citrus fruit, grapes, pineapples, pears, most berries, figs, most other fruit (except those listed as estrogen-promoting)
- Melons, squashes, cole crops such as cabbage, and most vegetables, except estrogen-promoting vegetables
- Onion, dill, thyme, and many other common herbs
- White rice, white flour, millet, buckwheat, tapioca, corn
- Soybean, which contains a natural anti-estrogen agent similar to tamoxifen.

Treating Menopause with Hormone Replacement Therapy -- Continuous, Daily, Oral, Micronized Estradiol and Progesterone [1]

(These are natural estrogens and progesterones)

Estrogen replacement therapy is beneficial for genital atrophy (dry vagina), osteoporosis, and for cardiovascular protection. Estrogen has an impact on many body organs: the brain, skin, heart, breasts, etc. Estrogen can add fat into the skin as well as moisture and collagen, giving skin a smoother, firm look and less opportunity to wrinkle. Estrogen can reverse the male pattern hair growth on face and body that some women experience. Many women fear using estrogen because of the increased risk of uterine and breast cancer. Also they do not want a withdrawal bleed which usually accompanies the cyclic administration of estrogen and progesterone replacement therapy. Most women now use the synthetic estrogens and progesterones for postmenopausal replacement therapy. The potential disadvantages of the synthetic estrogen and progesterone as compared with the natural estrogen and progesterone are numerous. Preparations containing estrogens that do not occur naturally in women have an increased metabolism in a woman's liver. In addition, the synthetic progesterones tend to increase a woman's cholesterol. Also, the synthetic progesterones can potentially increase testosterone, which can increase androgenicity (masculinity) for the woman.

The natural estradiol and progesterone, because they occur naturally in humans, (and are not foreign substances) are preferential to the synthetic counterparts for estrogen replacement therapy. The micronized natural progesterone preparation, when given orally, can produce excellent blood levels without the unwanted effects, such as fluid retention, breast tenderness, weight gain, and depression, as compared to the synthetics. In addition, natural estrogens and progesterones help relieve the flushing, genital atrophy and osteoporosis, and increase cardiovascular protection. In a study that was done at Vanderbilt Medical Center, of the women who were placed on the natural estrogen and progesterone, none had any evidence of endometrial cancer, that is uterine cancer, and, in addition to that, their overall cholesterol level was lowered! A further advantage was that the preparation only requires taking one pill a day. What was very affirming of the study was that all the patients on the natural estrogen and progesterone

continued on this therapy even after the study, which attests to the acceptability of this program.

In contrast, the women on the synthetic estrogen and progesterone had a 40 percent dropout rate after just one year. Over time, side effects from the synthetic hormones may worsen. The only side effect of the natural estrogen and progesterone was sleepiness, and usually that can be beneficial in some cases just by taking it before bedtime. The absolute contraindications for estrogen replacement therapy are acute liver disease, history of breast cancer, history of endometrial (uterine) cancer, undiagnosed genital bleeding, and active thrombophlebitis or thromboembolic disorder. The relative contraindications include a history of a thromboembolic event, chronic liver disease, a strong family history of breast cancer, fibrocystic disease, fibroid uterus, unstable hypertension, and poorly controlled glucose intolerance. In addition to that, it is required that a woman have a pap smear and a mammogram done before therapy, and that is to be continued once a year. Usually during perimenopause, that is, usually one year after one's menses stops, a woman can sometimes ovulate and experience some bleeding. This will occur even on the estrogen and progesterone, but if breakthrough bleeding occurs after one year while on hormonal therapy, sometimes an endometrial sampling is required. An endometrial sampling means that a small instrument is inserted into the uterus and a sample scraping is done of the lining of the uterus to rule out any cancer.

Recent studies suggest that estrogen keeps the brain young by stimulating neurotransmitters. Individuals who take natural estrogen frequently have improved mood and overall sense of well being.

To review some of the benefits of the natural estrogen and progesterone: they can relieve hot flashes, night sweats, insomnia, decreased libido, vaginal dryness, anxiety, and depression. In addition to that, they can prevent osteoporosis, decrease cholesterol and reduce risk for heart disease. Natural estrogen reduces the onset of diseases of aging.

---

1. Adapted from Hargrove, J., M.D.; Maxon, W., M.D.; Wentz, A., M.D.; Burnett, L., M. D., Menopausal Hormonal Replacement Therapy with Continuous, Daily, Oral, Micronized Estradiol and Progesterone, *American Journal of Obstet. & Gynecol.*, vol. 73:606, 1989.

Natural Hormone Preparations

NATURAL HORMONE PREPARATIONS AVAILABLE, DERIVED FROM YAMS		
Testosterone - 5 mg	Progesterone - 100 mg	Estradiol - .5 mg
Testosterone - 64 mg (can be taken every other day for male menopause, or male andropause)	Progesterone - 50 mg/Testosterone - 2.5 mg	Estradiol - .25 mg
	Progesterone - .5 mg/Estradiol - 100 mg	Estradiol - .5 mg/Testosterone - .5 mg

Women who are menopausal should use the 5 mg of testosterone as therapy. Women with PMS should use pure progesterone or a progesterone/testosterone combination. Hormone levels can be measured by blood tests.

Most Asked Questions About Natural Oral Progesterone [1]

QUESTION: What is the difference between natural and synthetic progesterone?

ANSWER: Progesterone was first crystallized in 1934, and today is available from plant sources. Natural micronized progesterone is an exact chemical duplicate of the progesterone that is normally produced by the ovary. Synthetic progesterone, called progestogen, mimics the action of the progesterone, but the body does not respond in the same way. Studies have shown that progestogen actually reduces the level of progesterone in the blood stream.

QUESTION: Are there side effects with natural progesterone?

ANSWER: Natural progesterone combines with progesterone receptor sites, and elicits biological effects without many of the undesirable side effects that are seen with the synthetic forms. Perhaps the only disadvantage to natural progesterone is that it is short-acting and to maintain adequate blood levels it has to be dosed four times daily. A small number of women may experience transient light-headedness or drowsiness.

QUESTION: How does oral natural progesterone work?

ANSWER: The oral route of progesterone administration has long been considered impractical because of poor absorption and short biological half life. Contrary to traditional teachings, recent reports[2] confirm that significant serum progesterone levels can be achieved with new modification in the preparation of progesterone for oral

---

1. The following information (pp. 279-284) is adapted from Dr. Katharina Dalton's handbook, *Once a Month* (1990) and her two booklets, *A Guide to Premenstrual Syndrome and its Treatment* (1984), and *A Guide to Prophylactic Progesterone for Postnatal Depression* (1981). For more information contact Madison Pharmacy Associates, 429 Gammon Place, P. O. Box 9641, Madison, WI 53715, 1-800-222-4PMS or 558-7046.

2. "Absorption of oral progesterone is influenced by vehicle and particle size," Joel T. Hargrove, M. D., Wayne S. Maxon, M. D. and Anne Colston Wentz, M. D., *American Journal of Obstetrics and Gynecology*, October 1989.

administration, including micronization and dissolution in oils consisting of principally long chain fatty acids.

QUESTION: **Is the oral form of natural progesterone approved by the FDA?**

ANSWER: Natural micronized progesterone has F. D. A. approval. The oral form of natural progesterone is compounded from a physician's prescription by a licensed pharmacist using F. D. A. approved ingredients. Therefore, it does not require separate F. D. A. approval.

QUESTION: **Isn't it true that natural progesterone taken orally is destroyed by stomach acid? How does the oral progesterone you compound achieve adequate blood levels?**

ANSWER: Natural progesterone *in powder form* is destroyed by stomach acid. But, when compounded in an oil base, the progesterone is so firmly held by the oil base that it is actually absorbed through the lymphatic system first, thereby allowing a couple of passes through the body before being cleared via the liver.

The Use of Progesterone
for Post-Partum (Postnatal) Depression

SYMPTOMS

It should be noted that depression may not be the first symptom, it may be present as:

anxiety, exhaustion, agitation, insomnia, irritability, confusion, delusions, hallucinations, rejection of the baby, unreality, mania, paranoia.

Depression is not necessarily the presenting symptom, and may be absent. If present, depression is manifested by loss of interest, enthusiasm, energy, an inability to cope or concentrate, extreme lethargy, a pessimistic outlook, or morbid suicidal thoughts. It differs from typical depression, (which may also occur in men, women, and children) in that there is marked irritability, increased appetite, weight gain, and a constant yearning for sleep. It occurs in some 10% of all new mothers and requires medical attention.

Postnatal psychosis may be characterized by agitation, confusion, delusions, aural or visual hallucinations, irrationality or rejection of the baby. It may occur suddenly or be preceded by a few days of insomnia, agitation or manic behavior. It is a life-threatening situation and hospitalization is required for the safety of the mother or her baby. Fortunately, it only occurs in about one in every 200 to 500 new mothers.

COURSE

Postnatal blues are self-limiting and the crying disappears within the first two weeks.

Postnatal depression and **psychosis** may end with the resumption of menstruation, or it may continue for years. As long ago as 1855, Marce, the French physician, noted among his hospital patients that as postnatal depression improved the improvement occurred after menstruation but tended to deteriorate before the next menstruation. This is known as the **second stage of postnatal depression**.

PRINCIPLES OF PROGESTERONE THERAPY

The principles of progesterone therapy requires an understanding of these three characteristics of progesterone receptors.

1. High doses will be required to overcome the protective resistance of progesterone receptors developed during pregnancy.

2. Progesterone enhances lactation, so lactation may be continued during progesterone therapy.

3. There are no drug interactions, so progesterone therapy may be combined with the patient's usual medication, be it antidepressants, tranquilizers, beta blockers, anticonvulsants, etc. When symptoms abate the other medication can be gradually reduced and stopped, always **reducing in the post menstruum**.

4. There are no absolute contraindications. If candidiasis is present then progesterone may cause an increase of symptoms. If it is present, the patient and her partner should be given antifungal treatment at the start of progesterone treatment.

5. It is impossible to overdose with progesterone. With our present methods of progesterone administration, the blood progesterone level reached rarely exceeds that normally present at the end of the first trimester of pregnancy.

RESULTS OF PROPHYLACTIC PROGESTERONE FOR POSTNATAL DEPRESSION

In 1989 a worldwide study of over 200 women, who had a history of previous postnatal depression, was reported in the *International Journal of Prenatal and Perinatal Studies* in which there was a 93% success rate among those receiving progesterone but only 33% in those who inquired about progesterone prophylaxis, but did not receive it.

Why Oral Progesterone?

Up until recently, the major forms of progesterone therapy have been via vaginal suppository, rectal suspension, or injection. The oral route of progesterone administration has long been considered impractical because of poor absorption. Contrary to traditional teaching, recent reports[1] confirm that significant serum progesterone levels can be achieved with a new modification in preparation of progesterone for oral administration. With the development of a formula of natural micronized progesterone compounded in a specific oil base by Women's International Pharmacy, an oral form of natural progesterone is now available, in which the progesterone is rapidly absorbed and reaches adequate blood levels.

Progesterone Administration

PMS is an endocrine disease which responds fully to progesterone replacement therapy.

The natural progesterone can be administered as:

Suppositories: Progesterone in pellets of inert wax inserted per rectum.

Pessaries: Progesterone in inert wax inserted per vagina.

Injections: Progesterone in oil administered intramuscularly.

Implants: Pellets of pure progesterone for implanting in the subcutaneous tissue of the anterior abdominal wall.

Oral: Micronized progesterone *may* bring a measure of relief to *some* sufferers of PMS, but is not available in Britain.

Natural Progesterone: New Ideas

Another alternative way, if you get a little too much bleeding from the natural progesterone, is to switch it from day 11 to day 20.

---

1. "Absorption of oral progesterone is influenced by vehicle and particle size," Joel T. Hargrove, M. D., Wayne S. Maxon, M. D. and Anne Colston Wentz, M. D., *American Journal of Obstetrics and Gynecology*, October 1989.

Progesterone Dosage

Starting dose: Nulliparous 400 mg pr or pv, (better give twice daily), or 50 mg im daily. Parous women 400 mg bd pr or pv, or 100 mg im daily. Those with a history of preeclampsia, postnatal depression or multigravida 400 mg pr or pv or 100 mg im daily.

Increasing dose: If no relief after first course increase at monthly intervals to 400 mg qid pr or pv, or 100 mg im supplemented by suppositories. Some women do not absorb efficiently pr or pv and require im.

Higher doses required by those of high parity, with a history of preeclampsia, postnatal depression or sterilization, also those of slim build. Dosage is not related to age, severity or multiplicity of symptoms.

Routes may be alternated, (e.g., 100 mg and 400 mg pr noct, or alternate days im or pr), or supplemented (e.g., pr and pv simultaneously). Do not insert two suppositories simultaneously into the same orifice as the melting wax prevents further absorption. Avoid using a tampon with pv administration as the tampon absorbs the progesterone.

Restabilization necessary after pregnancy, four months after sterilization and at times of stress. If pregnancy and puerperium normal, progesterone therapy may no longer be required.

Timing of Progesterone Course

Once symptomatic relief is achieved with progesterone, continue with the same dose for 3 more cycles, then gradually reduce either course or dose.

1. **Starting the course two days later each cycle**. If symptoms return the next month's course should be started at the shortest course producing complete symptomatic relief, and continued for at least 3 cycles.

2. **Reducing dose each cycle**, but continuing for the full 14 days. If symptoms recur start next course at lowest dose producing symptomatic relief for 3 cycles.

3. Women under 25 years may only need progesterone therapy for 6 - 9 months.

4. Women over 40 years are likely to need progesterone until menopause.

5. Women with history of high parity, preeclampsia, postnatal depression, or sterilization are likely to require prolonged progesterone therapy.

Drug Interactions with Progesterone

No drug interactions occur with progesterone.

When starting progesterone therapy continue with usual symptomatic medication (eg. anticonvulsants, antidepressants, tranquilizers, beta-blockers, steroids, bronchodilators) initially until optimum dosage and course is established.

Reduce other medication gradually in the postmenstruum.

Progesterone can be given simultaneously with progestogens (e.g., endometriosis) or with estrogens (e.g., menopause).

Side Effects of Progesterone Therapy

None are serious, but there may be:

1. **Lengthening of cycle.** Stop progesterone 2 days after time of expected menstruation; bleeding occurs within 48 hours.

2. **Shortening of cycle.** Start future courses 1 - 2 days later.

3. **Spotting in the premenstrum.** Stop progesterone for menstruation. Start next course 1 - 2 days later.

4. **Spotting at midcycle**, only occurs if progesterone is used in follicular phase, start course at ovulation or two days later.

5. **Erratic cycles**, an indication that progesterone has been forgotten for 1 - 2 days. Erratic takers have erratic cycles.

6. **Generalized urticarial rash** may occur as a reaction to the oily solution in which progesterone is dissolved for injections. Treatment should be continued with suppositories.

Overdose of Progesterone

The blood level of progesterone rises some fifty times higher during pregnancy, compared with the peak level reached during the luteal phase. In pregnancy the raised blood level of progesterone is maintained for nine months, compared with only two weeks during a menstrual cycle. With the best methods of progesterone administration available the blood level reached does not exceed that normally found in the fourth month of pregnancy; thus it is impossible to overdose a parous woman, or one capable of pregnancy. In immature nulliparous women signs of overdose are rarely seen; they include euphoria, restless energy, faintness, and dysmenorrhea.

Progesterone suppositories may be given to women known to have previously attempted drug overdoses. If more than one is used in the same orifice the melted wax prevents and lowers further absorption.

Synthetic Progestogens

Progestogens are not substitutes for progesterone, and are of no value in the treatment of PMS.

Progestogens are synthetic compounds, often testosterone analogues, alien to the human body, and are of value in gynecology and contraception.

Progestogens cannot be utilized by the progesterone receptors.

Progestogens are administered orally (medroxyprogesterone, norgesterol, norethisterone, dydrogesterone), or by long acting injections (medroxyprogesterone acetate, hydroxyprogesterone caproate or hexonate).

Progesterone Differs from Progestogens

It is important to know and recognize the difference between progesterone and progestogens because only progesterone is of value in the treatment of PMS.

1. Progesterone raises the blood level of progesterone, whereas progestogens lower the blood level of progesterone.

2. Progesterone is utilized by progesterone receptors in target cells, whereas progestogens are not utilized by progesterone receptors.

3. Progesterone is excreted as pregnanediol but progestogens are not excreted as pregnanediol.

4. Progesterone is not estrogenic; some progestogens are.

5. Progesterone is not androgenic; some progestogens are.

6. Progesterone is not anabolic; some progestogens are.

7. Progesterone is thermogenic and raises the basal body temperature; progestogens are not thermogenic.

8. Progesterone is not carcinogenic; some progestogens are.

9. Progesterone can be administered during pregnancy without harm to the foetus, but progestogens cause masculinization of the female foetus.

10. Progesterone lowers blood pressure; progestogens cause a rise in blood pressure.

11. Progesterone raises SHBG (sex hormone binding globulin); progestogens lower SHBG.

Conception on Progesterone

1. Start progesterone at least two days after ovulation.

2. Continue progesterone until menstruation or pregnancy has been confirmed.

3. Appreciate that progesterone is thermogenic; i.e., it raises the basal body temperature, which must not be mistaken for ovulation.

Update on Progesterone and Miscarriages

Twenty out of 100 women who have miscarriages have low levels of Progesterone. Other women with miscarriages have antiphospholipid antibodies, which is an autoimmune or lupus-like syndrome. A corpus luteal phase defect has been associated with progesterone deficiency. You can examine the uterine lining just before a period to determine if such a defect is present.

The Physiological Effects of Estrogen and Progesterone

Estrogen Effects

Breast stimulation
Creates proliferative endometrium
Salt and fluid retention
Increased fat in body
Depression and headaches
Interferes with thyroid hormone
Increased blood clotting
Decreases libido
Impairs blood sugar control
Loss of zinc and retention of copper
Reduced oxygen levels in all cells
Causes endometrial cancer
Increased risk of breast cancer
Slightly restrains osteoclast function

Progesterone Effects

Protects against fibrocysts
Maintains secretory endometrium
Natural diuretic
Helps use fat for energy
Natural antidepressant
Helps thyroid hormone action
Normalizes blood clotting
Restores libido
Normalizes blood sugar levels
Normalizes zinc and copper levels
restores proper cell oxygen levels
Prevents endometrial cancer
Helps prevent breast cancer
Stimulates osteoblast bone building
Necessary for survival of embryo
Precursor of cortisone synthesis

Premenstrual and Perimenstrual Tension

In most women, hormonal changes occur during the menstrual cycle with resulting anxiety, depression, edema, headache, and even on rare occasions, seizures and psychosis. Numerous biochemical factors make women more susceptible to these effects, such as preexisting hormonal deficiencies, e.g., estrogen, progesterone and thyroid; deficiencies in calcium, magnesium, zinc, manganese, or other trace metals, as well as elevated copper; deficiencies in amino acids and B-vitamins, excess weight or fluid retention.

Therefore, numerous factors can contribute and help with the treatment of PMS. A high protein diet will result in diuresis and reduce fluid retention. There are many benefits to diets low in salt, sugar, and refined carbohydrates. A diet high in B-6, which has a diuretic action as well as magnesium, and borage or primrose oil will also prevent fluid retention and may have beneficial effects on the endocrine imbalances associated with PMS. Numerous studies show the benefits of calcium and B-complex supplementation, as well as vitamin E and selenium in reducing cystic mastitis and overall symptoms of PMS. Ingestion of caffeine, tea, and empty calories -- from soft drinks, among other sources -- has been associated with the worsening of PMS symptoms. There also are endocrine factors that can be improved in PMS by using natural progesterone combinations and natural estrogen combinations now available in a new pill (micronized so it is properly absorbed), which have very little side effects, if any, compared to the synthetic estrogen/progesterone combinations. Natural hormones can contribute to a peaceful mind and mood for many women. Progesterone, in particular, is extremely calming and can be taken at night to help sleep. Natural progesterone supplements can modify and improve abnormalities revealed by brain mapping.

Rare factors involved in PMS are the effects of lead and other heavy metal poisonings and toxins in the environment which can be evaluated by hair testing. There are psychosocial factors which may be a factor in PMS, e.g., women seem to be more comfortable in their menstrual cycles in countries where they are less pressured to be the bread winners. This may be psychosocial to the extent that PMS reminds a woman that she is a woman. Therefore, there may be some negative impact (increased PMS) when traditional women's roles, e.g., homemaking and rearing children, are demeaned. PMS may respond to many other pharmacological approaches, e.g., lithium, Prozac, thyroid, Wellbutrin, antidepressants and anticonvulsants, etc.

PMS and BEAM

Studies by Dr. Joseph Martorano, a specialist in PMS, working with my colleague, Dr. Itell, at Valhalla, New York Medical College, have shown that the abnormalities on brain maps in PMS patients could improve with progesterone. Neurologists that we have worked with in the past have identified progesterone as a mild anti-seizure medicine, brain stabilizing, helpful to anxiety, which is why so many women feel well with progesterone.

PMS -- Current Research into Its Physical and Psychological Aspects [1]

After a history marked by a lack of funding and interest in PMS research, the proliferation within the past few years of a number of clinical drug trials and psychological studies reveals that PMS has been accepted by the medical community as a serious disorder, albeit a disorder difficult to define and treat.

One study, conducted at MIT, which looked at the link between nutrients and premenstrual depression, resulted in findings suggesting that D-fenfluramine (a drug

---

1. Derived from *PMS Access*, PMS Research Explores Physical, Psychological Links, 33: Sept/Oct 1991.

used to treat obesity) may reduce depression, anxiety and negative mood swings, as well as binge eating. This study has paved the way for research on an entire category of drugs which, like D-fenfluramine, increase the brain levels of the neurotransmitter serotonin.

Prozac is also being studied as a treatment for women with PMS suffering significant, persistent depression, but no conclusive research has been completed.

Hormonal studies have also been conducted exploring relief for PMS. For example, Danazol, a synthetic steroid, suppresses ovarian function; and while there has been some "good" response to the drug, there have also been significant side effects including depression and weight gain. For "severe and intractable" PMS, Canadian researchers have postulated that ovarian removal may provide last-resort relief.

Non-hormonal and non-drug therapies have also been researched. Painful menstruation has been successfully treated with prostaglandin inhibitors; and a double-blind, crossover study of calcium supplementation showed an impressive effect on symptoms of depression, irritability, headache and mood swings among others. In both kinds of research more investigation is needed.

Long-term follow-up of 100 women treated with different modalities for PMS has been undertaken by Dr. William Keye of William Beauman Hospital, Royal Oak, Michigan, to assess effects of treatment over time. Brain mapping as a research adjunct has also been used to show changes in brain activity, thus providing "immediate and direct confirmation of clinical changes," e.g., to document positive effects of oral micronized progesterone. Natural progesterone is a brain calmer and an anti-seizure and anti-cerebral dysrhythmia medicine.

Endometriosis

Dysmenorrhea, painful periods, dyspareunia, painful intercourse, infertility, pelvic pain, back pain, menstrual disorders, and spontaneous abortion are the typical problems.

Some of the complications include ruptured endometrium and/or ruptured ovaries or ectopic pregnancy. It can affect the stomach sites. Patients may suffer from vomiting, abdominal cramping, rectal pain, urgency to defecate, diarrhea, constipation, straining with bowel

movements, blood in the stool, low back pain, pain in the area of the pelvis, sharp gas pains, abdominal bloating, or rectal bleeding. In urinary tract sites, one can have pain or burning upon urination, possible blood in urine, urgency to urinate, fever, hypertension, headache, tenderness around the kidneys, and excessive fatigue. It also may affect the cervix. It may affect the pulmonary sites, manifesting itself by coughing of blood, shoulder pain, and shortness of breath.

Hair Loss in Women

Hair loss in women is common and is due to excess androgens, which can be demonstrated by an elevation of sex hormone binding globulin. Many of our female patients in their 40's and 50's have come in with pieces of hair missing and male pattern baldness, which seem to be helped with a combination of vitamins and Aldactone. It has been quite remarkable to see this happen. Their sex hormone binding globulin recovers afterwards.

Our new dosing for progesterone and PMS is going to be somewhere in the range of 200 mg in the morning and 300 mg at bedtime. The bedtime may be optional if it leaves the bloodstream.

Taking progesterone 10-14 days out of the month satisfies the requirement for protecting the uterus. If you take it 30 days you block endometrial hypoplasia regardless of the fact that you are not sloughing.

Using Natural Progesterone For Premenstrual Syndrome

First, I want to describe **what premenstrual syndrome is**. Basically, it is a hormonal disorder characterized by 1) a regularly recurring group of symptoms which occur from 2 to 14 days before a woman's menstrual period, usually disappearing after the period begins, followed by 2) a symptom-free time in each monthly cycle. These regularly recurring symptoms and their timing in the menstrual cycle typify PMS.

What PMS is not. PMS usually is not another name for menstrual cramps or premenstrual tension. The difference is that PMS occurs before the menstrual period and improves once the period begins. Menstrual cramps usually begin at the onset of the period, disappearing by the end of the flow. Premenstrual tension, which occurs before the period, may be a symptom of PMS but is usually just one of many symptoms a woman suffers. There are more than 150 symptoms which have been associated with PMS. Some of them include depression, fatigue, sudden anger and irritability, mood swings, crying and weeping jags, feelings of aggression or violence, headaches or migraines, breast tenderness, feelings of panic and frustration, mental and physical exhaustion, inability to concentrate, asthma, arthritis, leg and other muscle cramps, anxiety, joint and muscle pain, and cravings for certain foods, especially sweets. PMS sufferers are likely to have certain characteristics and experiences in common, including 1) adverse reactions to oral contraceptives, 2) absence of PMS symptoms during the last 6 months of pregnancy, 3) symptoms beginning at puberty while taking birth control pills or after pregnancy or with missed periods, 4) symptoms occurring or becoming more severe after tubal ligation or hysterectomy, 5) ordinarily pain-free menstrual periods, 6) pregnancy complications including miscarriage, toxemia, and post-partum depression, 7) acute symptoms (migraines, panic attacks, depression, even epileptic episodes occurring after long periods without food), 8) symptoms worsening with age, 9) changes in premenstrual sex drive, 10) increased premenstrual sensitivity to alcohol, 11) history of female family members with similar problems.

It has been estimated that 40 percent of all women between the ages of 14 and 50 experience PMS, and at least 10 percent of these women experience PMS symptoms severe enough to disrupt their lives. One way to find out if you have PMS is to keep a daily record of exactly when your symptoms occur for a minimum of three consecutive menstrual cycles.

What causes PMS? No one yet knows exactly what causes PMS. There are some suggested causes, including vitamin and mineral deficiencies, nutritional factors, progesterone deficiency, stress, or psychosomatic causes.

What can be done about PMS? There is as yet no single therapy for all women with PMS, and that is why it is necessary to try different treatments to see what is best for the individual patient. In terms of diet, some people recommend that you eat a high complex carbohydrate, high fiber diet, usually six small meals daily, and cut down on simple carbohydrates like refined sugar and soft drinks so that you maintain a steady glucose level. Also, avoiding caffeine, alcohol, and salt is important to reduce tension, fatigue, depression, and fluid retention. In terms of vitamin and mineral supplements, it is recommended that you take B-6, between 100 and 300 milligrams. Initially, two weeks before your period, you can start with 100 milligrams of B-6, and as you get closer to your period you can increase it to 300 milligrams. In addition to that, calcium and magnesium are also important. Exercise is helpful for PMS sufferers because it reduces stress and tension and provides a sense of well-being. At least three 20- to 60-minute sessions a week of aerobic exercise is usually recommended. In terms of prescription medications, one option is progesterone. There is a natural form of progesterone, and it comes in many different kinds of preparations. One is a rectal or vaginal suppository, and there is also natural progesterone in oral capsules, which are short-acting, usually requiring two to four times a day dosing. Now there is a progesterone even-release oral tablet, which is a natural progesterone. The usual dose of this is 300 milligrams at bedtime or twice a day. In addition, there is now a moisturizing cream with natural progesterone. The cream is rubbed on to your hands, face, chest, back, or abdomen about two to three times a day and the progesterone is absorbed through the skin in about three to five minutes. Natural progesterone does not appear to have the side effects that synthetics have, e.g., edema, breast tenderness, depression, and weight gain. In addition to progesterone, some women can benefit from Prozac, 20 milligrams a day. As you see, there are different modalities to use for PMS, and for each patient it has to be individualized.

Daily Symptom Record

MY DAILY SYMPTOM RECORD

SAMPLE: Date—October 7 (First day of menstrual flow is Day 1 of Cycle)

Examples of PMS symptoms:

Abdominal bloating, acne, anxiety, backache, breast tenderness, clumsiness, crying, depression, dizziness, fainting, fatigue, fluid retention, food cravings, forgetfulness, headache, hostility, irritability, joint swelling, mental confusion, migraine, mood swings, tension

Indicate symptom severity by filling in circle: ◯ No Symptom ◑ Moderate ● Severe   Menstrual Flow: M

Day of Cycle — 1 2 3 4 5 6 7 8 9 10 11 12 13 14 15 16 17 18 19 20 21 22 23 24 25 26 27 28 29 30 31 32 33 34 35 36 37 38 39 40

Irritability

Headache

Fluid Retention

Menses: M M M M

Date 10/7

MONTH 1

Day of Cycle — 1 2 3 4 5 6 7 8 9 10 11 12 13 14 15 16 17 18 19 20 21 22 23 24 25 26 27 28 29 30 31 32 33 34 35 36 37 38 39 40

Menses

Date

MONTH 2

Day of Cycle — 1 2 3 4 5 6 7 8 9 10 11 12 13 14 15 16 17 18 19 20 21 22 23 24 25 26 27 28 29 30 31 32 33 34 35 36 37 38 39 40

Menses

Date

MONTH 3

Day of Cycle — 1 2 3 4 5 6 7 8 9 10 11 12 13 14 15 16 17 18 19 20 21 22 23 24 25 26 27 28 29 30 31 32 33 34 35 36 37 38 39 40

Menses

Date

NOTE: In the interest of accuracy, it's important you keep this record on a daily basis. It may help to set aside a specific time each day — you'll need only a minute or two.

Pregnancy

Nutrition is the foundation for healthy children. If the mother is healthy, the baby will most likely be just as healthy. There are a lot of over-the-counter medications that are harmful to pregnant women, e.g., cigarettes, alcohol, Tylenol (may affect the hemoglobin of baby), pain relievers (may affect liver of baby, causing blood pressure to rise), laxatives (can affect stomach and kidneys of baby), sugar, antacids, sodium bicarbonate, use of certain chemical cleaners, and junk food.

To avoid unnecessary problems during pregnancy, it's important to be at an ideal weight before you get pregnant, avoiding as much stress as possible. Everything that is not nutritional is to be avoided during pregnancy. This is a time when a woman must look at her life-style and change the bad habits to protect the baby.

Maimonides, a famous Rabbi Physician, believed that food determined health in that it can determine whether a fetus will be healthy or sick. The mother's eating habits definitely affect the baby in the womb. The use of iron is beneficial during pregnancy as well as folic acid (protects against birth defects), vitamin B-12, vitamin D and calcium (all build bones) and zinc (protects against high blood pressure and birth defects). Most women who have a bad sense of taste and smell will find these improved through the use of zinc.

As the woman becomes closer to delivery, it's important to ingest enough magnesium because it lowers blood pressure. Fish oil may prevent premature births. Weight gain during pregnancy probably should be kept at 20 to 30 pounds. Weight gain of more than 30 pounds

usually means a junk-food eating woman. Her protein intake should be increased to 50 to 75 grams daily, and more may be necessary, i.e., a can and a half of tuna per day is essential but not necessarily sufficient.

Various nutrients affect the baby by decreasing the tendency for infection. Always breast-feed, even for six months or more, because it protects against the problem with vaccines that we hear so much about. Breast milk is actually protective and concentrated in vitamin A, D, zinc, and iron. If women don't make enough breast milk, niacin, taurine, potassium and other nutrients may increase a woman's capacity to produce milk. Once the baby has gone full term, it's important to keep up the good health through breast-feeding.

Infant formulas are often inadequate in taurine, biopterin, and other nutrients. Nutrition in premature babies is very critical. If you add more tryptophan to the soy protein formula, you may get a calmer baby with much less crying. They are also often vitamin E and zinc deficient. Prematurity may be a result of lead, cadmium, heavy metal toxicity, drug use, prior health and nutrition, etc. Congenital abnormalities have been linked to lead excess and zinc deficiency. Alcohol contributes to reduced birth weight, prematurity, and other abnormalities. Neural tube defects may be prevented by nutrients, particularly folic acid. Zinc supplements may also prevent birth defects but reduce iron absorption. Nutrient supplements feed the mother and baby and later feed the baby through the mother's milk.

Utilization by Pregnancy Trimester Markers for Gestational Health and Disease

Marker	First Trimester	Second Trimester	Third Trimester
Maternal serum alpha-fetoprotein	■ ■	■	+
Plasma estriol	+	■ ■	■ ■
Human chorionic gonadotropin	■	■ ■	
Progesterone	■		
Human placental lactogen		+	■ ■
Atrial natriuretic peptide		+	+ ■ ■
Plasma cystyl aminopeptidase		+	+ ■ ■

■   Major Use
■ ■   Potential or occasional use
+   Investigational stage

The abuse markers can be followed to evaluate the nutritional health and ability of the fetus.

Nutrition and Pregnancy

Pregnancy is the best time in your life to gain weight! You are supposed to gain about 25-35 lbs (unless you are obese -- then about 10-15 lbs) in order to ensure that your baby will be healthy and a good weight when he or she is born.

However, it is very important to eat the right foods. Remember, that your baby eats what you eat and its growth depends on your choosing healthful foods. The food that you eat daily should come from the following groups:

1) **Protein:** Examples: meat, fish, eggs, milk, chicken, cheese, beans, nuts, peanut butter. Protein builds strong muscles and helps the brain develop properly. Eat three or more servings each day.

2) **Milk and milk products:** Drink 4-5 glasses of milk each day or eat cheese, yogurt, or pudding. Milk provides calcium for building strong bones and protein for developing good muscles and organs.

3) **Fruits and vegetables:** These foods give you vitamins, minerals, energy, and fiber. Eat 4 or more servings each day.

4) **Breads and cereals:** These foods also provide vitamins, energy, and minerals. Select whole-grain or enriched breads and unsweetened cereals. Eat 5 or 6 servings each day.

Drinking 6-8 glasses of liquid including water, juice, and milk each day, is also necessary. Try to avoid "junk foods" such as coke, chips, and candy because they don't provide any vitamins, minerals, or protein for you or the baby. Don't use any over-the-counter medications without your doctor's permission. And, of course, don't smoke, drink alcohol, or use drugs during pregnancy.

If you would like additional nutrition information or a sample daily food guide, please ask the nurse or social worker assigned to your case. If you need help obtaining healthful foods, please talk with the social worker as he or she can connect you with the WIC program, Food Stamp Program, or the Commodity Supplemental Food Program.

Sex as a Mood Healer

According to a study by Barry R. Komisaruk, Rutgers University, vaginal stimulation is a potent analgesic for rats. Sexual stimulation is a remedy for pain. Adolescent sexual revolution and sexual use was due to the enormous amount of emotional, psychological, and medical brain pain. If we are going to restore a moral sexual society, we are going to have to reduce the pain through nutrients, drugs, etc.

Substance Abuse and Pregnancy

It is very important during your pregnancy to stay away from anything that might harm you or your baby. Drugs, alcohol, and smoking cigarettes will hurt you and your baby and can cause lifelong problems.

If you are addicted to alcohol or drugs such as marijuana, crack, cocaine or heroin, then your baby will also be born addicted to drugs or alcohol. The baby will have to go through painful withdrawal and could have permanent mental, physical, and emotional problems. Cigarette smoking is like poisoning your baby and should also be avoided.

Your Baby

Babies born to mothers who abuse drugs, alcohol, and cigarettes usually weigh less at birth than other babies. Low birth-weight babies often face many different problems including illness, developmental and emotional problems. Many of these babies grow into children who continue to face difficulties later on, especially in school.

You

Using drugs or alcohol during pregnancy (or anytime) also places your own health at risk. Pregnant women who use drugs or alcohol may develop a variety of medical problems such as diabetes, edema (swelling), hepatitis, high blood pressure, and urinary problems. Use of drugs or alcohol leads, as well, to social problems. When you are high, you will not be able to take good care of your baby even if you want to or think that you can. You will also spend your money on drugs or alcohol and may not have enough money left over to buy formula and diapers for your baby.

As you can see, the use of drugs and alcohol almost always results in problems for both you and your baby. Pregnancy lasts only 9 months so it is truly urgent that during this time you do everything that you can to avoid abusing drugs and alcohol. If you think that you have a substance abuse problem, please ask us for help right away. We have a number of agencies that are working with us to help you overcome your drug or alcohol problem, and we can make arrangements for you to receive help quickly.

Please remember that during your pregnancy you are responsible for two people, yourself and your unborn baby. Your baby is depending on you to take good care of yourself so that he or she can have a healthy and happy start in life with a healthy and happy Mom to help the child get through life!

Nutritional Needs of Your Infant

Once your baby is born, or if you are the mother of an infant, you will be spending a good deal of your time feeding your baby. Feeding can help develop a special closeness between you and your baby. Food also teaches babies new things about the world such as smells, tastes, shapes, and colors. You know that good nutrition is needed for growing up healthy and it is your responsibility as a parent to teach your baby good eating habits.

You will have a choice as to how to feed your newborn. You can either provide food with mother's milk, infant formula, or a combination of both. A newborn baby's diet is very simple. For the first four months of life, your baby needs only 5-10 feedings of mother's milk or formula per day. Your baby does not need any cereal at this time.

Mother's Milk

If you choose to nurse your baby, remember that you must eat a healthy diet and drink plenty of liquids (see Nutrition and Pregnancy Fact Sheet). Everything that you eat and drink will be passed through you to your baby. Therefore, it is very important to avoid smoking, drinking, and using drugs. Nursing provides the perfect balance of nutrients for your baby and also helps protect babies from some illnesses.

These are a few things to remember that might make breast feeding more comfortable:

1. At the beginning of a new feeding, begin at the breast where the last feeding was completed. (You can pin a safety pin to your bra to help you remember where to start.)

2. Make sure the baby has "latched on" correctly to avoid sore nipples. The baby should have the nipple and the areola (the dark part around the nipple) in his mouth; not just the nipple.

3. Try not to skip feedings as this might decrease your milk supply. If you must, try pumping your breasts with a breast pump or expressing (that is, pumping) milk by hand at the regular feeding time.

This is a very brief description of the process of breast feeding. Most mothers have a lot of questions and some mothers have problems with nursing, so be sure to talk to your doctor or nurse if you need more information about breast feeding.

Infant Formula

Infant formula will also provide good nutrition for your baby. (Remember that formula is not *cow's* milk that you buy at the grocery store. Babies can't digest regular milk at this age.) When using formula, you must carefully wash bottles, nipples and caps in hot, soapy water, rinse in hot water and let air dry. Follow the instructions on the can very carefully for preparing formula; after heating, test formula on your wrist to make sure that it isn't too hot. Bottle fed babies drink about 2-4 ounces at first. They will drink about 4-8 ounces by the time they are a few weeks old. Remember to throw away any formula left in the bottle after feeding.

At the beginning, it is recommended that you feed your baby "on demand" -- that is, whenever the baby is hungry. During the first few months your baby will eat somewhere between every 2-4 hours per day. Some feeding tips that are useful are:

1. Hold your baby with head raised during feeding.

2. Don't put your baby to bed with a bottle and avoid contact of baby's teeth with sweet liquids as these practices promote tooth decay.

3. Burp your baby frequently to get rid of any swallowed air.

As your baby gets older, new foods will slowly be added to his/her diet. Your nurse (or social worker) has a great deal more information on feeding your baby as he or she grows, and also has a very helpful infant feeding chart available for you. Remember to discuss any feeding problems with the nurse and to ask for any other nutritional information that you might need.

Protocol for Fibroids

The nasal spray Synarel (b.i.d.) often causes side effects and has poor compliance. A new natural peptide, Lupron, 3.75 mg injected monthly, can help shrink fibroids. At this time it is only used preoperatively but may have longer lasting value. Frequently individuals will not experience any problems with fibroids if their emotional state is controlled. If they take care of fatigue, depression, anxiety, and weight, they can often go years and years with large fibroids.

The Benefits of Iron Therapy

Iron deficiency is still the most common nutritional deficiency in this society. Low iron content manifests itself as deficiency in children, fatigue, etc. Full testing of blood iron measures ferritin, iron TIBC (total iron bonding capacity), per cent saturation and even red blood cell iron. This is the most accurate testing for iron.

For over one hundred years iron has been promoted as a remedy for female problems. Each woman in the menstrual years does need about 8 mg of iron each day, which often can be obtained from food. Ferrous salts of iron are better absorbed than the ferric salts, which are contained in the "so-called" iron-enriched white flour. Vitamin C promotes the absorption of all iron in both food

and supplements. Therefore, a patient on mega-nutrients who is found to have an iron level below 50 mcg should be given only one iron tablet per day. Larger doses may produce iron overload and depression of mood. Iron overload is a constant hazard in older males who have little iron loss except for hemorrhoids or bowel diseases. Therefore, the use of iron supplements should be based on the known presence of a low level of serum iron or percent saturation. PATH used to use Mol-Iron because we know that the tissues which produce hemoglobin also require molybdenum as a trace metal. Mol-Iron, by analysis, contains 1800 mcg of molybdenum. The body needs at least 500 mcg of molybdenum each day. Molybdenum, like zinc, is well absorbed orally but not conserved by the body. Molybdenum, however, can be given with a trace metal supplement; and Slow Fe, a very well-absorbed, nonconstipating form of iron, is probably the best supplement.

In rheumatoid arthritis the serum iron is invariably low but the tissue and joint iron is high. With nutrient treatment the iron slowly leaves the tissues and a more normal level is attained in the blood. Even small doses of iron given intravenously can cause a severe joint inflammation in rheumatoid arthritis. One should note that bacteria love iron so that the malnourished child may have increased infection when placed on iron therapy before the nutritional deficiency is corrected.

Understanding Pap Smears

Papanicolaou Classification	Descriptive Papanicolaou Classification	Cervical Intraepithelial neoplasia	Bethesda System
I Benign	Normal	None	Satisfactory/WNL
II Atypical benign	Atypical cells present but not dysplastic, usually due to cytotoxic atypia	None	Atypia of undetermined significance
III Suspicious	Cells consistent with: 1. mild dysplasia 2. moderate dysplasia	CIN I CIN II	Low grade SIL; either HPV or CIN I
IV Strongly suspicious for malignancy	Cells consistent with severe dysplasia or carcinoma in situ	CIN III	High grade SIL; includes CIN II, CIN III
V Malignancy	Cells consistent with invasive cancer	None	Squamous cell carcinoma

Patients with pap smears types III - V need aggressive treatment. Those with pap smears type II, and in some cases type III, can be treated with antioxidants, nutrients, and possibly Retin-A, and can be followed at 3-6 month intervals. Abnormal pap smears are linked to promiscuity, poor diet, smoking, birth control pills, etc.

Mammography

Mammography is an X-ray of the breast. It is of controversial value at this time. Generally the American Cancer Society recommends one every one to two years between ages 40 and 50 and annually after age 50. The problem arises from the fact that mammography may cause side effects such as increased cancer.

At this time we are following the American Cancer Society recommendation, although patients should be respected for making their own choices in this regard, due to the controversy surrounding the mammography issue.

Women and Heart Disease

Out of 550,000 people who die of heart disease each year, 250,000 are women. Heart attack is now the number one killer of American women. It is unfortunate since it's so easy to screen for heart disease and peripheral vascular disease with a cardiogram, a PET scan, or Doppler screening tests.

One in nine women ages 45 to 64 have some kind of form(s) of cardiovascular disease. Obvious risk factors are obesity, high blood pressure, and elevated cholesterol. 240,000 women die from these heart attacks. Almost 90,000 women die each year of stroke.

All of this can be prevented today if properly diagnosed by PET scanning and Doppler. What we need to do is measure the cholesterol levels, triglycerides, apolipoproteins, and fibrinogen. All of these are risk factors as well as poor nutrient status, antioxidants, and chromium.

Today women's health can be taken care of and transformed through these new preventative techniques. For further reading see:

Eysmam, Susan, Reperfusion and Revascularization Strategies for Coronary Artery Disease in Women, *JAMA*, 1992; 268:1903-1907.

Wenqer, Nannette K., Cardiovascular Health and Disease in Women, *NEJM* 329:247-256, 1993.

Douqlas, Pamela S., *Cardiovascular Health and Disease in Women*, W. B. Saunders & Company, 1993.

21. Osteoporosis and Bone Diseases

Bone Health

The fundamentals of bone health are nutrition, calcium, magnesium, vitamin D, strontium, boron, electrical stimulation and bioelectrical balancing.

Osteoporosis

Nearly 24 million people in the U.S. have some form of osteoporosis. Factors that contribute to the development of osteoporosis include: insufficient exercise, inadequate calcium and Vitamin D intake, excessive alcohol or caffeine consumption, a thin, light build, fair skin, white or Asian race.

Adequate dietary calcium and vitamin D are the cornerstones of therapy. Green vegetables are the best source of calcium. A 100 grams serving of collard or turnip greens provides over 20 mg of calcium and very little phosphorus (Ca: P ratio of 1 to 0.3). Such vegetables provide fiber and a host of other essential trace elements. To grow green vegetables, the farmer fertilizes the soil with lime and potash so both of these are nutritious green vegetables.

Postmenopausal women usually require at least 1500 mg of calcium; usually, a minimum of 1000 mg by means of supplementation. This is equivalent to about three extra glasses of milk daily. It would take about four or five glasses daily to provide the entire requirement. Some feel even this is not enough calcium and point out that familial hypercalcemia, where calcium levels are elevated above normal, is marked by virtually no osteoporosis. Most physicians are afraid to supplement with more calcium, fearing that in some individuals this may lead to kidney stone formation.

When should the good diet begin? Obviously, as soon as possible. A good high calcium diet includes greens, milk, salmon, sardines, cheese and yogurt. When should supplementation begin? The suggested age of

children has become younger and younger. Although prudent physicians used to suggest age 30, current evidence indicates long-term benefits from earlier calcium therapy. There are literally dozens of diseases for which claims for the benefits from calcium can be made.

What is the best form of supplementation? Calcium carbonate is the cheapest and easiest way to supplement calcium. Yet calcium citrate is better absorbed and does not produce constipation. Furthermore, there are brands which have no additives, or additives that are natural substances like amino acids, which help make a more solid pill.

The "dangerous" forms of supplementation may be dolomite, bone meal and oyster shells. Dolomite and bone meal can contain significant amounts of lead and aluminum.

Vitamin D (400 to 1800 units a day) is essential for calcium absorption. Many metals are essential for calcium absorption, e.g., fluoride, manganese and boron. Progress of bone loss is now easily studied by radiological testing. If the progress of osteoporosis is fast, supplementation with natural estrogens may be necessary as well as other hormone replacements.

Exercise regularly. We recommend performing a "weight-bearing" exercise at least 3 times a week for about 30-45 minutes each time. Tennis, weight training, running, low impact aerobics and stair climbing are all weight-bearing exercises.

Causes of Osteoporosis

Etiology of Osteoporosis

NUTRITIONAL FACTORS

- Calcium deficiency
- Phosphate deficiency
- Vitamin D deficiency
- Ascorbic acid deficiency
- Intestinal malabsorption
- High-protein diet

ENDOCRINE DISORDERS

- Hypogonadism
- Glucocorticoid excess (exogenous or endogenous)
- Hyperthyroidism
- Hyperparathyroidism
- Diabetes
- Growth hormone deficiency

DRUG-INDUCED (heparin, methotrexate)

GENETIC

- Osteogenesis imperfecta
- Homocystinuria

MISCELLANEOUS

- Metabolic and respiratory acidosis
- Rheumatoid arthritis
- Mastocytosis
- Malignancy
- Inactivity, immobilization, and disuse
- Deficient production of 1,25-dihydroxyvitamin D-3, with aging

Osteoporosis and Nutrients

What are the key nutrients and factors involved in osteoporosis? There are several important factors to consider in osteoporosis. The most important is estrogen. Without estrogen calcium is not absorbed. Nutrients such as boron and folic acid (20 mg doses) may have some estrogen effect.

Certainly every woman needs calcium after menopause. Some think calcium supplementation should be started somewhere after the age of thirty and most certainly after menopause. Calcium requires vitamin D and in some cases magnesium for proper absorption. Four micronutrients -- manganese, boron, strontium and fluoride -- also may have a role in the proper absorption of calcium. Magnesium is also important during calcium supplementation because it prevents constipation that can be caused by calcium carbonate. (Calcium citrate is less constipating.) Most other forms of calcium are really insufficient as supplements because they cannot be made into high potency tablets.

Osteoporosis and Diet

CALCIUM REQUIREMENT

Age	Requirement	Milk Servings/Day
Before Menopause	1,000 mg	3
During or After Menopause	1,500 mg	5

DAILY DIET

Calcium. The daily diet should include foods that are high in calcium. Food is the best source of calcium because calcium is better absorbed from food than from supplements. Milk and dairy products are the best sources of calcium. One cup of milk has about 300 mg. of calcium. Skim or low-fat milk products contain calcium but not the added fat or calories so these are your best sources. Plain low-fat yogurt is an excellent source of calcium and provides 415 mg. of calcium per cup. Hard cheeses, such as Swiss and Parmesan, are also good sources but are relatively high in fat. Cottage cheese and low-fat cottage cheese are the next best sources. Sardines and canned salmon eaten with bones are also good sources. To a lesser extent, broccoli and tofu also provide significant amounts of calcium.

Vitamin D. Vitamin D is essential for the absorption of calcium. The recommended dietary allowance for this vitamin is 400 I.U. per day. Vitamin-fortified milk and cereals, eggs and liver have this vitamin. One cup of milk provides 100 I.U. The body can manufacture its own Vitamin D. Fifteen minutes to one hour of midday sunshine will also meet the daily need for this vitamin.

Protein. Although protein is an important daily requirement, large quantities can lead to loss of calcium through the urine. Women whose diets are very high in protein should consider cutting back. Protein is found primarily in meats, poultry, fish and dairy products. (However, since dairy products also are important sources of calcium, that is not the place to cut back.) Forty-four grams of protein each day is the recommended dietary allowance for adult women; 56 grams is recommended for adult men. One chicken breast has 26 grams of protein; an eight ounce glass of milk has 9 grams.

Alcohol. Excessive use of alcohol increases the body's need for calcium. Drinking interferes with the intestinal absorption of calcium and it may be appropriate to avoid drinking any alcohol within 1 or 2 hours of eating your calcium-rich foods or taking your calcium supplements.

Smoking. It has been shown that smoking is associated with an accelerated loss of bone and a greater risk of osteoporosis. The negative effects on bone appear to be somewhat related to the number of cigarettes smoked. If you can not quit smoking here is another good reason to try and cut down. You may need to increase your intake of calcium somewhat in order to compensate for the amount you are losing. (Cigarette addiction is a brain chemistry disorder and responds to CES, nutrients and drugs when necessary.)

Caffeine. Excessive consumption of coffee (4-8 cups per day) can interfere with calcium absorption and increase the body's need for calcium. Caffeine-containing beverages (2-3 cups per day) appear to significantly increase calcium excretion. If you are drinking more than four caffeine-containing beverages a day you may want to cut down your intake or change to de-caffeinated beverages.

Oxalates. Oxalates are compounds found in large amounts in green vegetables such as asparagus, green beans, spinach, sorrel, dandelion greens and rhubarb. In the intestine, they combine with calcium to form large, insoluble complexes that can not be absorbed. You can continue to eat these foods but you should not depend upon them as primary sources of calcium. You also should try not to consume your calcium-rich foods (or calcium supplements) at the same time as you eat food containing oxalates.

Phytates. Phytates are phosphorus-containing compounds found principally in the outer husks of cereal grains, especially oatmeal and bran. These foods can interfere with calcium absorption by combining with calcium in the intestine. Again, you need not eliminate these foods from your diet but they may interfere with the absorption of calcium if eaten with dairy products.

Sodium. Most people consume ten to twenty times as much sodium as they a need. Try to limit the amount of sodium in your diet since the more sodium you consume the more calcium is excreted. You can reduce the salt in your diet by eating fewer processed foods. Reduce or eliminate the amount of salt you add to foods while eating or cooking. If you are on a low-sodium diet you may want to choose low-salt dairy products as well.

Magnesium. Magnesium -- as well as manganese, silicon and boron -- is often added to calcium supplements because magnesium increases calcium absorption.

Estrogen. Eat foods high in natural estrogens, progesterones and testosterones.

EATING A BALANCED OSTEOPOROSIS DIET:

1. Eat four or more servings of fresh fruits and vegetables per day.

2. Eat four or more servings of whole grain products such as bread, cereals, brown rice and pasta.

3 Limit your protein intake to two 4-ounce servings. The best sources of protein are chicken, turkey, fish, legumes and peanut butter. Reduce your consumption of beef products.

4. Reduce your overall intake of fat, specifically saturated fats found, mostly, in animal foods.

5. Reduce your overall consumption of foods high in sugar and salt.

22. Psychological Therapy, Problems and Factors in Disease

Anxiety

**Anxiety in a man's heart weighs him down,
but a good word makes him glad. (Prov. 12:25)**

Anxiety is one of the more difficult symptoms to treat. Patients describe a cluster of problems, e.g., shortness of breath, palpitations, chest discomfort, choking or smothering, dizziness, unreality, tingling hands and feet, hot or cold flashes, sweating, feeling faint, trembling or shaking, and fears of dying or going crazy. Other patients have motor tension, trembling, aches, fatigability, inability to relax, apprehensive expectation, i.e., worry, anticipation of misfortune, hyperattentiveness, or insomnia. Frequently, patients believe they have a physical malady -- and, indeed, there are many that cause anxiety -- but this is rarely the problem. Patients with acute anxiety often believe they are allergic to many things.

Anxiety can be the result of marked depression.

Hence, panic anxiety attacks are treated with antidepressants, e.g., Tofranil, Wellbutrin. Lactate, carbon dioxide, and oxygen each produce anxiety. Several nutrients are thought to decrease anxiety: serotonin agonists, (niacin, tryptophan, melatonin, lithium), inositol, and GABA (Valium-like effects). Certain nutrients that heighten depression can heighten anxiety. Patients with anxiety need psychological testing. Dietary considerations are important, especially removal of caffeine, cigarettes, and other stimulants (e.g., sugar). Many individuals with severe anxiety have organic brain diseases and need medications. The CES (Cranial Electrical Stimulation) device is FDA approved for marketing to treat anxiety. In depression-based anxiety, tyrosine and DL-phenylalanine can be helpful.

Hypochondriasis: Depression and Anxiety

Many individuals who suffer anxiety and depression present to the physician their concern about parts of their bodies, convinced that their headache is a brain tumor or their stomach pain is an ulcer or aching in the hands is arthritis. Sometimes, they even have a persistent delusion to the point that they are absolutely convinced that, despite all the medical evidence, the doctors are wrong -- that they do have cancer or heart disease. Most of these people are really the worried well, and they frequently undergo large medical evaluations. They may have a medical problem, but most likely it will be a biochemical imbalance in the brain contributing to their anxiety. For

other individuals it will be unresolved psychological tensions, which may only be approached through therapy and counseling. Nonetheless, the proper approach is to do a physical exam, routine blood tests, brain mapping, and psychodiagnostic evaluation. Remember, most people who excessively worry about their health are manifesting symptoms of anxiety and depression. The real key is to find out why they have so much anxiety and depression, how much is biochemical, how much is psychological, and how much is neurological. Most hypochondriacs will respond to antidepressants, anticonvulsants and/or less conventional approaches such as CES and amino acids.

Physical Causes of Anxiety-Like Symptoms

CATEGORY	SPECIFIC CAUSES
Cardiovascular:	Angina pectoris, arrhythmias, congestive heart failure, hypertension, hypovolemia myocardial infarction, syncope (of multiple causes), valvular disease, vascular collapse (shock)
Dietary:	Caffeinism, monosodium glutamate (Chinese-restaurant syndrome), vitamin deficiency diseases
Drug-related:	Akathisia (secondary to antipsychotic drugs), anticholinergic toxicity, digitalis toxicity, hypotensive agents, stimulants (amphetamines), withdrawal syndromes (alcohol or sedative-hypnotic), anemia
Immunologic:	Anaphylaxis, systemic lupus erythematosus
Metabolic:	Hyperadrenalism (Cushing's disease), hyperkalemia, hyperthermia, hyperthyroidism, hypocalcemia, hypoglycemia, hyponatremia, hypothyroidism, porphyria (acute intermittent)
Neurologic:	Encephalopathies (infectious, metabolic and toxic), essential tremor, intracranial mass lesions, postconcussion syndrome, seizure disorders (especially of the temporal lobe) vertigo, multiple sclerosis, cerebral dysrhythmia
Respiratory:	Asthma, chronic obstructive pulmonary disease, pneumonia, pneumothorax, pulmonary edema, pulmonary embolism
Secreting tumors:	Carcinoid, insulinoma, pheochromocytoma, small cell lung cancer and squamous cell lung cancer
Psychiatric:	Organic depressions, anxiety syndromes

In sum, virtually any physical disease may produce anxiety.

Depression and Manic Depression

Most physicians classify depression as monopolar (poor appetite, weight changes, insomnia or hypersomnia, restlessness, loss of interest in pleasure, loss of energy, feelings of worthlessness or guilt, loss of concentration, recurrent thoughts of death, suicide, etc.) or bipolar (same symptoms plus accompanied by agitation, anger, rage). Bipolar depression is distinguished from manic depression in that manic patients have increases in activity, are more talkative, have flight of ideas, inflated self-esteem, decreased need for sleep (days without sleep), distractibility, even choosing activities with a high potential for painful consequences and/or manifesting psychosis.

Most types of depression are treated with drugs which affect the neurotransmitters, e.g., dopamine, serotonin, and norepinephrine. Drugs are usually assigned without benefit of a medical analysis. Measurement of neurotransmitters and amino acids frequently indicates abnormalities in tryptophan (bipolar) or tyramine, methionine and phenylalanine (monopolar). Large doses of these nutrients

and supporting therapy are needed. For example, a bipolar patient deficient in tryptophan may need up to 10 grams of tryptophan, 3 grams of niacin, and 500 mg of B-6 and magnesium. Many other nutrients can be deficient and heavy metals can be in excess. Hence, additional supplementation with zinc, thiamine, folic acid, and B-12 may be necessary.

Monopolar patients often need 3-6 grams of methionine, tyrosine and phenylalanine. Other nutrients may be deficient as well. Monopolar patients are frequently constipated and can be treated with vitamin C, magnesium, or fiber. Norpramin, Prozac, and Wellbutrin are the best drugs for monopolar patients, while lithium, Tegretol, and Depakote are the best drugs for bipolar patients. The classification of depression into two categories is just a guideline. Drugs may be effective at lower doses when combined with amino acids, tryptophan, melatonin, niacin, and CES. Molybdenum, vanadium, and magnesium are nutrients that are often deficient in these patients. Other drugs useful for manic depression are calcium channel blockers which can be replaced by magnesium and antianxiety drugs which may be reduced by inositol. Diet is a big factor in all depressions. The use of stimulants (e.g., caffeine, sugar, carbohydrates, tyramine) and depressive foods (meat, cheese, fat, alcohol) are factors in mood disorders. Dietary adjustment must be made according to the form of depression.

Manic depression should be approached like bipolar depression, yet lithium and other nutrients are necessary. Lithium is usually effective at low doses, 1-3 tablets when combined with tryptophan and niacin. Most manic depression is probably temporal lobe epilepsy and is best treated with anticonvulsants like Tegretol, Depakote, phenobarbital, Diamox, and Dilantin.

MHPG Urine Test for Depression: Method and Explanation

MHPG urine test reveals the breakdown of neurotransmitters in the human brain. A value less than 2.5 reveals a need for Adrenalin-augmenting antidepressants, while values above suggest a need for serotonin-augmenting treatment. Below is a list of nutrients that can substitute partially for antidepressants.

Adrenalin	**Serotonin**
■ Tyrosine	■ Melatonin
■ Phenylalanine	■ Tryptophan
■ Methionine	■ Niacin
■ Copper	■ Zinc
■ Folic Acid	■ Manganese

Discard first void of the morning on the day you begin the test. Save all urine for 24 hours and keep refrigerated. On the following morning, include the first morning void before you bring the specimen in. Record the volume in ml on the label of the small white bottle. Invert the large orange bottle to mix all urine and pour into small white bottle. Only bring white bottle back to office.

Portrait of Aggressiveness

Probably all moral codes in history have been directed toward controlling aggression. Aggression occurs in many forms, and disorders of aggression are epidemic in our society.

Many syndromes are marked by primary problems of aggression. Drug toxicities which cause aggression provided the first data that there was a nutrient basis to aggression. Many drugs which cause aggression as a side effect probably do so by altering nutrient metabolism. Many nutrients and biochemical factors have subsequently been identified as factors in aggression. The analysis of nutritional tests, e.g., heavy metals (hair) and blood tests, can reveal causes of aggression.

Forms of Aggressiveness

Outer:

sadism	- perverse aggressiveness
murder	- violent aggressiveness
sports	- controlled aggressiveness
rape	- controlled violent aggressiveness
accidents	- uncontrolled, unaware aggressiveness
creativity	- aggression toward the old to make something new
love	- aggression matured toward affection
sex	- aggression merged

Inner: suicide   -   violent aggressiveness toward the self
              masochism   -   perverse self-aggressiveness
              depression   -   aggression turned inward
              anxiety   -   beginning of aggressiveness turned inward
              psychosis   -   an aggressive retreat from reality
              epilepsy   -   involving aggression against the body

Social: war   -   aggression of nation against nation
              sports   -   sublimated aggression
              riots   -   perverse violent aggression
              dances   -   diffused aggression

Medical Syndromes of Aggression

Premenstrual syndrome
Cerebral allergy (usually wheat, milk, corn)
Genetic XY syndrome - excessive height and violence in males
Temporal lobe epilepsy
Limbic encephalitis due to herpes or rabies virus
Experimental injury to ventromedial hypothalamus
Increased testosterone - rapists treated with progesterone injections
Lead and heavy metal poisoning
Psychiatric - see forms of aggressiveness

Aggression calming nutrients are B-complex, choline, tryptophan, zinc, etc.
Aggression calming drugs are anticonvulsants, lithium, beta blockers and tranquilizers.

Dissociation

Dissociation is a term we use to talk about divided consciousness or dissociation between conscious and unconscious activities. Dissociative states occur, for example, when people are at the cinema and are completely engrossed in the film they are viewing, unaware of being in an altered state (as if detached from their bodies). Only when the film hits a dull patch, they might wake up. Another instance is when you are reading a book that you have read before; all of a sudden you wake up and realize you are three pages ahead of where you were; you had blanked out and then returned to consciousness. These trancelike states also can occur when you are drowsy when driving at night on the road -- which can be dangerous if you actually go to sleep. These trancelike states also can be due to an injury or post-trance amnesia.

Other dissociative states can occur when you are talking on the telephone, scanning newspapers, or stirring the spaghetti sauce, without ceasing of the initial activity. Everyone daydreams, which is a dissociative state.

Altered states are induced by one's interaction with novels, magazines, movies, pornography, alcohol, cocaine, etc. Sexual experience is a dissociative state. Ultimately, these normal dissociative states could become pathological if they go out of control. Channeling, contacting altered personalities, and schizophrenia are typically permanently altered states. There are often other conditions and dissociative states, besides substance abuse, which can produce trances: sleepwalking, childhood companions, depersonalization, compulsive and unpredictable behavior, frequent mood swings, feeling uncomfortable and being alone, chronic feelings of emptiness and boredom, possession by demons, participation in cults, supernatural experiences, and others.

Being hypnotized easily is associated with the ability to dissociate. An example of hypoxic dissociation from brain trauma is, of course, amnesia following head trauma.

Out-of-body experiences, possession by souls of ancestors, taking on of a new personality, change in facial expressions, changing languages -- all these have been associated with "demons." This possession or dissociative state is either an obsession which results in internal dividedness of consciousness or the existence of incompatible emotional or ambivalent states. All dissociation begins in the lack of unity of the personality, which may be helped toward unification by a unified spiritual concept (i.e., one god). Dissociation plays itself out in day-to-day behavior in phrases like "I am not responsible for abuse." "I am not responsible for my own behavior." Certain language indicates that parts of the self are experienced as different selves; e.g., "It is wrong to show emotions, love/hate emotional experiences," etc. Frequently, the mind dissociates when it cannot handle bad memories, punishment or any other hurtful experience. Dissociations occur in individuals who have somatic symptoms but can not or refuse to relate them to emotional stress; for example, anxiety disorder (palpitations, backache, gastritis, numbness, etc.), eating disorders, panic disorders, psychosexual disorder, depression.

All these disorders have elements of dissociation. In dissociation, splittings or differences occur between the inward self and outward behavior. Unity of personality, therefore, is at the fundamental core of curing dissociation. Unity is probably best structurally symbolized by the idea of kneeling, praying hands, and monotheism. Christianity, in some individuals, has dissociated in that sexuality and emotion are frequently disconnected. Sexual energy is thought to be demonic. Hence, the common association of hyper-religiosity with an altered sexuality occurs at times in Christianity. It is felt that Greek dynamic dualism between mind and body, as well as dissociative romantic psychology, which projects abnormally sexualized religious and psychiatric ideas onto the body and unconscious mind, are especially dissociative. Christianity, actually, although Trinitarian, became a healing force for the worst form of dissociation -- Greek and Roman paganism. The concept of total health of mind, body, and spirit at work in medicine today, is, of course, a great unifying concept in healing. Monotheism heals the splitting of human consciousness and its dissociative disorders associated with disease

Organic Etiology of Psychotic Symptoms

Well Known

- Syphilis
- Pellagra
- Porphyria
- Hypothyroidism
- Drug abuse and intoxicants
- Homocystinuria
- Folate B12 deficiency
- Sleep deprivation
- Gold encephalopathy or any heavy metal
- sepsis, viral encephalitis

Less Well Known

- Hypoglycemia
- Psychomotor epilepsy and atypical seizures
- Cerebral allergy
- Wheat gluten sensitivity
- Histapenia-copper excess
- Histadelia
- Pyroluria
- Wilson's disease
- Chronic Candida infection
- Huntington's chorea

Being Studied

- Prostaglandins
- Dopamine excess
- Endorphins
- Serine excess
- Prolactin excess, cortisone excess
- Dialysis therapy
- Serotonin
- Leucine, histidine, serine, asparagine, excess
- Interferon, amantadine, antiviral drug toxicity
- Organic brain disease

Seasonal Affective Disorder

Seasonal Affective Disorder (SAD) is winter depression, winter "blahs." Victims of SAD can be from all races, ethnic groups, and ages. Many people know they have SAD when they have the following symptoms in the winter:

- Less energy then usual
- Less creative and less productive
- Feel sad, down, or depressed
- Feel less enthusiastic about the future and enjoy life less
- Need more sleep than usual
- No control over appetite or weight

The body releases a hormone called melatonin when it experiences long periods of darkness, and melatonin can cause adverse emotional effects. Bright light will suppress the secretion of the melatonin; hence it can be a useful therapy. It is usually necessary to begin the bright light therapy in the fall and continue until spring. Melatonin can also be given to the seasonal affective disorder patient early in the evening, thereby pushing the surge up earlier and suppressing the coming surge which is later and later with the wintertime and darkness. Melatonin is another way of treating seasonal affective disorder by usurping the body's natural melatonin cycle. For more information about Seasonal Affective Disorder, write to SAD Info., Department J, P.O. Box 10606, Rockville, MD 20849-0606. (See also Light as a Nutrient, Section 19, p. 334.)

Be Your Own Doctor?

Many patients are involved in self-diagnosis. This can be helpful in that a physician may be reminded by a patient about something they may have missed or neglected. A patient reading these handouts may remind a doctor about matters he may have forgotten or not emphasized adequately. Yet, self-diagnosis is frequently characteristic of a patient who tends to resist treatment. Oftentimes, this can be a symptom of a personality disorder, anxiety, hypochondria, or even schizophrenia. No patient can be healed by a physician unless he comes to listen and obey his doctor's advice. This first step of surrender and trust in a physician may be the most important step of your life. In vain, many patients call me doctor but don't listen to my advice.

Baseline Coping Repertoire

Balancing Skills

- Regular exercise
- Regular quality nutrition
- Self-kindness program -- being gentle to yourself
- Access to your own relaxation response

Revitalization and Reframing Skills

- Reframing -- creatively using stress
- Letting go -- of nonproductive attachments and incomplete goals
- Spiritual anchoring -- surrendering to your credo/faith
- Playfulness -- laughing and lightness
- Internal dialogue -- talking gently to yourself

Interpersonal Skills

- Empathetic listening and warmth
- Social connecting -- reaching out and receiving
- Affirmativeness and assertiveness -- saying no and yes
- Conflict resolution techniques -- knowing when to flee and when to fight
- Creating comfort in home and office
- Centering -- being dynamically relaxed
- Value clarification -- what are your values and priorities
- Goal setting -- setting and implementing goals
- Perseverance -- saying yes to discipline and no to procrastination
- Time management -- what is the best use of your time right now
- Autorhythm -- knowing your own circadian rhythm and pace

Cognitive Remediation: Brain Rehabilitation

Advanced Cognitive Remediation System

Cognitive remediation can now be accomplished with newly developed techniques that can improve and may restore premorbid operation of various brain functions or enhance complementary abilities that perform equivalent functions. This process enables the improvement of memory and other cognitive functions that have been impaired by traumatic accidents.

Advances in computer technology and neuroscience have made possible the development of computer-based exercises designed for recovery (in some cases, rapid) of memory, language, numerical, visuospatial, and intellectual processes. These are some of the advantages of the new computerized exercise programs:

More effective: The interactive computer display programs engage the interest and concentration of patients and intensify the beneficial effects of the exercises.

Versatility: The computer permits presentation of all types of exercise material, precisely designed, with exact exposure timing, and immediately scored. The instantaneous scoring allows changes to be made in the choice of exercises and difficulty levels during the session.

Measurable results: The patient's responses to the computer stimuli are automatically evaluated and scored, providing a measured indication of progress and remaining distance to premorbid levels, along with a prognosis of potential for further improvement in functioning.

Graded difficulty levels: Remediation for each of the cognitive skills is graded so that difficulty of the various exercises can be matched to each patient's improving ability at every stage of the remediation program.

Design and Content of the Remediation Program

The neuropsychological test batteries provide detailed information on measurement of specific cognitive deficits. This information is used in selecting the exercises designed to correct those deficits, starting at the ability level indicated by the test results. The selected exercises are then arranged in a program that produces the optimum results without taxing the patient's capacity. Continuous measurement provides for close monitoring of the patient's performance of the various cognitive functions, enabling exact grading of difficulty to advance his/her targeted abilities to higher levels.

Patients who do neuropsychological tests are often

found to have very diverse deficits, including deficits in attention and concentration, memory, hand-eye coordiation, categorization, learning strategies, etc. New comp- uter techniques, as well as new exercise techniques, have been shown to result in repair or recovery of these deficits, somewhat like physical rehabilitation -- one can engage in brain rehabilitation. A cognitive remediation program is now available on computer or in take-home form.

The Neuropsychological Examination

(See discussion, Section 18, p. 282.)

A New Science of Personality

There are new personality tests that are extraordinary in their ability to help an individual know thyself. Although the first principle in the Bible is that he who seeks himself will lose himself, he who seeks God will find himself. After seeking God, we must also see that God has many qualities, and that the better we understand how these qualities are reflected in us, the better we will be able to serve God and love our neighbor.

The two tests with the most incredible ability to contribute to this breakthrough are the Myers-Briggs Type Indicator and the Millon Clinical Multiaxial Inventory. The Myers-Briggs test identifies a basic strategy of personality based on four major categories: Whether you are extroverted or introverted, sensory oriented or intui- tive, thinking or feeling first in your approach to life, and perceptive or judgmental and orderly in your description. Having assessed those four categories and ending up with 16 different types, doctors can get all sorts of clues to basic personality: how the patient can be approached to maintain medications, and how personality type affects the entire cognitive style and approach to life.

The Myers-Briggs test coupled with the Millon test, the personality pathology work of Dr. Theodore Millon, who is charged with the *Diagnostic Statistical Manual of Psychiatry and Personality Disorders*, reveal a great deal about an individual's perception of disease, misconception of illness, etc.

Psychometric Testing

The *Psychosomatics Journal*, 1993, showed once again that patients with aggressive behavior, negative emotions, and negative self-image, are at higher risk for heart disease. They recommend Psychometric screening, the way that PATH does it with the Millon Profile, on all patients with heart disease problems, to alert the clinician concerning how to manage aggressive behavior, negative self-image, and other negative emotional factors that contribute to heart disease.

Psychotherapy

The first reports by researchers on the benefits of short term psychotherapy services on lowering the costs and utilization of medical and laboratory services were published in 1968. Eleven years later, a review of 58 research studies on the cost implications for short term psychotherapy reiterated that 85% of these studies confirmed the substantial reduction of medical and surgical costs for these patients.

PATH now offers seven different types of therapy because we know how critical therapy is to stress reduction. We have brain wave training cognitive remediation, psychoanalysis, cognitive psychotherapy, adaptive and career counseling, and marriage, pastoral, and addictions therapy offered to individuals, couples, and groups.

To meet your needs, ask what type of therapy you want. There is a whole strategy in picking a therapist. So do not allow yourself to idly page through a phone book to choose a therapist. Dr. Braverman studies each patient's medical needs and personal values in recommending a patient-therapist match. Great therapy can be great for your life.

The Psychodiagnostic Examination

The purpose of the psychodiagnostic examination is to provide the treating professional(s) with a comprehensive understanding of the patient's condition. The evaluation assesses current cognitive and psychological functioning, and provides information regarding the potential contributions of psychological and physiological factors to the patient's presenting problems. Such information is critical in terms of making accurate judgments and recommendations regarding treatment. The psycho-diagnostic evaluation also yields information regarding personality style and coping resources, which may be useful in devising an individualized treatment approach.

Typically, the examination lasts approximately three hours (but can be less or more, depending on the situation), during which a wide variety of objective and clinical tests are administered. Following the interpretation of examination results, a report will be prepared for the referring physician. A post-test consultation may be scheduled to discuss the evaluation's findings.

Please notify us of your insurance coverage so that we may work with you on how to pay the fees, and assist you with processing your claims.

Information About the
Myers-Briggs Type Indicator (MBTI)

The MBTI is not a test. It is a personality indicator designed to increase our understanding of an individual's beliefs and behavior. It was developed by the mother-daughter team of Isabel Myers and Katherine Briggs based on the psychological theories of Dr. Carl Jung.

You will be asked to answer a series of questions. Please remember that there are no right or wrong answers and no good or bad personality types. Some questions may be difficult to answer because you may want to pick both choices. Respond in the way that is most typical of you (do not answer as you'd like to be or as others would like you to be). It takes an average of 20 minutes to complete the questions.

After your indicator is scored you will be told which of the 16 personality types most closely corresponds with your answers. Only you can be the final judge of which type fits you the best. Some of the most common practical applications of the MBTI include:

- increased self awareness
- improved understanding of the similarities and differences between ourselves and others
- couple counseling
- career counseling
- team building and organization development
- spiritual guidance
- developing the skills associated with other personality types

The cost to take the MBTI is $200.00 [1] and this will include one brief interpretation with David Goldstein, Ph.D. Further interpretation is encouraged to get the full benefit of what the MBTI has to offer. If this fee is difficult for you, please let us know. We may be able to work with your insurance company to make this more affordable.

Please feel free to ask any additional questions you may have.

---

1. Subject to change without notice.

How the Myers-Briggs is Used for Evaluating Patient Compliance

Myers-Briggs is not really a test in the conventional sense, but a personality indicator designed to increase a physician's understanding of an individual's beliefs and behaviors in regard to their illness. Each person has a type made up of four components: E for extroverted or I for introverted, S for sensing or N for intuition, T for thinking or F for feeling, J for judging or P for perceiving. For example, a person with an ESTJ thinking pattern frequently does not take feeling values into account and overlooks feeling values and what other people care about. Therefore they build up pressure and find expression in inappropriate ways. Frequently this type of patient can be worked with to show how they might overly exaggerate their medical symptoms because of the building up of pressure and not be able to deal with their feelings in a more appropriate manner. This will enable the physician to guide medical care in a more appropriate way. ESTJ types are generally good at seeing what is illogical and inconsistent and this could be appealed to to help them diminish the pressure of their own feelings. Furthermore, this type may need help to reveal what they like, not merely what needs to be corrected, and therefore it should be elicited from the ESTJ what their medical choices are, and they will need more work by the doctor to elicit this.

ENTJ also need to work on feeling values, as they often rely on the logical approach and overlooking feeling values. They also can build up pressure which can find expression in inappropriate ways such as generalized anxiety, somatization, etc. These individuals, therefore, need to draw upon what is logical, and they can help diminish their medical symptoms and help themselves understand their medical care more appropriately. One must appeal to their logic and consistency when their feelings are overwhelming them. It is very important to help them learn an appreciation of the doctor's ideas and to give them adequate explanation. These types of patients need adequate explanation. They also need assistance in drawing out what they like about their medical care and what they do not like, rather than just dealing with what they want to correct in their health problems.

Individuals with ISTP temperaments on the Myers-Briggs Type Indicator frequently put off decisions or do not follow through. It is critical for a doctor to know this since he/she can predict ahead of time if a patient is going to follow advice. This can be extremely dangerous, of course, and in the long run can reduce the cost of medical care by a physician being alert to this trait immediately. These individuals also like economy of effort and therefore combining things and doing as much as possible at one time is very helpful. Frequently, if they do not have good judgement, they don't bother getting help and nothing important gets done. Therefore, it is critical for the physician to check the judgement and to realize if the patient is truly understanding of the problem.

INTP individuals rely so much on logic that they overlook what people care about and what they themselves care about. Therefore, they need help to realize the importance of their medical care. Frequently they are very logical and if you can appeal to logic, this sometimes can override some of their feelings. Logic frequently results in the suppression of their feeling values, and the feelings may build up pressure until expressed in inappropriate ways. Frequently they have difficulty in understanding how this got to this point and therefore it can help to explain that the neglect of their feelings resulted in an overexaggeration of health problems. Instead of analyzing what is wrong, you can appeal to their analyzing skills. It is hard for them to express appreciation so a physician must recognize that he/she may not get feedback in that manner and not to expect it.

The ESFJ type of personality has a hard time admitting the truth about problems with people or things they care about. They frequently will try to avoid, therefore you may have to work very hard as a doctor to explain to them directly and clearly how serious their problem is. They will try to avoid it, and you have to help them face disagreeable facts or criticism. They try to ignore their problems instead of searching for solutions. Therefore you need to enlist other family members to get compliance.

The ENFJ also finds it hard to admit the truth about problems with people or things they care about. Since they fail to face disagreeable facts, refuse to look at criticism when it hurts, and ignore problems instead of seeking solutions, again, confrontation and getting family support is very important. It requires a lot of work with them as well to help them understand their illness and problems and frequently you need to get family support.

The ISFP are often too sensitive and vulnerable and have dwindling confidence in life and in themselves. They are frequently weak and unable to go ahead and make the decisions they should make. They want to be needed and therefore have to get other people to help express that so they can get help. They have trouble being effective. They take for granted anything they do well and are the most modest of all the types. They underrate and understate themselves, therefore you have to be very careful with the ISFP that the severity of their problems will be understated. They will keep to themselves and will not let a person know and therefore you could have a time bomb.

The INFP also frequently have a sense of inadequacy and they keep dreaming of the impossible. They can be lost in a dream world and also not confront their illness. They become overly sensitive and vulnerable, have dwindling confidence in their life and themselves, and this is a type of person who will have inaction regarding their medical care.

The ESTP are effective if they have good judgement. They use their thinking principles to provide standards for their behavior and direction and purpose in their lives. When their judgement is not well-developed, they do not have stick-to-it-ness and they adapt mainly to a love of a good time and go from thing to thing and place to place. Frequently this person can be a very fickle patient and one has to be very careful that they do not continue having a case of doctoritis.

The ESFP success depends again on how much judgement they acquire. They need to develop their feelings so they can use their values to provide standards for their behavior. If judgement is not developed enough to give them character and stick-to-it-ness, they are also in danger of developing love of a good time and going from doctor to doctor and place to place.

The ISTJ sometimes retreat and feel that nothing of value has been produced. These individuals frequently withdraw and do not follow through. The physician must be very careful to enlist their thinking processes and get them to realize their problems. They are very suspicious of imagination and intuition and therefore they want just the facts from the doctor.

The ISFJ often is not effective in dealing with the world when their feeling preferences are not well-developed. They retreat and become absorbed in their own inner reactions and sense impressions and nothing of value comes out. They tend to be somewhat

suspicious of imagination and intuition, and they do not take it seriously enough. Therefore you have to stick with the facts and help them understand their feelings and not let them get overwhelmed by their medical problems.

The INTP are being drawn to exciting challenges of new possibilities. If their judgement is undeveloped, they commit themselves to ill-chosen projects and fail to finish anything. These individuals are the types who go from doctor to doctor, and one must be careful to settle them down and try to help them strengthen their judgement.

ENFP also goes from possibility to possibility. If their judgement is undeveloped, they commit themselves to ill-chosen projects and fail to finish anything. These are the people who love you as a doctor one minute and hate you the next.

INTJ are the types that do not listen to the opinions of others. These are the patients who will not listen to the doctor at all. You have to bang it home with this type of person. Without judgement, they are unable to shape their own inspirations and their own understanding into effective action. They need assistance. They need to get the family involved, and structure may need to be insisted upon by the doctor.

The INFJ individual sees the goal clearly but they fail to look for other things that might conflict with goals. When their judgement is undeveloped, they do not listen to feedback from others. Frequently a doctor has to get extra family members enlisted in this particular person's problems so they can hear the feedback. They try to regulate everything, small matters as well as great ones, according to their own ideas so little is accomplished. They can get overly involved with minutiae. They can be very good at taking medicine, but they may not follow your overall plan; therefore, you have to help them see the bigger picture.

In conclusion, the Myers-Briggs is an extraordinary instrument to help the physician get patients to follow the best advice for their own benefit. With such an instrument, a new era in medicine is available where a physician can change his/her behavior to meet the type of person he/she is dealing with so he/she can more effectively get the patient to follow advice. Without this information, it is a shot in the dark because the majority of problems that are faced in medicine today are a result of patients who do not follow medical advice. Without following medical advice, nothing can be accomplished. This test is a great way of giving us a strategy for helping patients proceed with their care.

Five Symptoms of Psychiatric Disorders

- Psychotic changes
- Affective changes
- Cognitive changes
- Behavioral changes
- Biological changes

The brain frequently presents itself as primarily biological changes.

The Millon Test and Heart Disease

Dr. Braverman's approach to screening all patients for Millon profile before seeing them was validated by a letter by Mark Ketterer, Ph.D., in the *Journal of Psychosomatics*. He was the consulting liaison psychiatrist at Henry Ford Hospital. He presented to the Academy of Psychosomatic Medicine that the amount of anger and distress was so critical a dimension of heart disease, and chronic negative emotions so much a risk factor, that the most cost effective means of alerting cardiologists and internists was through psychometric screening. The best profile is the Theodore Millon Profile.

Computerized Psychological Tests

The Millon Clinical Personality Inventory

Minnesota Multiphasic Personality Inventory

The holistic approach to health includes the belief that the whole person needs to be understood in order to select appropriate treatment. This means understanding the individual's personality, beliefs, ways of dealing with others, etc. The tests listed above are widely used to identify personality traits. Computers offer the additional advantage of being able to do comparisons and analyze the answers in a way no human examiner can. The results can also give clues about which medications and form of vitamins may be most effective and what health strategy will be best for your long term benefit.

Try to answer the questions as honestly as possible. Some questions will be easier to answer than others. It is the overall pattern that is important, not each individual answer. You will have opportunity to review the results with Dr. Braverman during your visit. Please feel free to ask any questions you may have.

Psychological testing is one part of the total health care of a patient; it helps the doctor to make better medical judgments as well as deal with psychological aspects of the patient's medical illness. A significant amount of your long-term health problems can be explained by this test.

Clozaril Dose Schedule

DAY	DATE	MORNING DOSE	BEDTIME DOSE	TOTAL
1. _____ _____		None	12.5 mg (1/2 - 25 mg tablet)	12.5 mg
2. _____ _____		None	25 mg (one 25 mg tablets)	25 mg
3. _____ _____		25 mg (one 25 mg tablet)	25 mg (one 25 mg tablets)	50 mg
4. _____ _____		25 mg (one 25 mg tablet)	50 mg (two 25 mg tablets)	75 mg
5. _____ _____		50 mg (two 25 mg tablet)	50 mg (two 25 mg tablets)	100 mg
6. _____ _____		50 mg (two 25 mg tablet)	75 mg (three 25 mg tablets)	125 mg
7. _____ _____		50 mg (two 25 mg tablet)	100 mg (one 100 mg tablets)	150 mg
8. _____ _____		50 mg (two 25 mg tablet)	100 mg (one 100 mg tablets)	150 mg
9. _____ _____		50 mg (two 25 mg tablet)	100 mg (one 100 mg tablets)	150 mg
10. _____ _____		100 mg (one 100 mg tablet)	100 mg (one 100 mg tablets)	200 mg
11. _____ _____		100 mg (one 100 mg tablet)	100 mg (one 100 mg tablets)	200 mg
12. _____ _____		50 mg (two 25 mg tablet)	100 mg (two 100 mg tablets)	250 mg
13. _____ _____		50 mg (two 25 mg tablet)	100 mg (two 100 mg tablets)	250 mg
14. _____ _____		100 mg (one 100 mg tablet)	100 mg (two 100 mg tablets)	300 mg
15. _____ _____		100 mg (one 100 mg tablet)	100 mg (two 100 mg tablets)	300 mg

Diary for Neurological/Somatization Disorders

DAY/DATE							

MEDICATION:

NAUSEA							
HEADACHE							
BURNING IN ARMS							
BURNING IN FEET							
BURNING IN HANDS							
BURNING IN LEGS							
BURNING IN BACK							
URINE URGENCY							
RUNDOWN							
WHOOSHING SOUND GOING TO SLEEP							
HEAVY ARMS AND HANDS							
OTHER							

COMMENTS:

Link Support Group Listing [1]

ALA-Call New Jersey	800-322-5525
AIDS Network	800-262-0733
Alcoholics Anonymous	908-668-1882
Alcoholics Anonymous South	609-888-3333
Cancer Information	800-4CANCER
Cocaine Helpline	800-COCAINE
Child Abuse Hotline	800-792-8610
Alzheimers Support Group	908-788-7580
CODA	800-OK4-CODA
Counsel on Compulsive Gambling	609-599-3299
Deaf Hearing Impaired	800-792-8339
Food Addicts Anonymous (FAA)	908-654-6223
Helpline	800-792-8600
Narcotics Anonymous	800-992-0401
New Jersey Drug Hotline	800-225-0196
Overeaters Anonymous	800-743-8703
Parents Anonymous	800-843-5437
Self Help Clearing House	800-367-6274
Suicide Hotline	800-272-4630
Women's Hotline	800-322-8092

---

1. From *The Recovery Link*, vol. 1, # 3, July 1994.

Personality Disorders [1]

Paranoid Personality Disorder

A pervasive and unwarranted tendency, beginning by early adulthood and present in a variety of contexts, to interpret the actions of people as deliberately demeaning or threatening, as indicated by at least four of the following:

(1)   expects, without sufficient basis, to be exploited or harmed by others
(2)   questions, without justification, the loyalty or trustworthiness of friends or associates
(3)   reads hidden demeaning or threatening meanings into benign remarks or events, e.g., suspects that a neighbor put out trash early to annoy him
(4)   bears grudges or is unforgiving of insults or slights
(5)   is reluctant to confide in others because of unwarranted fear that the information will be used against him or her
(6)   is easily slighted and quick to react with anger or to counterattack
(7)   questions, without justification, fidelity of spouse or sexual partner

Schizoid Personality Disorder

A pervasive pattern of indifference to social relationships and a restricted range of emotional experience and expression, beginning by early adulthood and present in a variety of contexts, as indicated by at least four of the following:

(1)   neither desires nor enjoys close relationships, including being part of a family
(2)   almost always chooses solitary activities
(3)   rarely, if ever, claims or appears to experience strong emotions, such as anger and joy
(4)   indicates little if any desire to have sexual experiences with another person (age being taken into account)
(5)   is indifferent to the praise and criticism of others
(6)   has no close friends or confidants (or only one) other than first-degree relatives
(7)   displays constricted affect, e.g., is aloof, cold, rarely reciprocates gestures or facial expressions, such as smiles or nods

Schizotypal Personality Disorder

A pervasive pattern of deficits in interpersonal relatedness and peculiarities of ideation, appearance, and behavior, beginning by early adulthood and present in a variety of contexts, as indicated by at least five of the following:

(1)   ideas of reference (excluding delusions of reference)
(2)   excessive social anxiety, e.g., extreme discomfort in social situations involving unfamiliar people
(3)   odd beliefs or magical thinking, influencing behavior and inconsistent with subcultural norms, e.g., superstitiousness, belief in clairvoyance, telepathy, or "sixth sense," "others can feel my feelings" (in children and adolescents, bizarre fantasies or preoccupations)
(4)   unusual perceptual experiences, e.g., illusions, sensing the presence of a force or person not actually present (e.g., "I felt as if my dead mother were in the room with me")
(5)   odd or eccentric behavior or appearance, e.g., unkempt, unusual mannerisms, talks to self
(6)   no close friends or confidants (or only one) other than first-degree relatives

---

1. These tables of personality disorders are reprinted with permission from the *Diagnostic and Statistical Manual of Mental Disorders, Third Edition, Revised,* Copyright 1987 American Psychiatric Association.

(7) odd speech (without loosening of associations or incoherence), e.g., speech that is impoverished, digressive, vague, or inappropriately abstract

(8) inappropriate or constricted affect, e.g., silly, aloof, rarely reciprocates gestures or facial expressions, such as smiles or nods

(9) suspiciousness or paranoid ideation

Antisocial Personality Disorder

A. Current age at least 18.

B. Evidence of Conduct Disorder with onset before age 15, as indicated by a history of three or more of the following:

(1) was often truant

(2) ran away from home overnight at least twice while living in parental or parental surrogate home (or once without returning)

(3) often initiated physical fights

(4) used a weapon in more than one fight

(5) forced someone into sexual activity with him or her

(6) was physically cruel to animals

(7) was physically cruel to other people

(8) deliberately destroyed others' property (other than by fire-setting)

(9) deliberately engaged in fire-setting

(10) often lied (other than to avoid physical or sexual abuse)

(11) has stolen without confrontation of a victim on more than one occasion (including forgery)

(12) has stolen with confrontation of a victim (e.g., mugging, purse-snatching, extortion, armed robbery)

C. A pattern of irresponsible and antisocial behavior since the age of 15, as indicated by at least four of the following:

(1) is unable to sustain consistent work behavior, as indicated by any of the following (including similar behavior in academic settings if the person is a student):

    (a) significant unemployment for six months or more within five years when expected to work and work was available

    (b) repeated absences from work unexplained by illness in self or family

    (c) abandonment of several jobs without realistic plans for others

(2) fails to conform to social norms with respect to lawful behavior, as indicated by repeatedly performing antisocial acts that are grounds for arrest (whether arrested or not), e.g., destroying property, harassing others, stealing, pursuing an illegal occupation

(3) is irritable and aggressive, as indicated by repeated physical fights or assaults (not required by one's job or to defend someone or oneself), including spouse- or child-beating

(4) repeatedly fails to honor financial obligations, as indicated by defaulting on debts or failing to provide child support or support for other dependents on a regular basis

(5) fails to plan ahead, or is impulsive, as indicated by one or both of the following:

    (a) traveling from place to place without a prearranged job or clear goal for the period of travel or clear idea about when the travel will terminate

    (b) lack of a fixed address for a month or more

(6) has no regard for the truth, as indicated by repeated lying, use of aliases, or "conning" others for personal profit or pleasure

(7) is reckless regarding his or her own or others' personal safety, as indicated by driving while intoxicated, or recurrent speeding

(8) if a parent or guardian, lacks ability to function as a responsible parent, as indicated by one or more of the following:

(a)   malnutrition of child
(b)   child's illness resulting from lack of minimal hygiene
(c)   failure to obtain medical care for a seriously ill child
(d)   child's dependence on neighbors or nonresident relatives for food or shelter
(e)   failure to arrange for a caretaker for young child when parent is away from home
(f)   repeated squandering, on personal items, of money required for household necessities

(9)   has never sustained a totally monogamous relationship for more than one year
(10) lacks remorse (feels justified in having hurt, mistreated, or stolen from another)

Borderline Personality Disorder

A pervasive pattern of instability of mood, interpersonal relationships, and self-image, beginning by early adulthood and present in a variety of contexts, as indicated by at least five of the following:

(1)   a pattern of unstable and intense interpersonal relationships characterized by alternating between extremes of overidealization and devaluation
(2)   impulsiveness in at least two areas that are potentially self-damaging, e.g., spending, sex, substance use, shoplifting, reckless driving, binge eating (Do not include suicidal or self-mutilating behavior covered in [5].)
(3)   affective instability: marked shifts from baseline mood to depression, irritability, or anxiety, usually lasting a few hours and only rarely more than a few days
(4)   inappropriate, intense anger or lack of control of anger, e.g., frequent displays of temper, constant anger, recurrent physical fights
(5)   recurrent suicidal threats, gestures, or behavior, or self-mutilating behavior
(6)   marked and persistent identity disturbance manifested by uncertainty about at least two of the following: self-image, sexual orientation, long-term goals or career choice, type of friends desired, preferred values
(7)   chronic feelings of emptiness or boredom
(7)   frantic efforts to avoid real or imagined abandonment (Do not include suicidal or self-mutilating behavior covered in [5].)

Histrionic Personality Disorder

A pervasive pattern of excessive emotionality and attention-seeking, beginning by early adulthood and present in a variety of contexts, as indicated by at least four of the following:

(1)   constantly seeks or demands reassurance, approval, or praise
(2)   is inappropriately sexually seductive in appearance or behavior
(3)   is overly concerned with physical attractiveness
(4)   expresses emotion with inappropriate exaggeration, e.g., embraces casual acquaintances with excessive ardor, uncontrollable sobbing on minor sentimental occasions, has temper tantrums
(5)   is uncomfortable in situations in which he or she is not the center of attention
(6)   displays rapidly shifting and shallow expression of emotions
(7)   is self-centered, actions being directed toward obtaining immediate satisfaction; has no tolerance for the frustration of delayed gratification
(8)   has a style of speech that is excessively impressionistic and lacking in detail, e.g., when asked to describe mother, can be no more specific than, "She was a beautiful person."

Narcissistic Personality Disorder

A pervasive pattern of grandiosity (in fantasy or behavior), lack of empathy, and hypersensitivity to the evaluation of others, beginning by early adulthood and present in a variety of contexts, as indicated by at least five of the following:

(1) reacts to criticism with feelings of rage, shame, or humiliation (even if not expressed)
(2) is interpersonally exploitative: takes advantage of others to achieve his or her own ends
(3) has a grandiose sense of self-importance, e.g., exaggerates achievements and talents, expects to be noticed as "special" without appropriate achievement
(4) believes that his or her problems are unique and can be understood only by other special people
(5) is preoccupied with fantasies of unlimited success, power, brilliance, beauty, or ideal love
(6) has a sense of entitlement: unreasonable expectation of especially favorable treatment, e.g., assumes that he or she does not have to wait in line when others must do so
(7) requires constant attention and admiration, e.g., keeps fishing for compliments
(8) lack of empathy: inability to recognize and experience how others feel, e.g., annoyance and surprise when a friend who is seriously ill cancels a date
(9) is preoccupied with feelings of envy

Avoidant Personality Disorder

A pervasive pattern of social discomfort, fear of negative evaluation, and timidity, beginning by early adulthood and present in a variety of contexts, as indicated by at least four of the following:

(1) is easily hurt by criticism or disapproval
(2) has no close friends or confidants (or only one) other than first-degree relatives
(3) is unwilling to get involved with people unless certain of being liked
(4) avoids social or occupational activities that involve significant interpersonal contact, e.g., refuses a promotion that will increase social demands
(5) is reticent in social situations because of a fear of saying something inappropriate or foolish, or of being unable to answer a question
(6) fears being embarrassed by blushing, crying, or showing signs of anxiety in front of other people
(7) exaggerates the potential difficulties, physical dangers, or risks involved in doing something ordinary but outside his or her usual routine, e.g., may cancel social plans because she anticipates being exhausted by the effort of getting there

Dependent Personality Disorder

A pervasive pattern of dependent and submissive behavior, beginning by early adulthood and present in a variety of contexts, as indicated by at east five of the following:

(1) is unable to make everyday decisions without an excessive amount of advice or reassurance from others
(2) allows others to make most of his or her important decisions, e.g., where to live, what job to take
(3) agrees with people even when he or she believes they are wrong, because of fear of being rejected
(4) has difficulty initiating projects or doing things on his or her own
(5) volunteers to do things that are unpleasant or demeaning in order to get other people to like him or her
(6) feels uncomfortable or helpless when alone, or goes to great lengths to avoid being alone
(7) feels devastated or helpless when close relationships end
(8) is frequently preoccupied with fears of being abandoned
(9) is easily hurt by criticism or disapproval

Obsessive Compulsive Personality Disorder

A pervasive pattern of perfectionism and inflexibility, beginning by early adulthood and present in a variety of contexts, as indicated by at least five of the following:

(1) perfectionism that interferes with task completion, e.g., inability to complete a project because own overly strict standards are not met

(2) preoccupation with details, rules, lists, order, organization, or schedules to the extent that the major point of the activity is lost

(3) unreasonable insistence that others submit to exactly his or her way of doing things, or unreasonable reluctance to allow others to do things because of the conviction that they will not do them correctly

(4) excessive devotion to work and productivity to the exclusion of leisure activities and friendships (not accounted for by obvious economic necessity)

(5) indecisiveness: decision making is either avoided, postponed, or protracted, e.g., the person cannot get assignments done on time because of ruminating about priorities (do not include if indecisiveness is due to excessive need for advice or reassurance from others)

(6) overconscientiousness, scrupulousness, and inflexibility about matters of morality, ethics, or values (not accounted for by cultural or religious identification)

(7) restricted expression of affection

(8) lack of generosity in giving time, money, or gifts when no personal gain is likely to result

(9) inability to discard worn-out or worthless objects even when they have no sentimental value

Multiple Personality Disorder

Multiple Personality disorder has been regarded by numerous philosophies and views as a dissociative disorder. Others view it as coming from a demon. Studies have shown that multiple personality disorder patients have borderline, avoidant, self-defeating, and schizoid personality types which are organic in nature.

We have seen brain maps of such patients that are somewhat similar to schizophrenia and temporal lobe disorder. Treatment often includes medication similar to those disorders. In some cases even attention deficit disorder is at the root.

Multiple personality disorder as a diagnosis should be avoided. More specific diagnosis in classical medicine should be established.

References Regarding Personality Disorders

Ross, C., *Multiple Personality Disorders: Diagnosis, Clinical Features and Treatment*, John Wiley, 1991.

Millon, T., *Disorders of Personality DMS-III; Axis II*, John Wiley, 1987.

Millon, T., *Millon Clinical Multiaxial Inventory-II*, sec. ed., National Computer Systems, 1987.

Neuropsycho-Spiritual Development

STAGES	PSYCHOSEXUAL STAGES FREUD'S & ERIKSON'S	MAHLER'S SEPARATION INDIVIDUATION PROCESS MODIFIED	PIAGETIAN PERIODS OF INTELLECTUAL DEVELOPMENT MODIFIED	KOHLBERG'S STAGES OF MORAL DEVELOPMENT	MILLON PERSONALITY DEVELOPMENT POSSIBLE STAGES	MYERS-BRIGGS TYPE
I	Oral-Respiratory, Sensory-Kinesthetic (Incorporative Modes) (1)	a) Normal Autism(0-2 mos) b) Symbiosis (as one with mother) (2-4 mos) Differentiation (separate identification, physical separation)(4-7)	Sensorimotor (1-2 yrs)	Precognitional Morality (Early Childhood) Obedience, punishment, submission	Dependent-Passive, Active-Histrionic	(NF) Intuitive feeling, Dependent closeness (SP) Sensory Perceiving, Joy of childhood
II	Anal-Urethral, Muscular(Retentive-Eliminative) (1-3)	Practicing a) moving away from mother b) free locomotion (7-15)	Symbolic (2-7) (pre-operational)	Hedonistic: personal gratification	Ambivalent-Independent-Dependent Compulsive-Passive-Aggressive	(SJ) Guardian, Protector of the family, Sensory protective-anal
III	Infantile-Phallic Locomotor (4-5)	Rapprochement (separation anxiety, return to mother) (16-24)	Concrete Operations (object relations and manipulation) (7-11)	Conventional role-conformity (Early childhood /Adolescence Compliance with social conventions and expectations of other (seeking personal approval by significant others, who serve as role models)	Independent-Narsistic-Aggressive	(NT) Oedipal, conquering
IV	Latency (6-13)	Consolidation (24-36)	Formal (propositional) Operations (11-) (abstract logic, concepts)	Extends #3 to larger context of society, involving regulation of social order by specific laws and standards (Adult)	Boundary Developmental Failure, Anti-social borderline, Self-defeating	(SJ) Dominant
V	Puberty (13-) (Adolescence)	Familial growth a) immediate family b) extended family c) work community	Daily abstraction and planning Weekly abstraction and planning	Self-accepted principles Duties and rights in abstract: legal and social laws and obligations prevail over individual rights in the best interests of all	Detached-Avoidance, Detached-Passive or Schizoid	(SP) Dominant
VI	Young Adulthood	d) local community e) national community f) world community	Monthly-yearly abstraction and planning	Individual principles of conscience	Detached with bound to failure, major potential personality deterioration, paranoid schizotypal	
VII	Adulthood	g) congregational-spiritual-world	Historical and Generational Abstractions	Individual principle of conscience in context with historical, cultural, religious, broader perspective	Resolution of all previous crisis in development	(NT) Dominant
VIII	Maturity		Lifetime Abstraction and Planning			Utilization of all four types

Adapted from the book *Stages of Faith* by James W. Fowler

Aspect: STAGE	A. Form of Logic (Piaget)	B. Perspective Taking (Selman)	C. Form of Moral Judgment (Kohlberg)	D. Bounds of Social Awareness	E. Locus of Authority	F. Form of World Coherence	G. Symbolic Function	EMERGENT STRENGTH OR VIRTUE OF EACH FAITH STAGE	CONVERSION-GIVING RISE TO RECAPITULATION OF PREVIOUS STAGES
I	Preoperational	Rudimentary empathy (egocentric)	Punishment - reward	Family, primal others	Attachment/dependence relationships. Size, power, visible symbols of authority	Episodic	Magical -Numinous	Infancy (Undifferentiated Faith)-Mutuality, trust, and pre-images of the Ground of Being	Reconstitution of pre-images of Ground of Being; re-establishment or deepening of basic trust
II	Concrete Operational	Simple perspective taking	Instrumental hedonism (Reciprocal fairness)	"Those like us" (in familial, ethnic, racial, class and religious terms)	Incumbents of authority roles, salience increased by personal relatedness	Narrative-Dramatic	One-Dimensional, literal	Early Childhood (Intuitive-Projective Faith) Rise of imagination; formation of images of Numinous and an Ultimate Environment	Transformed primal images of Numinous and the Ultimate Environment
III	Early Formal Operations	Mutual interpersonal	Interpersonal expectations & concordance	Composite of groups in which one has interpersonal relationships	Consensus of valued groups and in personally worthy representatives of belief-value traditions	Tacit system, felt meanings symbolically mediated, globally held	Symbols multi-dimensional, evocative power inheres in symbol	Childhood (Mythical-Literal Faith)-the rise of narrative and the forming of stories of faith	New stories, a new people, new community of faith
IV	Formal Operations (Dichotomizing)	Mutual, with self-selected group or class (societal)	Societal perspective, Reflective relativism or class-biased universalism	Ideologically compatible communities with congruence to self-chosen norms and insights	One's own judgement as informed by a self-ratified ideological perspective. Authorities and norms must be congruent with this	Explicit system, conceptually mediated clarity about boundaries and inner connections of system	Symbols separated from symbolized Translated (reduced) to ideations. Evocative power inheres in meaning conveyed by symbols	Adolescence (Synthetic-Conventional Faith)-The forming of identity and shaping of a personal faith	New identity in relation to new center of value, images of power, master story
V	Formal Operations	Mutual with groups,	Prior to society,	Extends beyond class	Dialectical joining of	Multisystemic symbolic and	Postcritical rejoining of	Young Adulthood (Individuative-	New vocational horizon; new

	A. Form of Logic (Piaget)	B. Perspective Taking (Selman)	C. Form of Moral Judgment (Kohlberg)	D. Bounds of Social Awareness	E. Locus of Authority	F. Form of World Coherence	G. Symbolic Function	EMERGENT STRENGTH OR VIRTUE OF EACH FAITH STAGE	CONVERSION-GIVING RISE TO RECAPITULATION OF PREVIOUS STAGES
	(Dialectical)	classes and traditions "other" than one's own	Principled higher law (Universal and critical)	norms and interests. Disciplined ideological vulnerability to "truths" and "claims" of outgroups and other traditions	judgment-experience processes with reflective claims of others and of various expressions of cumulative human wisdom.	conceptual mediation	irreducible symbolic power and ideational meaning. Evocative power inherent in the reality in and beyond symbol and in the power of unconscious processes in the self	Reflective Faith) Reflective construction of ideology; formation of a vocational dream	theology
VI	Formal Operations (Synthetic)	Mutual, with the commonwealth of being	Loyalty to being	Identification with the species, Trans-narcissistic love of being	In personal judgment informed by the experiences and truths of previous stages purified of egoic striving, and linked by disciplined intuition to the principle of being	Unitive actuality felt and participated unity of "One beyong the many	Evocative power of symbols actualized through unification of reality mediated by symbols and the self	Adulthood (Conjunctive Faith) Paradox, depth and intergenerational responsibility for the world	New quality of partnership with Being in and for the world
VII	Formal Operations (Teleological)	Mutuality of love of God and neighbor	Loyalty to God's commands	Serving God and the entire human family	The convicted (sinful) self	Part of the body of God "World coherence"	Resurrected self	Part of the tree of life	One with Messiah

For Further Reading

Gifts Differing by Isabel Meyers with Peter Meyers, Consulting Psychologists Press: Palo Alto, CA.

Working Together, A Personality Centered Approach to Management by Olaf Isachsen and Linda Berens, Neworld Management Press: Coronado, CA.

Work, Play and Type: Achieving Balance in Your Life by Judith Provost, Consulting Psychologists Press.

The 3 books above can be ordered through Consulting Psychologists Press, 1-800-624-1765

Please Understand Me by David Keirsey and Marilyn Bates, Prometheus Nemesis Books: Box 2748, Del Mar, CA. 92014, (619) 632-1575 (also available in local bookstores).

The Prayer and Temperament: Different Prayer Forms for Different Personality Types by Chester Michael and Marie Norrisey, The Open Door, Inc.: P.O. Box 855, Charlottesville, VA 22902, (804) 293-5068.

Type Talk: The 16 Personality Types That Determine How We Live, Love, and Work, Otto Kroeger and Janet M. Thuesen, Bantam Doubleday Dell Publishing Group, Inc.: New York, 1988.

Sixteen Men Understanding Masculine Personality Types, Loren Pedersen, Shambhala Press: Boston and London, 1993.

Life Types by S. Hirsh and G. Kummerow, Warner Books: Warner Communication, 1989

Blending Temperaments - Improving Relationships - Yours and Others by Ruth McRoberts Ward with John E McRoberts and Marvin A. MacRoberts, Baker Bookhouse: Grand Rapids, MI 49516, 1988.

Personality Type and Religious Leadership by Roy M. Oswald, Otto Kroeger, Alban Institute Publication, 1988.

Wholeness Lies Within by Terence Duniho, Type and Temperament, Inc.: 1986, 1987, 1991.

Portraits of Temperament by David Keirsey, Prometheus Nemesis Book Co., 1987.

Opposites: When ENFP & ISTJ Interact by William D. G. Murray and Rosalie R. Murray, Type Communications, 1988.

Discover The Power of Introversion by Cheryl N. W. Card, Type & Temperament Press, 1993.

Personalities at Risk: Addiction, Codependency and Psychological Type by Terence Duniho, Type & Temperament, Inc., 1989.

Who We Are is How We Pray by Dr. Charles J. Keating, Twenty Third Publications, 1991.

How We Belong, Fight and Pray by Lloyd Edwards. Alban Institute Publication. 1993.

Pygmaleon Project, Vol. III, *The Idealist* by Steven Montgomery, published by Prometheus Nemesis Book Company: P.O. Box 2748, Delmar, CA 92014.

23. *Pulmonary Disorders*

Spirometry or PFT

A Pulmonary Function Test (PFT) will measure the health of your pulmonary (lung) function. You will be asked to perform a variety of breathing maneuvers such as blowing out as hard as you can into a mouthpiece and then breathing in and out as fast as you can. The mouthpiece you will use is attached to a sophisticated instrument which will determine things such as your vital capacity, or the total amount of air you can breathe in and out as well as your airway resistance, which is increased in asthma and emphysema. Many other more technical measurements are made which determine the presence of early lung disease or abnormal performance.

The technician may give you a puff of a medicated inhaler to breathe and then repeat the test again. This is in order to determine if your breathing improves after a "bronchodilator." This is the case in some people with allergies, asthma or some types of emphysema.

PFT's should be done by any patient who smokes, has any lung disease, chronic cough, a shortness of breath, and generally any person over the age of 50. Total vital capacity predicts longevity and risk of lung cancer, especially in smokers. Hence spirometry is an important part of a total health analysis.

The Benefits of Spirometry

Office-based spirometry is an extremely useful test. The test is useful in asthma, smoking (e.g., individuals suspected of small airway disease due to smoking), bronchitis, allergy, chronic obstructive pulmonary disease, obesity, lung tumors, pneumonia, chest wall disease, and pleural effusions. Many dusts and chemicals can be associated with pulmonary function. Restrictive lung disorders can be found under the following conditions:

- Asbestos (insulation, construction, mining)
- Ceramic dust (talc, mica, kaolin)
- Fiberglass
- Metal dust (beryllium, iron, copper, rare earths)
- Lung disorders (usually pneumoconiosis)
- Silica mining and sandblasting, uranium mining, vermiculite-insulation, zeolite

Spirometry can be useful in occupational asthma which has many causes. Causes are ammonia fumes -- fertilizers, refrigeration -- anhydride dust, plastics and epoxy resins, animal protein dust from food processing and breeders, antibiotic powders, manufacture of pharmaceuticals, aluminum soldering flux, chlorine gas -- water purification, bleaching -- plastics, cotton dust-textile factories, di-isocyanide-spray painting, polyurethane foam, various dyes, enzyme dust from foods and detergents, flax dust from farmers and paper workers, grain dust -- farmers, grain handlers, food processors -- nitrogen oxides-air pollution, arc welding, fertilizers, organophosphates-pesticides, ozone air pollution, air welding, sewage and water treatment, phosgene gas, plant protein dust-food processing, iodine and fluoride/PVC fumes, plastic wrapping and heated plastic, smoke and fire chemicals, sulphur dioxide-air pollution, bleaching and paper manufacture, vegetable gums, and wood dust in lumber mills and carpentry shops.

Spirometry is also useful in any individual who is expecting to go for thoracic or upper abdominal surgery (age greater than seven years old), lengthy general anesthesia or history of cough, smoking, or wheezing. In acute asthma with FEV (forced expiratory volume), greater than 65% of predicted volume can be reasonably expected. Individuals with severe status asthmaticus usually have FEV-1 (one second) of one or less and less than 30% of predicted volume. FEV-1 or forced expiratory volume of one second is particularly useful for smokers and patients with asthma, bronchitis, allergies and COPD. FVC (forced vital capacity) usually indicates parenchymal diseases such as obesity, lung tumor, pneumonia, chest wall disease, pleural effusion. Early COPD in smokers will show up with an abnormal FEF or forced expiratory flow between 25% and 75%. This can be small airway disease.

Lung volume is restricted by many disorders -- of both intrinsic and extrinsic causes -- as well as neuromuscular disorders. Examples are as follows:

Intrinsic lung disorders

- Interstitial fibrosis
- Congestive heart failure with pulmonary edema
- Pneumonia
- Sarcoidosis
- Pneumoconiosis
- Tuberculosis
- Radiation-induced fibrosis
- Mitral stenosis with resulting lung disease
- Pneumonectomy or lobectomy
- Pneumothorax

Extrinsic disorders

- Gross obesity
- Spinal deformity/kyphosis/scoliosis
- Thoracoplasty
- Cushing syndrome
- Ankylosing spondylitis
- Pleural effusion
- Pleural fibrosis or tumor
- Pregnancy
- Ascites or abdominal masses
- Pain upon inhalation - pleurisy, rib fractures or incisions

Neuromuscular disorders

- Generalized weakness-malnutrition
- Paralysis in one or both diaphragms
- Myasthenia gravis
- Amyotrophic lateral sclerosis
- Muscular dystrophy
- Poliomyelitis

Also, poor effort upon inhalation, or tight clothing, can give false positive spirometry readings.

Common causes of upper airway obstruction which can affect spirometry are:

- Upper airway obstruction
- Vocal cord paralysis
- Postsurgical tracheal stenosis due to endotracheal tube
- Bronchial carcinoma near the carina
- Sleep apnea syndrome with macroglossia or excessive pharyngeal tissue
- Children with large tonsils or adenoids
- Thyroid masses obstructing the trachea

- Foreign bodies within the airway

The flow meter is particularly useful in making a diagnosis in the following conditions:

- Vocal cord paralysis which results in variable extrathoracic upper airway obstruction.
- Tracheal stenosis due to inflammation which causes a fixed extrathoracic upper airway obstruction.
- Polypoid tumor in the trachea which causes a variable intrathoracic upper airway obstruction.
- Squamous cell carcinoma of the right mainstem bronchus which would cause a fixed intrathoracic upper airway obstruction.
- Obese patients with sleep apnea demonstrate a fluttering plateau during forced exhalation or forced inhalation. This also can be found in Parkinson's disease.
- Non-reproducible or oddly-shaped inspiratory flows suggest submaximal efforts.

Asthma and Anxiety

A study by Clifford Bassett, M.D., Brooklyn, New York, Long Island College Hospital (1993), that patients who have asthma have more anxiety, fear, loneliness, insomnia, and depression, and that the brain controls the body and these are brain chemical imbalances. Therefore we do a brain electrical map on all patients to determine how much organic brain component is contributing to the medical condition. You cannot treat the body without dealing with the brain.

Asthma and Exercise

Asthmatics can do exercises for breathing rehabilitation. *How to Become a Former Asthmatic* by Paul Servino is a useful book for this. This book describes various chair exercises where, primarily, an individual sits on a chair and does an inhalation coming up and a forced exhalation going down. An extra bellow push out is another variation of this exercise which exercises the diaphragm.

Another technique is to put the proper hand position approximately on the waist, slightly above the belt, and to check the inflow of air as it comes in.

Also putting your hands on your knees while practicing posture on a chair can be another mechanism for getting proper breathing.

Singing exercises, diaphragmatic movement, all can help an asthmatic to some degree.

24. Rheumatological Disorders and Arthritis

Gout and Elevated Uric Acid

Gout is a disease in which uric acid (a breakdown product of DNA or purines) builds in the blood and tissues, and acute inflammatory joint pain develops. The arthritis is a response to uric acid crystals, which deposit in the synovial fluid of the joints. Some patients develop large, aggregated crystals called tophi. Patients with chronic gout are at risk for kidney disease and uric acid kidney stones.

Elevated uric acid levels without symptoms of gout are common, and about 20% (in the elderly) may progress to gout. Risks of drug treatment can be substantial, hence, a low purine diet with less red meat is the first approach. Uric acid is poorly soluble in urine, and some acids make this insolubility a clinical problem. Nicotinic acid and tartaric acid will precipitate gouty attacks, while ascorbic acid solubilizes uric acid. Tartaric acid is found in red wines.

High purine foods are: anchovies, asparagus, brains, kidney, liver, meat extracts, mincemeat, mushrooms, sardines, and sweetbreads.

Although gout and hyperuricemia are primarily of unknown origin, they can occur in the following conditions:

- Various drugs (e.g., thiazides, steroids)
- Chronic hemolysis
- Lesch-Nyhan syndrome
- Polycythemia vera
- Leukemia
- Von Gierke's disease
- Stress

In some cases of schizophrenia, and even cancer, elevated uric acid may be beneficial. This is because purines are inhibiting or calming neurotransmitters in the brain and have an antiarrhythmic action in the heart. Uric acid has antioxidant properties.

Treatment of elevated serum uric acid and acute gout is usually with anti-inflammatory agents or colchicine. Treatment for the chronic manifestations is usually with allopurinol or probenecid, the latter having fewer side effects. A regular daily aspirin dosage may also be effective.

Nutrition and Osteoarthritis

A low fat diet is essential for treating arthritis since saturated fat is the precursor of inflammatory substances (arachidonic acid). Refined carbohydrates and the night shade family (pepper, paprika, tomatoes, eggplant, and potatoes) are known to have possible implications in inflammatory processes. Similarly, other stimulants and depressant items such as caffeine, alcohol, dried fruit, etc. are eliminated since they may provoke anxiety which can cause a subjective sense of bone ache or arthritis.

Nutrients with proven therapeutic benefit for arthritis are omega 3 oils (1-2 capsules), methionine (1-3 grams),

and histidine (2-4 grams). Other nutrients with suspected therapeutic benefit in high doses include niacin, niacinamide, zinc, primrose oil, and antioxidants. All dosing should be done by a physician.

Nutrient treatments which may augment this therapy are the sulfur amino acids, vitamin C, zinc, and evening primrose oil (or borage oil). An optimal dose of vitamin C, two to three grams per day, can improve elevated serum uric acid level, and the patient slowly eliminates the excess uric acid. The scientific basis of this anecdotal finding is unclear.

Rheumatoid Arthritis

Rheumatoid arthritis is a persistent, serious disorder of unknown cause. Rheumatoid arthritic patients typically have a serum copper level twice the normal level and are low in zinc and manganese. Excess copper intake occurs from drinking water flowing through copper pipes, or use of commercial multivitamin-mineral formulas. In most cases of arthritis it probably reflects inflammation and/or mobilization of the body's natural estrogens.

Supplemental zinc and manganese along with vitamin C may help bring copper levels down to normal in 6 to 12 months, and joint symptoms may subside.

Occasionally, rheumatoid arthritis will occur after exposure to lead, cadmium, or other toxic metals. This can be detected by hair analysis. Zinc and vitamin C help remove most toxic metals.

Serum iron is frequently low while there is excess iron in joints and other tissues. With supplemental zinc and manganese, excess tissue iron may be displaced and serum iron may rise. Supplements of iron are often still necessary.

Many rheumatoid arthritic patients are deficient in sulfur, which is best supplied by antioxidant therapy.

Vitamin C, B-6, and niacin, or niacinamide, may be beneficial. Pantothenic acid helps in some cases, but in others it may worsen joint pains.

Arthritis sufferers may be sensitive to a chemical in plants of the nightshade family (potatoes, tomatoes, eggplants and peppers). By avoiding these foods as well as tobacco (also a nightshade) for at least three months, many arthritics, both rheumatoid and osteoid, have found relief. In certain cases, arthritis can be caused and aggravated by allergy to commonly eaten foods such as wheat, milk or pork, and improvement does not occur until these are avoided.

Rheumatoid arthritis can be helped by a variety of other nonconventional means such as antidepressants (Wellbutrin, desipramine). Antibiotics, especially tetracycline, and other drugs (nonsteroidal, and anti-inflammatory) as well as gold, methotrexate prednisone etc., may be necessary.

Fibromyalgia Syndrome (FMS)

Fibromyalgia Syndrome (FMS) is a musculoskeletal pain and fatigue disorder. Patients with FMS ache all over and sometimes have twitching and burning muscles. It is usually a mixed picture of both a medical disorder and anxiety symptoms. The aching all over can often be due to a postinfectious state similar to the way people feel after flu or chronic fatigue syndrome. FMS can be marked by elevations in sedimentation rates, C-reactive protein, T-helper/T-suppressor ratio, or even a positive ANA. Some of the twitching and burning symptoms are actually due to stress, worry, anxiety, and depression associated with the condition. To meet the strict criteria for FMS, one must have widespread pain in all four quadrants of the body for a minimum duration of three months, and at least 11 of 18 specified tender points. These 18 sites are used for diagnostic cluster, and are on the shoulder, neck, hip, chest, elbow, and knee region. The pain of FMS can be throughout the body, with deep muscular aching, burning, throbbing. Sometimes the FMS symptoms are due to brain burnout, and this will show up on a brain electrical map in an alpha-EEG anomaly. If a sleep EEG is done, there can also be abnormalities in sleep stages. Symptoms associated with FMS can be anxiety and brain arrhythmia symptoms, such as irritable bowel syndrome, constipation, diarrhea, abdominal pain, gas, nausea, chronic headaches, recurrent migraines, tension headaches, temporomandibular joint dysfunctions (TMJ), premenstrual syndrome, numbness, tingling sensation, muscle twitching, irritable bladder, feeling of swollen extremities, skin sensitivities, dry eyes and mouth, dizziness, etc. Change in weather and cold or drafty environments can worsen symptoms. The cause of FMS remains elusive, but can be due to infection, automobile accident, rheumatoid arthritis, lupus, hypothyroidism, psychological stress, brain chemical imbalances, particularly in serotonin levels; which is why Prozac, Zoloft, Anafranil, and tryptophan are thought to be beneficial. The symptoms of FMS may wax and wane due to stress.

Capsaicin

A good relief for arthritis is now available in a cream called Capsaicin (an extract from Cayenne pepper). This red pepper cream is great for arthritis and for neuropathies of the feet in diabetes. It was previously only available as Zostrix in small tubes, but is now available in a good size tube for about $10.

25. Sex

Sexual Brain Health and Increasing The Sex Drive

Integral to having a healthy brain is the presence of a healthy sex drive. It is no surprise that antidepressants like Wellbutrin and Nardil can impact sexual health in either a negative or positive manner. Usually Wellbutrin, tyrosine, DL-phenylalanine, and zinc increase sex drive. For some individuals -- both men and women -- Yocon (or yohimbine chloride, another adrenaline-producing herb) can be a tremendous sex stimulant and can be taken in doses as high as 40 mg per day safely (watch high blood pressure). Sex is a barometer of brain health and brain neurotransmitter function. Frequently, sex can be affected by numerous diseases which are the result of bad habits, such as diabetes due to sugar and carbohydrate addiction and vascular disease due to smoking. These bad habits (and therefore the disease) are avoidable if the brain rhythm is correct and addiction does not set in.

Sex, Infertility, and Impotence

Much has been said about sex, nutrition, and fertility, but very little is known. The role of zinc, calcium, carnitine, and arginine in sperm function has suggested possible roles for these nutrients in combatting infertility. A drug that inhibits phenylalanine metabolism can cause male infertility since it is possible that phenylalanine may promote fertility and sex drive. High fat and protein diet also may promote fertility since fat is converted to sex hormones.

Most infertility we see is due to marijuana abuse or occupational chemical exposure. Caffeine and nicotine may also have a negative effect on sperm.

An evaluation of various nutrients is important. A conventional endocrinology workup is essential for all cases of infertility. Infertility in women is easier to solve with use of various hormones (e.g., pergamol, LHRH, Clomid) than infertility in men.

Impotence in men is a common problem. Nutrients that increase circulation, e.g., niacin, EPA, vitamin E, have been suggested as useful. A drug, Yohimex (Yocon), increases catecholamines and sex drive, as may the amino acids, tyrosine and phenylalanine. (Methionine increases absorption.) Vitamin E therapy has been used to treat the unusual Peyronie disease (fibrous disease of the penis).

High doses of Yocon, up to 40 mg a day, can drastically increase sex drive but can raise blood pressure. Most impotence problems that will not respond to nutrients and yohimbine (Yocon) have an organic basis and require an external blood evaluation for hormone imbalance and diseases like diabetes and arteriosclerosis, which are often causes of impotence.

Prostate Problems

The following symptoms -- some or all -- may indicate a prostate problem:

1. Have you noticed a change in your urination pattern lasting for two weeks?

2. Is your urine flow weaker or interrupted?

3. Do you have difficulty urinating?

4. Do you need to urinate more frequently?

5. Does the need to urinate frequently wake you up at night?

6. Have you noticed any blood in your urine?

7. Do you have difficulty stopping the urine flow?

8. Do you feel a painful or slight burning sensation when you urinate?

9. Have you experienced lower back pain recently?

10. Do you have an achey feeling in your pelvic area or upper thighs?

Remember that prostate cancer and benign prostatic hypotrophy are easy to diagnose by PSA (prostatic specific antigen) and PAP (prostate acid phosphatase) in the blood, or by ultrasound. Zinc, saw palmetto herb, and the drug Proscar are all thought to be helpful in treating this problem.

Adapted from material compiled by American Medical Systems, 11001 Bren Road East, Minnetonka, Minnesota 55343.

Basic Rules of Sex Drive

1. Testosterone levels may increase in the morning.

2. Elevated testosterone is responsible for sex drive in both men and women.

3. Cut down on alcohol and cigarettes.

4. Exercise regularly.

5. Men who win sporting events or watch violence get aroused -- it is a sexual activity.

6. Be creative.

7. Go away together.

8. Think sex -- sex in the brain translates to sex in the bed.

Family Planning and Safe Sex

Family Planning

Now that your baby has been born, you will want to take some steps to prevent an unwanted pregnancy. There are many different types of birth control methods to choose from. Remember that the only way that these birth control methods will work is if you use them every time you have sex and if you use them correctly.

1) **Condoms** (rubbers): A condom is used by the male. It is placed over the erect penis prior to having sex and collects the man's semen. This prevents the sperm from entering the woman's vagina so that she cannot become pregnant. It is important to be careful not to let the condom slip off the penis when pulling out of the vagina. The condom is even safer when the woman also uses vaginal foam. However, do not use Vaseline or baby oil with a condom, as it weakens the condom.

2) **Vaginal foam**: Vaginal foam is inserted into the vagina with an applicant and prevents pregnancy by killing the sperm. It must be applied no more than a half an hour before sex and you must use more foam if you have sex again. You can purchase a foam kit at the drug store.

3) **Sponge**: The sponge is a small round piece of foam rubber with a strap across the bottom which can be purchased at the drug store. It prevents pregnancy by acting as a barrier and by killing sperm. The sponge is moistened with water before it is inserted into the vagina. It can be left in the vagina for up to 24 hours and you can have repeated sexual intercourse. You must leave it in place for at least six hours after you have sex. The sponge is removed by pulling on the strap. The sponge works best when used with something else, like condoms.

4) **Diaphragm**: The diaphragm is a round rubber cup that is used with sperm killing jelly or cream and is placed in the woman's vagina before intercourse. In order to obtain a diaphragm, you must be fitted for one by a doctor or midwife. The diaphragm can be put into the vagina up to six hours before intercourse and must be left in for eight hours after intercourse.

5) **Birth control pills**: The birth control pill is one of the best ways to prevent pregnancy. The pill must be prescribed by a doctor and it must be taken every day. You need to be on the pill for at least 10 days before it will prevent pregnancy. It is important to be in close contact with your doctor, as the pill may have some side effects.

6) **IUD**: The IUD is a small plastic device that is inserted into the uterus (womb) by a doctor and is left in place for at least one year. It has nylon strings attached; for three months after it is inserted you should check for the strings before intercourse. Then check strings after each period. The IUD may also have side effects; therefore, you should be followed closely by your doctor.

Methods such as withdrawal, rhythm, and douching are not going to keep you from getting pregnant. A great way to not get pregnant is to just say "NO!" Saying no delays sexual relationships until you are ready for them and allows you to develop strong friendships and make plans for your future.

Safe Sex

Another important issue today is to learn how to have safe sex. If you are sexually active, you may be at risk for sexually transmitted diseases, including AIDS. You don't have to give up sex altogether, but you may need to change your sexual habits. It is a fact that condoms do not insure safe sex. There is no safe sex except in a faithful marriage or in abstinence.

If you have sex, choose safer sex techniques such as using condoms with spermicide every time you have sex. Condoms will help prevent body fluids from entering your body, which is the primary way that sexually transmitted diseases (STD) are spread. Learn to talk with your partner about safe sex and to say "no" to unsafe sex. Also remember that alcohol and drugs affect your judgment, which increases your risk for engaging in unsafe sex.

We have a great deal more detailed information on both family planning and safe sex. Please Ask!

Birth Control Pills

Some birth control pills may help to prevent certain types of cancer but overall, birth control pills are known to lower beta carotene levels, all B-vitamin levels, especially folic acid and B-6, vitamin C, and E levels. Furthermore, they increase copper and iron levels and decrease zinc. Therefore they can aggravate schizophrenia, depression, cause migraine headaches, increase hypertension and formation of blood clots.

Women who smoke, are above age 35, and have type

A blood should not use the pill because blood clots can occur, and adversely affect sexual desire.

Frequently pills are made up of two synthetic hormones of estrogen and progesterone which negatively impact blood clotting. Birth control pills have also been shown to increase irritability, aggressiveness, anxiety, and possibly ovarian cysts.

I highly recommend other forms of birth control.

References:

Kirschmann JD, Dunne LJ, *Nutrition Almanac*, McGraw-Hill, 1984.

Masse PG, Roberge AG, Relationship between oral contraceptives, iron status and psychoaffective behavior, *Journal of Nutritional Medicine* 2:273-281, 1991.

Palan PR, Romney SL, et al., Effects of smoking and oral contraception on plasma Betacarotene levels in healthy women, Depts. of Obstetrics and Gyn and Epidemiology, Albert Einstein College of Medicine pp. 881-885, 1989.

Ovarian Cysts, *Prevention*, p. 16, 1989.

26. Surgery

Nutrition and Wound Healing [1]

Abstract

A review of the literature reveals that unfavorable surgical outcome, including problems with wound infection arid dehiscence, sepsis, and longer lengths of stay, correlates well with the determination of perioperative malnutrition as measured by a variety of indices. Increased malnutrition and more severe surgeries are individually predictive of poorer outcome. There is evidence that particular deficiencies of nutrients are likely to cause wound healing problems. Particularly important nutrients include amino acids (notably glycine, proline, and arginine) carbohydrates, fatty acids (especially linoleic and linolenic), vitamins (particularly C and A), minerals and the elements (particularly magnesium, copper, phosphorous and selenium). The postoperative feeding of seemingly large amounts of amino acids is correlated with positive nitrogen balance and shorter hospital stays. The enteral route is preferred unless there is disturbed absorption or other complications. Total parenteral nutrition (TPN) formulations should include all of the essential nutrients, especially trace elements which were formerly overlooked.

Introduction

With surgery, as with trauma there is an increase in the requirement for calories, amino acids, vitamins, minerals, water and oxygen.

This paper reviews the possible relationship between certain nutrients and wound healing, evidence pointing to a connection between perioperative nutritional status and surgical outcome (including wound healing), and information concerning route of administration and prevention of deficiencies of certain nutrients.

Nutrients Which May Affect Wound Healing

Wound healing is a biochemical process and that nutrition itself is really a clinical biochemistry, and an obvious relationship between these two areas exists . . . Nutrition has to be thought of by all clinicians as the specific nutrient substrates that are being delivered to the specific cells and tissues at a given) time. This is where nutrition really occurs, at the cell membrane and in the cell, and it is only when we realize this and practice surgery with this in the proper context that we will then achieve optimal wound healing to correlate with the technical and other aspects of wound healing in which we engage as surgeons. [1]

Protein and Amino Acid Balance

Surgery, trauma, and sepsis introduce a protein catabolic state. [2] Wound healing is in part dependent on the ability of the body to provide adequate amounts of amino acids. Animal studies conducted by Harvey and Gibson showed that simultaneous supplementation with glycine, proline, and arginine produced an increase of as much as 60-70% in nitrogen retained. [3] This effect may be reversed if glycine alone is used. [4]

Arginine, which can be converted to proline, is associated with more rapid wound healing and greater collagen synthesis in animal models and may even inhibit posttrauma weight loss. [5,6] Furthermore, arginine deficient rats rapidly lost collagen. [5] Glycine accounts for approximately one third of all amino acids found in most collagen alpha chains. [7] Glycine and arginine are shown to be necessary for the synthesis of creatinine and for optimal growth in experimental animals. [6] Furthermore, arginine detoxifies ammonia and detoxifies benzoic acid. Glycine may play a part in the repair of muscle fibers. [4] Arginine converts to ornithine glutamic semialdehyde and proline, leading to proline's conversion to collagen. Arginine can also be converted to lysine. [4] There are about 200 proline residues and thirty-five lysine residues in the alpha collagen strands. [7] Hypoalbuminism has been associated with impaired healing of forearm wounds in adults. [9] It is thought that the lower plasma albumin levels often observed following injury relate to slowed

1. Helen Rayner, M.P.H., Susan Lovelle Allen, M.D., and Eric R. Braverman, M.D. Reprinted from *The Journal of Orthomolecular Medicine*, first quarter, 1991, vol. 6, no. 1.

synthesis and increased deposition at wound sites. (An increase in absolute catabolism of albumin is not observed.[9] Plasma albumin is thought to act as an amino acid donor at wound sites and as a transporter of zinc, fatty acids, and sulfur-containing amino acids. [10]

Research suggests that nitrogen is more likely to be pulled from muscle tissue in surgical stress and the liver is likely to be spared. [9] Even the early stages of protein-calorie malnutrition have been correlated with impaired wound healing not unlike that of advanced malnutrition. [29] There is some evidence that slow scar formation in humans nevertheless results in normal scar tissue. [11]

Carbohydrates and Fats

Fatty acids are essential for the transport of substances across cell membranes. The optimal level of fat consumption for wound healing has not been determined but 20% or more is common in hospitals. Moderate liquid levels can reduce the potential hypoglycemic effect of high glucose feeding. A deficiency in essential fatty acids is associated with poor wound healing. [12] However, an experiment involving over 30% fat in a total parenteral formula yielded very unsatisfactory postsurgical results. It was thought that the fat inhibited the movement of leukocytes which are essential for the prevention of sepsis and stimulation of scar tissue formation. [13] Both carbohydrates and fats are important in that they provide calories, have a protein sparing effect and provide energy. Generally, it is necessary to use combinations of energy sources and proteins/amino acids in order to preserve or augment nitrogen balance, if less than caloric need of carbohydrate/lipid is given, it is also difficult to achieve positive nitrogen balance. [14] Usually carbohydrates provide the bulk of calories for perioperative patients regardless of route.

Water

Subcutaneous tissue is highly influenced by vasoconstriction and can be poorly hydrated while the brain, liver, heart, and kidney are well perfused. Studies show that dehydration is associated with low tissue pO_2 and increased catabolism. [15] Such patients are considered to be more susceptible to infection. One might postulate that supplies of other essential nutrients to wounds would be impaired as well by dehydration. When dialysis and heavy loads of water are used, the purity of water (i.e., low levels of aluminum and lead) is essential.

Oxygen

Subcutaneous hypoxia can be found in 33% to 80% of postoperative patients. [15] Most cases can be returned to normal tissue oxygen levels through vigorous hydration efforts and administration of a higher percent of oxygen. Medicine needs an easy, accurate way to measure tissue oxygen. Until this exists, aggressive measures to ensure hydration are essential to safeguard against hypoxia. [15]

A state of slight hyperoxia (obtainable usually with either normobaric or hyperbaric oxygen administration) can increase leukocyte bacterial-killing activity. This effect will be additive when done in conjunction with antibiotics. Hyperbaric oxygen treatment raising arterial pO_2 to over 1,000 - 2,000 mm Hg for one hour per day may be adequate to stimulate effective leukocyte bacterial killing. (Surgical manipulation of blood supply can also be used to create hyperoxia. [15]) Davis cites studies that showed that ischemia lowers local immunity and that, in one study, infections were found only in subjects with tissue pO_2 below 10 to 40 torr. Low pO_2 can result in poorly hydroxylated collagen which has less thermal stability. [1]

Vitamins, Minerals, and Wound Healing

Vitamins are essential for wound healing. Gerber found increased tensile strength in the wounds of rats fed supplemental retinylacetate, beta-carotene, or retinoic acid (all forms are precursors of vitamin A) with measurably stronger scar tissue. [16]

Vitamin A has also been shown to have a beneficial effect on the healing of colonic anastomoses. [17] Additionally, the increased risk of anastomotic breakdown, leakages, and spontaneous perforations seen both early and late after radiotherapy may be ameliorated by vitamin A therapy with significant mitigation of the decreased bursting strength and hydroxyproline content of the tissues which is seen after radiotherapy. [18] [19] [20]

Of interest, an actual deficiency of vitamin A may not be required for impaired wound healing. Niu reported increased hydroxyproline content at the site of arterial anastomoses and increased bursting strength at distant sites in rats supplemented with moderate levels of vitamin A over that seen in controls who were themselves on diets several times the National Research Council's RDA. [20]

Topical vitamin A appears also to have its uses; it may reverse the inhibitory effect of steroids on healing wounds, perhaps by affecting leukocyte numbers involved in the inflammatory and wound healing process. [19]

Vitamin A can restore epithelialization in the presence of glucocorticoids which would otherwise suppress macrophage activity and hence wound healing. It cannot, however, overcome the suppressive effect of glucocorticoids on wound contraction. [21]

Vitamin E is a free-radical scavenger which preserves macrophages and polynuclear leukocytes from the lipid peroxides that they make. [22] However, if a vitamin E deficiency exists, there may be some impairment of wound healing. [13]

Vitamin C is an essential cofactor in the formation of collagen. [17] One of the symptoms of scurvy is the weakening and dehiscence of old wounds. [23] Decreased tensile strength was found in the excised wounds of skin and facia lata in subjects deficient in vitamin C. [13] In a double blind study, vitamin C (500 mg) with meals and at bedtime produced a decrease of 43% versus 84% in patients with decubitus ulcers. [26]

The authors feel one striking anecdote concerning vitamin C and wound healing deserves telling. In a panel discussion by leading surgeons, one participant spoke of treating a cancer patient's infected maxillary wound in the pre-antibiotic era with vitamin C. He stated:

> I had read that in an individual who has infection, vitamin C is depleted, and although this man had no evidence of scurvy, I thought it might be a case of subclinical scurvy, so I gave him what I thought at that time was an enormous quantity of vitamin C, 1000 mg a day, and immediately the wound began to heal and the infection was controlled, and he got well, so this made an impression upon me. [13]

Vitamin E has just been added to the list of nutrients that can prevent side effects from surgery, particularly peritoneal adhesions. All those individuals going through laparoscopy, bowel surgery, and even colon surgery should be taking vitamin E prophylactically.

Thiamine deficiency interferes with collagen synthesis; granulation tissue was one fifth normal in thiamine-deficient rats. [24] Pantothenic acid may accelerate the wound healing process; when 20 mg/kg/day was given to rabbits, aponeurotic strength and number of fibroblasts increased. [25] Riboflavin is identified as an important mediator of wound healing. [9]

Zinc is a mineral which is important for the action of collagenase, the enzyme which breaks down collagen. [4]

Since 25% or more of the collagen formed in the first week of wound healing is normally broken down, [27] the importance of zinc can be inferred for the remodeling and strengthening of surgical wounds. One author suggests, however, that significant depletion of zinc stores must exist before it is an issue. Zinc metalloenzymes include DNA polymerase, superoxide dismutase, and reverse transcriptase. Zinc is depleted by stress and suppressed by the influence of ACTH and anabolic steroids which are elevated in the postsurgical patient. [22] Achieving the right balance is the issue. Pories and others found in 1967 that zinc sulfate given orally accelerated wound healing in one patient. Furthermore, Pories and colleagues found that zinc was important to the rapid reduction of wound cavity in excision of pilonidal cysts. [23]

Zinc will reduce copper stores if used in excess. Copper is also essential to proper wound healing as it is a cofactor for the action of lysylamine oxidase (LAO). It is the aldehyde reactions which generate strong covalent bonds in collagen. [7] [28] Selenium is also considered important for wound healing. Manganese is necessary for the glycosylation of hydroxyproline residues in the formation of collagen. [7]

Effects of Nutritional Status on Surgical Outcome and Wound Healing

It would be difficult to prove without a doubt that strong wounds are formed by providing adequate nutrition to patients or that they form faster. Most wound research involving tensile or bursting strength or even speed of wound healing has been done with animals and there are problems in assuming rat or guinea pig wound healing physiology sufficiently parallels that of humans.

Most of the evidence that nutritional status plays an important role in wound healing in humans is more indirect. There are many studies correlating nutritional status (pre- and/or postoperative) to surgical outcome (e.g., number of complications such as ruptured anastomoses, dehiscence, infection, sepsis, and length of stay).

Evaluating Patients At Risk

The prevalence of some degree of malnutrition (protein-calorie and/or vitamin deficiency) is high among medical and/or surgical patients. Buzby reviewed three studies and concluded that about 50% had some degree of protein-calorie malnutrition, regardless of medical specialty or socioeconomic background. [29] A table summarizing such epidemiologic surveys shows 30% to be the lowest rate among major surgery patients with 45-50%

the most common rate of protein-calorie malnutrition. Hypovitaminemia was found in 50% of medical and surgical patients at one New Jersey hospital. [30] Fortunately, serious malnutrition is found less frequently. Severity of complications correlate with the degree of malnutrition and with the seriousness of surgery. [30] The surgeon must take into account the type and extent of surgery to be performed in evaluating risk.

It is estimated that surgical patients lose 4-8% of their body weight for minor surgery and 15-25% for major surgery. [31] Experts advocate taking a very careful nutritional history for all surgical patients, covering weight loss and its time frame and possible causes; dietary habits; surgical history; unorthodox diets, use of medications, drugs or alcohol, food intolerance, functional capacity of the gastrointestinal tract; the presence of fever, tachycardia, catabolism, irritable bowel syndrome or short bowel syndrome. The physical examination can provide useful information on anthropometric measurements, edema, muscle wasting and various signs of deficiencies. Malnutrition is often accompanied by CNS depression, lowered ventilatory drive and blood pressure, bradycardia, achlorhydria, irritability, apathy, and inability to concentrate. [32] Growth hormone is depressed but thyrotrophic and adrenotrophic hormones are not. Objective criteria are used to determine degree of malnutrition, though few utilize all of these measurements: secretory proteins (albumin, transferrin, prealbumin, retinol binding protein), skeletal protein (24-hour urinary creatinine divided by height), muscle degradation (urinary 3-methylhistidine), and various anthropometric determinations (weight-for-height, triceps skinfold, midarm circumference). [32] Immunologic indications (skin test reactivity, complement levels and total leukocyte counts), metabolic profiles, and tests of critical organ function have all been associated with nutritional status. [33]

Correlating Nutritional Status With Surgical Outcome

To review some of the early research, Dr. Radin and others at the University of Pennsylvania produced a hypoproteinemic state in dog's dung in the 1930s and observed retarded gastric emptying times in animals which had gastroenterostomies. Moreover, there were several wound breakages which were attributed to delayed fibroplasia. [13] With human subjects, as early as 1936, Studley showed an association between poor nutrition and surgical outcome, describing how surgical risk increased eightfold (33.3 vs 3.5%) in patients with benign chronic peptic ulcer disease who had lost more than 20% of their body weight as compared with those who had no loss. [34] Controversy arose, however, over the implications of this study, is this association causal and, consequently, is perioperative nutritional supplementation warranted? [29]

Several other studies have answered in the affirmative. Muller randomized 125 surgical patients for ten days to either a typical hospital diet or total parenteral nutrition (TPN) preoperatively. Those on TPN had increased serum total protein, transferrin, albumin, and immunoglobulins as well as skin test responsiveness. Postoperative morbidity (intra-abdominal abscess, peritonitis, anastomotic leakage, ileus) was decreased albeit not significantly; however, the number of patients requiring artificial respiration was increased, again not significantly. [35]

Mughal (1987) studied thirty-two patients with clinical and laboratory evidence of malnutrition (serum albumin <3.5 and recent weight loss >10% plus any two of the following at or below the tenth percentile: weight for height, midarm circumference, triceps skinfold. They were found to have greater postoperative morbidity and mortality when compared to their well-nourished counterparts. In addition, if complications did occur, it took the malnourished patients twice as long to achieve satisfactory oral intake. [36]

The Cardiff study was able to demonstrate a significant decrease in the incidence of wound infections in those given parenteral nutritional support (40% vs 83%). [37] Gill and Mequid showed a correlation between complications (poor wound healing, increased fatality rates, longer hospitalization) and the severity of malnutrition to major surgery. [38] [39] Hospital duration was decreased as much as four to six days to two out of three studies of colorectal surgery. [40] [41] [42]

Dudrick said in a panel discussion that he and colleagues from the University of Texas Medical School (Houston) assessed ninety-six patients who were to have elective hip surgery. Twenty percent were found to be nutritionally deficient, especially ill protein status, when evaluated by fourteen indices. Protocol called for surgery to be done as planned. One year later 18% had significant complications (including infections and wobbling prostheses) and all of these patients had been judged malnourished at the time of surgery. Now they provide all such patients with one to three weeks of a preoperative repletional program (including occasional tube feeding) until normal nutritional status is regained. [15]

Dempsey and Mullen surveyed eighty studies dealing with nutritional status and surgical outcome. They point out that most (forty-five studies) had insufficient data to determine usefulness in terms of sensitivity, specificity, and efficiency. The percentage of patients with poor nutritional ratings who have poor outcomes ranged from 1% to 100% with a mean of 65%. The positive predictive value (which is the percentage of positive tests which are true indicators for outcome) ranged from 1% to 83% with a mean of 37%. Finally, the efficiency of nutritional predictors (or the ability of nutritional ratings to predict either a good or poor outcome) ranged from 27% to 94% with a mean of 68%. The conclusion of the paper is that more rigorous research methodology is needed to evaluate the efficacy of nutritional programs in improving surgical outcome. [33]

A review of the use of nutritional indicators concluded that predicting survival is possible 80% of the time and death 40% of the time. Use of serial measurements (made every 10 to 14 days) allows one to predict death accurately in 78% of all cases. [29] [43]

A set of simple predictive criteria used with elective surgery and other patients at M.D. Anderson Hospital and Hermann Hospital for several years is as follows: the patient is tested for three criteria -- a low serum albumin (less than 3.4 gr per dl), a low total lymphocyte count, and recent inadvertent weight loss of more than 10% body weight. The presence of one indicator corresponds with mild malnutrition, and rare wound disruption; two indicators correspond with moderate malnutrition and a 4-6% rate of wound disruption; three indicators are present in moderately severe to severe malnutrition and are associated with a 14% wound disruption rate. A patient who has lost 30% of their well weight in 30 to 60 days has a 30-50% chance of wound dehiscence. Tissue edema is expected in patients with serum protein below 5.5 gr percent. [13]

The superiority of any one plasma protein or formula as a predictor of surgical outcome is difficult to establish. Pomp and colleagues have summarized the strengths and weaknesses of various nutritional assessment tools. [44] [50] Significant underweight is an obvious and definite health risk. Changes in transferrin correlated significantly with changes in nitrogen balance (p = .02) but prealbumin did not in a study by Fletcher. [45] Transferrin may reduce the supply of iron to invasive organisms. [10]

Hill made a comparison of various studies and concluded that transferrin, prealbumin and the "Leeds Formula" yielded the most significant predictors. Changes in albumin are not rapid enough due to a long half-life; therefore, it is not the best protein for tracking patient progress. (It is useful for predictive outcome at the outset.) Simple determination of weight loss was quite specific for poor surgical outcome as were the Philadelphia and Boston formulas. The surgeon's assessment was 86% accurate for predicting good outcome in the presence of malnutrition but only 27% accurate for predicting a poor surgical outcome (positive predictive value). [10]

Buzby reports that patients having serum albumin levels of 2.6 g per dl or less have a less than 5% chance of survival. (Death is usually by sepsis.) The 50% chance occurs at 3.2 g per dl. [29] A rise in serum prealbumin taken weekly has been shown by Church and others to be predictive of positive nitrogen balance with a sensitivity of 88%, specificity of 70%, positive predictive value of 93%, and negative predictive value of 56%. In cases of death, dropping nitrogen balance was the best indicator. Of all the plasma proteins, prealbumin was the best indicator of poor outcome. [46] However, some consider it to reflect dietary intake more than nutritional status. [44]

Warnold found that malnourished, noncancerous surgery patients (having two or more abnormal values for percent weight loss, body weight relative to reference weight, midarm muscle circumference, or serum albumin) had an average length of stay of twenty-nine days versus fourteen days for normally nourished surgical patients. The malnourished group had a 31% rate of serious complications while the normals had 9% (p <.05). [47]

Patients showing negative response to a set of recall antigens in one study were later to have five times the normal rate of infection and mortality. Therefore when anergy is detected, physicians should assess nutritional risk carefully. [48] Many alterations in host immunity have been noted with malnutrition, including decreased intracellular bacterial killing, decreased C3 (which can in turn decrease opsonic function if the level falls to 30%), and fewer lymphocytes. [48]

Several formulas may be necessary to address all types of surgery. [10] More research is needed to confirm that the observed correlations are strictly nutritional. It is evident that nutritional status has considerable effect on surgical outcome which includes wound healing. Assumptions must be questioned. For example, there needs to be a way to determine in what way feeding will improve the surgical results or if the impact of the disease is mostly responsible for the condition. [49] Determination of the optimal nutritional prognosticators of surgical outcome would help determine more exactly how to do perioperative nutrition.

Protein-calorie malnutrition can occur in surgical and chronically ill patients. Predisposing factors are many, including anorexia, malabsorption due to various gastrointestinal disorders, hypermetabolism secondary to surgery, fever, infection, inflammation, trauma, and abnormal nutrient losses, e.g., after extensive burns. [10]

Perioperative Nutrition

Some considerations in providing perioperative nutrition are covered in this section. It is beyond the scope of this paper to fully describe the benefits and risks of enteral vs. parenteral feeding, the types of feeding arrangements, and possible formulas.

Method of Feeding

Briefly, it should be the principle of health care professionals to use the oral route when possible, followed by nasogastric tube, possibly jejunostomy or gastrostomy (for long-term use), then IV feeding. [10] Some feel a combination of enteral and peripheral parenteral nutrition (PPN) is less invasive than central parenteral nutrition (CPN). [32] However, CPN is the route of choice in severe malnutrition.

Enteral Feeding

Enteral feeding has the advantage of avoiding the accumulation of excess water, [50] encouraging crypt cell turnover and inhibiting villous atrophy in the gut. The stimulation of hormonal secretion may also have beneficial systemic effects. It is especially recommended in protein-calorie malnutrition with severe dysphasia, inadequate oral intake for the five successive days, massive small bowel resection (using TPN as well), and with low output enterocutaneous fistulas. [51]

Problems associated with enteral feeding include poor tolerance in very ill patients, diarrhea, and gastrointestinal intolerance, often due to bolus feedings. [51] Even depleted, stressed patients used only between 40 and 50 kcal/kg/day, the highest requirement going to the normally nourished, stressed patient. These patients have normal metabolic rates which have become somewhat catabolic. [10] [50] A careful calculation of calorie requirement can be made using a formula provided by Horowitz. [31] Protein needs perioperatively will run from 250 mg nitrogen/kg/day for depleted, unstressed patients to 400 mg nitrogen/kg/day for stressed patients. [10] A 70 kg man who has had uncomplicated surgery may need 70 gr/day of protein and a 55 kg woman, 57 gr protein.

Moss (1984) describes eighteen postcholecystectomy patients who were given full enteral nutrition with amino acids immediately postoperatively. Ten of these were given an elemental diet providing 132 gr amino acids/day, eight received 66 gr amino acids/day, and controls were fed with a standard hypocaloric solution. In the unfed controls, decreased branched chain amino acids (BCAAs) were observed; these increased after three or four days and normal levels were finally restored after five to ten days. Patients receiving the higher amount of protein maintained their basal levels immediately postoperatively, then had increased levels. Intermediate amino acid feedings (66 gr) had lower BCAAs for twenty-four hours and then rapidly returned to normal. Moss correlates this positive protein balance and increased serum amino acid levels with enhanced wound healing, resistance to sepsis, and shortened hospital duration. [52] Other studies have confirmed the positive nitrogen balance and reduced hospital duration, but failed to show any decrease in postoperative complications. [53] [55]

Parenteral Nutrition

Direct delivery of calories and nutrients to the bloodstream was first done in 1656 by Sir Christopher Wren who infused ale and wine into the veins of dogs. Various improvements over the next 300 years ensued, but it wasn't until 1967 when Dudrick and associates first developed the use of central venous lines that long-term survival on parenteral fluids was feasible. [56] [57] Now, 5400 mOsm of nutritionally complete, fat-free solution can be provided, supplying 3600 kcal/day and far outdistancing the previous limits of 1800 mOsm and 1000 kcal possible by the peripheral venous route.

Total parental nutrition (TPN) is indicated in patients who cannot absorb through the gastrointestinal tract, have severe diarrhea, disease of small bowel, major surgery, enterocutaneous fistulas, and extremely catabolic states, to name a few indications. [50]

Minor surgery patients are generally considered to need less aggressive nutritional support (e.g., no parenteral nutrition unless severely malnourished). Within seven days of surgery they should be ingesting a maintenance diet orally. [31] Elective colectomy patients, however, were studied for postoperative eating patterns and were shown to have an average 1,155 kcal of calorie deficit daily in the first fourteen days post surgery. [59] Patients with major surgery or injury usually need two to three times the RDA postoperatively to avoid significant weight loss. This is a fascinating example of stress producing a need for mega-nutrition. If patients have protein-calorie malnutrition, they need aggressive preoperative therapy as well. [31]

Glucose and lipid, though both partially protein sparing, are insufficient to maintain a positive nitrogen balance in the absence of exogenous amino acids. [60] However, use of dextrose-free amino acid IV solution has shown no clear benefit. [43] A full range of nutrients including carbohydrates, lipids, and protein have been shown to be more effective. [61]

A fairly standard IV feeding formula today may consist of two solutions, one of amino acids, dextrose, electrolytes, vitamins, and trace elements, and another, lipid emulsion, are used in total parenteral nutrition (TPN); they are infused simultaneously. The standard first solution contains 25% dextrose and 5% amino acids in equal volumes. [23] 115-120 mmol sodium, 80-100 mmol potassium, 10 mmol calcium, 12-15 mmol magnesium, and 12-20 mmol phosphorus are routinely added. Vitamins and trace elements are introduced as required. In the average adult, 1.5-2 L/day of IV solution are given. 1.0 to 1.5 liters of lipid are infused concurrently. These two solutions provide 100 grams of amino acids, 1250-1700 kcal glucose, and 1100-1650 kcal lipid for a total of 2350-3550 kcal/day. [62] [63]

There are many commercially available formulas allowing for accommodation of requirements imposed by specific diseases, and having the advantages of "known composition, controlled osmolality and consistency, ease in preparation and storage, and cosat." One must know when to add vitamin and mineral or amino acid packages which are also prepackaged. [32] [64] It is becoming more widely recognized that steroids, sedatives, antibiotics and anticonvulsants create an additional need for vitamins. [10]

The fat portion of an IV feeding has often been administered separately. However, at least one study shows excellent results with a mixture of 20% fat emulsion, 8% amino acids, dextrose, electrolytes, vitamins, and trace minerals. [63] It was used from 2% to 35% with no adverse results. [70] The lipid portion can be useful in insulin resistant patients, decreasing fatty infiltration of the liver, and because it does not increase osmolality of the solution and may decrease pulmonary diffusion. [12] As much as 20% and even 30% in the IV solution are not uncommon. [50] [65]

Complications of intravenous hyperalimentation (IVH) are not uncommon and include mechanical (pneumo-, hemo-, and hydrothorax, arterial or nerve injury, embolism), septic (contaminants in solution or line, sepsis, especially with Staph aureus and Candida, septic embolism and thromboembophlebitis), and metabolic (hyper- and hypoglycemia, hyperammonemia, increased lipids, and deficiencies of essential fatty acids electrolytes, minerals, trace elements, and vitamins). Continuous TPN is associated with less diarrhea than with intermittent. Bolus feedings are discouraged. [54] Only some of the more important deficiency states will be discussed.

Potential Nutrient Deficiencies

Deficiencies of certain nutrients have occurred over the years in association with perioperative nutrition. A review of them reveals interesting information about deficiency states.

Essential Fatty Acids

One of the first deficiencies to be discovered was the essential fatty acids (EFA). In 1972, Caldwell, et al., described infants on TPN for five or more months. They noted dermatitis, alopecia, thrombocytopenia, and impaired wound healing, all of which improved upon addition of a linoleic acid solution. [66] Other regimens have resulted in increased liver function enzymes, fatty liver and inclusion bodies in hepatocytes, as early as 6-8 weeks after institution of TPN. [12] In addition, Freund has found that an increase in intraocular pressure is a useful early sign in detecting EFA deficiency. [67] This may have relevance to glaucoma. The authors have seen several patients obtain lower intraocular pressures with high dose polyunsaturates.

The optimal amount of linoleic acid is believed to be that which keeps the thrienoic:tetraenoic ratio less than 0.4; in adults being repleted, this is approximately 4% of total calorie intake. [68]

A deficiency state for linolenic acid has likewise been described by Holman, et al., who noted neurological symptoms including paresthesia, numbness, inability to walk, leg pain, and blurring of vision. Others have challenged this report.

Phosphate

As with several other nutrients, a deficiency syndrome for phosphate was not discovered until the 1970's; until this time, TPN solutions had routinely included the anion. With the advent of "new and improved" crystalline amino acid solutions lacking phosphate, however, an acute syndrome of hypophosphatemia was seen to develop within days of starting on TPN.

Lichiman, et al., [70] Silvis and Paragus, [71] and Travis, et al., [72] all reported acute, marked hypophosphatemia (<1.0 mg/dl) in patients on intravenous hyperalimentation;

they noted decreased 2,3-DPG and ATP (both of which require the anion for phosphorylation) with increased hemoglobin affinity for oxygen and resultant respiratory difficulty. The full syndrome includes paresthesia, muscle weakness, encephalopathy, coma, and death. [32] Deficiency of phosphate is also associated with impaired glycolysis, impaired phagocyte function, hemolysis, rhabdomyolysis, and congestive cardiomyopathy. [73] Since phosphate-free IV solutions have been given for years without development of this syndrome, it is believed the problem is an intracellular shift of phosphate caused by the hypercaloric or anabolic effect of the solution.

Phosphate has a role in intermediary metabolism and in cellular/skeletal structure as phospholipids and hydroxyapatite. Parenteral solutions should provide 0.5-1.0 mmol/kg/day in stable patients without renal failure; serum levels are the optimal way to monitor treatment. [73] Clinicians should be aware of phosphate deficiency caused by excess calcium intake.

Zinc

In 1976, Kay, et al., described four patients who after approximately two weeks on TPN developed diarrhea, dermatitis, alopecia, and mental depression concurrent with low serum zinc (<20 mcg/dl, down form 80-150 mcg/dl pre-TPN). [74] They recovered rapidly after zinc supplementation. Fawaz also reported four stressed patients with serum zinc levels between 25-56 mcg/dl; he noted eczematoid dermatitis in all, and decreased hematocrit and albumin in three of the four patients. [75] Arakawa found decreased alkaline phosphate levels associated with subnormal zinc. [76]

Zinc is involved in production of alkaline phosphatase and other enzymes and in protein synthesis. Poor wound healing, impaired immunological function, ageusia, alopecia, acrodermatitis, and anosmia are associated with low levels. There are increased losses of zinc, with GI fistulas, diarrhea, zincuria during amino acid infusions, and rapid weight gain. [32] [67] [73] Supplementation with 2.5 to 4 mg/day in TPN is thought to be sufficient, with an additional 2 mg in acute catabolic states and 6-12 mg with diarrhea or other intestinal losses. [77]

It is possible that higher doses of zinc may produce other benefits in surgical patients.

Copper

As with zinc, copper deficiency related to TPN Solutions was not discovered until the 1970's when the crystalline amino acid mixtures, now free of several trace elements, were first introduced. Karpel and Peden described an infant on prolonged TPN with markedly low serum copper and ceruloplasmin. Microcytic hypochromic anemia, hypoplastic bone marrow, retarded bone age, and metaphyseal bone lesions that corrected with copper were seen. [78] Deficiency is also associated with neutropenia and bacterial infection, and normocytic normochromic anemia. [32] Copper is a cofactor of ceruloplasmin and is involved in the synthesis of oxidative metalloenzymes and elastin. Excreted in bile, these requirements increase with diarrhea, and decrease with liver diseases which block or reduce biliary excretion. Replacement with 0.5-1.5 mg/day is standard. [68]

Chromium

Jeejeebhoy reported a woman in 1977 who presented after three and a half years on TPN with 10% weight loss and peripheral neuropathy with slow nerve conduction. Her glucose tolerance test was abnormal and she had moderate hyperglycemia in the fasting state. Free fatty acids were elevated and her respiratory quotient (RQ) was low. Both serum and hair levels of chromium were low: all symptoms corrected with supplemental chromium. [79]

Chromium is part of the glucose tolerance factor; it is involved in the potentiation of insulin. Standard supplementation is provided in a trace elements package which includes zinc, copper, chromium (10-15 mcg/day) and manganese (0.15-0.8 mg/day). [23] Chromium's role in sugar metabolism has been confirmed.

Selenium

Although "white muscle disease" (loss of myocytes and replacement with connective tissue) has been recognized in New Zealand sheep raised in selenium-deficient soil, it was not until 1979 that van Rij reported TPN patients with a clinical myopathy that corrected on 100 mcg/day of selenomethionine. [80] An earlier report by Fleming, et al., in 1976 described a fatal cardiomyopathy culminating in ventricular fibrillation in a twenty-four year old man on TPN for six years. [81]

Selenium is involved in glutathione peroxidase and vitamin E metabolism with a vulnerability to deficiency being associated with low vitamin E levels. [68] Decreased enzyme levels without clinical manifestations were seen by Baptista; replacement with 100 mcg/day of selenium (as selenious acid) improved selenium levels while RBC glutathione peroxidase remained impaired. [82]

Recommendation for standard replacement has been for 0.04-0.16 mg/day as a toxicity syndrome has been described at higher levels. For depleted patients, 200-400 mcg/day is suggested. [73]

Rare Deficiency Syndromes

Other, more rare deficiency syndromes have been reported: molybdenum, with headache, visual disturbances, and mental changes; biotin, with dermatitis, blepharitis, alopecia, and delirium; and carnitine, with jaundice, muscle weakness, and hypoglycemia. [68] These differences point out the need for a complete balance of nutrients from amino acids to trace elements.

Conclusion

Wound healing requires a complete nutritional effort. The nutritional influences on wound healing are approached in humans mostly from the context of overall surgical outcome. Several studies indicate needs for specific nutrients. Many studies were cited correlating poor surgical outcome with poor nutritional status. Determinants for nutritional status are generally agreed to include anthropometric, serum proteins, immune status, nutritional measurements, and many other indicators but investigators disagree widely as to which ones serve as the most reliable predictors of surgical outcome. Deficiencies of nutrients once manifested during TPN are now more easily avoided with the addition of more fatty acids, amino acids, vitamins, minerals and trace elements. In the future we expect to identify more nutrients, trace metals, peptides, and oils that need to be added to TPN.

References

1. Polk H: In: Sparkman RS, ed. *The healing of surgical wounds: state of the art in the ninth decade of the 20th century.* American Cyanamid Co., 1985:79.

2. Wolfe BM, Ruderman RL, Rollard A: Basic principles of surgical nutrition: metabolic responses to starvation, trauma and sepsis. In: Deital M, ed., *Nutrition in clinical surgery.* Baltimore: Williams and Wilkins, 1985:17.

3. Harvey SG, Gibson JR: The effects on wound healing of three amino acids -- a comparison of two models. *Br. J. Derm.,* 1984; 111(27):171-173.

4. Braverman ER, Pfeiffer CC: *The healing nutrients within: facts, findings and new research on amino acids,* New Canaan: Keats Publishing Inc., 1987:176, 181, 243, 244.

5. Barbul A, Rettura G, Levensen SM, Seifter E: Arginine: a thymotrophic and wound healing promoting agent. *Surg. Forum* XVIII, 1977; (Oct.):101-103.

6. Seifter E, et al.: Arginine: an essential amino acid for injured rats. *Surgery* 1978; 84:224-230.

7. Miller EJ: Chemistry, structure and function of collagen. In: Menaker L, ed., *Biologic basis of wound healing,* New York: Harper and Row, 1975:164-169.

8. Lindstedt E, Sandblom P: Wound healing in man: tensile strength of healing wounds in some patient groups, *Ann. Surg.* 1975; 181:842-846.

9. Navia JM: Nutrition and wound healing. In: Menaker L, ed., *Biologic basis of wound healing,* New York: Harper and Row, 1975:164-169.

10. Hill GL: The perioperative patient. In: Kinney JM, Jeejeebhoy MB, Hill GL, Owen OE, *Nutrition and metabolism in patient care,* Philadelphia, 1988: Harcourt, Brace and Jovanovich, 643-655.

11. Temple WJ, Voitk AJ, Snelling FE: Effect of nutrition, diet and suture material on long term wound healing, *Ann Surg.,* 1975, 182:93-97.

12. Dowling RJ, Alexander MAJ, Mullen JL: Use of fat emulsions. In: Deitel M, ed. Nutrition in clinical surgery, Baltimore: Williams and Wilkins, 1985:139-147.

13. Sparkman RS, ed: The healing of surgical wounds: state of the art in the ninth decade of the 20th Century, American Cyanamid Co., 1985, (Panel discussion transcript) 75-80, 119.

14. Jeejeebhoy KN: Carbohydrate-lipid utilization: mixed fuel delivery for total parenteral nutrition. In: Dietel M, ed., *Nutrition in clinical surgery.* Baltimore: Williams & Wilkins, 1985:121.130.

15. Davis JC, Hunt TK: *Problem wounds; the role of oxygen,* New York: Elsevier.

16. Gerber LE: Wound healing in rats fed small supplement acetate, beta-carotene, or retinoic acid, *Fed. Proceeding* #3543:838, March 1, 1981.

17. Bark S, Rettura G., Goldman D, et al.: Effects of supplemental vitamin A on the healing of colon anastomoses, *J. Surg. Res.* 36:470-474, 1984.

18. Wellwood JM, Jackson BT: The intestinal complications of radiotherapy, *Br. J. Surg.* 60:814-818, 1973.

19. Winsey K., Simon RJ, Levenson SM, et al.: Effect of supplemental vitamin A on colon anastomotic healing in rats given preoperative irradiation, *Am. J. Surg.* 153(2):153--156, Feb. 1987.

20. Levenson SM, Gruber CA, Rettura G, et al.: Supplemental vitamin A prevents the acute radiation-induced defect on wound healing, *Ann. Surg.* 200:106-124, 1984.

21. Ahonen J, Jiborn H, Zederfeldt B: Hormone influence on wound healing. In: Hunt TK, ed., Wound healing and wound infection: theory and surgical practice, New York: Appleton, Century and Crofts, 1980:99-105.

22. Chavpril M: Zone and other factors of the pharmacology of wound healing. In: Hunt TK, ed., Wound healing and wound infection: theory and surgical practice, New York: Appleton, Century and Crofts 1980:135-149.

23. Williams Sr: Nutrition and diet therapy, St. Louis: Times Mirror/Mosby College Publishing, 1985:343, 735.

24. Alvarez OM: Thiamine influence on collagen during granulation of skin wounds. *J. Surg. Res.* 32:24-31, 1982.

25. Aprahamian M, Dentinger A, Stock-Damge C, Kouassi J-C: *J. Clin. Nutr.* 1985:578-589.

26. Haydock DA, Hill GL: Improved wound healing response in surgical patients receiving intravenous nutrition, *Br. J. Surg.* 1987, 74:320-323.

27. Hunt TK commentary: In: Hunt TK, ed., *Wound healing and wound infection: theory and surgical practice*, Appleton, Century and Crofts, 1980:43.

28. Schwartz KJ, Ryan RF: *Wound healing: a programmed surgery manual*, New York: Appleton, Century and Crofts, 1975.

29. Buzby GP, Mullen JL, Matthews DC, Hobbs CL, Rosato EF: Prognostic nutritional index in gastrointestinal surgery, *Am. J. Surg.* 1980: 160-167.

30. Horowitz J, Roongrisuthipong C, Zibida J, Heymsfield SB: Nutritional management of the surgical patient, introduction. In: Lubin M, Walker HK, Smith RB, ed., *Medical management of the surgical patient*, Boston: Butterworths, 1988:3-5.

31. Horowitz J, Roongrisuthipong C. Zibida J, Heymsfield SB: Nutritional consideration in the surgical patient. In: Lubin M, Walker HK, Smith RB, eds., *Medical management of the surgical patient*, Boston: Butterworths 1988:7-24.

32. Fleming CR, Nelson J: Nutritional Options. Kinney JM, Jeejeebhoy MB, Hill GL, Own OE, eds., *Nutrition and metabolism in patient care*, Philadelphia: Harcourt, Brace and Jovenovich, 1988:752-776.

33. Dempsey DI, Mullen JI: Prognostic value of nutritional indices, *JPEN* 1987:11:No.5 supplement: 1095-1145.

34. Studley HO: Percentage of weight loss, *JAMA* 106:458-460.

35. Muller JM, Brenner U, Dienst C. Pichlmaier H: *Preoperative parenteral feeding in patients with gastrointestinal carcinoma*, Lancet 1982, 1:68-72.

36. Mughal MM, Mequid MM: The effect of nutritional status on morbidity after elective surgery for benign gastrointestinal disease, *JPEN* 1987, 11(2):140-143.

37. Heatley RV, Williams RHP, Lewis MH: Preoperative intravenous feeding -- a controlled trial, *Postgrad. Med. J.* 1979, 55:541-545.

38. Gill GL, Blackett RL, Pickford I, et al.: Malnutrition in general surgical patients, *Lancet* 1977, 1:689-692.

39. Meguid MM, Debonis D, Meguid V, Terz JJ: Nutritional support in cancer, *Lancet* 1983, 2:230-231.

40. Collins JP, Oxby CB, Hill GL: Intravenous amino acids and intravenous hyperalimentation as protein-sparing therapy after major surgery, *Lancet* 1978, 1:188-191.

41. Preshaw RM, Attisha RP, Hollingsworth WJ, Todd JD: Randomized sequential trial of parenteral nutrition in healing of colonic anastomoses in man, *Can. J. Surg.* 1979, 22:437-439.

42. Jensen S: Parenteral nutrition and cancer surgery, *JPEN* 1982, 6:335.

43. Blackburn CL, Flait JP, Clowes GH: Peripheral intravenous feeding with isotonic amino acid solutions, *Am. J. Surg.* 1973, 125:447-454.

44. Pomp A, Bates M, Alboner JE: Specialized nutritional support in surgical patients, *Prob. Gen. Surg.* 1988, 5:271-295.

45. Fletcher JP, Little JM, Guest PK: A comparison of serum transferrin and serum prealbumin as nutritional parameters, *JPEN* 1987, 11:144-148.

46. Church JM, Graham IH: Assessing the efficacy of intravenous nutrients in general surgical patients: dynamic nutritional assessment with plasma protein, *JPEN* 1987, 11:135-139.

47. Warnold I, Lundholm K: Clinical significance of preoperative nutritional status in 215 noncancerous patients.

48. Chandra R: Immunity and infection. In: Kinney JM, Jeejeebboy MB, Hill GL, Own OE: *Nutrition and metabolism in patient care*, Philadelphia 1988, Harcourt, Brace and Jevanovich, 600-602.

49. Bozztti F: Nutritional assessment from the perspective of a clinician, *JPEN* 1987, 11:1155-1215.

50. Yeung CK, Smith RC, Hill GL: Effect of an elemental diet on body composition; a comparison on intravenous nutrition, *Gastroenterology* 1979, 77:652-657.

51. ASPEN Board of Directors: Guidelines for the use on enteral nutrition in the adult patient, *JPEN* 1987, 11:435-439.

52. Moss C: Elevation of postoperative plasma amino acid concentrations by immediate full enteral nutrition, *J. Am. Coll. Nutr.* 1984, 3:335-342.

53. Sagar S, Harland P, Shields R: Early postoperative feeding with elemental diet, *Br. Med. J.* 1979, 1:293-295.

54. Hoover HC, Ryan JA, Anderson EJ, Fischer Je: Nutritional benefits of immediate postoperative jejunal feeding of an elemental diet, *Am. J. Surg.* 1980, 139:153-159.

55. Fairfull-Smith RJ, Freeman JB: Immediate postoperative enteral nutrition with a nonelemental diet, *J. Surg. Res.* 1980, 29:236-239.

56. Sanderson I, Basi SS, Deitel M: History of nutrition in surgery. In: Dietel M, ed., Nutrition in clinical surgery, Baltimore: Williams & Wilkins, 1985:139-147.

57. Dudrick SJ, Wilmore DW, Vars HM, Rbcades JE: Long-term total parenteral nutrition with growth, development, and positive nitrogen balance, *Surgery* 1968, 64:142-113.

58. ASPEN Board of Directors: Guidelines for the use of total parenteral nutrition in the hospitalized patient, *JPEN* 1986, 10:441-445.

59. Hackett GF, Yeung CK, Hill GL: Eating patterns in patients recovering from major surgery -- a study of voluntary food intake and energy balance. *Br. J. Surg.* 1979, 66:415-418.

60. Zlotkin SH, Anderson GH: Amino-acid requirements and sources during total parenteral nutrition. In: Dietel M, ed., Nutrition in clinical surgery. Baltimore: Williams & Wilkins, 1985:139-147.

61. Irvin TT, Hunt TK: Effect of malnutrition on colonic healing, *Am. Surg.* 1974, 180:765-772.

62. Steiger E, Gurndfest-Bioniatoruske S, Misny T: Intravenous hyperalimentation: temporary and permanent vascular access and administration. In: Dietel M, ed., *Nutrition in clinical surgery*, Baltimore: Williams & Wilkins, 1985:139-147.

63. Ang SD, Canham JE, Daly JM: Parenteral infusion with an admixture of amino acids, dextrose, and fat emulsion solution: compatibility and clinical safety, JPEN 1987, 11:23-27.

64. Horowitz J, Roongrisuthipong C, Zibida J, Heymsfield SB: Methods of nutritional support. In: Lubin M, Walker HK, Smith RB, eds., *Medical management of the surgical patient*, Boston: Butterworths, 1988:25-40.

65. Alexander JW: Nutritional management of the infected patient. In: Kenney.

66. Caldwell MD, Jonsson HT, Othersen HB: Essential fatty acid deficiency in an infant receiving prolonged parenteral alimentation, *J. Pediatr.* 1972, 81:894-898.

67. Freund HR: Acute renal failure. In: Dietel M, ed., *Nutrition in clinical surgery*, Baltimore: Williams & Wilkins, 1985:348-356.

68. Rudman D and Williams RJ: Nutrient deficiencies during total parenteral nutrition, *Nutr. Rev.* 1985;43(1)1-13.

69. Holman RT, Honson SB, Hatch TF: A case of human linolenic acid deficiency involving neurological abnormalities, *Am. J. Clin. Nutr.* 1982, 35:617-623.

70. Lichtman MA, Miller DR, Cohen J, Waterhouse C: Reduced red-cell glycolysis, 2,3-diphosphoglycerate, and adenosine triphosphate concentration, and increased hemoglobin-oxygen affinity caused by hypophosphatemia, *Ann. Intern. Med.* 1971, 74: 562-568.

71. Silvis SE and Paragus PD: Paresthesias, weakness. seizures, and hypophosphatemia in patients receiving hyperalimentation, *Gastroenter.* 1972, 62:513-520.

72. Travis SF, Sugerman HJ, Ruberg RL, et al.: Alterations red-cell glycolytic intermediates and oxygen transport as a consequence of hypophosphatemia in patients receiving intravenous hyperalimentation, *NEJM* 1971, 285:763-768.

73. Reilly JJ and Gerhardt C: Surgical nutrition, *Current Problems in Surgery* 1985, 22(10):4-81.

74. Kay RG, Tasman-Jones J, Pybus R, et al.: A syndrome of acute zinc deficiency during total parenteral alimentation in man, *Annals Surg.* 1976, 183:331-340.

75. Fawaz F: Zinc deficiency in surgical patients: a clinical study, *J. Paren. Enter. Nutr.* 1985, 9(3):364-369.

76. Arakawa T. Tamura T, Igarishi Y, et al.: Zinc deficiency in two infants during total parenteral alimentation for diarrhea, *Am. J. Clin. Nutr.* 1976, 29:197-204.

77. Mills CB, Gray DS, Freed BA, Kaminski MV: Trace element requirements. In: Dietel M, ed., *Nutrition in clinical surgery*, Baltimore: Williams & Wilkins, 1985:169-184.

78. Karpel JT and Penden VH: Copper deficiency in long-term parenteral nutrition, *J. Pediatr.* 1972, 80:32-36.

79. Jeejeebhoy KN, Chu RC. Marliss EB, et al.: Chromium deficiency, glucose intolerance, and neuropathy reversed by chromium supplements in a patient receiving long-term total parenteral nutrition, *Am. J. Clin. Nutr.* 1977, 30:530-538.

80. Van Rij AM. Thomson CD, McKeniie JM, and Robinson ME: Selenium deficiencies in total parenteral nutrition, *Am. J. Clin. Nutr.* 1979, 32:2076-2085.

81. Fleming CR, Smith LM, Hodges RE: Essential fatty acid deficiency in adults receiving total parenteral nutrition, *Am. J. Clin. Nutr.* 1976, 29:976-983.

82. Baptista RJ, Bistrian BR, Blackburn GI, et al.: Utilizing selenious acid to reverse selenium deficiency in total parenteral nutrition patients, *Am. J. Clin. Nutr.* 1984, 39:816-820.

27. Sports and Exercise

Sports and Exercise:
Nutritional Augmentation
and
Health Benefits [1]

Benefits of Exercise

The Historical Benefits of Exercise

Athletic prowess and strength have always been values respected by our society, even in Biblical times. Jacob wrestled with an angel and prevailed, and rolled a large stone off the mouth of the well, and was marvelled at for his strength (Genesis 25:27; 32:36; 29:10). Exercise was recognized as the great soporific, and sleep of the laboring man was described as sweet (Psalm 27). Strength as the glory of young men was praised (Proverbs 20:29), and even God is characterized as strong and mighty (Psalm 24:8). Learning the sport of archery at 20 years of age is described in Numbers 1:4 and 2 Samuel 1:18. And men were trained to be equally adept in shooting arrows using the right and left hands (1 Chronicles 12:2). Many athletes, as described in the Bible, were able to sling stones at a hairbreadth and not miss, (Judges 20:16) and shoot arrows and great stones from towers (2 Chronicles 26:15). Shooting arrows at specific targets is described in 1 Samuel 20:20, as is the bending of the bow in Lamentations 1:12, thrusting one's enemy with a sword (2 Samuel 2:15), and scaling walls (Psalms 18:80), which were probably part of the sports/war training process.

In Christian and Talmudic times (Rosner, 1989), it is well described that oil rubs and light massage were employed to improve physical performance and relaxation. Numerous examples of the benefits of great running feats, dancing, walking, ball playing, and swimming can be found throughout the Bible. This led the great physicians Moses Maimonides and Hippocrates to recognize the benefits of moderate and severe exercise to and describe both great physical and mental health benefits. Hypocates

stated that the maintenance of health lies in forsaking the disinclination to exertion: "Nothing is to be found that can substitute for exercise in any way because in exercise the natural heat flames up and all the superfluities (impurities) are expelled. Exercise will expel the harm done by most of the bad (dietary) regimens that most men follow." Maimonides also concluded that exercise, because of its impact on the brain's neurotransmitters and the body's metabolism and human moods, can cover, at least for a while, a multitude of dietary sins.

Maimonides termed exercise as powerful or rapid motion or a combination of both that is vigorous with which the respiration alters and one begins to heave sighs. Whatever exceeds that is exertion. That is to say that very strong exercise is called exertion. Although not everyone can endure exertion or needs it, it is nonetheless better in the preservation of health than the omission of exercise. Maimonides described adequate warm-up and cooling down phases as part of exercise regimens. Even Paul of Tarsus wrote that physical fitness had benefits (of course not equal to spiritual fitness) and that the body was a temple; thereby worthy (and even required by God) to be maintained. Hence, Western and Judeo-Christian traditions have a long history of describing sports and exercise (war training in some cases) as beneficial to health.

Health Benefits of Exercise

The health benefits of exercise are numerous, i.e., cancer prevention, lower cholesterol, regulation of sugar metabolism, antianxiety or depression, improved quality of

---

1. Reprinted from *The Journal of Orthomolecular Medicine*, vol. 6, no. 3 & 4, 1991.

life with age, and anti-degenerative diseases such as arthritis. Exercise is not a panacea, but any technique that reduces stress will have benefits in virtually all categories of disease. Hence, exercise has many benefits because it improves overall health and brain chemistry. Researchers theorize that physical activity may cause food by-products and carcinogens to be removed more quickly through the colon. Recently it was shown that men and women who exercise have a reduced colon cancer incidence in a study that interviewed 229 men and women with colon cancer and compared them to their healthy controls. Another recent study suggests the benefits of exercise in preventing breast cancer in young women (Kritchevsky, 1990) because exercise reduces caloric intake and appetite. Exercise produces more health and healthy people feel more motivated for exercise.

Other studies suggest that exercise has benefits on lipid levels, and this benefit can probably be augmented by the addition of nutrients. There is an improvement in MDL, as well as cholesterol and triglyceride lowering as much as 30 percent in body builders (Baldo-Enzi, et al., 1990).

Exercise, Sugar Metabolism and Weight Loss

Another benefit of exercise may be to improve sugar metabolism. Glucose tolerance was found to improve over an 18-week study in individuals undergoing aerobic exercise. Three out of four prediabetic people who had strength training saw their glucose tolerance return to normal. Exercise itself may include individual requirements for nutrients but has benefits to contribute to better sugar metabolism which is particularly relevant to long-term training. Exercise may even improve the efficiency of absorption of nutrients from food and may be beneficial for weight loss as well (King, et al, 1989).

Benefits of Exercise for All Age Groups

It is suggested that both strength training in children and strength training in the elderly has beneficial effects. The best approach to teach exercise in society is to start exercise education at a very early age and continue to a very late age. There are benefits to preserving muscle mass with age if exercise is continued. Exercise in the young and elderly builds confidence, and in the elderly probably slows the progression of osteoporosis and other degenerative diseases, e.g., arthritis. Walking with hand-held weights can be a beneficial form of exercise for the elderly. The elderly can continue to build muscle with exercise and thereby have a more vigorous geriatric life. Furthermore, severe illness is better tolerated in the

conditioned athlete or individual with better fitness (Webb, 1990).

Studies suggest that "young" old people (age 60-72) can increase their thigh muscle strength by almost 200 percent and their muscle mass by 15 percent with exercise. At Tufts University, researchers have shown that weight training can occur in young old men and women aged 60 to 72 and even in men and women aged 86 to 96 to improve body muscle. Medical wisdom in this area seems to show us once again that we underestimate what things are possible (White, et al., 1987; Ekelund, et al., 1988; Blackburn, et al., 1988; Blair, et al., 1989; Leon, et al., 1987; Paffenbarger, et al., 1986; Powell, et al., 1987; Blair, et al., 1984).

Psychiatric Benefits of Exercise

A Stanford University study showed that the mental state of juvenile delinquents is improved by exercise. Those who exercised three times a week improved their scores in measures of depression and self-esteem. Obviously exercise can be a distraction from worries and social pressures, and using your body can provide a sense of greater mastery and control over life. During exercise, changes may occur in the levels of circulating endorphins and other neurotransmitters. It was suggested by a study at the National Institute of Mental Health that exercise increases noropenepherine, serotonin, dopamine, endorphins (high or euphoria effect), and possibly all neurotransmitters thought to be low in depressed people. The beneficial effects of exercise on mood may not be long-lasting but primarily short-term. Exercise is a mild antidepressant (and antianxiety) and is often the driving force behind highly motivated athletes. These athletes frequently need to add neurotransmitter precursors when not in training to maintain optimum mental health. Cranial electrical stimulation of the brain may simulate some of the brain chemistry effects of exercise (MacMahon, et al., 1980; Lennox, et al., 1990).

Dangers of Strenuous Exercise and Their Prevention

Lack of stretching, taut muscles, and long-term, high intensity, high mileage running is a potential risk factor for premature osteoarthritis. It may be true that any regular exercise without exercise rotation (running one day, swimming the next day, tennis the next day, etc., or running in the summer, swimming in the winter) puts an individual at high risk for various injuries. The fears about aerobic exercise during pregnancy are not warranted (Sumida, et al., 1989; Marti, et al., 1989; Kleiner, et al,

1989).

Insufficient Exercise in America

It is concluded that 79 percent of all Americans do not get enough exercise to have any significant beneficial effect upon heart function and disease. Therefore, possibly the most important question we have to ask is what is required to motivate an individual to do exercise? Such an answer would probably be found primarily in brain chemistry and the depletion of various neurotransmitters which can motivate an individual. It is certainly now well recognized that a low level of physical fitness is associated with a high risk of death from coronary heart disease. Not to exercise is self-destructive, even suicidal behavior! Depletion of neurotransmitters, especially the adrenaline builders, e.g., tyrosine, methionine, and DL phenylalanine, may lead to low energy and lack of motivation for exercise. In a sense, a vicious circle is often created, i.e., low mood leads to reduced frequency of exercise, which in turn leads to less exercise, which further promotes low mood. Cranial electrical stimulation may be another natural way to break this cycle (Grinenko, et al., 1988; Braverman, et al., 1990).

Nutrition and Athletic Performance

Athletes Use Supplements

According to a recent study at Johns Hopkins reviewed in *Prevention* magazine, athletes, marathon runners in particular, believe that supplements can be beneficial. As many as 48 percent report use of at least one type of supplement within a 3-day period. Athletes are already using supplements but are not yet aware that scientific testing can contribute a fine tuning of their nutritional programs (Hickson, et al., 1989; Nieman, et al., 1989).

Nutritional Deficiencies in Athletes

One thing for certain, according to Keith and colleagues (1989), is that trained female cyclists take in RDA's well below the appropriate level, such as 76 percent reduction in folic acid, 81 percent reduction in magnesium, 59 percent iron, 48 percent zinc, compared to normal. Many athletes have nutritional deficiencies but have not been educated about how easy it is to identify the deficiencies and treat them (Van Erp-Baart, et al., 1989; Keith, et al., 1989).

Increased Nutritional Requirements of Heavy Exercise

It is clear that the body requires more nutrients during exercise and the body responds to intense aerobic exercise by preserving and reducing excretion of magnesium, zinc, and copper. Vlcek (1989) studied thirteen healthy men, ages 17 to 35. There was a rapid drop in plasma magnesium following significant exercise and a rapid increase in copper. These studies suggest the need for nutritional supplements during the process of exercise.

According to Hood and colleagues (1990), branch chain amino acids, particularly leucine, increase metabolism during rigorous exercise. In fact, their work is probably the strongest that clearly documented that the dietary intake of leucine be increased to a level commensurate with whole body rate oxidation. Possibly all strenuous exercise requires supplementation of leucine and other branch chain amino acids. Leucine may be as close as we can come to a natural steroid inducer. As high as 11 percent of high school athletes have tried anabolic steroids (Zuliani, et al., 1988). There is clear evidence that branch chain amino acids are increasingly utilized by exercise. This should be no surprise since numerous studies document the fact that branch chain amino acids are the most important amino acids utilized during trauma, sepsis, surgery, and any acute stress on the body (Braverman, et al., 1990). Branched chain amino acids, particularly leucine, are already proven to preserve muscle mass during acute stress. Body building and strenuous exercise are catabolic events similar to trauma, surgery, etc.; hence, branched chain amino acids are likely to be beneficial supplements, especially in high doses. Leucine and to a lesser extent isoleucine are uniquely metabolized amino acids through the fat oxidation pathway. Eating leucine is like getting the energy benefits of fat without eating fat! These principles regarding sports nutrition can also be applied to the stress of war and post-traumatic illnesses of many types. The nutrient carnitine (in conjunction with branched chain amino acids) may also improve muscle functioning and, although controversial, has potential benefits to endurance. Carnitine levels also can be measured in the blood to optimize supplement levels (Soop, et al., 1988; Jaspers, et al, 1989; Elam, et al, 1989; Jacobson, 1990; Maes, et al., 1990).

Benefits of B-complex

Athletes throughout the world, according to a study in the *Journal of Obesity*, suggest that B-complex, particularly B-1, B-6, and B-12, have a calming effect and reduce slight, almost unnoticeable tremor in pistol shooting, possibly by inducing natural neurotransmitters in the brain. It has even been suggested that caffeine be banned by the International Olympic Committee because of its ability to increase basal metabolic rate, work as a diuretic, and produce slight tremor, possibly because it increases excretion and utilization of B vitamins. B complex supplementation is certainly a reasonable idea for athletes of many types that require steadiness of hands. Vitamin B complex supplementation, according to Maretti, particularly B-6, will increase the plasma levels of growth hormone induced by exercise. Hence, exercise is probably a good growth hormone releaser by itself, possibly even better than arginine or branch chain amino acids (Braverman, 1987). B-complex may augment the effect of exercise on growth hormones.

B-6 and exercise increase growth hormone and low glutamine, and high glutamic acid increases muscle synthesis. B-6 decarboxylases glutamine to glutamic acid. Pantothenic acid may increase endurance; in one mice exercise study (swimming in water) nonsupplemented mice sank to the bottom of the jar quicker than those who received extra pantothenic acid.

Magnesium and Endurance Athletes

According to Goodman and information gathered in 1985 at the University of Oregon from a group of elite, all long-distance athletes including Alberto Salazar (former world record holder in the marathon), runners lose magnesium in perspiration. Because long-distance runners perspire a great deal more than sprinters, long-distance runners' magnesium levels tended to be lower. On the other hand, sprinters can normally possess elevated calcium readings and, because of the need for calcium in muscle contraction, they require more of it than long-distance runners. The question of whether or not magnesium supplementation could improve athletic performance and endurance has been suggested by numerous studies. A convincing example of the benefits of magnesium was provided by Matt Biondi, one of the world's fastest swimmers and holder of the 50 meter and 100 meter free-style records. From 1985 through 1987, while a student at Berkeley, Biondi underwent mineral analysis which showed a definite magnesium deficiency. He handled sprinting races easily but had been experiencing difficulty in the 200 meter free-style, an

event which required considerable endurance. After several weeks of magnesium supplements, Biondi's strength and endurance improved significantly during long-distance performance. Possibly other athletes can benefit from magnesium supplements. Red blood cell and white blood cell magnesium tests can easily identify subtle deficiencies.

Other Trace Elements in Endurance Athletes

Other athletes provide evidence similar to that of Biondi, not only about macroelements like magnesium, but also a range of trace minerals including but not limited to zinc, iron, copper, and chromium. Mac Wilkins, Olympic athlete and former world record holder in discus, has stated that the benefits of chemical element analysis in athletes and their supplementation can be so dramatic he is amazed it is legal! Athletes typically report that nutritional supplements improve their leg cramps and reduced or eliminated their time in competitions where shaving 1/10 of a second off a time can spell the difference between winning and not placing at all. Obviously the effects can be very subtle (Keen, et al, 1984; Vlcek, et al, 1989).

The Department of Agriculture suggests that as much as 90 percent of the United States population may not be getting adequate chromium, zinc, or magnesium. A recent study of U.S. Navy Seal trainees showed that during training they also had a reduced intake of magnesium, zinc, and copper (34, 44, and 37 percent respectively). Supplementation of these nutrients to maintain baseline levels may not be a bad idea. Obviously athletes may benefit from macro- and microelement supplements, especially if deficiencies can be identified by red blood cell testing. Recent studies by Campbell suggested that increased levels of dietary chromium may have beneficial effects of glycogen and glycogen synthesis. This effect may hot be limited to athletes that are deficient, but there may be benefits to even higher levels of supplementation. Chromium supplementation may be one of the most important factors in weight control and may be one of the key dimensions of why most diets for weight loss fail. Chromium, which is also frequently deficient in diabetics, may be a necessary supplement for maintaining level sugar metabolism and lean body mass (Campbell, et al., 1989; Siugh, et al., 1989; Goodmati, 1990).

Iron Deficiency

According to Chigo, the problem of iron deficiency is confusing since recent articles by Drs. Goldstein and Lofler suggest that lower iron might actually benefit athletes and that rigorous exercise results in substantial blood loss through the gastrointestinal tract and sweat. Many women athletes in particular have low iron levels. If low iron were beneficial, blood donation may help certain athletes, although most of these benefits will be transitory. The overwhelming amount of data suggests that long-term iron deficiency will result in very significant cognitive problems, coldness, fatigue, and depression. Many athletes have sub par performance due to even borderline iron deficiency. In addition, excess iron can lead to fatigue (Dallongeville, et al., 1989; Rowland, et al., 1989; O'Tolle, et al., 1989; Clarnette, et al., 1990).

Importance of Potassium

It is important not to neglect potassium. Some studies suggest that highly trained women compensate for increased utilization of potassium by having a higher intake of potassium. This increase in potassium may be beneficial. It is very easy to give 10 milliequivalents of Klotrix every other day in athletes without noticing any toxicity problem whatsoever in terms of elevation of the potassium. Furthermore, this supplementation will probably guarantee greater reserves during high performance stress.

Role of Sodium

No review of sports nutrition is complete without mention of sodium. Low sodium levels can result in altered mentation, seizures, and pulmonary edema. Water intake can be a problem without adequate sodium and electrolytes. Water should be thought of as a nutrient, and water high in trace minerals should be ingested. By increasing potassium, this may increase sodium loss. Careful electrolyte balance must be maintained in athletes. The problem is quite similar to very ill patients where proper electrolyte balance can make the difference between life and death.

Nutritional Supplements That Benefit Athletes: Amino Acids

Branch chain amino acids are not the only amino acids that can benefit athletic performance. Tyrosine, one of the amino acids that builds Adrenalin, also has other benefits according to U.S. Army Research Institute of Environmental Medicine in Nadic, Massachusetts. In this study, 23 men aged 18 to 26 were exposed to altitude changes. The subjects who received 600 milligrams each of tyrosine were better able to tolerate 40 minutes of exposure to mountainous terrain. Tyrosine significantly

reduced the adverse effects produced by exposure to cold, decreased oxygen, headache, coldness, distress, fatigue, muscular discomfort, and sleepiness in simulated mountain climbing stresses. Many similar studies have also repeated the use of tyrosine with benefit in military stress conditions. Recent research has linked stress-caused impairments of performance with depletion of brain stores of the neurotransmitter norepinephrine, which functions in neural tracts responding to stress. The amino acid tyrosine is the dietary precursor for norepinephrine, and supplementation with tyrosine has been demonstrated in the laboratory to alleviate declines in both neural norepinephrine and performance during stress. Thus, tyrosine supplementation might help to prevent and treat stress casualties in sports or combat.

In acutely stressful situations, one may benefit from tyrosine ingestion along with branched chain amino acids. Branched chain amino acids like steroids may reduce tyrosine and tryptophane absorption. Taking methionine with tyrosine may result in increased absorption of tyrosine, according to Braverman, 1987. In general, tyrosine and methionine supplements are best taken during the morning and afternoon, while branched chain amino acids are best taken before dinner, bedtime, or a workout (Banderet, et al, 1989; Salter, 1989).

Segura and Ventura (1988) suggest that L-tryptophan supplementation may benefit exercise performance. Twelve healthy sportsmen were subjected to a work load corresponding to 80% of their maximal oxygen uptake on two separate trials, after receiving a placebo and after receiving the same amount of L-tryptophan. The subjects ran on a treadmill until exhaustion. Total exercise time, perceived exertion rate, maximum heart rate, peak oxygen consumption, pulse recovery rate, and excess post-exercise oxygen consumption were determined during the two trials. The total exercise time was 49.4% greater after receiving L-tryptophan than after receiving the placebo. The longer exercise time as well as the total work load performed could be due to an increased pain tolerance as a result of L-tryptophan ingestion, which is best taken at night. (L-tryptophan will be back on the market as soon as proper protection from contamination of the product is assured.)

The performance of strenuous physical exercise is associated with discomfort and pain, the tolerance for that being modulated by the activity of the endogenous opioid systems. 5-hydroxytryptamine (5HT) affects nociception through its effects on the enkephalin-endorphin system. Tryptophan and possibly cranial electrical stimulation (CES) may raise serotonin levels, increase pain tolerance, and thereby increase exercise tolerance. After all, no pain, no gain, or according to the suffering is the reward!

Growth Hormone

Increasing evidence suggests that growth hormone can restore muscle health very late in life, and increase muscle development early in life. Increases in growth hormone can probably occur from many amino acids (i.e., tryptophan, leucine, isoleucine, arginine, ornithine). These increases are greatest when the amino acids are given intravenously. Possibly amino acid loading prior to strenuous exercise (this has already proven benefits for trauma, the catabolic state most similar to severe exercise) may be beneficial. At this time it is unclear if oral amino acids can really elevate growth hormone and its mediators significantly. Growth hormone injections may be practical in the very near future, according to recent studies (Moretti, et al., 1982).

Possible Benefits of Choline

Studies on 17 healthy athletes who ran the Boston Marathon, as published October 2, 1986 in The New England Journal of Medicine, showed that this exercise was associated with a major fall (i.e., about 40%) in plasma choline levels; all of the subjects showed at least some reduction in the choline levels. A second study conducted on 16 additional subjects the following year confirmed this observation: mean plasma choline levels fell by 35%, and all but 2 of the subjects exhibited some reduction. Plasma choline fulfills two major functions: all of the cells in the body use it to produce constituents of their own membranes (like phosphatidyl choline and sphingomyelin); moreover, particular nerve cells, or neurons, all over the body use it to make acetylcholine, the chemical signal that they release to transmit instructions to the cells that they innervate. Among such cholinergic neurons are all of the nerves that determine whether muscles will contract. Other studies, using pieces of muscle with their nerve intact, incubated in the presence of fluids containing varying amounts of choline and stimulated electrically, have clearly shown that when choline levels are reduced, the amounts of acetylcholine that the nerves release are reduced in parallel. Thus, it is not unlikely that a major reduction in plasma choline levels in the body would also diminish the ability of the nervous system to "instruct" muscles to contract, potentially affecting performance. Plasma choline levels can be raised at will by taking purified phosphatidyl choline orally. In general, it takes 7-9 grams to approximately double plasma choline, and it can be anticipated that a like amount would be able to sustain plasma choline levels in the exercising athletes. Choline also has benefits in brain function which may help concentration and overall performance (Ghigo, et al, 1989; Safford, et al, 1989).

Management of Soft-Tissue Injuries with Nutritional Therapies

Management of soft-tissue injuries in sports has taken some interesting turns with the natural agent 5'-methylthioadenosine, a naturally occurring nucleoside which has anti-inflammatory and analgesic activity. The usual approaches to sports soft-tissue injuries have used the concept of RICE (rest, ice application, compression bandage, and elevation) and the use of NSAID's, or nonsteroidal anti-inflammatory drugs (fish oil can often replace the use of these). The natural compound is a derivative of adenosine, which has also been used as an antiarrhythmic and probably anticonvulsant, has some anti-inflammatory properties, and holds promise for natural treatment of sports injuries and may even be beneficial as a compound for massage in very high stress athletic competition. At this point the use of lotions or creams for the benefits of sports is not clear. It does seem though that contusions, sprains, tendinitis, epicondylitis, and strain may be treated by 5'methylthioadenosine (Anselmi, et al., 1990).

Optimizing
Athletic Performance

The Optimal Diet for Athletes

The proper diet for an athlete depends on what stage he or she is in in terms of performance. Numerous studies suggest the importance of an adequate calorie content for various athletes and that carbohydrate loading is essential to adequate endurance, especially right before sporting events. Frequently athletes eat a big macaroni or pasta meal before an important event. During periods where training is not as intense, increased protein intake may be necessary to build lean muscle. High protein diets are also adequate defenses against fluid retention. Long-term use of high protein diets probably will result in reduced endurance but increased muscle development (Ballor, et al., 1990; Ballor, et al., 1988).

Resistance weight training during caloric restriction enhances lean body weight maintenance. It also increases HDL and lowers LDL. If one wishes to improve lean body mass, there can be benefits of being on a high protein diet and doing resistance weight training. There is a time for a complex carbohydrate diet and a time for a high protein diet in athletics. Another possible diet in theory is the Princeton Plan which alternates high carbohydrate and high protein. On the high carbohydrate day, aerobics are used to burn body fat as fuel. The next day, resistance training utilizes the glycogen stored in the muscles and liver from the day before. You eat based on your exercise needs for the next day (Heleniak, et al., 1990; Ratz, et al., 1989).

Reaching Maximum Performance: The Use of Diet

Complex carbohydrate loading regimens have been reported in many studies to benefit high-intensity, strenuous exercise (i.e., marathons). Through exercise, glucagon can be depleted by nearly 35 percent. Moderate intensity, long duration exercise and even short intensity exercise may be helped by complex carbohydrate loading. According to some studies, there are glucose polymers that will assist this carbohydrate loading and are available in drink form. Glucose polymers with nutrients given intravenously may result in even greater athletic performance benefits. Maximum manipulation of performance in athletes will probably continue to improve with the use of peptides and other natural hormonelike substances. Loading athletes through superintravenous nutrition prior to marathons or sporting events would seem to be the most striking way of impacting athletic performance naturally. For example, intra-arterial infusion of PgE2 (prostaglandin E2) produces increased skeletal muscle protein degradation. PgE1 increases growth hormone secretion and decreases insulin secretion, while insulin is antagonistic to growth hormone. Fish oil, vitamin E hormones, PGE1, and other prostaglandins might be infused to impact muscle growth. Furthermore, intravenous arginine is probably the only way in which arginine can significantly increase peak performance by increasing growth hormone. Intravenous loading of nutrients (particularly amino acids, prostaglandins) a day prior to athletic performance, as well as carbohydrate loading, may produce outstanding effects in athletic performance (Pressler, et al., 1984).

Arriving at a Supplement Program

A review by Brouns (1989) suggests that numerous vitamins can benefit exercise performance when deficiency is established. It is clear that poor vitamin status is harmful and that any given individual might suffer from a mild deficiency at any given time. Rigorous athletic performance is marked by nutrient deficiencies if looked for. Although no recommendation for megadoses can be made solidly, it can be concluded that any nutrient deficiencies, induced by either low intakes or losses during performance (both are extremely common), can impair physical performance. The concept of low level of protective supplementation certainly seems prudent considering the numerous studies documenting nutrient losses. Testing of athletes in most cases should document some treatable deficiency or tendency (Singh, et al, 1990).

Ways of Improving Muscle Strength and Performance

General muscle weakness and atrophy is a common feature of hyperthyroidism. Proximal muscles seem to be much more affected than distal muscles. Neuromuscular abnormalities also occur in hypothyroidism in the contractile mechanism of the muscle. Hyperthyroid patients that are treated have an absolute increase in muscle strength, and this is probably also true of hypothyroidism patients. Through thyroid stress testing it may be determined that a small percentage of athletes may have borderline hypothyroidism and thereby benefit from thyroid supplements. Another technique to augment athletic performance might include the use of Cytomel (or T3) (Celsing, et al., 1990).

Tests for Athletes: Nutritional Status

It would seem appropriate for all determined athletes to have regular body composition tests and complete trace element, fatty acid, amino acid, and vitamin diagnostic testing along with routine blood testing. Even neurotransmitter profiles might be evaluated. Correcting marginal nutritional imbalances would probably contribute a small but sometimes very significant amount to overall athletic performance. It might also be important to study brain mapping (brain electrical activity map or BEAM) and amino acids and neurotransmitters pre- and post-exercise since we know that running releases endorphins, increases neurotransmitters, etc. New brain scanning techniques such as positron emission tomography (PET) or single photo emission computerized tomography (SPEGF) along with BEAM should document the biochemical nature of the runner's highs such as love, spirituality, etc. Exercise is a great natural antidepressant and is probably critical to good mental health. Below is an outline of potential, beneficial testing for athletes.

Recommended Nutritional Testing for High Performance Athletes

- Routine blood tests (i.e., ESR, thyroid, etc.)
- Essential fatty acids, plasma
- Essential plasma amino acids
- CoQ1O
- Carnitine
- Vitamin diagnostics profile
- Complete trace metal screening in red blood cell

Other Low Yield Possible Tests for High Performance Athletes

- Hair test for toxins
- Immune testing
- Endorphin and neurotransmitter levels
- Brain mapping (to follow changes in the brain before and after strenuous exercise)
- Trace elements in white blood cells
- Allergy testing

References

1. Keen CL, Hackman RM: Trace elements in athletic performance. *Sport, Health and Nutrition.* Katch Fl (ed). Olympic Scientific Congress Proceedings, 2:51-65, 1984.

2. Sop M, Bjorkman O, Cederblad G, Hagenfeldt L, Wahren J: Influence of carnitine supplementation on muscle substrate and carnitine metabolism during exercise. *Amer. Physiological Society*, 2394-2399, 1988.

3. King AC, Frey-Hewitt B, Dreon DM, Wood PD: Diet vs. exercise in weight maintenance: The effects of minimal intervention strategies on long-term outcomes in men. *Arch. Intern. Med.*, 149:2741-2746, 1989.

4. Zuliani U, Bernardini B, Catapano A, Campana M, Cerioli G, Spattini M: Effects of anabolic steroids, testosterone, and HGH on blood lipids and echocardiographic parameters in body builders. *Int. J. Sports Med.*, 10:62-66, 1988.

5. Ballor DL, Smith DB, Tommerup LR, Thomas DP: Neither high-nor low-intensity exercise promotes whole-body conservation of protein during severe dietary restrictions. *Int. J. Obesity*, 14: 279-287, 1990.

6. Sumida S, Tanaka K, Kitao H, Nakadomo F: Exercise-induced lipid peroxidation and leakage of enzymes before and after vitamin E supplementation. *Int. J. Biochem.*, 21:835-838, 1989.

7. Campbell W, Polansky M, Bryden N, Soares J, Anderson R: Exercise training and dietary chromium effects on glycogen, glycogen synthase, phosphorylase, and total protein in rats. *J. Nutr.*, 119:653-660, 1989.

8. Ballor DL, Catch VL, Becque MD, Marks CR: Resistance weight training during caloric restriction enhances lean body weight maintenance. *Am. J. Clin. Nutr.*, 47:19-25, 1988.

9. You can do it: How to grow muscles in your golden years (You're only as old as your biomarkers!). *Men's Health*, 6, 1989.

10. Dallongeville J, Ledoux M, Brisson G: Iron deficiency among active men. *J. Amer. Coll. Nutr.*, 8(3):195-202, 1989.

11. Owens SG, Al-Ahned A, Moffati RJ: Physiological effects of walking and running with hand-held weights. *I. Sports Med. & Phys. Fit.*, 29(4):384-387, 1989.

12. Webb DR: Strength Training in children and adolescents. *Ped. Clin. N. Amer.*, 37(5): 1187-1210, 1990.

13. Singh A, Day BA, DeBolt JE, Trostmann UH, Bernier LL, Deuster PA: Magnesium, zinc, and copper status of US Navy SEAL trainees. *Am. J. Clin. Nutr.*, 49:695-700, 1989.

14. Gerster H: The role of vitamin C in athletic performance. *I. Amer. Coll. Nutr.*, 8(6):636-643, 1989.

15. Incidental (sexual) intelligence. *Med. Aspects Hum. Sex.*, July 1989.

16. Jaspers S, Henriksen EJ, Satarug S, Tischler M: Effects of stretching and disuse on amino acids in muscles of rat hind limbs. *Metabolism*, 38(4):303-310, 1989.

17. Marti B, Knobloch M, Tschopp A, Jucker A, Howald H: Is excessive running predictive of degenerative hip disease? Controlled study of former elite athletes. *Br. Med. J.*, 299:9193, 1989.

18. Ratz SR, Pettigrew FP, Noble EG, Taylor AW: Effect of dietary manipulation on a high intensity performance test. *J. Sports Med. Phys. Fitness*, 29:129-135, 1989.

19. Barr SI, Costill DL: Water: Can the endurance athlete get too much of a good thing? *J. Am. Diet. Assoc.*, 89:1629-1635, 1989.

20. Frankel T: Walking may protect hips. Healthfront. *Prevention*, 8, Feb. 1990.

21. Moretti C, Fabbri A, Gnessi L, Bonifacto V, Fraioli F, Isodori A: Pyridoxine (B-6) suppresses the rise in prolactin and increases the rise in growth hormone induced by exercise. *NE J. Med.*, 444, Aug. 12, 1982.

22. Rosner F, Weg IL: Exercise in Judaism. *Bull. NY Acad. Med.*, 65(8):842-850, 1989.

23. Pressler VM, Fagan JM, Scott TE, McMillen A, Wilmore DW: Intra-arterial infusion of PGE2 produces increased skeletal muscle protein degradation in rats. *Metabolism & Nutr.*, 52-53, 1984.

24. Baldo-Enzi G, Giada F, Zuliani G, Baroni L, Vitale E, Enzi G, Magnanini P, Fellin R: Lipid and apoprotein modifications in body builders during and after self-administration of anabolic steroids. *Metabolism*, 39(2):203-208, 1990.

25. O'Tolle ML, Iwane H, Douglas PS, Applegate EA, Hiller DB: Iron status in ultraendurance triathletes. *Physician & Sports Med.*, 17(12):90-102, 1989.

26. MacMahonJ, Gross R: Delinquents' mental state improved by exercise. *Amer. J. Diseases of Children*, 142:1361-1366, 1989.

27. Rowland TW, Kelleher JF: Many female swimmers shown to have low iron level. *Amer. J. Diseases of Children*, Feb. 1989.

28. White CG, et al.: Behavior risk factors surveys: The descriptive epidemiology of exercise. *Amer. J. Prev. Med.*, 3:304-310,1987.

29. Ekelund L, Haskell WL, Johnson JL, Whaley FS, Driqui MH, Sheps DS: Physical fitness as a predictor of cardiovascular mortality in asymptomatic North American men. *N. Engl. J. Med.*, 319:1379-1384, 1988.

30. Blackburn H, Jacobs, DR: Physical activity and the risk of coronary heart disease. *N. Engl. J. Med.*, 319:1217-1219, 1988.

31. Kleiner SM, Calabrese LH, Fielder KM, Naito HK, Skibinski CI: Dietary influences on cardiovascular disease risk in anabolic steroid-using and nonusing bodybuilders. *Amer. Coll. Nutr.*, 8(2):109-119, 1989.

32. Hood DA, Terjung RL: Amino acid metabolism during exercise and following endurance training. *Sports Med.*, 9(1):23-35, 1990.

33. Vlcek J, Stemberk V, Koupil P: Serum concentrations and urinary excretion of Mg, Zn, and Cu during high-intensity exercise in healthy men. *Trace Elements in Med.*, 6(4):150-153, 1989.

34. Blair SN, Kohl HW, Paffenbarger RS, Clark DG, Cooper KH, Gibbons LW: Physical fitness and all-cause mortality: A prospective study of healthy men and women. *JAMA*, 262:2395-2401, 1989.

35. Hickson JF, Wolinsky I (eds): Nutrition in exercise and sport. Boca Raton, Florida, FL, CRC Press, 1989.

36. Nieman DC, Gates JR, Butler JV, Polleti LM, Dietrich SJ, Lutz RD: Supplementation patterns in marathon runners. *I. Amer. Diet. Assoc.*, 89(11):1615-1619, 1989.

37. Ghigo E, Mazza E, Corrias A, Imperiale E, Goffi S, Arvat E, Bellone J, De Sanctis C, Muller EE, Camanni F: Effect of cholinergic enhancement by pyridostigmine on growth hormone secretion in obese adults and chil dren. *Metabolism*, 38(7):631-633, 1989.

38. Does pumping iron deflate diabetes? Healthfront. *Prevention*, 9, March 1990.

39. Goodman RA: The atomic level athletic frontier. *The World and I*, 286-291, February 1990.

40. Leon AS, Connett J, Jacobs DR, et al: Leisure-time physical activity levels and risk of coronary heart disease and death: The Multiple Risk Factor Inwrnational Trial. *JAMA*, 258:2388-2395, 1987.

41. Paffenbarger RD, Hyde RT, Wing AL, et al.: Physical activity, all-cause mortality, and longevity of college alumni. *N. Engl. J. Med.*, 314:605-613, 1986.

42. Powell KE, Thompson PD, Caspersen CJ, et al.: Physical activity and the incidence of coronary heart disease. *Ann. Rev. Public Health*, 8:253-287, 1987.

43. Blair SN, Goodyear NN, Gibbons LW, et al.: Physical fitness and incidence of hypertension in healthy normotensive men and women. *JAMA*, 252:487-490, 1984.

44. Ekelund LG, Haskell WL., Johnson JL, et al.: Physical fitness as a predictor of cardiovascular mortality in asymptomatic North American men: The Lipid Research Clinics Mortality Follow-up Study. *N. Engl. J. Med.*, 319:1379-1384, 1988.

45. Elam RP, Hardin DH, Sutton RAL, Hagen L: Effects of arginine and ornithine on strength, lean body mass and urinary hydroxyproline in adult males. *J. Sports Med. arn Phys. Fitness*, 29(1), 1989.

46. Singh A, Deuster PA, Day BA, Moser-Veillon PB: Dietary intakes and biochemical markers of selected minerals: Comparison of highly trained runners and untrained women. *J. Amer. Coll. Nutr.*, 9(1):65-75, 1990.

47. Clarnetie RM, Tampi R, Choo P: Red cell ferritin: Its role in the assessment of iron stores in endurance runners. *Aust. NZ J. Med.*, 20:263-264, 1990.

48. Brouns F, Saris W: How vitamins affect performance. J. *Sports Med. and Phys. Fitness*, 29(4):4O0-404, 1989.

49. Van ERp-Baart A, Saris W, Binkhorst R, et al.: Nationwide survey on nutritional habits in elite athletes: Part I. energy, carbohydrate, protein, and fat intake. *Int. J. Sports Med.*, 10:S3-S10, 1989.

50. Somerset Medical Center: Regarding Women and Health Care. Amer. J. Obstetrics and Gynecology, 161(6), 1989.

51. Banderet L, Lieberman H: Treatment with tyrosine, a neurotransmitter precursor, reduces environmental stress in humans. *Brain Res. B.*, 22:759-762, 1989.

52. Keith RE, O'Keeffe KA, Alt LA, Young DL: Dietary status of trained female cyclists. *J. Am. Diet. Assoc.*, 89:1620-1623, 1989.

53. Jacobson BH: Effect of amino acids on growth hormone release. *Physicians and Sportsmedicine*, 18(1), 1990.

54. Anselmi B, Caroli GC, Costa CM, Di Fraia G, Moratti EM: Topical 5'-methylthioadenosine for the treatment of sports-related acute soft-tissue injuries. *Drug Invst.*, 2(4):249-254, 1990.

55. Celsing F, Westing SH, Adamson U, Ekblom B: Muscle strength in hyperthyroid patients before and after medical treatment. *Clin. Psycho.*, 10:545-550, 1990.

56. Grinenko A, Krupitskiy EM, Lebedev VP, et al.: Metabolism of biogenic amines during the treatment of alcohol withdrawal syndrome by transcranial electric treatment. *Biogenic Amines*, 5(6):427-436, 1988.

57. Segura R, Ventura JL: Effect of L-tryptophan supplementation on exercise performance. *Int. J. Sports Med.*, 9(5):301-305, 1988.

58. Heleniak F, Aston B: The Princeton Plan. New York: St. Martin's Press, 1990.

59. Kritchevsky D: Nutrition and breast cancer. *Cancer*, 66(6):1321-1324, 1990.

60. Salter CA: Dietary tyrosine as an aid to stress resistance among troops. Military Med., 154(3):114, 1989.

61. Maes NI, Jacobs MP, Soy F, Minner B, Leclercq C, Christiaens F, Raus J: Suppressant effects of dexamethasone on the availability of plasma L-tryptophan and tyrosine in healthy controls and in depressed patients, *Acta. Psychiatr. Scand.*, 81:19-23, 1990.

62. Braverman ER, Pfeiffer CC: *The Healing Nutrients Within.* New Canaan, CT: Keats Publishing, 1987.

63. Braverman ER, Blum K, Smayda RJ: A commentary on brain mapping in 60 substance abusers: can the potential for drug abuse be predicted and prevented by treatment? *Curr. Ther. Res.*, 48(4):569-585, 1990.

64. Braverman E, Smith R, Smayda R, Blum D: Modification of P300 amplitude and other electrophysiological parameters of drug abuse by cranial electrical stimulation. *Curr. Ther. Res.*, 48(4):586-596, 1990.

65. Lennox SS, Bedell FR, Stone AA: The effect of exercise on normal mood. *J. Psychosomatic Res.*, 34(6):629-636, 1990.

66. Sifford F, Baumel B: An exploratory study of the effects of dietary lecithin on mental function of healthy older adults. Summary of Poster Presentation, Gerontological Society, San Francisco, CA, Nov. 20, 1989.

67. Wurtman RJ: Decreased plasma choline concentrations in marathon runners, *NE J. Med.*, 315(14):892, 1986.

28. *Spirituality*y

Although this is a medical book, we would be remiss if we failed to acknowledge that much of the wisdom in the previous medical sections are also found in the wisdom of the ages in the Christian-Judaic tradition. Below are some additional spiritual selections for those who are interested.

Psychoneuroimmunology

Recently, there have been many books about Psychoneuro-immunology: how the mind's attitudes affect the nervous system and body. The best-seller, *Love, Medicine and Miracles* by Bernie Seigel, M.D. shows how exceptional patients can be cured of AIDS and cancer through a change of attitude. Their immune systems are restored by inner spiritual transformation. The implication of Dr. Seigel's work and that of many other researchers is that faith can heal. The spiritual dimension and attitudes toward disease are relevant to the entire holistic medicine approach.

If indeed spiritual attitudes can build the immune system and health, each person must ask, how can I evaluate my spiritual health? *What's Your Spiritual Health* is an inventory and questionnaire that can help you develop spiritual attitudes which can contribute to your total health. Your well-developed spiritual life may be your best defense against disease. It is not a total guarantee, yet developing your spiritual health is a key way to total health. (See more about psychoneuro-immunology, Section 18, p. 226.)

Abridged Spiritual Behavior Inventory

I devised this short version of the Inventory, which contains one main representative question for each of the twenty behavioral categories of spiritual health listed in an upcoming book. While only some possible responses are set forth in this short version, they are all discussed fully in the main text.

Answer the following questions according to the grading system below:

1 = strongly agree
2 = somewhat agree
3 = neither agree nor disagree
4 = somewhat disagree
5 = strongly disagree

Circle the 1, 2, 3, 4, or 5 next to the answer which best suits you.

1.   I can give to others possessions that are valuable to me, even a kidney to a loved one if necessary.   1 2 3 4 5

2.   I sing and dance to the Lord.   1 2 3 4 5

3.   Everyone has spiritual needs; some needs are the same and some are different.   1 2 3 4 5

4.   My home is a small temple of godliness.   1 2 3 4 5

5. My family's religious history is an asset to my spirituality today.

1   2   3   4   5

6. I have a relationship with the Lord because I am in His image.

1   2   3   4   5

7. Repentance is one way to find the Kingdom of Heaven.

1   2   3   4   5

8. God has a divine purpose for my life and for the world.

1   2   3   4   5

9. My choice of clothing can be part of service to God.

1   2   3   4   5

10. God has a divine purpose for my life and for the world.

1   2   3   4   5

11. I can find peace in prayer and everything I do can be a prayer.

1   2   3   4   5

12. Unjust things do not happen to just people.

1   2   3   4   5

13. I need a community to reach my full spiritual potential.

1   2   3   4   5

14. There are many apparent contradictions and difficulties in interpreting the scripture, which is why there are so many different religions.

1   2   3   4   5

15. I believe in a commitment to serve all mankind according to the Lord's ways.

1   2   3   4   5

16. I do careful evaluation of my thoughts and actions daily or weekly concerning my service to the Lord.

1   2   3   4   5

17. He who desires to reach the Lord will eventually develop a relationship with Him and learn to love neighbors as himself.

1   2   3   4   5

18. The messianic era is already here in part, and I have a role in its fulfillment.

1   2   3   4   5

19. The Lord has a relationship with me that He has with no one else.

1   2   3   4   5

20. A proper balance of God's love and discipline is important in my understanding of all aspects of my life.

1   2   3   4   5

Spiritual Distress Diagnosis

Many patients suffer from anxiety and depression that are brought on by spiritual distress. Frequently, death in the family, crisis at work, or illness can raise questions of the meaning and the purpose of life. Most patients in our secular society have no way of coping with spiritual problems without a sense of divine purpose or afterlife. A belief system of some kind is necessary to deal with crisis.

In our secular world, patients tend to retreat into allergy, depression, paranoia, anger, and hypochondriasis. Hypochondria (obsession with health is a sign of the denial of holiness) is one of the most frequent escapes from dealing with spiritual issues. To begin to address these issues, one must begin to read the Scriptures and to explore inner thoughts and feelings. The Naves Bible is particularly helpful in that it presents issues of love and death, family and children topically so that it can generate

spiritual discussion. Some key chapters of Scripture, and their topical allusions, are:

- Danger -- Psalm 91
- Forgiveness -- Psalm 51
- Companionship -- Psalm 23
- Blue -- Psalm 34
- Friends Fail -- Psalm 27
- Sleeplessness -- Psalm 4
- Love -- 1 John 3 and 1 Cor. 13
- Peace -- John 1-4
- Heaven -- Rev. 21
- Faith -- Heb. 11.

Once Scripture begins to comfort an individual, progress toward the next stage, doing God's will with joyful obedience, begins to occur.

Proverbs and Healthy Emotions

The Book of Proverbs has much to say about the connection between emotions and health. Below are excerpts from Proverbs on this subject, quoted from the *Revised Standard Version*.

Be not wise in your own eyes; fear the Lord, and turn away from evil. It will be healing to your flesh and refreshment to your bones (3:7, 8).

A man who is kind benefits himself, but a cruel man hurts himself (AV: troubleth his own flesh) (11:17).

There is one whose rash words are like sword thrusts, but the tongue of the wise brings healing (12:18).

Anxiety in a man's heart weighs him down, but a good word makes him glad (12:25).

A tranquil mind gives life to the flesh, but passion (AV: envy) makes the bones rot (14:30).

Better is a dinner of herbs where love is than a fatted ox and hatred with it (15:17).

The light of the eyes rejoices the heart, and good news refreshes the bones (15:30).

Pleasant words are like a honeycomb, sweetness to the soul and health to the body (16:24).

Better is a dry morsel with quiet than a house full of feasting with strife (17:1).

A cheerful heart is a good medicine, but a downcast spirit dries up the bones (17:22).

A man's spirit will endure sickness; but a broken spirit who can bear? (18:14).

A man without self-control is like a city broken into and left without walls (25:28).

The Biological, Psychological, and Spiritual Bases of Death

A National Institute of Health study indicates a single EEG recording of electrocerebral silence six hours after acute hemorrhage or damage to the brain is sufficient indication of death, or two recordings six hours apart. Also required is the absence of brain stem reflexes and the absence of spontaneous respiration. These criteria will not apply, though, to patients with severe hypothermia, metabolic disorders, or drug overdose, all of which can produce an apparently isoelectric record. Therefore, EEG alone is never adequate to diagnose brain death.

DETERMINING BRAIN DEATH

Basically, brain death will produce primarily a flat line, except for cardiac activity that will bleed through the record. Euthanasia issues became particularly germane in medicine when lifesaving technology became prevalent, i.e., the ability to substitute artificial lungs or an artificial heart to maintain a human being alive. It became obvious that medicine was operating without judgment as it moved towards preserving life by extraordinary means. There was not a parallel move by the medical community towards any evaluation whatsoever of the quality of life being preserved. Religious people have a blanket belief, although not biblically grounded, that euthanasia is not appropriate. Obviously, there are numerous examples of euthanasia in the Bible, such as Saul, and in a sense, Jesus, who willingly chose death rather than life in its current form. We now have situations where we rectify the problem by having DNR (Do not Resuscitate) orders in hospitals, and living wills which permit individuals the option of death with dignity. It is certainly an unstated goal and purpose behind almost all modern medicine to defeat death and to eventually achieve greater longevity for human beings, whether it means replacing organ parts one by one, making a new body for man, or using chemicals, injections, and other techniques to prolong life. This generation has come to recognize that the medical basis of life is located in the brain, and the medical basis of death is also the brain. Throughout history it has not always been clear to people that the brain was the source of quality life. Descartes thought the pineal gland, and others thought the heart, could actually think. However, now we have sometimes gone too far in another direction and called the heart a dumb pump when it is actually a complicated gland.

STAGES OF DYING -- PSYCHOLOGY

Elizabeth Kubler Ross and other psychiatrists have come up with basic stages of dying: first, the impact or numbness stage; second, the recoil or depression stage; third, the recovery stage. Symptoms during the depressed period are well-known to most people in the following order: crying being most prevalent, followed by sleep disturbance, low mood, loss of appetite, fatigue, poor memory, loss of interest, difficulty with concentration, weight loss, guilt, restlessness, irritability, reverse diurnal variation, death wishes, hopelessness, hallucinations, suicidal thoughts, fear of losing one's mind. Physical symptoms also accompany the stages of dying, such as headache, dysmenorrhea, other pains, urinary frequency, constipation, abdominal pain, blurred vision, anxiety attacks, etc.

RELIGIOUS VIEWS OF DEATH.

The ability to convert psychological symptoms into physical symptoms is very common in our society and accounts for most of the visits made to doctors. Religion, like psychotherapy, has offered numerous healing approaches to death. Jewish healing approaches we know about are the seven-day grieving period, the 30-day grieving period, the yearly grieving period, and special prayers. Other coping mechanisms are spiritism, the belief in life after death. Other approaches to defeating death occur during a lifetime, e.g., the born again concept of being saved. Others defeat death through intergenerational contacts and family contacts tied to the tree of life of a nation or a people, or by connecting to the eternal, or by imagining that the dead know what the living are doing.

Other religious approaches to death are washing the dead, watching the dead, participating in wakes, and building monuments. These are all therapeutic processes and rituals meant to help a person through the stages of grieving. All religious structures have psychological strategies for healing.

MATERIALISTIC RELIGION

Another perspective is that death is part of life and that all of us are constantly killing cells and removing them, and therefore one must believe that there is constantly a connection to life even when there is death. Possibly the parable of the newborn fetus approaches the subject best by describing the medical answer to the question, "Is there life after birth?"

There is a song, The Kindertodtenlieder (song for the death of a child), by Gustav Mahler, which is an attempt at healing the pain of death and loss. In section one is presented the concept that the sun shines on everyone else and grief came only to him, the singer. This represents a famous biblical statement in Midrash, in which God is viewed as shining even upon the wicked; His light continues even in the face of darkness; and only a little light has been extinguished. This symbolism appears in the Jewish Kaddish when God's Kingdom is declared, meaning that we are given the light that brightens the world, whether it be God or Christ, and regardless of the darkness in our own lives. The singer's anger in the first stage, is because God does not appear to be grieved. But, in the second section, he seems to accept that fate has deluded him; he sees God as Greco-Roman in nature, a God that sets up a fate he, the singer, cannot control. The biblical perspective is that we have both determinism and nondeterminism. In identifying God as fate, the singer, in my opinion, is expressing rage at God.

Section three of the lieder (song) expresses the singer's remembrance of the parent's joy at being together with their child. The memories that linger are not reality, however; but this, too, is part of the recovery stage: the belief developing in this stage that the light was extinguished (the light being a metaphor here for the holy spirit of God dwelling within people); and the delusion developing as well that death is unreal and temporary. The usual religious antidote arising from such ideas is that loved ones will meet again in heaven or in the resurrection, thus avoiding the reality of loss and the eventual healing process.

Finally, in the song's fifth section, recrimination and guilt remain because God's authority is not fully accepted. Some reconciliation is reached, however, as the child rests in the mother's arms, with God Himself looking over them. Such a reconciliation with God as parent between Judaism and Christianity is indeed an answer to death.

Breaking Addictions: 12 Steps on the Path to Wellness

1. Admitted we were powerless, and that our lives had become unmanageable.

2. Came to believe that a Power greater than ourselves could restore us to sanity.

3. Made a decision to turn our will and our lives over to the care of God as we understood Him.

4. Made a searching and fearless moral inventory of ourselves.

5. Admitted to God, to ourselves and to another human being the exact nature of our wrongs.

6. Were entirely ready to have God remove all these defects of character.

7. Humbly asked Him to remove our shortcomings.

8. Made a list of all persons we had harmed and became willing to make amends to them all.

9. Made direct amends to such people wherever possible, except when to do so would injure them or others.

10. Continued to take personal inventory, and when we were wrong, promptly admitted it.

11. Sought through prayer and meditation to improve our conscious contact with God, as we understood Him, praying only for knowledge of His will for us, and the power to carry that out.

12. Having had a spiritual awakening as the result of these steps, we tried to carry this message to others, and to practice these principles in all our affairs.

Controlling Appetite with the Word of the Lord

Avoid sweets and all wickedness

Put a knife to your throat, if you be a man given to appetite. Be not desirous of pastries for they are deceitful meat (Prov. 23:2, 3).

Set a watch, O Lord, before my mouth; keep the door of my lips. Incline not my heart to any evil thing (unhealthy food), to practice wicked works with men that work iniquity; and let me not eat of their pastries (Psa. 141:3, 4).

Pray to the Lord for new desires

O Lord, I beseech, let now Your ear be attentive to the prayer of Your servant, and to the prayer of Your servants who desire to revere Your name (Neh. 11:1).

Therefore I say to you, what things you desire, when ye pray, believe that you will receive them and you shall have them (Mark 11:24).

Desire spiritual gifts and you will receive your own desires

Follow after charity, and desire spiritual gifts (1 Cor. 14:1).

Delight yourself in the Lord; and He shall give you the desires of your heart (Psa. 37:4).

All the world, from babes to nations, called to desire the will of the Lord

As newborn babies, desire the sincere milk of the word, that you may grow (1 Peter 2:2).

For the Lord of Commandments says, I will shake the heavens, and the earth, and the sea, and the dry land; and I will shake all nations, and the desire of all nations shall come; and I will fill this house with glory, says the Lord of Commandments (Haggai 2:6, 7).

Nutritional Ten Commandments

And the Word of the Lord God, the Nurturer and Sustainer of life, came unto me:

Thou shall eat only the natural foods, for they are holy and do not contain food additives, preservatives, and chemicals.

Thou shall eat tropical fruits, for they are rich with minerals and manganese.

Thou shall eat quality protein, for it provides the building blocks of the amino acids.

Thou shall eat milk, seeds, eggs and nuts, for they contain the complete energy of development.

Thou shall eat vegetables, for they fight cancer and heart disease.

Thou shall eat fermented foods, for they contain the potential life-giving power of bacteria.

Thou shall eat the foods of the sea, for their oils are essential to life.

Thou shall drink living spring water, for it contains the minerals of the earth.

Thou shall use only nutrients as food preservatives, colors, and flavorers.

Thou shall sanctify and enrich thy food to build holiness and health.

And when you eat these and be sated, you shall bless Me.

And if you keep these commandments, I will dwell with you all the days of your life.

Verses of Peace and Healing

Peace through Love of God and Neighbor

Rabbi, which is the great commandment in the Scriptures? Yeshua said unto him, Thou shalt love the Lord thy God with all thy heart, and with all thy soul, and with all thy mind. This is the first and greatest commandment. And the second is like unto it, Thou shalt love thy neighbor as thyself. On these two commandments hang all the Torah and the prophets. (Matt. 22:36-40).

Thou wilt keep him in perfect peace, whose mind is focused on you, because he trusts in you (Isa. 26:3).

Peace Ordained by God

Lord, Thou wilt ordain peace for us, for He has created greatness within us (Isa. 26:12).

Behold, I will bring them health and healing and I will cure them, and will reveal to them the abundance of peace and truth (Jer. 33:6).

The Lord will give strength to His people; the Lord will bless His people with peace (Psa. 29:11).

Healing is the Forgiveness of Sin

And, behold, they brought to him a man sick of the palsy, lying on a bed: and Jesus seeing their faith said unto the sick of the palsy; Son, be of good cheer; your sins are forgiven you. And behold, certain of the scribes said to themselves, This man blasphemeth. And Jesus knowing their thoughts said, Why do you think evil in your hearts? Is it easier to say, your sins be forgiven you; or to say, Arise, and walk? (Matt. 9:2-5).

The Application of Intelligence to the Development of Character: Breaking the Cycle of Anxiety and Anger

The development of inner peace and emotional stability is one of the purposes of the Scriptures. The cycle of anxiety and anger begins with expectation and judgment of others. Expectation leads to judgment and judgment leads to blame, then anger, depression, and finally, overall instability of character.

Scripture says to judge yourself, to trust, to expect nothing from this world, and to love and forgive your neighbor. Mightiness is the ability to control passions, and a man's glory is in overlooking an offense. A perfect man has no error in his speech. Learning to love better is the key source of defeating anger.

Anxiety is cured by prayer to God and by reaping the fruits of the spirit. The fruits of the spirit are joy, long suffering, kindness, gentleness, patience, love, and peace. They are cultivated by daily discipline, vigilance, and careful self-judgment. The laws of God are a defense against losing the presence of the Holy Spirit, which is the source of spiritual motivation. To begin the task, repent -- that is, apologize to God and to men for judging them. Repent and believe the Scriptures, for the Kingdom of God is at hand. Read and live the Scriptures, and your character will develop whether you are a genius or whether you are a simple person. He who develops this kind of character, the character of Christ, will glow in the light of the Lord. The development of this character is the result of the greatest application of intelligence.

The Three Paths to Healing Model

	PROBLEM	SOLUTION	TRUTH	ERROR
MEDICAL DISEASE	Biochemical and Biochemical imbalance	Treatment by a professional	Heart is deceptive -- who can know it	No personal responsibility
RELIGION	Sin Behavioral disobedience	Obedience	Choice sinful nature	Shallow view of sin and repentance -- legalistic
PSYCHO-LOGICAL	Loneliness	Affirmation	High value on people	No God relationship

Holy Medicine

Treatment of Disease by Jesus

Multiple methods of healing were used by Jesus in the Bible.

- Laying on of hands (Mark 6:5; 16:9-19)
- Bible instruction (Matt. 23:23-33)
- Gift of the Holy Spirit (Acts)
- Baptism
- Obedience to the Commandments (Matt 19:16-30; 7:21; John 20:19-23)
- Forgiveness of sin (John 20:19-23)
- Example and Parable (Luke 15:8-32)

All these "ways" given to us by God through Jesus, in order to release the healing power of the spirit into the body, are important foundations to a complete medical healing practice.

Character and Communication

Intelligence is important, but it is character, which is both important and more critical to have. Practice of the basic 12 rules of good communication will further development of those elements of character important to success in a social setting -- no matter how difficult such a process may be for the highly intellectual individual.

1. When there is a problem, be willing to admit that you are part of the problem.

2. Be willing to change.

3. Do not use emotionally charged expressions like "You do not really care," "You don't do anything right" etc.

4. Be responsible for your own emotions, words, actions, and reactions. Do not blame them on other people. Accept the

blame.

5. Refrain from having reruns of old problems.

6. Deal with one problem at a time.

7. Deal in the present, not in the past. Hang a "no fishing" sign over previous problems.

8. Measure the positive instead of the negative.

9. Learn to communicate in nonverbal ways.

10. Express your thoughts and concerns, but also listen, understand and respond to the meaning behind what people are saying. When people fly off the handle, remember that it is often because they want attention and not because they are trying intentionally to be disrespectful or destructive.

11. Practice the golden rule. Treat people as you would like to be treated.

12. Do the best you can to help others, not expecting to receive in return.

Conventional Medicine and Foolishness

Conventional medicine has a long history of foolishness, e.g., x-ray treatments for acne, ringworm and thyroid disease. Untested so-called miracle drugs, DES and thalidomide, are still ruining lives. Many current treatments your doctor now brags about will be proven dangerous, such as beta blockers (already considered dangerous if taken more than three years after heart attack) and diuretics. Consider the history of medicine before you accept the explanations of conventional medicine. The same problems have occurred in the use of environmental treatments such as DDT and strychnine -- these drugs are now thought to have done more to damage than to help. The use of natural agents, e.g., in nutrition, and electrical approaches, will lead to the best pharmacological treatment for human health and environmental problems.

What can this generation of doctors -- impaired by their tunnel vision -- be compared to? They can be compared to an auto mechanic who, having only knowledge of the muffler system, thinks that the way to solve all the engine's problems is by dealing with the tail pipe.

Faith in Medicine

A recent study in *American Medical News*, December 20, 1993, said that physicians are obligated to deal, at least to some degree, with issues of faith because it affects patients and their judgment of how they are going to be treated.

AMA News said that knowing patients' religious beliefs helped physicians understand how they cope with serious illnesses. For example, Harold Vanderpool, Ph.D., University of Texas Medical Branch, has found patient, family, and medical team extremely important in managing the overall care.

Turning a blind eye to a patient's faith or lack of faith is turning a blind eye to the whole realm of the doctor/patient interrelationship. There are religious, questions according to the *American Medical News*, that even nonreligious physicians have to acknowledge in order to be a whole physician.

Of course, a physician's religious convictions should never be forced on a patient, and he can't become a clergyman and a doctor at the same time, but he can provide the opportunities for pastoral growth, which we are now providing though Rev. Charles Rush and Rabbi Aryeh Alpern, as well as the 12 step programs of Bob Moss.

Family Matters

A recent article in the *American Congress Rehabilitation Medicine, American Academy of Physical Medicine*, showed that one year following a traumatic brain injury, that the better a family is able to cope with the stress of a child's head trauma, or probably any injury for that matter, has been able to be linked to overall recovery.

Therefore, we have come to recognize that family generational issues and family cutoffs, where people don't talk to each other, don't speak to each other, or hold grudges, are critical aspects to each patient's total recovery.

We have experts in family counseling that are trained in the Bowen method. These critical issues should be addressed in the long run.

Vaccines, Medicines, and Religion

The federal government agreed to pay the claims of the pharmaceutical companies which would have to stop doing vaccinations. This ironically is representation of church and state since religion also bears on the issue of health. Many of the practices, rituals and customs of modern medicine actually now would be well defined as religious practices, in that modern medicine, as it is currently practiced, is a religion and its consequences have divine effects.

Religious Addiction

There are many ways to be addicted. As we have talked, there is chocolate addiction, alcohol addiction, marijuana and illicit drug addiction, carbohydrate addiction, sugar addiction, white flour addiction, fat addiction through cheeses and meats, even meat addiction. One area that surprises that can become a drug is religious addiction, where the qualities can be inability to think, doubt, or question information or authority except for religious authority; overly black and white simplistic thinking; shame-based belief systems, you're never good enough, never doing it right; magical thinking that God can fix everything without people utilizing worldly resources; scrupulosity; rigid, obsessive adherence to rules, codes, ethics, or guidelines to the point of forgetting some of the deeper meanings of life; compulsive praying; compulsive quoting of scripture; compulsive church attendance without bringing the effects into daily life; unrealistic financial contributions that can't be sustained; judgmental attitudes that are completely closed or never reviewed again; belief that sex is inherently dirty even between spouses; compulsive fasting; conflict with all forms of science, medicine, education; detachment from the world; manipulating scripture or text; feeling chosen; claiming special messages from God without backing it up with contributions to our neighbors; trancelike religious highs or states. Like all addictions, it is accompanied by somatic illnesses, from sleeplessness, back pain, headaches to high blood pressure.

Reference: When God Becomes a Drug: Breaking the Chain of Religious Addiction Abuse, 1991, Leo Booth.

Some Signs of Inner Peace

A tendency to think and act spontaneously rather than from fear based on past experiences.

Living in the moment.

Vulnerable to love extended by others as well as a desire to extend love.

Extending appreciation, affirming people.

Trouble worrying, finding it easier to take life as it is.

Some smiling through the eyes from the deepness of the heart.

Diminishing in judging other people, condemning other people, blaming other people, interpreting the actions of others as attacks or conflicting with others.

Letting life happen rather than trying to control life and make it happen.

Dedication of the P.A.T.H. Wellness Manual

The PATH Wellness Manual is dedicated to seizing the holistic truths of the world for the purposes and sake of God's kingdom.

The use of conventional terminology in the translations of scripture used nor the juxtaposition of Jewish or Christian concepts is no way put in acceptance by the author of the correctness of typical Bible translations or those views but is presented as material that can be useful for those who are starting to utilize the spiritual dimension in their life.

Scriptures on Abortion

The Lord said to Moses, "Consecrate to me every firstborn male. The first offspring of every womb among the Israelites belongs to me, whether man or animal" (Ex. 13:1).

Naked I came from my mother's womb, and naked I will depart (Job 1:2).

He did not shut the doors of the womb on me to hide trouble from my eyes (Job 3:10).

Did not he who made me in the womb make them? Did not the same one form us both within our mothers? (Job 31).

As one whom his mother comforteth, so will I comfort you (Isa. 66:13).

When Rachel saw that she was not bearing Jacob any children, she became jealous of her sister. So she said to Jacob, "Give me children, or I will die." Jacob became angry with her and said, "Am I in the place of God, who has kept you from having children?" (Gen. 30:1-2).

Ephraim's glory will fly away like a bird -- no birth, no pregnancy, no conception (Hos. 9:11).

Yet you brought me out of the womb; you made me trust in you even at my mother's breast. From birth I was cast upon you; from my mother's womb you have been my God (Psa. 22:9-10).

From whose womb comes the ice? Who gives birth to the frost from the heavens? (Job 38).

Give them, O Lord -- what will you give them? Give them wombs that miscarry and breasts that are dry (Hos. 9:14).

Why then did you bring me out of the womb? I wish I had died before any eye saw me (Job 10:18).

Even from birth the wicked go astray; from the womb they are wayward and speak lies (Isa. 58:3).

Moses, "Please, my lord, do not hold against us the sin we have so foolishly committed. Do not let her be like a stillborn infant coming from its mother's womb with its flesh half eaten away" (Num. 12:12).

Can a mother forget the baby at her breast and have no compassion on the child she has borne? Though she may forget, I will not forget you! (Isa. 49:15).

If men who are fighting hit a pregnant woman and she give birth prematurely but there is no serious injury, the offender must be fined whatever the woman's husband demands and the court allows. But if there is a serious injury [abortion], you are to take life for life, tooth for tooth, hand for hand, foot for foot, burn for burn, wound for wound, bruise for bruise (Ex. 21:22-25).

Then God remembered Rachel; he listened to her and opened her womb. She became pregnant and gave birth to a son and said, "God has taken away my disgrace." She named him Joseph, and said, "May the Lord add to me another son" (Gen. 30:22-24).

Relationships Between Biofeedback and Religious Terminology

1. Imagery -- the religious equivalent is prophetic imagination and books.

2. Meditative quiet -- be still and know the Lord is God.

3. Repetitive thought processing and cognitive drilling are equivalent to repetitive, incessant prayer, contemplative prayer.

4. Alpha waves or creative brain waves -- getting the right resonance with the Creator's will.

5. Relaxation -- experiencing the Peace of the Shabbas.

6. Breathing control -- His Holy Spirit can be inspired with every breath.

7. Pain control -- in God there is no more pain, nor death, nor sorrow in the Lord; He has conquered all pain.

8. Blood pressure -- the brain controls the body as the heavens control the earth; therefore, the heart, pulse, BP rate can be controlled.

9. Immune system -- the Lord is my shield; His word is my sword.

10. Getting answers from the inner self or from higher consciousness. Ask the higher power of God and He will open the door and answer you. Find spiritual discernment through the holy spirit.

11. Brain wave training -- learn self-control over one's thoughts. God has given us the spirit of self-control.

12. Attention training -- learning to focus in on the higher power. Reading and meditating on the Word day and night.

For additional material on biofeedback, see p. 179ff.

The Brain Controls the Body as the Mind and Spirit Control Health

The aging brain needs to be rehabilitated. Intravenous choline, amino acids, B-vitamins, as well as electrical stimulation, and light therapies may rejuvenate the aging brain and help restore taste and smell in the elderly and, probably to some degree, intellectual capacity. The brain is the master of the body and therefore the attitudes of the mind and the spirit affect health greatly. It is manipulation of the brain's chemistry that can help us direct our mind and spirit toward the proper development. The brain is the master endocrine organ of the body, which, through its biochemical products, the spinal cord and its connections, rules the body. It is the electrical impulses of the brain that are most dominant, even over its biochemistry. True brain rehabilitation and brain healing require electrical stimulation as well as nutritional building of the neurotransmitters. These basic neurotransmitters are acetyl choline from choline, the adrenalines from tyrosine and DL-phenylalanine, the enkephalins from methionine and branched chain amino acids, and the glutathione from N-acetylcysteine. Other amino acid precursors, like taurine and GABA, also make up important neurotransmitters which link amino acids as the key environmental nutrients for the brain. The essential amino acids are the key neurotransmitters for the brain and body.

Medicine

We have presented to us everyday a conventional medicine blind to the brain and blind to holistic health. We have also the pantheists who love nature's medicine, but do not respect man's medical creations because they do not know that man, made in the image of God, is also capable of creating wonderful things through God's will.

So, we have modern medicine split in two; but there is only one path between the two -- a path that honors God as the Creator of heaven and earth, honors His creation and honors man and his contribution, whatever he can make, design and conceive, as long as it is according to God's will.

Biofeedback

Many states of illness tend to occur following major stressful events in our lives. Some examples include loss of a job or death of a loved one. In addition, preexisting diseases may worsen, such as an increase in high blood pressure or more frequent attacks of colitis or irritable bowel. This is because the state of our mind contributes to the state of our physical health. Modern medicine is beginning to recognize that all disease is partly psychosomatic -- that is, our outlook and anticipation of the future strongly influence the course of our wellness or sickness.

The ability to deal with stress is an important tool in maintaining our sense of mental proportion. If we "fall apart" under pressure we may be subject to frequent anxiety attacks, hyperventilation, painful muscle spasms, heart palpitations, or even the more long term side effects such as high blood pressure, chronic headaches, diabetes, or heart attack. On the other hand, if we "keep cool" under stress we may avoid all the above problems and be much happier persons.

The skills to deal with stress can be learned, in fact, quite easily. Biofeedback is a form of self-awareness training whose goal is to help you become more in control of your emotions and body functions. With the assistance of our trained nurse or biofeedback technician you will learn how to lower your heart rate and blood pressure, improve your circulation, "cool down" nervous perspiration, and thoroughly loosen your muscles. Relaxation exercises will be demonstrated which you can practice at home to help you achieve these goals. With continued practice and with the opportunity to learn from watching your responses, you can achieve a level of self-control and peace of mind you may not have thought possible. This technique can then be called upon in prayer or to help provide support in a variety of everyday stressful situations, e.g., when in a traffic jam. CES combined with biofeedback is even more effective.

Biofeedback training has already proven very helpful in treating many conditions including high blood pressure, heart disease, asthma, headaches (migraine and tension), certain forms of poor circulation (Raynaud's pheno-menon), impotence, peptic ulcer, irritable bowel and muscle spasms. In addition, it is an essential aid in achieving smoking cessation and modifying chronic anxiety states.

PATH'S Guide to Biofeedback

Training Brain Waves to Maximize Health, Heal Illness, and Help Individuals Increase Their Ability to Think, Relax, Meditate, or Pray

Biofeedback - General Introduction

Relaxation usually generalizes to the rest of the body. Our ability to control certain relaxation techniques in circulation, in the hands or the pulse, can generalize to the whole system. Most of all, relaxation techniques that focus in on brain wave training have the widest benefits, because the nervous system and the brain are involved with more aspects of body functions than any other body system. Biofeedback has been useful in the following disorders: migraine headache, gastrointestinal and muscular disorders, anxiety, epilepsy, and cerebral palsy.

Biofeedback is a tool for releasing potential, similar to prayer and meditation, except that it makes use of medical technology to give an individual more feedback. Brain wave training is particularly useful because the brain has no sensory processes by which it can detect its own brainwave activity. Your hands may feel cold, but you may not know that you are in theta wave rather than alpha wave. You can get a sense of the brain's control through the technique of biofeedback. It is a dreamlike state and is particularly useful for increasing imagery. One of the goals of biofeedback training is to increase the normal alpha frequency, which normally decreases with age and enable you to have the flexibility to go into the fringe of consciousness and theta states. Ultimately, theta is easier to suppress under the control of the conscious individual and alpha frequency can be increased.

This is the way in which the sounds are made audible: the lower limit of hearing is 25 hertz, but the average alpha frequency is 10 hertz, which is inaudible without amplification. By multiplying it by 200, the average alpha feedback tone goes to 2,000 hertz, which lies within the range of the human hearing spectrum and generates a series of musical tones which can sound like flute music. Theta feedback sounds are more like an oboe. Imagery can help induce these kinds of states. Visualization and imagery may be the best way of programming the body and reaching the body's immune system. In fact, there have been some studies suggesting visualization as an aid to cancer and immune disorder recovery.

In Christian mysticism the path has been called Jacob's ladder. In China the path is called Tao. In Sanskrit the path is called Antakarana. The power of biofeedback lies in its effect on stress. Every individual facing a disease has a triple stress: the stress that predated the disease and which was a factor leading to its onset; the stress of having the disease with all its threats to self-image, identity, and personal security; and the stress of the treatment -- painful, frightening and depleting. Biofeedback can lead to quiet emotions, and quiet emotions can promote a quiet body and inner peace. Self-regulation is at the core; but really regulation by the higher power is ultimately what is accomplished in biofeedback. Let go, let God, is what is accomplished in the biofeedback session: getting on the PATH.

In epilepsy, another potential rhythm for treating biofeedback is 12-14 hertz, or mu rhythm, also recorded from the rolandic cortex. Some studies have suggested that a mu rhythm is often described as an abnormal rhythm because of its appearance. Reverie is designated as 7-9 hertz and can also help reduce seizure frequency. Many muscular-skeletal problems have been amenable to biofeedback treatment:

- prolonged immobilization
- myositis ossificans
- joint repair
- elevated activity following back strain
- frozen shoulder

- muscle tendon transfer
- substitution movements
- muscle strengthening and relaxation
- whiplash
- muscle shortening
- asymmetry and homologous trunk or back muscles

Biofeedback can also be used for neuromuscular reeducation, stretch reflex, and tactile stimulation, among other activities.

The idea behind biofeedback training is to use sensitive detectors to tell you what is happening inside your own body so you can have a better sense of changes occurring in your body which are associated with various emotions. This will ultimately give you a sense of assisted relaxation, assisted prayer, and assisted meditation.

In human history, unconscious, involuntary processes formally sent feedback signals only to the hypothalamus. We can now give feedback signals to the cortex. Closing the biocybernetics loop means bridging the normal gap between conscious and unconscious and voluntary and involuntary processes. It is accomplishing voluntary self-regulation through imagination and visualization. There are also many dimensions used in biofeedback which include not only regular biofeedback techniques, but also verbal and medical biofeedback techniques as well; such as measuring urinary conicotine levels, salivary cyanide, expired carbon monoxide, etc. in smokers. With biofeedback, people learn to recognize essential stress cues that they might not normally recognize.

Basic Rules for Establishing Good Biofeedback

Biofeedback attempts to connect the mind to the body. Some basic work between temperature, heart training, EMG, or smooth muscle training, such as pelvic, bladder, or bowel control, may be useful. Attention deficit disorders and memory/concentration problems use the beta-theta approach, and relaxation uses the alpha-theta approach. Usually 6 skin temperature training sessions are done to maintain digit skin temperature of 95 degrees for 10 minutes.

Alpha feedback training can be done using the 01 monopolar placement, OZ or P2 (even the T3 electrode can be placed on the basis of the BEAM abnormality), with auditory feedback on alpha when alpha percent is greater than 40 percent. When alpha reaches 50 percent,

theta training can replace alpha. When theta reaches 50 percent, biofeedback for both alpha and theta feedback can be done with a different bell for each. For certain kinds of disorganization and cloudy consciousness, beta training is not done until relaxation is learned.

Biofeedback from the Living God

Biofeedback is sometimes a very confusing topic. Biofeedback refers to the use of electronic medical devices to give more auditory, verbal, and visual information back to the body about how it is working. For example, during biofeedback, when one tries to relax one's muscles, one can hear a sound telling the degree of relaxation. Or if one aims to slow one's pulse, one can hear or see one's pulse more easily than by just feeling the pulse. By hearing the pulse, it is easier to try to manipulate it with one's conscious control. This is also done with temperature control. When people are nervous, their hands might get colder or sweaty and warmer. With biofeedback we learn to control our vascular and nervous system.

During biofeedback, by giving auditory and/or visual signals, individuals are able to better direct their conscious thoughts and thus control what would normally be outside their control. Everyday our nervous systems interact with our bodies. In Peace and/or in Christ, in healthiness and Godliness, both our minds and our bodies are one; they are the temples of the Holy Spirit. In many illnesses, this connection is severed.

For many individuals the consequence of anxiety is a decreased immune system, manifested by increased colds and disease. They may also experience anxiety in one or some of these forms:

- palpitations
- sweaty hands or cold hands
- shortness of breath
- light headedness
- headache
- eye strain
- difficulty swallowing
- diarrhea
- constipation
- frequent urination
- numbness in the hands and toes
- acne

There are vital ways in which the mind or brain's chemistry affects the body's health. This is the connection that we are trying to make for people with biofeedback. Helping individuals to understand this connection between the mind and the body and how their emotions impact their temperature and vascular system, pulse rate, bowel, and bladder habits is the first step.

Biofeedback has been used by proponents of the new age movement to access what is known as lower consciousness, and what is sometimes thought of as demonic, unconscious, psychic or channeling processes. Biofeedback can now be used to access higher consciousness by altering the drowsiness states of certain individuals who have abnormal brain chemistry or abnormal neurological states on brain mapping, such as a low P300 wave. (A positive brain wave which occurs at about 1/3 of a second). These individuals can learn brain exercises in order to move from the theta state or drowsiness state to a more alert, creative mind frame in the alpha state. These individuals can also reduce anxiety and all its manifestations, which include ulcers, palpitations, smoking, overeating, irritability, anger, etc., in both their emotional and physical components.

Biofeedback can easily become a biblical or meditative experience depending on patient choice. For example:

1. The use of imagery in biofeedback can be selected from prophetic images: God and His chariot (Ezekiel); the scroll extended from heaven to earth (Revelation); the talking donkey (Numbers); turning water into wine (John); clock turning backwards (Chronicles); sun standing still (Joshua); walking on water (Gospels); dead coming back to life (Revelation). God provides prophetic imagery in the Bible because of its relaxing, beneficial effect on the brain. By using prophetic imagery in the context of biofeedback, one can maximize the healing effect of imagery on the brain's physical nervous system.

2. The use of a form of biofeedback which emphasizes meditative quiet. The Biblical principle here is "Be still and know that the Lord is God." This principle applies to both meditation and good concentration. There is a time during which a person must be still in order to experience his/her connection to a higher power (for example, the Lord God Jesus Christ - LGJC/Yahweh), however one may know it.

3. The use of an aspect of biofeedback which works on repetitive thought processing and cognitive drilling. This is equivalent to repetitive, incessant or contemplative prayer. Various prayers can be used during the biofeedback process as an attempt to increase the alpha-theta transition state, a state in which we can dream and see visions, in an attempt

to gain greater emotional and intellectual flexibility.

4. Many individuals want to use biofeedback to increase their alpha waves because the alpha state is more creative.   There is no greater source of creativity than being in touch with the Creator or Higher Power Himself.

5. Use of still another form of biofeedback -- relaxation and experiencing the Sabbath peace (which surpasses all understanding); evidence suggests that this is an important part of total holiness. The practice of biofeedback can improve one's ability to willfully relax and therefore makes it easier to "turn off" one day per week in a society that never turns off and never stops. Relaxation training, therefore, is an important part of the Biblical path.

6. Biofeedback can be used to help an individual learn to control the vascular and nervous system in his/her body. In God there is no pain, no death, no sorrow. Pain control is achieved when one is able to shut off certain neural circuits as pain's pathways. This becomes a Biblical tool for greater self-control which is a gift of God's Holy Spirit - who teaches a reality far greater than a higher power, greater and more important than any power known in this world.

7. Biofeedback has also been used to control blood pressure. The biblical principle here is that the brain controls the body as the heavens control the earth; therefore, the heart and pulse rate and other bodily functions can be controlled by the brain. We need to look at biofeedback as a way of extending the heavenly and spiritual control of the brain into the body. If the spirit of God controls one's brain, one will have better total health overall. When the brain truly has control, it can control various bodily functions such as acidity in the stomach, diarrhea, palpitations, etc. What we try to accomplish with biofeedback is to break the circuitry if the brain has irregular rhythms, before they cause disease. We combine biofeedback with Cranial Electrical Stimulation to maximize effectiveness.

8. Everyone doing the biofeedback is a prayerful spirit and is actually building up their immune systems.

9. Scientists claim that by using biofeedback one can gain answers to one's problems from one's inner self. Believers in God know that the Kingdom of God is within them -- the source of all truth. This connection to God, or Higher Consciousness, can be achieved by increasing the alpha state, which is the goal of biofeedback.

God has given us the spirit of self-control and any

technique that helps us master self-control is moving us along the path toward total holiness. By reading and meditating on the Word in conjunction with special biofeedback techniques one can reach a higher state of consciousness/Godliness.

Biofeedback Imagery for Christians

The lion shall dwell with the lamb. When Christ comes there will be no more pain nor suffering nor death, and every tear will be wiped from our eyes. The old order of things will pass away. The dwelling of God will be with men, and He will live with them. And the holy city New Jerusalem will come down from heaven from God as a bride beautifully dressed in white for her husband Christ. The first heaven and the first earth will pass away and there will be a new earth and a new heaven in glory. And the world will not need a sun or a moon to shine, for the glory of God and the lamb of God will give it light. And all nations will walk by that light.

The Word of God and the kings of the earth will bring their splendor to the city of Christ. Nothing impure will be in this world. Nothing shameful nor deceitful. No fear of abandonment or loss; no fear at all, but only freedom. God's love will have cast out fear forever. And the spirit of the lamb will dwell in Jerusalem, and peace will reign all over the world. But the cowardly, the unbelieving, the vile, the murderers, the immoral, those who practice magic and drugs will not have a place in this Kingdom.

There will be a spring of Water of Life from which all the thirsty can drink, and the dry bones of the righteous will stand up and walk on that day, and the River of Life will be there for them to drink. And the throne of God and the lamb will be on this earth to the glory of God the Creator. Its light will burn as a seven-candle lamp stand, and his cross will be not a cross of blood but a cross of stars. And all demons will be cast into the Abyss with their father the devil.

God is coming in His clouds and with His armies of angels and every eye will see Him. His head and hair are white as snow, and His eyes are like a blazing fire. His feet are like bronze glowing in the furnace, and His voice is like the sound of rushing water with the power of thunder. In His right hand He holds seven stars, and the power of the seven spirits of God is with the law. And He brings with Him peace for all, love and goodwill to all men and women.

Biofeedback and Imagery

Biofeedback is a useful way to exercise the brain. It can be used to augment alpha and theta brain waves, which can help individuals with headaches, irritable bowel syndrome, stomach problems, palpitations, and other brain chemically-mediated stress conditions. To help the doctor develop the best images to use during the biofeedback training system, 3-4 images of the following subjects should be written down: images of peace related to family, images of peace related to the world, images of peace related to finances, images of peace related to self, images of peace related to work, images of peace related to the community or society. These images should be numbered in order of importance.

Biofeedback and Meditation

With biofeedback, many people ultimately come in touch with the inner path of their life. In the West, it is called the source, talent and strength of each person, the source of their creativity, sometimes called the ego, the transpersonal spiritual self of every person. This ego is distinct from the ego of psychology and psychiatry -- it is an extension of the personality and frequently called the soul. The personality is sometimes defined as the sum total of our physical, emotional, mental, and stereotypical characteristics, limited by heredity, conditioning, culture, experience, and education. It is an ego often thought to be the immortal self which transcends the personality, opens the door to the genuinely creative, unpredictable, undeduced solution of the body, emotions, and mind. In China, this source of the soul is called the Tao, or the path. In Zen it is called true self. In India it is called true self or Jiva. The path concept is common both in China and in Christianity and Judaism. In the book of Acts, early Christians were called to be on the path. Derech, or the path to God, has been the great tradition in Judaism.

Biofeedback shows us that there is control over the body and the soul or self. Even single muscle cells can be controlled by volition. There can be autogenic training of the bladder, muscles. Our bodies are equipped with regulating mechanisms that work automatically. Thank God we don't have to think and say, "Heart, start beating," nor do we have to remind our lungs to breath. But we do impact these automatic mechanisms when we catch our breath after being startled, when we blush due to embarrassment, or when our mouths water when we smell food. It is important to have some sense that your body is impacted by your mind, and biofeedback helps individuals who have numerous mind-body connection problems, such as allergies and immune system disorders. The brain regulates all these systems, for example, the bowel, the bladder; and what biofeedback can do help reconnect the brain's control of these areas.

Biofeedback Techniques at PATH

One of the biofeedback techniques at PATH is autogenic training of the heart. Patients are taught to hear their heart rate: their heart beat is put on a loud speaker and they try to relax and slow down their heart rate. They use the beat as an indication of their progress. They can do this with their hand, electrodes or with a Doppler device. Cardiac patients have been able to study the behavior of their hearts by watching and/or hearing their EKG signals. In some cases they have reduced the frequency of their PVC's, which can be induced by anxiety.

Diseases that occur without our realizing it, like Raynaud's and poor circulation, frequently occur with anxiety. Many individuals can learn to control their hand temperature ten to twenty degrees, which can make it possible to overcome this problem. There is a king cell or primary neuro-nucleus in the primary subcortical structures that can help control this. Mind-body duality as a healing concept can be achieved through biofeedback before the brain makes the body critically sick; for example, when the irritable bowel syndrome of anxiety progresses to diverticulosis because of the combination of poor food choices and stress.

Biofeedback and Stress

Biofeedback can help numerous conditions which are a result of stress, such as psychiatric conditions, anxiety, depression, substance abuse disorders, sleep disorders, learning disabilities, hyperactivity, tinnitus, agoraphobia, and neurological conditions such as temporal lobe epilepsy and manic-depression. Biofeedback can also help allergic conditions such as asthma by reducing reactivity, as well as helping immune disorders and skin disorders. Other conditions in which stress is probably the major contributor are PMS, colitis, Raynaud's Syndrome (cold extremities), palpitations, and other cardiovascular disorders such as high blood pressure. Biofeedback techniques also can help a person learn to avoid stress.

Biblical or PATH [1] Therapy Versus Conventional or Freudian Psychotherapy: Their Differences and Similarities, Their Strengths and Weaknesses

Counseling and good advice are essential to life, hence we must understand the basis of good counseling. Freud is at the core of all modern psychiatry, while Christ and the Torah are at the core of all Biblical counseling. Freudian psychotherapy is the theory of personality espoused by Sigmund Freud. Biblical counseling is the theory of personality and life itself as set forth by the Author and Creator of all life. Christian counselors believe that the Bible is sufficient to provide a framework for thinking about every personality issue. Freudian personality theorists believe that their method is purely scientific, that it does not rely on a higher power or outside source.

Nonetheless, ironically, at times Biblical concept and Freudian theory can and do come to some similar conclusions. Freud proposes that the bases of life and health are love and work; the Bible teaches faith and God's works as the foundation. Faith is symbolized by love, and the works of God are love in action. The emphasis on work and love is grounded in the unity of their source. The Bible refers to prophets like Joseph and Daniel, who were interpreters of dreams, to some degree in the same way as Freud, who also was an interpreter of dreams. Freud saw dreams as an access to the lower and higher unconscious. The Bible sees dreams in the same light, but focuses more on the higher conscious mind.

---

1. The Bible describes the disciples' work as the Way. A better translation is the Path which implies a journey toward God -- a journey which approaches Him from many directions, which may never reach its goal, but can still be in accordance with God's will. Acts 24:14, 22; 22:4; 19:19, 23; 9:2; 16:17, and 15:25, 26; 2 Peter 2:2; John 14:6.

Thus, the big difference between these therapies is the recognition of a higher power, biblical authority, and biblical sufficiency as opposed to scientific authority and scientific sufficiency. The PATH, or biblical counselor, himself claims not only to have the scientific method, but he claims to have the extra advantage of being led by the holy spirit, as opposed to Freud who feels there is no higher power than man's own vision.

Virtually all psychiatrists were called Freudian in their method for the first 40 or 50 years of psychoanalysis. This is similar to the way all Christians were called Christians until they later became Franciscans, Lutherans, and Calvinists. Freudians also have broken into denominations, e.g., Ericksonians, Jungians, Rogerians, etc. Ultimately, all modern psychiatry is a religion with denominations originating from Sigmund Freud. Christ is the core of Christian faith and denominations of him are called by the name of some of his followers.

To heal in the name of Sigmund Freud, or to be a Freudian, does not mean to put your hands on someone and say, "In the name of Sigmund Freud, I heal you," but to lay people on the couch or just to use Freud's scientific method of personality to heal them. To heal in the name of Christ is to lay on hands, use anointing oil and follow biblical counseling techniques such as fasting, prayer, diet, etc. Obviously, laying hands on the patient is not going to heal him instantly of anorexia, bulimia, and other psychiatric conditions. We must use, however, the method of healing that can be derived from the scripture's teachings. It may be that the counselor has to work very hard to utilize the bible for presenting problems such as anorexia, obsessive compulsive disorder, etc.. But one can see that these disorders actually have some similar spiritual basis. For example, obsessive compulsive disorder is a repetitive ritual that is destructive in the practice of scrupulosity; yet we must be "scrupulous" in our dealings with people and God (not, however, in our dealings related to our own cleanliness and by making our body an idol). We must not be picking at our fingers all the time, but picking at our behavior. Anorexics and bulimics who are punishing themselves by denying themselves food are also violating biblical commandments. Disobedience to God is at the root of bad habits.

Bad behavior is rooted in fundamental disobedience to, or ignorance of, scripture. As Jesus said, not knowing the scripture, we do greatly err. We can find biblical answers to all questions by exploring the process of communication and reflection within the Bible. We must come to recognize as a Christian or PATH counselor that there is a certain advantage in regard to transference.

Transference to a Freudian counselor in all modern psychiatry is transference to a man and is a transference that has been documented as difficult to break. Transference to a PATH counselor is not to the counselor, but to God, through Christ's example.

The fundamental message of counseling is not just the message taught by counselors; but the message and beliefs within the counselor also will penetrate others even more deeply. So the Christian counselor's strength (as well as his duty to his patient) lies in living the truth and growing consistently in relationship with God, thus equipping himself to communicate with the power flowing from that relationship. The source of Freudian strength is in living scientifically and rationally. Unfortunately, this leads only to living by one's own willpower and not by a power from on high (in many ways it is a doctrine of works only).

The biblical personality concept is that man is sick due to irresponsibility and sin. Freud's personality theory turns irresponsibility and sin into neuroses. PATH therapy gives the patient hope of a higher power to strengthen the individual in his effort to change his behavior. Paul makes the conclusion that within him, despite his desire to do well, is another being (possibly his id) seeking to do evil; that mankind must overcome this self.

Freudian and PATH therapy have relational model concepts in that the Bible and Freud both recognize that loneliness is a problem of all mankind and that affirmation and self-expression are important as counters to this condition. Both recognize the dynamic model that fundamentally mankind is sick and that treatment is required. Fundamental to PATH Christian counseling is the concept that man bears the image of God. Freudian psychology divides the personality into superego, ego, and id. Actually, the core of the Freudian personality theory is the unconscious (id) which symbolizes man as bearing an image to an animal rather than the divine image. Psychology seeks as its goal independence to distribute and dispose animal and psychic energy to sublimate the repressed negative desires into positive desires. Although biblical counseling also sublimates, Freud's idea that repression has led to illness has resulted in Freud becoming the father of sexual liberation and sexual promiscuity, abortion, etc. Men and woman can get sick because they repress sex and sexual feelings, but Freud and his followers have espoused the domination of the unrepressed sexual desire contrary to God's laws.

The biblical concept of personality is fundamental to the health of the personality and recognition of complete dependency on God. Ultimately, it is in accepting dependency on others that mankind becomes fundamentally independent. Man is a personal being who longs deeply to feel valuable. Man is a passionate being who thinks, a volitional being who chooses, an emotional being who feels. The tools which Freudian psychology eventually developed were tools of measurement, such as the Millon test, MMPI, Caliper profile, neuropsychological testing, etc. These tools are the outcome of the Freudian theory of personality and the scientific method. Christian counseling, now in its infancy, also has come to a theory of personality. The next logical development is to develop tools for testing the state of being in Christ. These are spiritual measurements, or christo-metrics rather than psychometrics. Here at PATH we strive to have all patients see biblical PATH counselors, who in turn, have taken the spiritual behavior inventory to evaluate their own spirituality.

Human distress, according to Christian-Jewish counseling or PATH counseling, is a steadfast determination to remain independent of God and still make life work. While for Freudian theorists, the core of human distress is a dependency on one's parents, manifested by a resolve to marry one's parent of the opposite sex. Freudian and PATH therapies both liberate adults from destructive childhood dependencies. Trying to remain independent of God is actually at the core of why people remain too dependent on their parents. Christ on the cross, God's son offering his life before God, actually is the resolution of the Oedipus conflict (the son trying to steal his mother from his father). All sons who unite with Christ end disobedience to their fathers -- meaning that the son, or the man, who submits to the authority of God his father, thereby becomes independent of his worldly father. He is, instead, dependent on God as God's born again son. Resolution of the Oedipus conflict for man in biblically based counseling is in Christ and in a symbolic act of total submission in which biblical followers share the cross with Christ (rather than a couch). Man is crucified and recreated in his submission to God.

Freud, after developing his personality theory, went further and developed a total religious view of life in the books *Moses and Monotheism* and *Totem and Taboo*, in which he wrote his own Genesis. He concluded that the origin of mankind was not a biblical type of inception, but an opposite one, in which God was created when brothers rose up and killed their father and set up a totem called God. Focus on God (he said) was a neurosis; that really the ultimate person focuses on himself. Thus, Freud's ideas became the basis of the age of narcissism in our society.

It would be no surprise that Sigmund Freud, late in his life, instead of laying down his life, ended it in cocaine dependency. Also in some sense, he is the father of the age of drug abuse. Jesus taught that to lose yourself in God is to find yourself -- in an addiction to the Word. Ironically, Freudians dependent on self, have become dependent on drugs in the age of narcissism. According to the Christian concept, or the PATH concept, the condition for intimacy of relationship is obedience to God. This relationship to God is based on what Jesus calls the greatest commandment which is "Hear O Israel, the Lord our God, the Lord is one." The oneness of God as a person enables us in our oneness of personality to merge with Him. God's wife is the Holy Spirit; his children are symbolized by Christ our leader and brother.

The biblical concept of healing is the renewal of the mind, while the Freudian concept teaches the transformation of the instincts into productivity and work. These concepts are similar in their emphasis on healing, except that biblical therapy results in a renewal of the mind. The ideal in psychology is the stabilized individual; this is also PATH psychology. (Please note that the word "path" is what early Christians were called, not Christians.) This ideal is reached when individuals have defeated competitive compulsion and developed repetitive productivity (on the path of God repetitive productivity is natural). For Freud, psychic energy is useful for the performance of valuable psychological work. The desire to behave destructively, which is in human beings, has been transformed into productive psychology rather than into spiritual and religious creativity. PATH, or biblical psychology, perceives man differently: man, in order to become a stabilized personality, must engage in repetitive rituals and disciplines, such as prayer, study, love, meditation, phylacteries, spiritual clothing (Cranial Electrical Stimulation) and special diets. The biblical system recognizes that there is a higher source and a higher power, and therefore the breaking of the destructive force, the pleasure principle, can be accomplished through his work. The Bible also scoffs at the eat, drink, and be merry principle. The destructive force according to Freud is just called the animal instincts or id, while the Bible calls it Satan. Freud dilutes the badness of evil and the greatness of good by eliminating sacred terminology completely from his man-centered vocabulary.

The goal of PATH counseling is to live totally in the higher spiritual realm in a closer relationship with God. The Bible's conclusion is the beginning of wisdom, that is, the fear of the Lord and the love of the Lord. As it is written, let those who love the Lord hate evil. The fool says in his heart there is no God. Freudian psychology, by biblical definition, has many tenets and practices which can be utilized by a wise person to some degree; but, ultimately, he who rejects God will end up in foolishness. It is written there are two paths, the path that leads to destruction and the path that leads to life. The path that leads to life is narrow; few enter upon it and of those many perish. The Christians and Jews who go through the biblical counseling path (PATH counseling encompasses Christian Counseling) are urged to become like Christ, offering their bodies as living sacrifice. Freud teaches ultimately that independence from the past leads to life; but it is actually this teaching plus acknowledgment of dependence upon God that leads to life.

PATH counseling continues to share with Freudian therapy, at least in part, a belief in the unconscious -- that certain beliefs, images and pain are under the conscious line. Consciousness includes in its substance the understanding of behavior, beliefs and emotions. PATH counseling, and Freud to some degree, says Satan or evil can masquerade as an angel of light, that things of the mind and heart are not always as they appear.

There are three methods of self-exposure for the believer in God: the word of God, the spirit of God, the people of God. Freud, on the other hand, sees self-exposure as coming from the id -- childhood; the ego -- adult maturity; and the superego -- conscience. A biblically based personality theory views confusion as the opportunity for development and trust in God. Basic simple conclusions can often be useful, e.g., bad behaviors are dynamically related to bad emotions; bad goals relate to bad emotions; bad thinking is dynamically related to bad emotions; and bad faith is dynamically related to bad emotions. Working on thinking right, getting spiritual and redirecting one's life are the fundamentals of PATH Christian counseling.

The counseling of both PATH and Freudian psychology to some degree recognizes the organic basis of many brain chemical conditions -- that the mind, the body and the spirit are all connected, and, therefore, a complete healing must deal with biochemical imbalances associated with both spiritual and psychological distress. The principles of Christian healing share some similarity with Freud in that both say to fully experience your emotions; use your emotions; evaluate what they reveal about your beliefs and purposes; and be free to express every emotion, but limit such expressions by the purposes of love. While scripture becomes the container through which we express emotions from a PATH Christian circle,

Freudian psychology uses just the principles of work and love, which are secular but similar of course, to encourage the individual to live faithfully and do good works.

Darwin wrote a new Genesis, saying that man was a creation who evolved from apes, not a creation from heaven. Freud wrote about the natural result of this new Genesis: that inside man is an animal which he must learn to control. Biblical counseling says that inside man is also the Holy Spirit, and one must learn to express it. PATH interfaith counseling looks at the entire scripture as a resource and foundation for our direct relationship to God. The resolution of PATH Christian counseling is to make all men brothers in that all men are brothers interdependent on each other and dependent on the same holy father; thus God is both father and mother to all mankind. Freudian counseling aims to make all mankind brothers but still separate individuals, a condition which probably leads to a community of anarchy. Freud ultimately rests his case on the belief that man has an ability and nobility of his own and does not need God's nobility or ability. He is optimistic about the human being's ability to overcome his own instincts without help from a higher being, believing that man can determine his own fate. This has been the heart of Freud's teaching -- that the wise man believes he is above God's law, that he *is* the law. Hence, the Freudian man lives without a relationship to God.

When Freud is combined with Darwin and Marx we can see the anti-Christ: Freud says that man is an animal (beast); Darwin says man is descended from animals (beasts); and Marx says that man can make a society of animals (beasts) without God. They all shape the anti-Christ on a doctrinal level in varying ways, yet still partaking of many of the biblical truths. Mainstream christianity says God is in three persons; Freud says man is in three persons. And Freud's philosophy, although not integrated spiritually, actually serves as an antitrinitarian model of God. His conclusion was that religion was a universal obsessional neurosis. In some sense he might be right. For example, Mary worship is the typical Oedipus complex attachment to the mother and a death wish to the father; with the result that God is usurped by a mother-of-God image. Religiosity may be an obsessional neurosis, but biblical faith is not. If Jesus is not Son of God but God the Son, then he should have a grandson, and we should all be anticipating the coming of the grandson of God! The conclusion is that religion fulfills the illusions of the oldest, strongest and most urgent wishes of mankind.

Freud tried to replace religion with psychology, which is why all psychology actually becomes psycho/religious heresy. Yet, ironically, nothing but Christ's true religion can fulfill man's destiny with God.

Freud's religion, of course, was science, and he concluded that science is not an illusion. But it would be an illusion to suppose that what science can not give us we can get elsewhere. Ironically, Freud's idea that psychoanalysis was a replacement for religion was of course the most unscientific of ideas, since no tribe, nation, or people has ever been found in the history of the world without religion! Ultimately, everyone has a psychology and a religion, a basic viewpoint of the world at the core of their lives. Will your philosophy be about a higher power, biblical in its traditions, or will it be your own?

It is foolish for a child to think he knows better than his parents. Do we dare think the children of this generation know better than the parents of the previous generations, with all their previous experiences. Get the experience of PATH counseling; get on the path of total holiness. Get born again. In the born again state, the superego, the parent, becomes one with God and the id is sublimated under the Holy Spirit, creating an ego that submits to the superego with an id childlike creativity. Rebirth is unity of ego, id and superego with the Holy Spirit. Born again is the goal of all counseling, since it corrects the past and gives us new life in the present. Of course, counselors should be chosen for patients with congruent values while secular counseling should be appropriately chosen for secular patients.

The Electrical Basis of the Holy Spirit Rauch Ha Kodesh

In his book, *Depression and the Body*, Alexander Lowen, M.D., mentions the biological basis of faith and reality, ironically quoting Ashley Montagu:

> In his book, *Touching*, Ashley Montagu develops the thesis that skin contact of a pleasurable kind between mother and child is essential to the development of the child's personality. Body contact reaffirms the mother's tangible presence. It provides the security on which the child can build stable object-relationships. The mother's tangibility, which the child experiences as he touches her with hands, mouth and body, is the "absolute reassurance." And Montagu remarks, "Even faith rests ultimately upon a belief in the substance of things to come or of past events experienced." The touchstone of faith is touch itself.

CES's touch is an electrical experience which indeed has a spiritual or faith component to it which similarly reaffirms stability, i.e., binding it to the wrist and to the forehead (Deut. 6).

Appendices

Eric R. Braverman, M.D.
An Autobiographical Note

Eric R. Braverman, M.D., is the founder and medical director of The Place for Achieving Total Health (PATH Medical) with offices in New York, Pennsylvania, and Florida.

In addition to his clinical practice, Dr. Braverman conducts research on diagnosing and treating brain illness, epilepsy, head trauma, substance abuse, anxiety, and other psychiatric disorders.

His recent studies on brain activity indicate that it is possible to identify individuals who are at high-risk of becoming substance abusers. His research shows that brain activity dysfunctions can be treated effectively (alone or in combination with other treatments) with gentle, prescribed electrical therapy -- cranial electrical stimulation (CES).

Dr. Braverman serves on the editorial boards of the *Journal of Applied Nutrition* and *Journal of Brain Dysfunction*. He has contributed more than 50 scientific publications, and is the author of *The Healing Nutrients Within: Facts, Findings and New Research on Amino Acids*, New Canaan: Keats Publishing, 1997 [1987].

Dr. Braverman earned his B. A. degree from Brandeis University; he was graduated summa cum laude and was elected to Phi Beta Kappa. He received his M.D. degree with honors from New York University and did research at Harvard University and New York University Medical Schools. Following his training at a Yale Medical School-affiliate hospital, he received the American Medical Association's Physician's Recognition Award.

Curriculum Vitae

Name: **Eric R. Braverman, M. D.**

Birthdate: December 28, 1957, New York, New York

Directorships

Office Address: The Place for Achieving Total Health (PATH Medical), Director

274 Madison Avenue, Suite 402

New York, NY 10016

(212) 213-6155 / (888) 231-PATH

Private Practice/Director

PATH Foundation (non-profit research foundation), Director

Academic Career

College: Brandeis University Graduate B. A. 1979
             Summa Cum Laude - High Honors General Science
             PHI BETA KAPPA

Medical School: New York University Medical School -- M. D. 1983
             Honors in Physiology

Post Graduate: Internal Medicine 1983-1984 Yale Medical School Affiliate
Greenwich Hospital Association

Advanced Cardiac Life Support: Certified 10/83 to 10/85

BEAM Certification: Certified in the clinical aspect of the BEAM technique Charter Peachtree Neuropsychiatric Diagnostic Center, Atlanta GA, 7/90

Previous Employment

- Princeton Brain Bio Center
  Skillman, New Jersey

- Atkins Center For Alternative Therapies
  New York, New York

- Paramus Medical Nutrition Center
  Paramus, New Jersey

- Earth House, Canal Road
  East Millstone, N.J. 08873
  Affiliate Physician

Board Certification and Licenses

- National Board of Medical Examiners - Passed Parts I, II, III

Maintains Active Medical Licenses in the Following States:
- Alabama
- Arizona
- New Jersey
- New York
- Pennsylvania
- Florida

Memberships

- Mensa
- International Academy of Preventive Medicine
- American Medical Association
- Academy of Medicine of New Jersey
- Somerset County Medical Society
- New Jersey and New York State Medical Society
- Advisory Board, Oasi Mental Retardation Institute, Troina, Italy
- Charter Member, The American Society of Hypertension Inc.
- International University of Nutrition Education, California Board of Advisors.
- Board of Directors, Schizophrenia Foundation of New Jersey
- Fellow, American College of Nutrition

Faculty Appointments

- Post-Graduate Faculty, Life College
- Consulting Staff, Family Practice, Helene Fuld Medical Center

- Instructor of Psychiatry, New York University Medical School
- Affiliate of Robert Wood Johnson Medical School
- Adjunct Instructor in Research for Elective Course to Robert Wood Johnson Medical School
- Family Practice tutorial, University of New England College of Osteopathic Medicine

Editorial Positions

- Editorial Board, *Journal of Applied Nutrition*
- Editorial Board, *Total Health: Body, Mind & Spirit, California.* Writer of bi-monthly column.
- Editorial Board, *Journal of Brain Dysfunction*
- Consulting Editor, *Biological Psychiatry*
- Board of Editors, *The Journal of Applied Nutrition*
- Consulting Editor, *Journal of Neurotherapy*

Medical Research Publications [1]

1. Braverman, Eric R., "Porphyrin Metabolic Pathways," *Proc. 2nd. Int'l Conf. on Hum. Funct.*, Biocom. Press: Wichita, 1978.
2. Braverman, Eric R., "Sperm Fusion," *Science News*, 1979.
3. Braverman, Eric R., "Biochemistry of Zinc," *Proc. 3rd Int'l Conf. on Hum. Funct.*, Biocom. Press: Wichita, 1979.
4. Braverman, Eric R., "Orthomolecular Medicine and Megavitamin Therapy: Future and Philosophy," *J. Ortho. Psych.*, 3(4): 265-272, 1979.
5. Pfeiffer, Carl C. and Braverman, Eric R., "Oral Zinc in Normal Subjects," *Federation Proceedings*, 38(3):680, 1979.
6. Pfeiffer, Carl C. and Braverman, Eric R., "Folic Acid and Vitamin B12 Therapy for the Low Histamine, High Copper Biotype of Schizophrenia," in Botez, M., and Reynold, H., *Folic Acid in Neurology, Psychiatry and Internal Medicine*, New York: Raven Press, 1979.
7. Pfeiffer, Carl C. and Braverman, Eric R., "Epochal Trace Elements and Evolution," *Agents and Actions*, vol. 12(3):412-415, 1982.
8. Braverman, Eric R. and Pfeiffer, Carl C., "Essential Trace Elements and Cancer," *The Journal of Orthomolecular Psychiatry*, vol. 11(1):28-40, 1982.
9. Pfeiffer, Carl C. and Braverman, Eric R., "Zinc, the Brain and Behavior," *Biological Psychiatry*, 1982.
10. Braverman, Eric R. and Pfeiffer, Carl C., "Suicide and Biochemistry," *Biological Psychiatry*, 20:123-124, 1985.
11. Braverman Eric R., Lamola, Scott and Pfeiffer, Carl C., "Comparison of Acute and Chronic L-tryptophan Loading," *Advances in Clinical Nutrition*, July 21, 1985.
12. Braverman, Eric R., Lamola, Scott and Pfeiffer, Carl C., "Low Plasma Tryptophan in Depressed Out-patients," *Abstracts, 4th World Congress of Biological Psychiatry*, Sept. 9, 1985, Philadelphia, Pa.
13. Braverman, Eric R., Lamola, Scott and Pfeiffer, Carl C., "Pharmacology of Chronic Supplementation of Amino Acids," *Journal of Clinical Pharmacology* 25:455-474, 1985.
14. Braverman, Eric R., "Amino Acids and Ketogenic Diet," *Proceedings of 2nd International Conference on Diet and Obesity*, Sept. 17, 1986, Israel.
15. Braverman, Eric R., M. D., and Weissberg, Edward, B. A., "Hypertension: Magnesium Deficiency and Nutritional Therapy," *Journal of the American Society of Hypertension*, Dec. 5, 1986.
16. Braverman, Eric R., "Acute and Chronic Supplementation of Amino Acids," *Journal of Orthomolecular Medicine*, 1986.
17. Braverman, Eric R., "T-cell Ratios: Modulation by Nutrition," *Journal of Orthomolecular Medicine* 2(1), 1987.
18. Braverman, Eric R., M. D. and Weissberg, Edward, B. A., "Reduction in Plasma Tyrosine Associated with

---

1. Articles are available at Path for approximately $2.00.

Improvement of Psychosis," *6th International Catecholamine Symposium*, June 14, 1987.

19. Braverman, Eric R. and Ivovich, B., "Nutrient Profile of Hypothermics," *The Journal of Orthomolecular Medicine*, vol. 2(3), 1987.

20. Braverman, Eric R., M. D. and Weissberg, Edward, B. A. "Elevated IGE Levels in Patients With Low Whole Blood Histamine," *The Journal of Orthomolecular Medicine*, 2(4), 1987.

21. Braverman, Eric R., M. D. and Weissberg, Edward, B. A., "Fish Oil As One Therapy in Cardiovascular Risk Factor Reduction," *The Journal of Orthomolecular Medicine*, 3(1), 1987.

22. Braverman, Eric R., "Behavior Pathologies: Pharmacology of Acute and Chronic Amino Acid Supplementation: Clinical Implications," *Nutrients and Brain Function*, 1987.

23. Braverman, Eric R., M. D. and Rayner, Helen, M. P. H., "Plasma Fatty Acids in HTN Patients Before and After EPA Supplements," *Journal of the American Society of Hypertension*, Dec., 1988.

24. Braverman, Eric R., "Medical History and the Holistic Perspective," *The Journal of Orthomolecular Medicine*, 3(4), 1988.

25. Braverman, Eric R., Sohler, A., Pfeiffer, Carl. C., "Cesium Chloride: Preventive Medicine for Radioactive Cesium Exposure?", *Medical Hypothesis* 26:93-95, 1988.

26. Braverman, Eric R., "Memories of Carl C. Pfeiffer, M. D., Ph. D., Physician, Scientist, Teacher, and Philanthropist," *The Journal of Orthomolecular Medicine*, 4 (1), 1989.

27. Shafer, Robert W., M. D., and Braverman, Eric R., M. D., "Q Fever Endocarditis: Delay in Diagnosis Due to an Apparent Clinical Response to Corticosteroids," *American Journal of Medicine*, vol. 86, 1989.

28. Braverman, Eric R., "Case Histories in Psychoneuroimmunology," *Psychosomatics*, review, 1989.

29. Braverman, Eric R., "Carl C. Pfeiffer, Ph. D., M. D., A Life of Scientific Exploration and Conquest," *Canadian Schizophrenia Foundation*, review, 1989.

30. Braverman, Eric R., "Phenylketonuria in an 8-Year-Old Hyperactive Child," *Pediatrics* 2:217-218, 1989.

31. Braverman, Eric R., "Remission of Forty Years of Headaches with Divalproex Sodium," *Brain Dysfunction* 2:55, 1989.

32. Braverman, Eric R., Smith, R, Smayda, R., Blum, K., "Modification of P300 Amplitude and Other Electro-physiological Parameters of Drug Abuse by Cranial Electrical Stimulation," *Current Therapeutic Research*, 48:586-596, 1990.

33. Braverman, Eric R., Blum, K., Smayda, R., "A Commentary on Brain Mapping in 60 Substance Abusers: Can the Potential for Drug Abuse be Predicted and Prevented by Treatment?", *Current Therapeutic Research*, 48:569-585, 1990.

34. Braverman, Eric R., "Brain Mapping: A Short Guide to Interpretation, Philosophy and Future," *The Journal of Orthomolecular Medicine* 5:1-12, 1990.

35. Braverman, Eric R., "Brain Electrical Activity Mapping in Treatment Resistant Schizophrenics," *The Journal of Orthomolecular Medicine* 5:46-48, 1990.

36. Braverman, Eric R., "Fish Oil Lowers Fibrinogen," *Journal of Applied Nutrition* 42, 1990.

37. Braverman, Eric R., "Brain Mapping," *Townsend Letter for Doctors* 1991, pp. 254-255.

38. Rayner, H., Lovelle, S., Braverman, E., "Nutrition and Wound Healing," *Journal of Orthomolecular Medicine* 1991, pp. 31-43.

39. Braverman, Eric R., "Olfactory Hallucinations Remit with Alprazolam: Usefulness of Brain Mapping in Diagnosis," *Journal of Orthomolecular Medicine* 6:110-111, 1991.

40. Braverman, Eric R., "Psychoneuroimmunology," *Health and Nutrition*, vol. 6 (2):6-8, 1991.

41. Braverman, Eric R., "Reversal of Pre-leukaemia with Antioxidants," *Journal of Nutritional Medicine* 1991, pp. 313-315.

42. Braverman, Eric R., and Swartz, Kristin, "Cranial Electrotheraphy Stimulation," *Townsend Letter for Doctors*, 1991.

43. Braverman, Eric R., "Sports and Exercise: Nutritional Augmentation and Health Benefits," *Journal of Orthomolecular Medicine* 6:191-201, 1991.

44. Braverman, Eric R., "Addiction: The Most Critical Dimension of Nutrition and Preventive Medicine," *Townsend Letter for Doctors*, 1992.

45. Braverman, Eric R., "Brain Mapping and Electro Stimulation: Summary of a Presentation," *New York City Health Newsletter*, April 1992.

46. Braverman, Eric R., "Brain Mapping in 100 Substance Abusers," Abstract 1, *American Society of Addiction Medicine*, *23rd Annual Medical-Scientific Conference*, April 2-5, 1992.

47. Braverman, Eric R., "Modification of P300," Abstract 2, *American Society of Addiction Medicine, 23rd Annual Medical-Scientific Conference*, April 2-5, 1992.

48. Braverman, Eric R., Smayda, Richard J., "Chronic Lead Poisoning as a Cause of Bulimia: Hair Analysis and Brain Electrical Activity Mapping (BEAM) as Diagnostic Aid," *Journal of Orthomolecular Medicine* 7:53-55, 1992.

49. Braverman, Eric R., Swartz, Kristin, Blum, Kenneth, Ph. D., Moss, R, C. A. C., "Electrotherapy for Addictions," *Addiction and Recovery*, May/June 1992, pp. 34-36.

50. Braverman, Eric R., Electromagnetic Pollution: is there an Electromagnetic Antidote?, *Townsend Letter for Doctors*, August/September 1992; 710-712.

51. Blum K., Braverman E., et al.: Neurogenetics of Compulsive Disease: Nuronutrients as Adjuncts to Recovery. In: Wallace BC, ed., *The Chemically Dependent*, New york: Brunner/Mazel, 1992:187-231.

52. Braverman E., Weissberg E., Nutritional Treatments for Hypertension, *journal of Orthomolecular Medicine*, 1992; 7(4):221-244.

53   Braverman E., Smith R., CES Efficacy Evaluation, *Townsend Letter for Doctors*, April 1993; 324-325.

54. Braverman E., Brain Electrical Activity Mapping (BEAM) in Patients Who Commit Violent Crimes: Are Bitemporal Abnormalities a Characteristic? *Journal of Orthomolecular Medicine*, 1993;8(3):154-156.

55. Braverman E., Addiction: The Most Critical Dimension of Nutrition and Preventive Medicine, *Journal of Orthomolecular Medicine*, in press.

56. Blum K., Braverman E., Wood R., Sheridan P., The D2 Dopamine Receptor Gene as a Predictor of Compulsive Disease: Bayes' Theorem, *Istituto Neurologico "C. Mondino*," in press.

57. Blum K., Sheridan P., Wood R., Braverman E., Utilization of Bayes' Theorem to Estimate the Predictive Value of the A1 Allele of the D2 Dopamine Receptor Gene in Compulsive Disease, *European Brain and Behavior Society* and the *Meeting of the Austrian Neuroscience Association*, 2nd annual meeting, September 4-8, 1994. (In press, *Integrative Psychiatry* 1994).

58. Blum K., Braverman E., Dinardo M., Wood R., Sheridan P., Prolonged P300 Latency in a Neuropsychiatric Population with the D2 Dopamine Receptor A1 Allele," *American Psychiatric Electrophysiology Association*, 2nd annual meeting, Philadelphia, PA., May 20, 1994. *Pharmacogenetics*, 1994; 4:313-322.

59. Braverman, E., Blum K., Thaper R., Wood R., Sheridan P., Abnormalities in Obesity, *American Psychiatric Electrophysiology Association*, 2nd annual meeting, Philadelphia, PA., May 20, 1994. (In press, *Integrative psychiatry*, 1994).

60. Defrance J., Hymel C., Trachtenberg M., Ginsberg L., Braverman E., Blum K., Enkephalinase-inhibition and Precursor Aamino Acid Loading Enhances Attention Processing and P300 in Healthy Humans," *American Psychiatric Electrophysiology Association*, 2nd annual meeting, Philadelphia, PA., May 20, 1994.

61. Blum K., Sheridan P., Wood R., Braverman E., Comings D., Multiple-independent Meta-analyses Confirm Association of RFLPS at the Dopamine D2 Receptor Gene Locus in Impulsive-addictive-compulsive Behaviors, in press.

62. Braverman, E. There is Hope for Depression: Try These Holistic Alternatives, Doctors' forum, *Health News and Review*, 1993; 3(4):12.

63. Blum K., Braverman E., Wood R., Sheridan P., Increased Prevalence of the TAQ I A1 Allele of the Dopamine D2 Receptor Gene in Obesity with Comorbid Polysubstance Abuse, *International Journal of Obesity*, in press review.

64. Blum k., Braverman E., Wood R., Sheridan P., Comings D., DRD2 A1 Allele and P300 Abnormalities in Obesity. *American Society of Human Genetics*, Montical, Canada, October 18, 1994.

65. Blum K., Sheridan P., Wood R., Braverman E., Dopamine D2 Receptor Gene Polymorphisms in Scandinavian Chronic Alcoholics: A Reappraisal, *Eur Arch Psychiatry Clin Neurosci*, Schneider Druck GMBH, Rotherburg, November 3, 1994.

66. Braverman, Eric R., Handbook of Pediatric Nutrition, *The Journal of Applied Nutrition*, 46(3):95, 1994.

67. Braverman, Eric R., Handbook of Pediatric Nutrition, *The Journal of Applied Nutrition*, 46(3):95, 1994

68. Blum, K., Wood, R.C., Braverman, E.R., Chen, T.J.H., Chridan, P.J., The D2 Dopamine Receptor Gene as a predictor of Compulsive Disease: Baye's Theorem, *Functional Neurology*, X(1), 1995.

Research: Laboratory Experience

Harvard Medical School 1978-79

Science Thesis, "Dihydroreductase Deficiency in Fibroblast and Other Cell Cultures."

**New York University
Medical School 1982-83**

"Hypothermia and Insulin Coma as Methods in the Preparation of the Mammalian in Vitro Brain."

Lectures

Elective Instructor at Columbia School of Medicine (Physicians and Surgeons); January, 1988.

Elective Instructor for Broadlawns Medical Center, Des Moines, Iowa, Nutritional Medicine, April, 1989.

Guest Lecturer for University of Medicine and Dentistry of NJ at NJ Dental School, "Novel Approaches for TMJ" 1985.

Guest Lecturer for Princeton Brain Bio Center, on the following topic: "Hypertension, Amino Acids and Holistic Medical History" 1984-1986.

Guest Lecturer for Schizophrenia Association of Greater Washington, Wheaton, MD, "The Healing Nutrients Within: The Amazing Amino Acids," April, 1987.

Guest Lecturer for Foundation for Alternative Cancer Therapies in Wynnewood, PA, "N-acetylcysteine in Chemotherapy Protection" October 1987.

Guest Lecturer for North American Nutrition and Preventive Medical Association in Atlanta, GA, "Hypertension and Nutrition," and "Amino Acids and Diseases," April 1988.

Guest Lecturer for Denville Hospital, NJ, Grand Rounds, "Amino Acids in Psychiatry," 1988.

Guest Lecturer for Robert Wood Johnson Medical School, NJ, Rehab Center, "New Treatments of Multiple Sclerosis," 1988.

Guest Lecturer for Academy of Integrated Medicine, Lenox, MA, "A Weekend with Dr. Braverman," February 1989.

Guest Lecturer for State of New Jersey - Department of Law and Public Safety Division of State Police, "Prevention of Heart Disease," March, 1989.

Guest Lecturer for University of Medicine and Dentistry of NJ at Robert Wood Johnson Medical School, "Nutrition, Lifestyle, and the Immune System," March 1989.

Guest Lecturer for the Princeton Bio Center, NJ, 4th Useful Longevity Symposium, "New Horizons in Medicine, Nutrition and Brain Mapping," May 1989.

Guest Lecturer for Fair Oaks Hospital, NJ, "Clinical Uses of Brain Mapping," June 1989.

Guest Lecturer for VA Lyons Medical Center, "Clinical Uses of Brain Mapping," October 1989.

Guest Lecturer for Rutgers Center for Alcohol Studies, "Brain Mapping in Drug Abuse," June 17, 1991.

Guest Lecturer at the National Institute on Drug Abuse, "Electrotherapy in Drug Addiction: Is Drug Addiction Primarily Cerebral Dysrhythmia?," February 19, 1993.

Guest Lecturer at Children's Hospital of Philadelphia, "Applications of BEAM Testing to Neurology and Psychiatry," June 24, 1993.

Guest Lecturer at American Psychiatric Electrophysiology Association (APEA), 2nd Annual Meeting, May 20-21, 1994.

Prizes and Honors

1978 - 1st prize $1,000, student research paper, "Biochemistry of Zinc," awarded each year by the Biomedical Syn. Inst., Wichita, KS.

1979 - 1st prize $1,000 student research paper, "Porphyrin Metabolic Pathways," awarded each year by the Biomedical Syn. Inst., Wichita, KS.

1980 - Selected by Jay Cees to *Who's Who of Outstanding Men in America*.

1986 - Physician's Recognition Award in continuing medical education, American Medical Association.

1992 - Physician's Recognition Award in Psychiatry, American Medical Association

Medical Books

The Healing Nutrients Within: Facts, Findings and New Research on Amino Acids, New Canaan, CT: Keats Publishing, 1987.

Path Wellness Manual, Princeton, NJ: Princeton Publications for Achieving Total Health, second edition, 1995.

How to Lower Your Blood Pressure and Reverse Heart Disease Naturally, Princeton, NJ: Princeton Publications for Achieving Total Health, 1995.

Contributions to Other Publications

Brandeis University and the Core Curriculum, Brandeis Press, 1977.

Zinc and Other Micro-nutrients, Pfeiffer, Carl C., 1978.

"Orthomolecular Psychiatry," *Arista Science Encyclopedia*, 1978.

Television and Radio

Guest speaker: Health Line, WDVT, Philadelphia, PA.

Guest speaker: Carlton Fredericks Show, WOR, NY, NY.

Guest speaker: Pat McCann Show, WMCA, NY, NY.

Guest speaker: WIP Healthline, Philadelphia, PA.

Guest speaker: Gary Null's cable TV show, NY, NY.

Commentator: ABC talk radio, WABC, NY, NY. Every Sunday 2 pm to 4 pm, July 1986 to January 1987.

Host: Total Health radio show, simulcast:

WTTM (Trenton, NJ),

WMCA (New York, NY)

Saturdays 5 pm to 6 pm

Also: WOR (New York, NY) Saturdays 8:30 - 9:00 pm

Columnist

Health News and Review, bi-monthly, "Ask Dr. Braverman," 1988.

Total Health Magazine, bi-monthly, "Total Health of Body, Mind and Spirit," 1987 to 1989.

Medical School Work:
Extracurricular

Science Writer, Brandeis *Justice*; editor-writer 1979-1983.

Ideas and News in Medicine; New York University Medical Student Journal.

Member of New York University Medical Student championship basketball team, the *Blades*, 1979-1983.

Periodicals [1]

The Brandeis Justice

1. "The Much Maligned Egg," 10/11/77.
2. "Growing Older Gracefully," 9/19/78, p. 3.
3. "My Life: I Think I'll Stretch It," 10/17/78, p. 3.
4. "Despair -- The Agony of the Psychotic," 10/14/78, p. 8.
5. "Saturday Night Sickness," 11/14/78, p. 4.

Washington Square News

6 . "'Gifts' to the School of Medicine Could be an Example of Influence Buying," 2/6/80.

Ideas and News in Medicine

7. "Life in the Womb Revealed," vol. 1 (1): 9-11, 12/18/79.
8. "Hypochondria and Depression," 1 (1):33-35, 12/18/79.
9. "Life as a Neuron: Man, Cell, and Society," 1 (1):9-11, 2/3/80.
10. "On Wisdom - The Seven Sins of Medicine," 9 (2): 25-30, 2/3/80.
11. "The Best of the NYU Tradition," 9(2): 38-40.
12. "Nutrition Notes: Food Dyes and Lab Tests," 1 (3):4, 4/28/80.
13. "Medical Models of 'Immortality': Regeneration as Machine," 1 (3): 4/28/80.
14. "Wisdom in Medical Education," 1 (3):18-20, 4/28/80.
15. "The Cholesterol Controversy," 1 (3):6-8, 4/28/80.
16. "Wisdom in Medicine," 1 (4): 7-9, 5/26/80.
17. "An Interview with Sigmund Fraud," 9 (4):9-15, 5/26/80.
18. "The Concept of Diet," 2 (1): 1, 10/1/80.
19. "Magnesium and the Pathogenesis of Disease," 2(1): 5-8, 10/1/80.
20. "Narcissism: World Perspectives," 2 (1) 16-18, 10/1/80.
21. "Miss American Tomography," 2 (1): 19-21, 10/1/80.
22. "Medicine Past and Future in Growth," 2 (2):1-2, 1/16/80.
23. "Blades Roll," 2 (2): 3-4, 1/15/80.
24. "Life as a Medical Student," 2 (2): 8, 1/15/80.

---

1. Articles are available from PATH for approximately $2.00 each.

25. "Who Gets Cancer," 2 (2):9, 1/15/80.
26. "Medical Futures: New Ideas," 2 (2): 14-17, 1/15/80.
27. "Looking for Wisdom in Medical History," 2 (2): 18, 1/15/80.
28. "What Does Medicine Really Do?," 2 (2): 19-20, 1/15/80.
29. "Homo Ludens," 2 (2): 21-22, 1/15/80.
30. "Sickness unto Death," 2 (3): 1, 4/6/81.
31. "Social Factors and Disease," 2 (3): 7-9, 4/6/81.
32. "Liberal Arts and the Medical Curriculum," 2 (3): 4, 4/6/81.
33. "Vitamins, Drugs and Faith," 2 (3): 10-11, 4/6/81.
34. "Curiosity and Physician Performance," 3 (1), 12/81.
35. "Aesthetics and the Physical Exam," (1): 1, 12/1/81.
36. "On the Nature of the Natural," (1): 3-5, 12/1/81.
37. "Historical Notes," (1): 6, 12/1/81.
38. "Diseases Come and Go, but Illness is Constant," (1): 7-8, 12/2/81.
39. "Ontogeny, Phylogeny and Ecology of Fever," (1): 9, 12/1/81.
40. "Images of Death," (1): 10-11, 12/1/81.
41. "Medicine De-mythed," (2): 12, 12/1/81.
42. "Medicine and Society," (2): 13, 12;/1/81.
43. "Medicine Reviews its Own Tests and Procedures," (2): 15-21, 12/1/81.
44. "Future Headlines," (3):22, 12/1/81.
45. "On the Question of Authorship," (i):1, 3/1/82.
46. "How Literature Prepares the Mind for Scientific Discovery," (i):3-5, 3/1/82.
47. "G. B. Shaw's Doctor's Dilemma," (i): 6-8, 3/1/82.
48. "Dickens and Doctors," (i):9, 3/1/82.
49. "O'Neill: the Doctor Who Sells What People Want," (i): 10-11, 3/1/82.
50. "Chekhov: Ward 6 and the Residency," (i):12, 3/1/82.
51. "Narrative Medicine: Two Examples," (i): 13-16, 3/1/82.
52. "The Observed Fetus," (ii): 17-22, 3/1/82.
53. "Birth and Religion," (ii): 23-26, 3/1/82.
54. "Future Birth," (ii): 27, 3/1/82.
55. "Psychoanalytic Obstetrician," (ii): 28-29, 3/1/82.
56. "Congenital Malformations: Photo Essay," (ii): 30, 3/1/82.
57. "Ethnology of Birth," (ii): 31-34, 3/1/82.
58. "Birth Metaphors in Great Fiction," (ii): 35-44, 3/1/82.
59. "Future Headlines: the Fanciful and Bizarre," (iii): 45, 3/1/82.
60. "Lessons from the Surgery Clerkship: Laws of Human Anatomy," (i): 1-4, 6/15/82.
61. "Lessons from the Surgery Clerkship: Anatomy Through History," (i): 5, 6/15/82.
62. "Lessons from the Surgery Clerkship: 5-year Residency," (i): 6, 6/15/82.
63. "Lessons from the Surgery Clerkship: Shaw on Surgeons," (i): 7, 6/15/82.
64. "Lessons from the Surgery Clerkship: Psychoanalysis and Surgery," (i): 8-9, 6/15/82.
65. "Lessons from the Surgery Clerkship: Life in the Operating Room," (i): 10-12, 6/15/82.
66. "Lessons from the Surgery Clerkship: The Children of ICU/Death of a Lady," (i): 13, 6/15/82.
67. "Lessons from the Neurology Clerkship: Medicine and Poetry/Farewell to the Cat Scan," (i): 14, 6/15/82.
68. "Lessons from the Neurology Clerkship: The Stethoscope Song, by Oliver Wendell Holmes," (i): 15-16, 6/15/82.
69. "Lessons from the Neurology Clerkship: Symmetric and Asymmetric Patterns of the Nervous System," (i): 17-19, 6/15/82.
70. "Lessons from the Psychiatry Clerkship: The Flying Mind," (i): 20-21, 6/15/82.
71. "S. Vaisrub Essays, Master of the Metaphor: Meaning and Interpretation of Science," (ii): 22, 6/15/82.
72. "Decision and Contemplation: The Choice of Life," (iii): 33-38, 6/15/82.
73. "Decision and Contemplation: The Fanciful and the Bizarre," (iii): 39-41, 6/15/82.
74. "Parable of the Heart and the Brain - or You Gotta Have Heart," 2-4, 3/1/83.

75. "Medical Thinking - No Solution but Begins With Self-judgment," 5-7, 3/1/83.
76. "Gods and Goddesses of Medicine - Pagan Origins of Modern Medicine!" 8-9, 3/1/83.
77. "Thoughts on Monotheism, Medicine and Science - An Ironic Fate of Sublimation," 10-18, 3/1/83.
78. "Psychoanalysis and Medicine - An Ironic Fate of Sublimation," 19, 3/1/83.
79. "Metaphors in Medicine - Boundaries of Thought Breaking Down," 20-24, 3/1/83.
80. "Diet and Drugs - From Prevention to Kosher," 25-27, 3/1/83.
81. "Errors in Medical Reasoning - Mistakes I Make," 28, 3/1/83.
82. "Thoughts on Economics and Medicine - White Coat in the White House?," 29-30, 3/1/83.
83. "Religion and Medicine - Bishop Moves to Pk4," 31-33, 3/1/83.
84. "Fanciful and the Bizarre," 34, 3/1/83.
85. "Parable of the Eye and Ear - for Optometrists Only," 35-36, 3/1/83.
86. "Sermon from the Genome - a Talk with DNA," 36, 3/1/83.
87. "Religion and Medicine: The Rabbi Doctor as a Profession of the Future," 1-5, 5/20/83.
88. "Priest and Doctor in Literature: Camus, the Plague, Greene, a Burnt-out Case, Problems in the Professional Separation of the Spiritual and the Physical," 6-7, 5/20/83.
89. "Gospel According to Science - the Spiritual Content of Science Revealed," 8-9, 5/20/83.
90. "Medical Halacha: Spiritual Law for a Lawless Profession," 10, 5/20/83.
91. "Medicine in Bible and Talmud: Ancient Fundamental Laws of Good Health," 11-14, 5/20/83.
92. "From Pills to Peace: Drugs vs. Vitamins vs. Prayer," 15-17, 5/20/83.
93. "Physician as Messenger: Physician as God's Right-hand Man," 18, 5/20/83.
94. "Bizarre and Fanciful Prophecies: From Off the Wall to Off the Wall Street Journal," 20-24, 5/20/83.
95. "The Last Act: Or Thoughts on Death in the Hospital," 24, 5/20/83.
96. "God vs. God, Love vs. Fear," 25, 5/20/83.
97. "Carlton Fredericks: A Voice Crying in the Wilderness," *Update*, 1987.

The Place for Achieving Total Health
Multimedia Projects

Total Health Radio Program

Total Health with Dr. Eric Braverman currently is broadcast live in the New York City area on WEVD 1050 AM Radio. Please call the PATH Medical office or visit our website for the broadcast time.

To find out if a radio station in your listening area broadcasts *Total Health,* please call the PATH Medical office or visit our website.

Internet

Visit PATH Medical on the Internet at http://www.pathmed.com. The website includes the following features:

- Descriptions of diagnostic and treatment techniques
- On-line articles about current medical subjects
- Audio clips from *Total Health* (see above)
- Staff biographies
- List of Dr. Braverman's latest publications
- List of supplements available from PATH Medical
- Interactive Quizzes – they will keep you informed about important medical issues

Subject Index

Notes: Diets: references to various types of diets are listed in alphabetical order under the word Diet.
Oils: references to oils are listed under oil.
Recipes: references to recipes are listed under recipe.

A1 Allele 32
Abdomen, cramps 217
Abdomen, distended 215
Abdomen, bloating 350
Abdomen, cramping 350
Abdomen, masses 390
Abdomen, pain 87, 394
ABI (Ankle Brachial Index) test 229
Abnormal fears 173
Abortion, Scriptures on 434
Abortion, spontaneous 350
Abscess 45
Abscess, intra-abdominal 404
Abuse, physical 37
Acanthosis nigricans 76
Accutane 73, 74, 76, 77, 78, 267, 270
Acetyl-carnitine 237
Acetylcholine 50, 171, 172, 253, 261, 320, 321, 337
Acetylcholine in the brain 237
Acetylcysteine 308, 321
Aches 365
Aches or pains 283
Achlorhydria 404
Aciduria 309
Acne 73, 74, 76, 189, 326, 329, 339, 431, 438
Acne, McDonald's 74
Acne, risk factors for 74
Acne Rosacea 74
Acne, treatments 73
ACTH 183, 403
Actigall 220
Acupuncture 311
Addiction, carbohydrates 79
Addiction, cocaine 34
Addiction, food 1
Addiction, gambling 28
Addiction, hierarchy of addiction 90
Addiction, the most critical dimension 91
Addiction 433
Addiction, breaking, 12 steps on the path to wellness 427
Additives to be avoided 129
Adenosine 48, 195
Adipex 48
Adrenal and sex hormones 339
Adrenal glands 31, 183, 184, 186, 187, 188
Adrenal glands, stress tests 183
Adrenal hormone called DHEA 187
Adrenal hormones 189
Adrenal stress tests 187
Adrenalin 182, 272, 314, 367
Adrenalin and the brain 12
Adrenalin system and the CES device 182
Adrenopause 11, 187, 189
Adrenopause, males and females have 183
Advil 48, 221, 336
Age of narcissism 443
Aggression 313
Aggressiveness, forms of 367
Aggressiveness, portrait of 367
Aging 62, 187, 305
Aging, breaking the aging barrier 185
Aging, Eldepryl, anti-aging compound 27, 48
Aging, Eldepryl and brain aging 185

Aging, estrogen, natural, reduces the onset of diseases of 342
Aging, reversal 183
Aging, see Memory
Aging, signs of 184
Agitation 36
Agnosia 291
Agoraphobia 441
Aggression, medical syndromes of 368
AIDS 33, 45, 253, 255, 256, 267, 271, 273, 274, 285, 399, 423
Air cleaners 205
Air conditioners 205
Air pollutants 201
Akineton 292
Alanine 301, 304, 312
Albumin 404, 405
Albuterol 3
Alcohol 182, 200, 240, 243, 259, 319, 329, 333
Alcohol 353, 356, 361, 363, 367, 393, 398
Alcohol 12, 26, 32, 59, 84, 89, 90, 91, 113, 131
Alcohol abuse 170, 301
Alcohol consumption 339
Alcohol, cravings for 11
Alcohol gastritis 315
Alcoholics 11, 43, 92, 171, 172, 173, 183, 315, 328
Alcoholics Anonymous 11
Alcoholism 92, 144, 148, 171, 258, 287, 291, 305, 321
Alcoholism, "dry drunks" 11
Aldactone 321
Alertness, decreased alertness and performance 334
Alkylamines 7, 8
Allelic sulfides 61
Allergic/Atopic disorders 272
Allergic disorders 198
Allergic encephalomyelitis 291
Allergic reactions, classification 7
Allergic reactions, four types of 263
Allergic rhinitis 3, 7, 75
Allergic symptoms 210
Allergies 264, 270, 272, 288, 310, 336, 339
Allergy 144, 220, 305, 308, 315, 394, 425
Allergy, cat 5
Allergy, cerebral 22
Allergy, conditions 187
Allergy, corn 210
Allergy, discover a food 1
Allergy, dust precautions for 5
Allergy, food 138, 253, 296
Allergy, food allergy testing 76
Allergy, food, concomitant and synergistic foods 6
Allergy, gastrointestinal 139
Allergy, low histamine diet 2
Allergy, milk 7, 79
Allergy, mold 5
Allergy, patients 301
Allergy, reducing allergy to protein 125
Allergy, references 8
Allergy, seasonal rhinitis 2
Allergy, soy protein 7
Allergy, tests 1
Allergy, treatments 2, 31
Allergy, wool intolerance 75
Allopurinol 393
Aloe vera 77, 79

Alopecia areata 77
Alpha activity 49
Alpha-adrenergic antagonists 88
Alpha 14
Alpha waves 14, 15, 25, 43, 168, 439
Alphahydroxy-acids, etc. 75
Aluminum 164, 196, 201, 212, 221, 235, 280, 325, 339, 361
Aluminum cookware utensils 299
Aluminum intoxication. 280
Alzheimer's disease 183, 185, 187, 188, 189, 221
Alzheimer's disease 13, 22, 26-28, 31, 37, 43, 45, 91
Alzheimer's disease 234, 257, 281, 289, 337
Alzheimer's/Parkinson's disease 193
Amalgams 201, 202, 330
Amantadine 292
Amino acid blood test 11, 301
Amino acid, supplements 300
Amino acids 12, 14, 34, 88, 280, 290
Amino acids 302, 361, 331, 365, 397, 401
Amino acids, as precursors of neurotransmitters 136, 302
Amino acids, as neurotransmitters 136, 316
Amino acids, essential, requirements 300
Amino acids, essential 111, 124, 320
Amino acids, levels, abnormal 301
Amino acids, may be the most fundamental to brain chemistry . 302
Amino acids, nonessential 111, 300
Amino acids, significant increases in plasma 304, 305
Amino Acids, supplementation 302
Amino Stim. 27, 246, 319, 331
Ammonia 401
Amnesia 291
Amnesia, following head trauma. 368
Amnesia, post-traumatic 36
Amphetamines 14, 91
Amyloid 253, 314
Amyotrophic lateral sclerosis 307, 390
Anafranil 394
Anaprox 173
Androgens 74
Anemia 31, 59, 79, 280, 350
Anesthesia 15, 25
Aneurysm 45
Anger 238 425, 439
Anger, breaking the cycle of anxiety and anger 429
Angina 2, 120, 197, 228, 236, 245, 315, 336
Angina, reduction of 186
Angiograms 296
Angioplasty 236
Aniline 259
Ankylosing spondylitis 128, 147
Anus, rectal fissure and pruritus 128, 147
Anorexia 282, 287, 301, 305, 319, 326, 406, 442
Anorexia, causes and origin 87
Anorexia, most has an organic brain disease basis 87
Anorexia, symptoms, women who suffer from 87
Anorexia, treatment of 87
Antabuse 11
Antacids 221
Anti-clotting drugs 239
Anti-DNA 259
Anti-idiotypes 253
Antianxiety drugs 296
Antiarrhythmic 328
Antibiotic toxicity 280
Antibiotics 128, 217, 254
Anticonvulsants 295, 281, 296, 302, 349
Antidepressants 87, 295, 296, 305, 308, 311, 320, 349
Antifungal cream 200
Antihistamines 2, 7, 203, 296, 311, 320
Antihistamines, spectrum of 8
Antihypertensive medications 246
Antimalignant antibodies screening (AMAS) 59
Antimania 321
Antioxidant BHT 240
Antioxidant formula for detoxification 319
Antioxidant sulfur amino acids 296
Antioxidants 34, 75, 164, 203, 221, 237, 240, 243, 255, 292
Antioxidants 338, 337, 393
Antiplatelet agents, natural 238
Antipsychotic drugs 25, 87
Antisocial feelings 173
Antisocial personality disorder 381
Anxiety 196, 197, 202, 217, 288, 295
Anxiety 90, 92, 112, 167, 168, 169, 171-173, 178
Anxiety 1, 12, 14, 15, 22, 25, 36, 45
Anxiety 326, 336, 342, 349, 350, 394, 429, 437
Anxiety, antianxiety compounds in the brain. 321
Anxiety, antianxiety drugs 367
Anxiety, antianxiety drugs 296, 367
Anxiety attacks 436
Anxiety is one of the more difficult symptoms to treat 365
Anxiety neurosis 171
Anxiety, physical causes of anxiety-like symptoms 366
Anxiety, severe 365
Anxiety states 313
Anxiety symptoms 394
Apathy 404
Aphasia 291
Aphrodisiac 314
Aphthous stomatitis, healing 271
Apolipoproteins 359
Appendectomy 253
Appendicitis 93, 218
Appetite control, ... 15
Appetite, controlling, with the Word of the Lord 428
Appetite, loss of 202, 321, 336
Appetite suppressants that may alter brain chemistry 88
Appetite suppression 320, 336
Apraxia 291
Arachidonic acid 239, 240, 393
Arachidonic-linoleic acid ratio 239
Arginine 304, 305, 315, 397
Arginine 60, 62, 77, 134, 243, 259, 270, 280, 401, 418
Armour thyroid 184
Aroma therapy 201
Arrhythmia 87, 246, 247, 281, 309
Arrhythmia, antiarrhythmic 328
Arrhythmias, severe atrial 246
Arsenic poisoning 201
Artane 292
Arterial disease 229
Arteriograms 236
Arteriosclerosis 84, 93, 141, 225, 234, 246, 333
Arthralgia 259
Arthritis 301, 311, 320, 321, 331, 332, 336, 339, 393, 395
Arthritis 3, 7, 48, 98, 187, 192, 217, 241, 259, 264, 272, 285
Arthritis, case of 285
Arthritis, alleviating 308
Arthritis, Methionine Complex - the Arthritis Formula 320
Ascites or abdominal masses 390
Asendin 218
Asparagine 302, 304
Aspartate 237
Aspartic acid 310
Aspirin 3, 48, 64, 78, 87, 221, 238, 240, 247, 318, 393
Aspirin derivatives 254
Asthma 3, 7, 75, 197, 203, 204, 286, 310, 334, 339, 441
Asthma, acupuncture has been recommended for 3
Asthma, anxiety 391
Asthma, case of 286
Asthma, chlorine associated with the asthma 4
Asthma, exercise for 391
Asthma, occupational 4
Asthma, well known to be a brain disorder 3
Asthma, white wine can sometimes help 3
Asthmatics 308
Asymptomatic carotid bruits 226
Ataxia 25, 307, 309, 337

Ataxia telangiectasia . . . 262
Atherosclerotic disease . . . 339
Athletes . . . 310
Athletes, magnesium and endurance . . . 416
Athletes, nutrition and performance . . . 415
Athletes, nutritional deficiencies in . . . 415
Athletes, nutritional supplements that benefit . . . 417
Athletes, optimal diet for . . . 418
Athletes, recommended nutritional testing for high performance . 420
Athletes, tests for nutritional status . . . 419
Athletic competition, extreme . . . 328
Athletic training . . . 307
Atrial fibrillation . . . 246
Atrophic vaginitis . . . 339
Attention deficit . . . 308
Attention deficit and depression . . . 70
Attention deficit individuals . . . 183
Attention Deficit Disorder with hyperactivity symptoms . . . 69
Attention Deficit Disorder, in adults . . . 38
Attention Deficit Disorder (ADD) . . . 26, 32
Attention Deficit Disorder, resources . . . 39
Attention difficulties . . . 36
Attitudes . . . 145
Autism . . . 70
Autoantibodies . . . 253
Autoimmune disease . . . 3, 85, 198, 217, 254, 261
262, 267, 271, 272, 273
Automobile accident . . . 394
Avocados . . . 99
Avoidant Personality Disorder . . . 383
Azathioprine . . . 59, 78, 254, 259
Azulfidine . . . 292
B-cells . . . 267
B-endorphin . . . 253, 261
B-estradiol . . . 340
Babies, preterm . . . 309
Baby, Tylenol may affect the hemoglobin of . . . 353
Baby, your . . . 355
Back pain . . . 220, 286, 350, 369
Back Pain, case of . . . 286
Back pain, low . . . 336, 350
Back problems . . . 98, 329
Back, strain and sprain . . . 161
Back strain, elevated activity following . . . 437
Backache can suggest kidney involvement . . . 279
Bad behavior . . . 442, 444
Bad thoughts . . . 285
Baker's yeast . . . 88
Baldness . . . 308
Barbecue sauces . . . 80
Barbiturates . . . 296
Barium enema . . . 328
Bartter's syndrome . . . 328
Baseline coping repertoire . . . 370
Breast feed, always . . . 353
BEAM (see also Brain) . 13, 15, 22, 28, 48, 161, 167, 173, 281, 290
BEAM, and head injury references . . . 36
BEAM, and nutrition references . . . 24
BEAM, and temporal lobe abnormalities . . . 22, 40
BEAM, auditory evoked responses . . . 22
BEAM EEG (electroencephalography) . . . 22, 23
BEAM, hypoglycemia and diabetes impact . . . 183
BEAM, P300 diagnosis and testing . . . 26, 27
BEAM, P300 wave . . . 13, 26, 33, 48, 84, 183, 320, 321
BEAM spectral analysis . . . 22
BEAM testing . . . 183, 195, 215
BEAM testing, information about disorders . . . 22
BEAM topography . . . 24
Behavior, change in . . . 22
Behavior, destructive . . . 90
Behavior, disorders . . . 28
Behavior, testing . . . 55
Behavior, violent . . . 287
Benadryl . . . 292, 336
Benign prostatic hypotrophy . . . 398
Benzenes . . . 164
Benzodiazepines . . . 12, 14, 27, 336
Benzoic acid . . . 401
Berger's disease . . . 226
Beri-Beri . . . 92
Beta activity . . . 49
Beta adrenergic agonist (amphetamines) . . . 88
Beta agonist drugs . . . 3
Beta blockers . . . 37, 58, 246, 334
Beta carotene . . . 60, 66, 73, 76, 124, 164, 221, 237, 238
Beta carotene . . . 259, 264, 270, 274, 319, 331, 337
Beta lipoprotein . . . 339
Beta waves . . . 15, 25
Betagan . . . 58, 334
Betoptic . . . 58, 334
Beverages . . . 103, 112, 131
Biafrans . . . 112
Biblical or PATH therapy vs. conventional or Freudian Psyc . . . 441
Bile . . . 312
Bile acid therapy . . . 220
Biliary gastrointestinal fistula . . . 220
Biliary obstruction . . . 220
Bilirubin . . . 312
Binge eating . . . 350
Biochemical depression . . . 314
Biochemical imbalance . . . 336
Bioelectrical devices . . . 15
Biofeedback . . . 3, 27, 28, 202, 225, 285, 436, 439
Biofeedback, and stress . . . 441
Biofeedback, basic rules for establishing good . . . 438
Biofeedback, combined with CES . . . 436
Biofeedback, exercises . . . 85
Biofeedback, from the living God . . . 438
Biofeedback, general introduction . . . 437
Biofeedback, imagery for Christians . . . 440
Biofeedback, Imagery in . . . 439
Biofeedback, PATH'S guide to . . . 437
Biofeedback, techniques at PATH . . . 441
Biofeedback, training . . . 57
Biofeedback, training, idea behind . . . 438
Bioflavonoids . . . 4, 57, 60, 71, 134, 143, 337
Bioguar . . . 117
Biological psychiatry . . . 46
Biological rhythms . . . 4, 48, 195
Biopterin . . . 311
Bipolar depression . . . 366
Bipolar patient . . . 366
Bipolar traits, individuals with . . . 287
Birch . . . 83
Birth control pills . . . 87, 197, 308, 313, 330, 399, 340, 400
Birth control pills, and irritability . . . 400
Birth defects, folic acid protects against . . . 353
Birth defects in offspring . . . 202
Birth events . . . 281
Blastomycosis . . . 259
Bleeding disorder . . . 197
Bloating . . . 29, 128, 150, 217, 221
Blocadren . . . 173
Blood-brain barrier . . . 70
Blood, circulation troubles . . . 225
Blood clots . . . 239
Blood clotting . . . 120, 246
Blood clotting disorders . . . 339
Blood flow in arteries and veins . . . 225
Blood in the stool . . . 350
Blood pressure . . . 186, 212, 320, 439
Blood pressure, DHEA deficiency, a factor . . . 186
Blood pressure, higher . . . 127
Blood pressure, low or high . . . 197
Blood pressure, lower . . . 321, 325
Blood pressure, lowering . . . 120
Blood pressure, twenty-four hour monitor . . . 251, 252
Blood sugar, control of . . . 320

Blood sugar, lowering 120
Blood sugar, regulation of 320
Blood sugar tolerance, new testing for 183
Blood, thin the 320
Blood, type A 400
Blood vessels 184
Body building 315
Body composition, addendum 250
Body composition analysis, pretest instructions 251
Body composition analysis 98, 249, 251
Body fat, excess of 98
Body fat, percentage of 249
Body hair, coarse 329
Body mass, lean 98
Body size, slender 339
Bombesin 88
Bone, fractures, hard-to-heal 168
Bone fragility 326
Bone health 361
Bone-marrow transplantation 273
Bone meal 361
Bone spurs 102
Bones 184
Borderline Personality Disorder 382
Boron 73, 319, 361, 362, 364
Bowel cleaner 319
Bowel diseases 357
Bowel disorders 150
Bowel distention 94
Bowel motility 217, 218
Bowel movement, trouble holding one's 292
Bowel movement, urgency to defecate 350
Bowel movements, straining with 350
Bowel, short bowel syndrome 404
Bowels, control of the 320
Bradycardia 404
Brain, see also BEAM
Brain 237
Brain, aging, and Eldepryl 185
Brain, area of battle for weight control 87
Brain, arrhythmia 281, 394
Brain Beats on the Path 57
Brain biochemical imbalances 11
Brain biofeedback exercises and training 57
Brain blood-brain barrier 70
Brain/body connection 246
Brain catecholamine synthesis 183
Brain chemistry, appetite suppressants that may alter .. 88
Brain chemical imbalances 161, 394
Brain controls body, as mind and spirit control 436
Brain controls the body as the heavens control the earth .. 439
Brain death, determining 426
Brain disease, organic. 178, 289
Brain diseases 11
Brain dysfunction 171
Brain dysrhythmia 336
Brain electrical activity mapping 12, 13, 22, 29, 36
Brain electrical map 394
Brain fatigue 11
Brain function, improving 193
Brain, imaging the 25
Brain, impaired judgment 36
Brain, injury 53, 70
Brain mapping 295, 349
Brain mapping, philosophy of 15
Brain mapping, references for healing your abnormal ... 46
Brain monamines 116
Brain, neurotransmitters 50-52
Brain, P300 diagnosis and testing 26, 27
Brain, P300 wave 13, 26, 33, 48, 84, 183, 320, 321
Brain, poor development 309
Brain, rehabilitation. 12
Brain, rejuvenation 14, 15
Brain, rhythm 167, 217, 244, 245, 281

Brain, stimulants 48
Brain, tumor risk 246
Brain waves and states of consciousness 49
Brain waves, training to max. health, heal illness and ... 437
Bran 277, 278
Branch chain amino acids 133, 199, 255, 264, 305, 314, 415
Branch chain amino acid complex 319
Branch chain amino acid (BCAA), anabolic properties ... 307
Branchial blood pressure differences 226
Bread, high-fiber breads and cereals 330
Breads 89
Breast cancer 68
Breast feeding 7, 85, 196, 353, 356
Breast feeding, progesterone enhances lactation 344
Breast milk, make enough 353
Breast tenderness or enlargement 340
Breasts, cystic 67
Breasts, enlarged 221
Breath, odor 329
Breath, shortness of 283, 350, 365
Breath, shortness of 438
Breathing difficulty 336
Brewer's yeast 88, 330
Brittleness of bones and teeth 328
Bromelin 57
Bromides 74
Bromocriptine 313
Bronchitis 3
Bronchitis, chronic 204, 315
Brown fat 117
Bruit 228
Bulimia 29, 201
Bulimics 442
Burn damage 189
Burning sensation 228
Burping 94
Bursitis 161, 270
Butter 114
Butyric acid 219
Bypass surgery 328
C-peptide 84
Cadaverine 62
Cadmium 196, 247, 280, 325
Cadmium from smoking and 330
Cadmium poisoning 201, 329
Cafergot 173
Caffeinated beverages 278
Caffeine 361, 362, 363, 365, 367, 393, 397
Caffeine 12, 62, 78, 90, 91, 144, 182, 221, 296
Cakes 89
Calan 173
Calcitonin (thyrocalcitonin) 88
Calcium 203, 219, 234, 237, 242, 259, 279, 291, 295
Calcium 7, 60, 64, 114, 117, 124, 127, 134, 141, 143, 144, 173
Calcium 311, 312, 325, 326, 331, 339, 349
Calcium after menopause 362
Calcium - Bone Formula 319
Calcium carbonate 361, 362
Calcium channel blockers 3, 234, 367
Calcium citrate 362
Calcium deposits 328
Calcium/magnesium ratio 277
Calcium requirement 363
Caliper profile 443
Cancer 270, 301, 305, 308, 311, 315, 318, 319, 326, 330, 339, 423
Cancer 67, 92, 94, 134, 187, 192, 197, 218, 248, 254, 258, 264, 267
Cancer, anticancer diet & nutrients 60
Cancer, anticancer polyamine diet 62
Cancer, breast 91, 200, 342
Cancer, bronchial 390
Cancer, cervical 67, 340
Cancer, colon 60, 66, 93, 134, 248
Cancer, DHEA slows 184
Cancer, endometrial (uterine) 342

Cancer, gastrointestinal . . . 59, 219
Cancer, heart . . . 194
Cancer, hematological . . . 67
Cancer, information . . . 67
Cancer, liver . . . 308
Cancer, lung . . . 66, 248
Cancer, musculoskeletal . . . 248
Cancer, natural therapies . . . 63
Cancer, new era diagnosis and prevention . . . 66
Cancer, ovarian . . . 248
Cancer, pancreatic . . . 91, 144
Cancer, prevention. . . . 134
Cancer, prostate . . . 67, 398
Cancer, referrals, where to check the promises . . . 68
Cancer related pain . . . 311
Cancer research . . . 337
Cancer, reversal of preleukemia with antioxidants . . . 65
Cancer, skin . . . 66, 76
Cancer, smokers . . . 337
Cancer, spermidine (a cancer maker) . . . 310
Cancer, technique that finds . . . 248
Cancer, testicular, screening for . . . 64
Cancer, tests . . . 67
Cancer treatments, shark cartilage . . . 64
Cancer, uterine . . . 342
Candida . . . 279
Candy, Hershey Bars . . . 80
Capsaicin . . . 79, 85, 395
Capsilum . . . 117
Carbachol . . . 58, 334
Carbamazepine . . . 288, 296
Carbohydrate addiction . . . 397
Carbohydrate addicts . . . 12
Carbohydrate, complex carbohydrate loading regimens . . . 419
Carbohydrate craving . . . 313, 320, 334
Carbohydrates . . . 88, 91, 148, 298, 401
Carbohydrates, addiction to . . . 79
Carbohydrates, and fats . . . 402
Carbohydrates, burn first . . . 112
Carbohydrates, complex . . . 114, 133, 217
Carbohydrates, complex carbohydrate diet . . . 85
Carbohydrates, grains . . . 130
Carbohydrates, refined . . . 124, 338, 393
Carbohydrates, simple . . . 351
Carbohydrates, vegetables . . . 130
Carbohydratism . . . 92
Carbohydtates, anticarbohydrate craving action . . . 320
Carbon dioxide . . . 365
Carbon tetrachloride . . . 164
Carbonic anhydrase . . . 334
Carcinoid syndrome . . . 44
Carcinomas . . . 59, 223
Cardiac arrhythmia . . . 328
Cardiac disease, reduction of . . . 319
Cardiac disease reversal program . . . 225
Cardiac function . . . 328
Cardiac rhythm . . . 244, 245
Cardiac spasms . . . 48
Cardiogram . . . 359
Cardiogram, 24-hour . . . 246
Cardiograms . . . 238
Cardiolipin antibodies . . . 259
Cardiomyopathy . . . 247, 309
Cardiovascular disease . . . 45, 100, 148, 234, 326
Career testing . . . 55
Carnitine . . . 80, 84, 197, 237, 243, 280, 310, 320, 397
Carnitine deficiency . . . 280
Carnitine metabolism . . . 309
Carotenoids . . . 61
Carotid and leg circulation . . . 244, 245
Carotid artery scanning . . . 237
Carotid artery stenosis . . . 226
Carotid bruits . . . 237
Carotid cerebral studies . . . 226
Carotid, yearly checks . . . 238
Carpal tunnel . . . 134
Carrots . . . 99
Cat allergy . . . 5
CAT scans . . . 25
Catabolism . . . 404
Cataracts . . . 75, 198, 308, 332, 333
Catechins . . . 61
Catecholamine effect . . . 311
Catecholamines . . . 310, 311, 314, 397
Cayenne . . . 88
Cayenne pepper . . . 238, 321, 395
Celiac disease . . . 7
Celiac disease and immunoglobulins . . . 262
Cellulitis . . . 228
Cereals, high-fiber breads and cereals . . . 330
Cerebellar disease . . . 262
Cerebral dysrhythmia . . . 281, 290
Cerebral palsy . . . 437
Cerebral thrombosis . . . 226
Cerebral vascular circulation . . . 321
Cerebrovascular disorders . . . 13, 44
Cerulean . . . 88
Cervical cancer . . . 67
Cervical pain . . . 178
Cervix . . . 350
CES . . . 3, 12, 14, 27, 31, 34, 37, 58, 75, 79, 80
CES . . . 87, 88, 90, 92, 100, 161, 164, 169-172, 178
CES . . . 179, 182, 184, 216, 257, 264, 281, 283, 290
CES . . . 292, 295, 296, 309, 338, 365, 366, 417, 445
CES, adrenalin system and device . . . 182
CES, and methadone . . . 172
CES, brief summary of . . . 167
CES, case histories, treatment of resistant headaches . . . 173
CES, combined with biofeedback . . . 436
CES, electrical parameters . . . 179
CES, Liss device . . . 311
CES, placement . . . 177
CES, pulsing brain hormones by? . . . 169
CES, use of 3M Corporation device . . . 178
Cesium . . . 203
Channeling . . . 368, 439
Character and communication . . . 430
Character, application of intelligence to the development of . . . 429
Cheese . . . 112
Cheese, moldy and aged . . . 89
Chelated magnesium . . . 328
Chelating agents . . . 164
Chelation, EDTA . . . 201
Chelation, heavy metal toxicity . . . 201
Chelation therapy . . . 225, 234, 235, 236
Chelation therapy, monitoring renal function . . . 279
Chelation therapy, side effect . . . 201, 237
Chemical intolerance . . . 326
Chemotherapy . . . 77, 78, 254, 308
Chemotherapy, side-effects . . . 134
Chest discomfort . . . 365
Chest wall disease . . . 389, 390
Chicken pox . . . 268
Chicken soup . . . 308
Childhood dependencies . . . 443
Children and childhood diseases and nutrition . . . 70
Children, homemaking and rearing . . . 349
Children, hyperactive . . . 301
Children, neglect of . . . 299
Children who watch television . . . 182
Children, young, slow to walk, may require extra manganese . . . 329
Chinese herbal tea . . . 76
Chiropractic . . . 289
Chlamydia . . . 217, 270, 279
Chlorine . . . 204
Chlorine, associated with the asthma . . . 4
Chocolate addiction . . . 32
Cholangitis . . . 220

Cholecystectomy 220
Cholecystitis 220, 340
Cholecystokinin 88, 316, 317
Cholelithiasis 340
Cholesterol 82, 126, 127, 186, 197, 212, 234, 237
Cholesterol 245, 253, 280, 310, 312, 320, 339, 342
Cholesterol, and sex hormones 245
Cholesterol, elevated 196, 247, 310, 312, 321 359
Cholesterol, high levels, causes 244
Cholesterol, levels are predictive 244
Cholesterol, lowering 186, 315, 320, 321, 331
Cholesterol, lowering LDL levels 93
Cholesterol, update 244
Choline 7, 27, 216, 237, 241, 280, 290, 320, 321, 337
Choline, possible benefits of 418
Choriocarcinoma 340
Christ 444
Christian-Jewish counseling 444
Chromatic color vision 58
Chromium 84, 90, 148, 241, 243, 247, 319, 320, 325, 326, 408
Chronic fatigue 319, 320, 328
Chronic fatigue, and brain biochemistry 257
Chronic fatigue syndrome (CFS) 31, 48, 217, 257, 394
Chronic headaches or migraines 25
Chronic lymphocytic leukemia 271
Chronic macular edema 58
Chronic or subacute cutaneous dentoid lupus erythmetosis 259
Chronic renal failure 280
Chronoset 48, 195, 296, 313, 320
Cigarette smoke 308
Cigarette smoking 202, 355
Cigarettes 12, 62, 90, 91, 92, 221, 353, 365, 398
Cigarettes, drug withdrawal from 336
Cinnamon 83
Circulation, carotid and leg 244, 245
Circulation, improving 331
Cirrhosis 98, 307, 309, 315
Claudication, ischemic 226, 228
Cleocin 73
Clindamycin 73
Clinoril 292
Clomid 397
Clonazepam 12, 291
Clonidine 172, 202, 226, 240, 290, 336
Clotting, copper deficiency can affect 240
Clotting, trace metals and 239
Clozapine (Clozaril) 173, 290
Clozaril dose schedule 377
CNS depression 404
Cobalt 280
Cobalt toxicity 308
Coca Cola 80
Cocaine 90, 91, 172, 314
Cocaine abuse 12, 26, 32, 34, 306
Cockcroft-Gault equation 279
Cocoa 296
Cod liver oil 84, 318
Codeine 171
Coffee 87, 92, 216, 243, 296
Coffee consumption 3, 80
Coffee, tea, cola drinks, cocoa (all caffeine) 296
Cogentin 292
Cognitex 238, 320
Cognitive brain dysfunction 173
Cognitive deficits 187
Cognitive function 201
Cognitive functioning, improving 172
Cognitive remediation 56, 85
Cognitive remediation, brain rehabilitation 371
Coherin 321
Cola drinks 243, 296
Colchicine 291, 393
Cold hands or feet 225

Cold virus 255
Colds 254, 270
Colitis 128, 135, 150, 441
Colitis, ulcerative 218
Collagen 315, 403
Collagen synthesis 403
Collagenase 403
Colon 93
Colon cancer 60, 66, 414
Colon, polyps 93
Colorectal surgery 404
Complaining, tendency to 36
Complex carbohydrate diet 85
Compulsive and unpredictable behavior 368
Compulsive, destructive behavior 91
Compulsive person 25
Computer monitor screens 164
Concentratation, inability 404
Concentration 308
Concentration difficulty 173
Conception on progesterone 348
Condoms do not insure safe sex 399
Confusion 36
Congenital abnormalities 25, 353
Congenital disorders 262
Congestive cardiomyopathy 312
Congestive heart failure with pulmonary edema 390
Congestive heart failure 120, 312, 334
Conjugated estrogens 340
Conjunctivitis 58, 74, 75, 262
Connective tissue weakness 326
Consciousness, analysis of 15, 25
Consciousness-raising 25
Constipation 87, 93, 128, 135
Constipation 196, 215, 218, 219, 282
Constipation 319, 328, 330, 336, 350, 361, 394, 438
Contraceptives, oral 228, 313, 329
Convulsions 292, 315
Convulsions, anticonvulsants 3, 27, 296
Cooking 299
Cooking, tips for 212
Coordination, fine motor, difficulties 36
Copolymer 292
Copper 142, 239, 240, 247, 280, 309, 310, 311
Copper 314, 326, 331, 340, 394, 400, 401, 403, 408
Copper anemia 60
Copper deficiency can also affect clotting 240
Copper, elevated 305, 349
Copper, elevated levels contribute to depression 201
Copper, excess 240
Copper, high 309, 310, 394
Copper toxicity from plumbing 329, 330
CoQ10 .... 111, 114, 320, 332, 420
Corgard 173
Corn 210
Corneal vascularization 74
Coronary artery disease, correlation of low testosterone 186
Coronary artery disease 247
Cortef 183, 254
Corticosteroids 74
Cortisol 253
Cough 204, 205
Coughing of blood 350
Cognitive Remediation System 56
Coumadin 225
Counseling 441
Crack 91
Cramps, daytime 242
Cramps, muscle 1
Cramps, night 242
Cranberry juice 279
Cravings 135
Craving for alcohol 11
Craving for fat, Galamin affects 246

Craving for sweets and salt . . . 29
Creatinine . . . 279, 401
Creatinine clearance, for kidney function . . . 235, 278, 279
Creatinine versus creatinine clearance . . . 279
Creativity, lack of . . . 15, 25
Crohn's disease . . . 93, 135, 218
CT scanning . . . 13, 36, 289
Cults . . . 368
Cushing syndrome . . . 301, 390
Cyanosis . . . 228
Cyclooxygenase . . . 318
Cyclophosphamide . . . 254, 259
Cyclosporin . . . 76, 80, 84, 280
Cylert . . . 38, 69
Cyst, parasitic . . . 45
Cysteamine . . . 308
Cysteine . . . 60, 76, 77, 134, 164, 202, 221, 237
Cysteine . . . 240, 255, 264, 301, 309, 310, 312, 319
Cystic breasts . . . 67
Cystic fibrosis and nutrition . . . 215
Cystitis . . . 136, 279
Cytomegalovirus . . . 270
Cytotec . . . 221, 267
Cytoxan . . . 292
D-fenfluramine . . . 88, 349
D-L phenylalanine . . . 311
D-penicillamine . . . 308
D-phenylalanine . . . 182
Daily symptom record . . . 352
Dairy products . . . 130
Dalmane . . . 12
Danazol . . . 350
Dandelion . . . 83
Dandruff . . . 77, 338
Dandruff shampoos . . . 77
Danazol . . . 59
Darwin . . . 444
Darwin and Marx . . . 444
DDT . . . 340, 431
Deafness . . . 291
Deanol . . . 290, 310, 337
Death, biological, psychological and spiritual bases of . . . 426
Degenerative diseases . . . 161
Dehiscence . . . 401
Dehydration . . . 402
Delirium . . . 328
Delta . . . 14
Delta and theta waves . . . 25
Delta waves . . . 15
Dementia . . . 25, 313
Demon possession . . . 368
Denial . . . 36
Dental cavities . . . 308
Dental profession . . . 202
Dentistry . . . 71
Dentistry, amalgams . . . 201, 202
Dentistry, filling-related mercury toxicity . . . 202
Depakote . . . 173, 174, 309, 366, 366
Dependency . . . 36
Dependent Personality Disorder . . . 383
Depressed patients . . . 301
Depression . . . 3, 12, 13, 14, 15, 22, 25, 29, 36, 43
Depression . . . 185, 187, 196, 197, 201, 202, 215, 217
Depression . . . 87, 90, 98, 100, 112, 136, 167, 168, 169
Depression . . . 171-173, 178, 270, 286, 287, 288, 291
Depression . . . 295, 296, 336, 340, 342, 366, 367, 369
Depression . . . 301, 302, 305, 306, 320, 334, 414, 425
Depression, addiction and anticonvulsants . . . 281
Depression, aggression in diabetics . . . 85
Depression, antidepressants . . . 27
Depression, at the menopause . . . 339
Depression, attention deficit and . . . 70
Depression, atypical . . . 194
Depression-based anxiety . . . 365
Depression, biochemical . . . 296
Depression, bipolar . . . 366
Depression, chronic organic . . . 26
Depression, elevated copper levels . . . 201
Depression, feel sad, down, or depressed . . . 370
Depression, manic . . . 366
Depression, medication-resistant . . . 314
Depression, postnatal, progesterone, prophylactic for . . . 345
Depression, progesterone for postpartum (postnatal) . . . 344
Depression, treatment-resistant . . . 173, 319
Depth perception impairment . . . 312
Dermabrasion . . . 73
Dermatitis . . . 7, 313
Dermatitis, atopic . . . 75, 76
Dermatitis, contact . . . 75
Dermatitis, exfoliative . . . 77
Dermatitis herpetiformis . . . 76
Dermatographism on the hands . . . 75
Dermatology . . . 73
Dermatology, diet update . . . 76
Dermatology, new studies in . . . 76
Dermatology, nutrition . . . 75
DES . . . 431
Desipramine . . . 259, 394
Desserts and sweeteners . . . 131
Desserts, mastering . . . 100
Desyrel . . . 87, 267, 271
Detergents . . . 340
Detoxification, antioxidant formula for . . . 319
Devil Club tea . . . 79, 84
Dexedrine . . . 38
Dextrose . . . 307
DHEA (dehydroepoendostrione) . . . 11, 183, 184, 185, 186
187, 191, 200, 254, 270
DHEA, and adrenopause, protecting your brain . . . 187
DHEA, availability . . . 190
DHEA, deficiency, factor in control of blood pressure . . . 186
DHEA, level . . . 244, 245
DHEA, low in people with declining memory and aging . . . 187
DHEA, references . . . 192
DHEA, slows cancer . . . 184
DHEA, supplements . . . 189
DHEA, treatment for obesity and adrenopause . . . 189
Diabetes . . . 226, 228, 237, 246, 258, 259
Diabetes . . . 183, 187-189, 192, 198, 216
Diabetes . . . 2, 31, 79, 85, 91, 93, 98, 100, 137
Diabetes . . . 301, 308, 312, 320, 326, 329, 397, 436
Diabetes, adult-onset . . . 325
Diabetes, adult-type . . . 148
Diabetes, depression and aggression in . . . 85
Diabetes, foods and insulin control . . . 83
Diabetes, hypoglycemic attacks in . . . 84
Diabetes, juvenile . . . 84, 85
Diabetes, long-standing . . . 226
Diabetes, neuropathies of the feet in . . . 395
Diabetes, non-insulin dependent . . . 84
Diabetic gangrene . . . 234
Diabetic neuropathy . . . 84
Dialysis and transplantation . . . 280
Dialysis machines . . . 280
Diamox . . . 28, 58, 334, 367
Diaphragm . . . 399
Diarrhea . . . 79, 94, 128, 137, 202, 217, 218, 219, 281
Diarrhea . . . 313, 330, 336, 350, 394, 408, 438
Diary for neurological/somatization disorders . . . 378
Diet, acne rosacea . . . 132
Diet, adrenoleukodystrophy diet . . . 132
Diet, allergy or low histamine diet . . . 132
Diet, almanac . . . 129
Diet, and anticoagulants . . . 243
Diet, antiaggression . . . 132
Diet, anti-hyperactivity . . . 87
Diet, anti-inflammation . . . 142
Diet, anticancer & nutrients . . . 134

Diet, anticancer diet & nutrients . . . 60
Diet, anticancer polyamine diet . . . 62
Diet, anxiety diet . . . 132
Diet, appendicitis diet . . . 132
Diet, arthritis diet . . . 132
Diet, athletes, optimal for . . . 418
Diet, basic health and diet rules . . . 89
Diet, basic health diet guidance . . . 129
Diet, beauty diet . . . 132
Diet, Bezoars . . . 133
Diet, biliary atresia . . . 133
Diet, biologic classification of foods, rotation . . . 207
Diet, body builder's . . . 133
Diet, breaking bad habits . . . 133
Diet, Buerger's disease . . . 133
Diet, cardiac patients and a vegetarian diet . . . 126
Diet, cardiomyopathy . . . 134
Diet, cardiovascular . . . 134
Diet, carpal tunnel . . . 134
Diet, cataract . . . 134
Diet, cholesterol-lowering . . . 134
Diet, Chron's disease . . . 135
Diet, chronic bronchitis . . . 134
Diet, cirrhosis . . . 135
Diet, claudication . . . 135
Diet, cold and citrus . . . 135
Diet, colitis . . . 135
Diet, complex carbohydrate diet . . . 85
Diet, constipation . . . 135
Diet, cravings . . . 135
Diet, cystitis . . . 136
Diet, depression . . . 111, 136
Diet, dermatology and diet update . . . 76
Diet, diabetic . . . 137, 149
Diet, diarrhea . . . 137
Diet, Dr. Fuhrman's Strict Vegetarian . . . 126
Diet, eating a balanced osteoporosis diet . . . 364
Diet, edema diet . . . 137
Diet, embolus . . . 137
Diet, epilepsy . . . 137
Diet, ethnicity . . . 137
Diet, fast-eating . . . 138
Diet, Fast-PATH . . . 120
Diet, Feingold Anti-Hyperactivity . . . 101
Diet, flatulence or gas . . . 138
Diet, food allergy . . . 138
Diet, future . . . 138
Diet, gall bladder . . . 138
Diet, gout . . . 139
Diet, hair . . . 139
Diet, headache (low tyramine) . . . 139
Diet, heart arrhythmia . . . 140
Diet, heart attacks, to prevent . . . 140
Diet, hemorrhoid . . . 140
Diet, hepatitis . . . 140
Diet, herpes . . . 115, 140
Diet, high blood pressure . . . 112
Diet, high complex carbohydrate . . . 241
Diet, high fat . . . 92, 280
Diet, high fat and protein . . . 397
Diet, high fiber . . . 212
Diet, high protein (protein sparing), low carbohydrate, high fiber 102
Diet, high protein . . . 80, 87, 112
Diet, high triglyceride . . . 149
Diet, high-vegetable . . . 124
Diet, high vegetable, low fat, reduced meat . . . 247
Diet, hives . . . 140
Diet, hormone diet, influencing foods and herbs . . . 341
Diet, hypertension . . . 114, 140
Diet, hyperthyroid . . . 141
Diet, hypoglycemic . . . 141
Diet, ichthyosis . . . 141
Diet, immune-building/anti-infection . . . 141
Diet, infection and hepatitis . . . 142
Diet, keloid . . . 142
Diet, ketogenic . . . 144
Diet, kidney stone . . . 142
Diet, liver failure . . . 143
Diet, low-calorie . . . 144
Diet, low carbohydrate . . . 112
Diet, low carbohydrate and high blood pressure diet . . . 112
Diet, low fat, high fiber . . . 199
Diet, low fat diet . . . 138
Diet, low monamine . . . 116
Diet, low sodium . . . 277
Diet, low sugar . . . 148
Diet, low tyramine . . . 139
Diet, low tyramine (low headache) . . . 115
Diet, memory loss . . . 143
Diet, migraine headache . . . 143
Diet, moderate protein, moderate complex carbohydrate high fiber 118
Diet, motion sickness and nausea . . . 143
Diet, multiple sclerosis (MS) . . . 143
Diet, nephrotic syndrome . . . 143
Diet, obesity . . . 144
Diet, oligoallergenic . . . 77
Diet, osteoporosis . . . 144
Diet, otitis media ear infections (chronic) . . . 144
Diet, pancreatic cancer . . . 144
Diet, Parkinson's disease . . . 144
Diet, peace and well-being . . . 144
Diet, photosensitivity . . . 146
Diet, polyp . . . 146
Diet, prayer and salvation . . . 146
Diet, premenstrual tension . . . 146
Diet, prostate . . . 147
Diet, pseudogout . . . 147
Diet, reaching maximum performance . . . 419
Diet, rectal fissure . . . 147
Diet, religion . . . 147
Diet, respiratory failure . . . 147
Diet, sample menus for general high protein diet . . . 104
Diet, schizophrenia diet . . . 147
Diet, sex . . . 147
Diet, Sjogren's syndrome . . . 148
Diet, sleep . . . 148
Diet, spice . . . 148
Diet, sugar craver's, breaking addiction to . . . 148
Diet, tanning . . . 149
Diet, The Fast PATH to Dieting . . . 111
Diet, The Princeton Plan Diet . . . 117
Diet, thrombosis . . . 149
Diet, tic douloureux . . . 149
Diet, Tourette . . . 149
Diet, trigeminal neuralgia . . . 149
Diet, tyramine diet # 3 . . . 116
Diet, tyramine diet # 2 . . . 116
Diet, vegetarian diet . . . 149
Diet, weight gain . . . 150
Diet, yeast . . . 150
Dietary information for meats, fish and poultry . . . 96
Dietary information for salad dressings . . . 97
Dieters . . . 301
Difficulty swallowing . . . 438
Digital test . . . 232
Digoxin . . . 328
Dihomogamma linoleic acid . . . 239
Dilantin . . . 3, 4, 28, 79, 84, 173, 238, 281, 283, 296, 367
Diltiazem . . . 247
Dimethyl Succimer, DMSA . . . 201
Dimethylcysteine . . . 308
Dioxin exposure . . . 271
Diplopia . . . 291
Discs between the vertebrae . . . 329
Disease, treatment of by Jesus . . . 430
Disorientation . . . 36
Dissociation . . . 368, 369
Disulfiram . . . 11

Diuretics 246, 247, 320, 321
Diuretics deplete potassium, magnesium and zinc as well as . . . 247
Diverticulosis 93, 219
Dizziness 36, 124, 173, 282, 336, 394
Dizziness, unexplained 237
DL-phenylalanine 34, 365, 397
DLPA 27
DNA 393
DNA polymerase 403
Doctor, be your own? 370
Doldrums 334
Dolomite 328, 361
Dopa 292
Dopamine 3, 48, 50, 84, 253, 261, 271
Dopamine 302, 313, 314, 316, 317, 366
Dopamine compounds 185
Dopamine, D2 dopamine receptor gene 32
Dopamine metabolic control 336
Dopaminergic neurons 185
Doppler carotid testing 226
Doppler screening tests 359
Doppler test 184, 225, 226, 229, 238, 244, 245, 247, 271
Double vision 291, 292
Down's syndrome 313
Doxepin 202, 296, 309
Doxycycline 73, 74, 76, 200
DPT 268
Dream recall 296
Dried fruit 393
Drowsiness during the day 334
Drug abuse 15, 43, 178
Drug abusers 271
Drug addiction 314
Drug-related vasculitis 280
Drugs, detoxification from 34
Drugs for many purposes 336
Drugs, nutritional detoxification from 34
Drugs, side effects due to 3
Dry mouth 216
Dumping syndrome 93
Dwarfism 329
Dydrogesterone 347
Dying, stages of dying -- psychology 426
Dynorphins 317
Dyslexia 22, 295
Dysmenorrhea 178, 182, 336, 347, 350
Dysmenorrhea PMS 161
Dyspareunia 350
Dyspepsia, chronic 220
Dysplasia 66, 76
Dysrhythmia, following 328
Dystropic epidermal lysis bullosa 76
E-coli 216
Ear, middle ear infections 254
Ear, otitis media ear infections 144
Ear, pus discharge 254
Eating disorders 369
Eating out tips 123
Echocardiogram 241
Ecotrin 225
ECT 170, 292
Ectopic pregnancy 340
Eczema 3, 77, 148, 187
Eczema, atopic 77
Eczema with peeling 75
Edema 137, 226, 228, 280, 349, 404
Edema of face and legs 202
EDTA 234, 279
EDTA, ethylene diamine tetra acetic acid (an amino acid) 234
EDTA, oral 234
EEG 13, 14, 22, 36, 58, 173, 295, 334
EEG, abnormal 22
Estrogen and progesterone, synthetic 342
Eggs 60, 113, 117, 124, 127, 129, 134, 143

Eggs, best amino acid food 127
Ego 444
Egocentricity 36
EKG 246
EKG and echocardiogram 241
Elavil 84, 85, 173, 309
Eldepryl 291, 292
Eldepryl and brain aging 185
Eldepryl, anti-aging compound 27, 48
Electric blankets 195
Electrical imbalances 281
Electrolytes and nutrients 182
Electromagnetic fields 164
Electromagnetic pollution 48, 162, 169, 195
Electromedicine 180
Electromedicine at Path 161
Electronic ionizers 201
Elements 298
Elements of good nutrition and malnutrition 298
Elevated copper levels 296
ELF EMF 164
ELF EMF cancer link 162
ELF-EMF, ten observed sources of 165
Embolic clots 239, 407
Embolic strokes 238
Embolus 137
Emotional instability 309
Emotional trauma 285
Emotionality, severe 292
Emotions 145
Emotions and thoughts 284
Emphysema 3, 197
EMS (Eosinophilia Myalgia Syndrome) 254
Encephalitis 292
Encephalopathy 31, 199, 257
Encephalopathy, generalized 290
Endocrine disorders 329, 362
Endocrine hormones 285
Endocrinology 183
Endocrinology, nutrition and 199
Endometrial hyperplasia 339
Endometrial hypoplasia 350
Endometriosis 350
Endorphin-mediated pain relief theory 182
Endorphin receptor sites 171
Endorphins 12, 32, 164, 168, 171, 172, 241, 316, 317
Endorphins, natural endogenous 182
Enduracin 331
Endurance, lack of 98
Energy 321
Energy level, low 320, 334
Energy levels 255
Energy metabolism 308
Enkephalin-endorphin system 417
Enkephalins 314
Enteritis 128
Enterogastrone 88
Environmental pollution 3
Environmental sensitivities 203, 288
Enzyme CoQ10 . . . . 111, 114, 320, 332
Enzyme, essential cofactor 52
Enzymes 71
EPA 243, 311, 397
EPA, eicosapentaenoic acid 239
Ephedrine 88
Epilepsy 13, 15, 44, 137, 288, 312, 329, 340, 437
Epilepsy, international classification of epileptic seizures . . . 293, 294
Epilepsy, temporal lobe 441
Epinephrine 12, 314, 316, 317
Epinephrine/norepinephrine (adrenaline) 50
Epogen 80
Epstein-Barr virus 270, 271, 286, 291
Epstein-Barr virus, case of 286
Erratic cycles 347

Erythema 76
Erythremia Nodosum Leprosum (ENL) 271
Erythrocyte sedimentation rate 79
Erythromycin 73, 74, 200
Erythropoietin 80
Eskalith 287
Eskimos 239
Essential Amino Acids 300
Estradiol 191, 199, 200, 340
Estradiol and progesterone, natural 342
Estradiol/estriol 191
Estradiol/progesterone 191
Estrogen 64, 73, 88, 147, 184, 187, 189, 191, 197
Estrogen 199, 200, 314, 340, 349, 362, 394
Estrogen and testosterone therapy at the menopause 339
Estrogen deficiency 187
Estrogen, effects of 319, 340, 348
Estrogen has an impact on many body organs 342
Estrogen hormone therapy, new age in natural 340
Estrogen-intolerant individuals 188
Estrogen keeps the brain young 342
Estrogen may increase seizures 14
Estrogen, natural, reduces the onset of diseases of aging 342
Estrogen, only natural should be used 340
Estrogen producing and/or imitating pesticides 186
Estrogen, prolongs life 339
Estrogen-promoting foods and herbs 341
Estrogen replacement therapy 342
Estrogen treatment in males 339
Estrogens, progesterones and testosterones, natural 364
Estrone 340
Estrone/progesterone 191
Ethanolamines . . . . -. . . 7, 8
Ethylenediamines 8
Euphoria 197
Exercise 79, 131, 241, 339, 361, 398, 414
Exercise, aerobic 241
Exercise, benefits 242
Exercise, benefits for all age groups 414
Exercise, body building 315
Exercise, dangers of strenuous 414
Exercise, health benefits of 413
Exercise, heavy, increased nutritional requirements 415
Exercise, how much? 242
Exercise, marathon 321
Exercise, marathon running 241
Exercise, muscle building 319
Exercise, psychiatric benefits of 414
Exercise, reduces hypertension 241
Exercise, some preparation tips for 241
Exercise, sugar metabolism and weight loss 414
Exercise, summary 242
Exercise, the historical benefits of 413
Exercise, weight-lifting 241
Exfoliation syndrome 58
Extremities, thin 215
Extroverted 372
Eye disease 312
Eye drops 333
Eye examinations, routine 333
Eye exercise 333
Eye strain 438
Eyebright 58, 333
Eyes, blurring in 283
Eyes, darkening around the 75
Eyes, diseases 57
Eyes, dry 394
Eyes, dry eyes and mouth 394
Eyes, health 57
Eyes, hemorrhage 57
Eyes, itchy, scratchy 2
Eyes, poor focus 196
Facial paleness 75
Facial paralysis 291

Faith 91
Falls, unsteadiness or falls 237
Familial hypercalcemia 361
Familial polyposis 219
Family matters 432
Family planning and safe sex 399
Fast Path formula - the diet formula 320
Fast Path ingredients 301
Fastin 48, 254, 290, 254, 290
Fasting, benefits of 120
Fasting, therapeutic 120
Fat 367
Fat, dietary 99
Fat, saturated fat 243, 247
Fat, trimming the 95
Fat, utilization 310
Fatigability 312, 365
Fatigue 189, 196, 197, 203, 220, 259, 282
Fatigue 311, 326, 336, 357
Fatigue 1, 34, 36, 48, 80, 173
Fatigue, chronic 198, 217
Fatigue disorder 394
Fatigue, excessive 350
Fatigue, severe 292
Fats 298
Fats and oils 113
Fatty acids 401, 402
Fatty acids, essential 407
Fear of people 29, 173
Fears, irrational 203
Feel Good Response (FGR) 49
Feeling faint 365
Feeling of swollen extremities 394
Feelings, chronic, of emptiness and boredom 368
Feelings of unimportantance 29
Felbamate 28, 281
Felbamate, a new anticonvulsant 282
Felbatol 282
Fenfluramines 84
Fenoterol 3
Fenugreek seeds 84
Fertility 241
Fever 254, 301, 305, 307, 330, 350, 404, 406
Feverfew 173
Fiber 61, 82, 88, 93, 94, 124, 134, 217, 219, 361, 366
Fiber, can help reduce health problems 94
Fiber Complex 320
Fiber, disease states beneficial for 93
Fiber, guar gum 79, 84
Fiber, guar gum the most valuable fiber 82
Fiber, types of 93
Fiber, water-insoluble 93
Fiber, water-soluble 93
Fibrillation, atrial 246
Fibrinogen 340, 359
Fibroblasts 403
Fibrocystic disease 342
Fibroid uterus 342
Fibroids 340
Fibroids, protocol for 357
Fibromyalgia syndrome (FMS) 217, 394
Fibroplasia 404
Fibrositis 336
Fibrous tissue 68
Fine motor coordination difficulties 36
Fish 134, 212, 243, 247, 321
Fish, contaminated 299
Fish lowers triglycerides 149
Fish oil 75, 76
Fish oil (EPA) 3, 60, 73, 79
Fish protein 125
Five, 5-hydroxytryptamine 417
Five, 5-hydroxytryptophan 27, 69, 308, 311
Flagyl 73, 200

Flatulence 128, 138
Flatulence or gas 216, 217, 220
Flatulex 216
Flavonoids 61
Flexible sigmoidoscopy 222
Flour, white 330, 338
Flu 254, 394
Flu shots 254
Fluid retention 340
Fluid retention, prevent 349
Fluorescent lighting 48, 195
Fluoride 71, 361
Flushing 331
Folliculitis 301
Food 207
Food acquisitions 299
Food cravings, no control over appetite or weight 370
Food intolerance and the IGE 262
Food processing 299
Food storage 299
Foods, animal 207
Foods, canned 212
Foods, certain contain estrogen, such as black cohosh and yams . 199
Foods, concomitant 6
Foods, fortified 89
Foods, fried 114, 142
Foods, insulin control 83
Foods, potential cancer fighters in 61
Foods, processed 89
Foods, processing of 330
Foods, protein 112, 129
Foods, radiated, makes certain toxic amino acids 213
Foods rich in manganese 329
Foods, synergistic 6
Foods to prevent clotting, strokes, heart attacks 240
Foods with monamine oxidase inhibitors to be avoided 116, 121
Foods, with monamine oxidase inhibitors, avoid 210
Foot ulcers 79
Forgetfulness 291
Formula milk 312
Fractured ribs 3
Frequent PAC's 246
Freud, Sigmund 442-444
Freud's religion 445
Freudian counseling 444
Freudian personality theorists 441
Fructosamine 79, 84
Fructose 84
Fruit yogurts 80
Fruits 113, 130
Frustration 238
Full spectrum lighting 48, 195
Fungal infections 44
Fungicides 308
Fungus, antifungal cream 200
Fungus, avoiding 88
Fungus, nail, and Sporonox 259
GABA 11, 12, 28, 48, 51, 195, 237, 281, 296
GABA 301, 312, 315, 316, 317, 365
GABA and GABA Plus 321
Gall bladder 218, 307
Gall bladder disease 98
Gall bladder disorders 302, 340
Gall stones 93, 138, 218, 220, 312, 318
Gallstone pancreatitis 220
Galamin, affects fat craving 246
Gambling 28
Gamma glutamyl cystine 308
Gammalinoleic acid 320
Gangrene 228
Garlic 134, 173, 212, 216, 219, 221, 237, 319, 340
Garlic 238, 239, 240, 242, 243, 247
Gas 79, 94, 138, 150, 394
Gas or flatulence 216, 217, 220, 221

Gas pains, sharp 350
Gastrin-releasing peptide 88
Gastritis 369
Gastroenterology 215
Gastroenterostomies 404
Gastrointestinal and muscular disorders 437
Gastrointestinal diseases and nutrition 218
Gastrointestinal dysbiosis 216
Gastrointestinal symptoms 221
Genistein 61
Genital bleeding, undiagnosed 342
Geriatric patients 226
Gilbert's syndrome 218
Ginger 114, 143, 218, 237-240
Ginkgo biloba 238
Ginseng 147
Girls, teenage 339
Girls with fat localized predominantly in the hips 199
Girls with predominantly abdominal fat 199
Glands, etc. 244
Glaucoma 57, 58
Glaucoma and other eye diseases 333
Glaucoma, congenital 58
Glaucoma, drugs that worsen it 58, 334
Glaucoma, pigmentary 58
Glucagon 84, 88
Glucagonoma 301
Glucocorticoids 198, 403
Glucose 307
Glucose intolerance 326
Glucose tolerance factor 90, 100, 148
Glucose tolerance test 82, 183
Glutamate 237
Glutamic acid 312, 416
Glutamic acid-taurine 312
Glutamine 100, 416
Glutamine/glutamate 50
Glutathione 3, 134, 255, 305, 308, 313, 315, 316
Glutathione peroxidase 330
Glutathione, the body's strongest antioxidant 308
Glycemic index of foods 80
Glycerol 88
Glycine 301, 302, 305, 401
Glycine/taurine/alanine 51
Glycogen levels 321
Glycohemoglobin 84
God 439
Goitrogen foods such as cabbage, spinach and kale 196
Gold 240, 394
Goldenrod 2
Gonadotrophins 199
Gout 139, 393
Gout, acute 393
Gout and elevated uric acid 393
Gout patients. 301
Gout-related stones 277, 278
Grains 112, 208
Grapefruit 99
Greenhouses 5
Growing hair shaft 325
Growing pains 329
Growth 328
Growth hormone 404, 418
Growth hormone release 199
Guaiac card or hemoccult stool blood test 223
Guanosine 292
Guar gum 79, 84, 88, 320
Guar gum, the most valuable fiber 82
Guillain-Barre syndrome 291
Gynecology 339
Habit, bad dietary, techniques for breaking 91
Habits, breaking 90, 91
Hair 77, 139
Hair analysis 326, 394

Hair, coarse body hair 329
Hair loss 77, 308, 336
Hair loss due to vegetarianism 77
Hair loss in women 350
Hair test 29, 201
Hair thinning 220
Halcion 12
Haldol 290, 296, 337
Hallucinations 124, 334
Haloperidol 74
Hands, itching 75
Hard water 247
Hartnup's 313
Hay fever 2
HDL 112, 243, 318, 339, 418
HDL (the good cholesterol) 247
HDL/cholesterol ratio 243, 244
HDL, lowered 196
Head injuries, minor and severe 36
Head injury 13, 36
Head trauma 22, 40, 44, 295
Head trauma BEAM bibliography 41
Head trauma BEAM, bibliography for head trauma 41
Headache 189, 202, 203, 220, 336, 339, 349, 350, 438
Headache 1, 13, 36, 139, 168, 228, 242, 282, 283, 436
Headache, chronic 286
Headache, chronic sufferer, case of 286
Headache, migraine 25, 45, 143, 306, 311, 336, 339, 340, 400
Headaches, chronic 394
Headaches, tension 329, 394
Healing is the forgiveness of sin 429
Healing, slow healing 326
Health Spa 110
Healthy choice shopping list 160
Hearing 25, 184, 437
Hearing loss 292
Heart 184, 196
Heart arrhythmia 140, 328
Heart attack 140, 241, 246, 295, 328, 436
Heart attack, nutrients to prevent 247
Heart attacks, prevent 320
Heart attacks, the physical link between stress and 246
Heart beat, irregular 197
Heart, bypass surgery 236
Heart disease 2, 92, 98, 186, 187, 196, 197
Heart disease 225, 240, 320, 321, 326, 340
Heart disease, prevention 245
Heart, enlarged or hypertrophied 241
Heart failure 3
Heart failure, congestive 120
Heart Formula 319
Heart muscle disease 309
Heart palpitations 436
Heart-rhythm problems 328
Heart rhythms 167
Heartburn 216
Heavy metal detoxification 315
Heavy metal poisoning 301, 308, 310
Heavy metal toxicity and chelation 201
Heavy metals 280
Heavy metals, intoxification 234
Heidelberg test 221
Hemadrin 292
Hematologic disorder 259
Hematological cancers 67
Hematuria 330
Hemiplegia 291
Hemolysis, chronic 393
Hemolytic 59
Hemolytic anemia 259
Hemolytic streptococci 216
Hemophilus influenza B vaccine 268
Hemorrhoids 140, 223, 357
Hemorrhoids, varicose 93

Heparin 362
Hepatic and renal disorders 43
Hepatitis 140, 142, 270
Hepatitis B vaccine 268
Hepatitis, chronic 219
Hepatitis, lupoid 271
Hepatitis vaccine 268
Hepatolenticular degeneration (Wilson's disease) 44
Herbal plant therapeutics 83
Herbal substitute for salt 212
Herbal teas 131
Herbicides 308
Herbs, hormone diet, influencing foods and herbs 341
Hernias 98
Heroin 12, 90, 91, 172, 336
Heroin addicts 314
Herpes 140, 279, 291
Herpes 1, 2 and 6 270
Herpes, antiherpes-like effects 320
Herpes simplex virus 271
Herpetiformis 7
Hiatal hernia 93
High blood pressure 2, 225, 234, 247, 319, 320
High blood pressure 326, 359, 397, 436, 441
High-fiber breads and cereals 330
High protein diets 80
High purine foods 393
High triglycerides 280
Histamine 50, 302, 305
Histamines, antihistamines 2, 7
Histidine 199, 280, 301, 302, 393
Histidine, vasodilator and antirheumatism 309
Histone antibodies 259
Histoplasmosis 259
Histrionic Personality Disorder 382
HIV 270
HIV patients 315
Hives 140
Holiness 439, 440
Holter monitors 252
Holy Spirit, ... 444
Holy Spirit, electrical basis of 445
Homemaking and rearing children 349
Homeostasis 253
Homeostasis, immune system as regulator of 261
Homocysteine 310, 312, 333
Homocystinuria 362
Homosexuality 33
Hormonal factors 285
Hormonal, nutritional and metabolic disorders 44
Hormone imbalance 59
Hormone levels 244
Hormone replacement 200, 361
Hormones 183, 244, 285
Hormones, female 340
Hormones, fetal and placental 339
Hormones, growth receptors for 285
Hormones, natural 349
Hormones, natural, preparations available, derived from yams .. 343
Hormones, side effects from the synthetic 342
Hormones, sources for purchase 190
Hot flashes 342
Hot or cold flashes 365
Household appliances 204
Human papilloma virus 279
HTLV viruses 292
Humidifiers 205
Huntington's chorea 307, 337
Hydergine 43
Hydrazine derivatives 259
Hydrochloroprine 254
Hydrogen peroxide solution 71
Hydroxy cortisone 187
Hydroxy-indol-o-methyl transferase 194

Hydroxychloroquine 259
Hydroxycortisone 184
Hydroxycortisone, for allergies, depression, and chronic fatigue . 198
Hydroxyprogesterone caproate 347
Hydroxyproline 315, 402
Hydroxyproline residues 403
Hydroxytryptophan 70, 313, 320
Hydroxyzine 75
Hyperacidity 170
Hyperactive children 301
Hyperactivity 15, 25, 48, 70, 170, 195, 310, 441
Hyperactivity and ADD 69
Hyperactivity, childhood 69
Hyperammonemia 407
Hyperbaric oxygen 292
Hyperbaric oxygen treatment 402
Hyperbilirubinemia 312
Hyperchlorhydria 222
Hypercholesterolemia 93
Hypergammaglobulinemia 271
Hyperlipidemia 228, 309
Hyperoxia 402
Hypertension 3, 85, 90, 91, 93, 98, 112, 140, 216, 226, 246
Hypertension 280, 309, 312, 313, 320, 330, 333, 336, 350, 400
Hypertension, ginger, garlic and onions lower 114
Hypertension of pregnancy 328
Hypertension, program for 114
Hyperthyroid patients 419
Hyperthyroidism 141, 196
Hyperthyroidism 419
Hypertriglyceridemia 93
Hyperuricemia 393
Hyperventilation 436
Hypnosis 202, 285
Hypnotized 368
Hypoalbuminism 401
Hypochlorhydria 222
Hypochondria 365, 425
Hypochondriasis, depression and anxiety 365
Hypoglycemia 301, 307, 309, 326, 328, 329, 407
Hypoglycemia 11, 43, 62, 80, 89, 100, 112, 141, 173, 183
Hypoglycemia and diabetes, impact BEAM 183
Hypoglycemia, glucose tolerance test 82
Hypoglycemia, insulin resistance 84
Hypoglycemic attacks in diabetics 84
Hypogonadism 329
Hypomania 287
Hypotension 314
Hypothalamus 172, 184, 186, 197
Hypothermia 305
Hypothyroid disease 196, 197
Hypothyroid individuals 310
Hypothyroidism 43, 77, 394
Hypothyroidism, notes on iodine and thyroid 196
Hypovitaminemia 404
Hypoxia 402
I.Q. 291
Ibuprofen 320
Ichthyosis 75, 141
Id 444
Idiopathic edema 120
Idiopathic Thrombocytopenic Purpura (ITP) 59
IgA 265
IgA, deficiency 253
IgA, low 262
IgE 75, 265
IgE, levels in disease 272
IgE-RAST testing, ... 1
IgG 265
IgG or IgE response. 7
IgM 265
Ileus 404
Imagery 285
Imagination 25

Imidazole 309
Imipramine 38
Immune disorders 441
Immune dysfunction 326
Immune regulation nutrients 264
Immune response 253
Immune suppressants 271
Immune suppressing drugs 259
Immune suppression 325, 326
Immune suppression, diseases of 270
Immune system 15, 37, 79, 168, 197, 244, 245, 253, 285
Immune system, as regulator of homeostasis 261
Immune system, balancing 270
Immune system, building and maintaining 264
Immune system, enhancement 192
Immune system, imbalance of autoimmune disorders 272
Immune system, lowered 187
Immune system, proteins 261
Immune system, ways to improve when ill 270
Immunoglobulin and disease, references 263
Immunoglobulin, the life of an 263
Immunoglobulins 253, 261, 265, 301, 404
Immunoglobulins and celiac disease 262
Immunoglobulins and disease 262
Immunologic disorder 259
Immunologic disorders of uncertain pathogenesis 272
Immunology 253
Immunosuppressive drugs 259
Impatience 36
Impotence 226, 292, 329, 336, 437
Impotence in men 397
Impotence, sex, infertility and 397
Impotence test 233
Impulsivity 38, 69
Inattention 69
Indigestion 128, 336
Indoles 61
Infant formulas 196, 353, 357
Infants, calmer baby 353
Infants, premature 312
Infarct 237
Infection 44, 142, 193, 254, 281, 305, 307, 394, 406
Infection, and nutrients 255
Infection, modification by food, nutrients and behavior 255
Infection, protozoal 44
Infection, recurrent 326
Infections, viral 332
Infectious causes 31
Infectious disease 253, 301
Infertility 221, 350
Infertility, impotence, sex, and 397
Infertility in men 310, 397
Infertility in women 397
Inflammation 326, 406
Inflammatory bowel disease 217, 223
Inflammatory disease 270
Inflexibility 36
Influenza 292
Initiative, decreased 36
Injuries, management of soft-tissue 418
Inositol 281, 296, 365
Inotrope 302
Insomnia 282, 295, 302, 334, 342, 365
Insomnia 14, 167, 169, 171, 172, 173, 178, 202
Insulin 253, 261
Insulin regulation 320
Insulin release 307
Insulin resistance 84, 340
Intelligence 430
Intercourse, painful 350
Interferon 62, 285
Interferon injections 270
Interferons, natural 264
Interleukin 255, 318, 331

Interpersonal skills 371
Interstitial fibrosis 390
Intestinal flora 128
Intestinal problems 98
Intraocular pressure 333
Intravenous lidocaine 296
Introverted 372
Intuitive 372
Involuntary movements 290
Iodine 147, 196, 197, 320, 331
Iodine, thyroid hormones and 197
Ions, positive and negative 182
Iron 120, 280, 302, 311, 325, 331, 353, 357, 394, 400
Iron, Slow Fe 321, 358
Iron therapy, benefits of 357
Iron, too much iron can promote infection 255
Irregular bleeding 340
Irritability 1, 15, 25, 29, 171, 196, 197, 326, 340, 404, 439
Irritable bladder 394
Irritable bowel syndrome 93, 218, 221, 326, 394, 404, 437
Irritable colon 336
Ischemia 15, 25
Ischemia 402
Isoleucine 87, 199, 255, 280, 301, 307, 418
Isoniazid 259, 313
Isothiocyanates 61
Itching hands 75
Itraconazole 259
IUD 399
Jello 80
Jesus 443
Jesus, treatment of disease by 430
Jet lag 48, 194, 195, 320
Joint injuries 161
Joint pain 189, 329, 394
Joint repair 437
Junk food 92
Juvenile delinquents 414
Juvenile diabetes 84, 85
Keloid 142
Ketchup 80
Ketosis 112
Kidney dialysis 280
Kidney dialysis patients 309
Kidney disease 84, 277, 393
Kidney disease (proteinuria or casts) 259
Kidney failure 79, 120, 143, 225, 258, 280, 301, 305, 313, 315
Kidney function 111
Kidney stone formation 361
Kidney stones 142, 234, 277
Kidney stones, calcium oxalate 277, 278
Kidney stones, questions and answers 277
Kidney stones, silicate 328
Kidney stones, uric acid 393
Kidney transplant 280
Kidneys 300, 340
Kidneys, calcium oxalate in urine 279
Kidneys, chronic renal failure 280
Kidneys, excess of protein 280
Klebsiella 216
Klonopin 11, 28, 84, 85, 185, 281, 283, 296
Korsakoff's psychosis 171
Kwashiorkor 309
L-canavanine 259
L-carnitine, oxidizer of fat 309
L-cysteine 308
L-dopa 43, 267, 310, 311, 314, 320
L-tryptophan 417
L-tyrosine 32
L. Bifidus 128
Lactate 88, 365
Lactic acid 128
Lactobacillus 128
Lactobacillus for antibiotic 128

Lactose intolerance 217
Larodopa 292
Laser sclerostomy 334
Lasix 225
Laughter 285
Laxative 336
Laxative, natural 319
Laxatives, can affect stomach and kidneys of baby 353
LDL 101, 418
LDL levels 243
Lead 15, 30, 164, 196, 201, 234, 235
Lead 247, 308, 310, 325, 349, 361
Lead, cadmium, or other toxic metals 394
Lead poisoning 29, 87, 329
Lead toxicity 201, 330
Learning disabilities 15, 170, 315, 325, 441
Lecithin 73, 77, 78, 127, 280, 290, 337
Lecithin in viral hepatitis 255
Leg cramps 242
Leg edema 225
Leg gangrene 225
Leg swelling 226
Legionnaires' disease 44
Legumes 99
Lengthening of cycle 347
Lennox Gastaut Syndrome 282
Leprosy 270, 273
Leprosy, non-ENL (skin) 271
Lesch-Nyhan syndrome 393
Lesions, mass 13
Lethargy 312
Leucine 87, 199, 255, 280, 301, 302, 305, 307, 415, 418
Leukemia 59, 67, 393
Leukemia, chronic lymphocytic 271
Leukocyte bacterial-killing activity 402
Leukocytes 402
Leukopenia 259
Leukopenic anergy 271
Leukoplakia 66
Levamisole 309
Levsin 292
LHRH 397
Libido, decreased 342
Librax 216
Librium 11, 12, 34, 92
Lichen Planus 143
Light 48, 194, 195
Light as a nutrient 334
Light, full spectrum lighting 48, 195
Light headedness 438
Light, impact of daylight deprivation 334
Light, levels in our environment 335
Light, ultrabright light systems 335
Light, UV 334
Limbic system 11
Limonoids 61
Link support group listing 379
Linoleic 401
Linoleic acid 61, 84101, 114, 239, 247
Linolenic 401
Lioresal 291
Liss device 311
Listlessness 334
Lithium 4, 11, 69, 71, 78, 87, 90, 92, 100
Lithium 146, 149, 197, 287, 349, 336, 365, 367
Lithium citrate 287
Liver 342
Liver, chronic disease 342
Liver cirrhosis 308
Liver damage 319
Liver disease 301
Liver enzymes 243, 331
Liver failure 143, 307
Liver, metabolic disease 309

Liver trauma	319
Lobectomy	390
Locus ceruleus	172
Loneliness	285
Long-distance running	241
Longevity	183
Lonopin	336
Love	285
Low calorie diets	120
Low fat diets	277
Low serum albumin	405
Lower cholesterol	413
LSD	90, 91, 92
Lung, intrinsic lung disorders	390
Lung tumor	389, 390
Lung volume	390
Lungs	184
Lupoid hepatitis	271
Lupus	59, 187, 201, 254, 264, 270, 285, 280, 394
Lupus, systemic	259, 271
Luteinizing hormone	199
Lycopene	61
Lyme disease	31, 44, 256, 257
Lyme disease, testing for	256
Lymphocytes	405
Lymphoma	59
Lymphopenia	259
Lysine	115, 124, 280, 301, 302, 305, 401
Lysine requirement	300
Macrophage activity	403
Macula	334
Macular degeneration	234
Macular edema, chronic	333
Magnesium	4, 11, 28, 70, 79, 82, 85, 114, 141, 144
Magnesium	146, 173, 182, 216, 235, 241, 242, 243
Magnesium	247, 259, 277, 295, 312, 319, 325, 326
Magnesium	328, 336, 339, 349, 362, 364, 366, 367, 401
Magnesium deficiency	301
Magnesium Formula	319
Magnesium found to aid bypass patients	328
Magnesium orotate	328
Magnesium oxide	328
Magnesium silicate	328
Magnesium-to-calcium ratio	278
Malar or discoid rash	259
Male menopause	186, 187, 200
Male pattern baldness	350
Males and females have adrenopause	183
Mammogram	67, 340, 342, 359
Manganese	48, 60, 125, 134, 195, 197, 296, 311, 312, 319
Manganese	325, 326, 329, 330, 349, 361, 364, 394, 403
Manganese deficient farmlands	329
Mania	302, 336
Manic	309
Manic depression	195, 288, 336, 366, 367
Manic-depression	441
Manic depression, post-traumatic	287
MAO inhibitors	84
Marathon running	241
Marathons	419
Marijuana	12, 32, 90, 397
Marital instability	38
Massage	285
MAX-EPA	239, 240
Measles	319
Measles vaccine	268
Meclomen	173
Medications, symptoms and side effects of	336
Medicine	436
Medicine, conventional, and foolishness	431
Medicine, faith in	432
Medicine, holy	430
Medifast	111, 120
Meditation	285, 437
Medroxy	34
Medroxyprogesterone	347
Medroxyprogesterone acetate	347
Mega amino acid therapy	306
Megace	62, 64
Melancholia	336
Melanin	48, 314
Melanomas	311
Melatonin	4, 28, 34, 48, 69, 88, 195, 281
Melatonin	296, 313, 320, 338, 365, 370
Melatonin, a modified amino acid	194
Melatonin deficiency	195
Melatonin production	194
Mellaril	7, 87, 296, 336
Memory	184, 334, 337
Memory, aging problems	187
Memory, difficulties	11, 36, 173
Memory, improved, and concentration	321
Memory, loss	143, 187, 201, 234, 334
Memory, rejuvenation of	15
Memory, short term	173
Meningitis	258
Menopause	187, 339, 341
Menopause, depression at	339
Menopause, male	186, 187, 200
Menopause, osteoporosis in menopausal women	341
Menopause, post, women	339, 361
Menopause, prevention of hot flashes	339
Menopause, treating with hormone replacement therapy	342
Menstrual cramps	182
Menstrual disorders	350
Menstruation, painful	350
Menstruation, spotting at midcycle	347
Mental disorder	169
Mental functioning	325
Menus, additional ideas	109
Mercury	15, 280, 308, 325
Mercury, amalgams	201, 202
Mercury from fillings	330
Mercury poisoning	201, 202
Mercury poisoning, symptomatology	202
Mercury vapor test	202
Mesmer	168
Metabolism, regulation	320
Metabolites	51
Metaplasias	66
Methadone	90, 172, 314, 336
Methdilazine	7
Methionine	199, 202, 203, 216, 218
Methionine	2, 27, 34, 43, 71, 77, 124, 133, 243, 279, 280, 292
Methionine	301, 302, 311, 312, 314, 319, 320, 340, 366, 393, 397
Methionine Complex - the Arthritis Formula	320
Methionine, for arthritis, Parkinson's and depression	310
Methotrexate	3, 78, 362, 394
Methyl-sphenidate	14
MetroGel	200
Metronidazole	74
MHPG urine test for depression, method and explanation	367
Microalbuminerin	84
Microwave radiation	213
Migraine	25, 45
Migraine headaches	306, 311, 336, 339, 340, 394, 400, 437
Migraine patients	301
Milk	89, 124, 148, 198, 243
Milk allergy	7, 79
Milk, formula	312
Milk intolerance	217
Milk of magnesia	221, 328
Milk, soy and cow's	85
Millon Clinical Multiaxial Inventory	372
Millon Clinical Personality Inventory	376
Millon test	443
Millon test and heart disease	376
Mind	145

Mind dissociates when it cannot handle bad memories 369
Mind racing 173
Mineral analysis 325, 326
Mineral deficiency 325
Mineral deficiency, affects health 325
Mineral deficiency, symptoms associated with 326
Mineral levels, testing 325
Minnesota Multiphasic Personality Inventory 376
Minoxidil 77
Miotic drops 58, 334
Miscarriages 348
Miscarriages and progesterone, update on 348
Mitral stenosis with resulting lung disease 390
Mitral valve prolapse 197, 312
MMPI 443
Mold allergy 5
Molds 88
Moles 77
Molybdenum 60, 71, 134, 296, 330, 357, 358, 366
Monoamine oxidase enzyme, MAO-B inhibitor enzyme 185
Monopolar patients 366
Monosaturated fats 79
Monoterpenes 61
Mood and infection 255
Mood disorders 52, 148
Mood elevation 285
Mood foods 111
Mood stabilization 320, 321
Mood swings 11, 22, 38, 48, 148, 196, 217, 288, 320, 350
Mood swings, frequent 368
Moodiness 195, 203, 334
Morphine 312
Mother's milk 353, 356
Motion Sickness 143, 218, 220
Motor slowness 36
Motrin 3, 182, 221, 267, 311, 338
Movements, excessive 307
MRI, Magnetic Resonance Imaging 13, 22, 25, 237, 289, 292
Mucopolysaccharides 64
Multiple sclerosis . . 15, 35, 45, 143, 187, 234, 264, 270, 286, 289, 291
Multiple Sclerosis (MS), case of 286
Multivitamin and Mineral Formula 319
Mumps 270
Murmur 197
Muscle cramping 326
Muscle function 328
Muscle shortening 438
Muscle spasm, potassium deficiency can cause 242
Muscle spasms 437
Muscle spasms, painful 436
Muscle strength, ways of improving, and performance 419
Muscle strengthening and relaxation 438
Muscle tendon transfer 438
Muscle tissue 249, 402
Muscle tone 320
Muscle twitching 394
Muscle wasting 404
Muscle weakness and atrophy 419
Muscles 184
Muscles, cramps 1
Muscles, healing 167
Muscles, twitching and burning 394
Muscular degeneration 307
Muscular dystrophy 390
Muscular pain 178
Muscular tremors 202
Musculoskeletal pain 394
Mushrooms 62
Mustard oils 3
Myalgia 254
Myasthenia gravis 59, 264, 270, 271, 337, 390
Myasthenia syndrome 337
Mycoplasma 217
Myeloid leukemia 162

Myers-Briggs, how used for evaluating patient compliance 374
Myers-Briggs testing 55
Myers-Briggs Type Indicator (MBTI) 372, 373
Mylicon 216
Myocardial infarctions 240
Myopia 58
Myositis ossificans 437
Mysoline 28, 281
N-acetyl-carnitine 27
N-acetyl-cysteine 3, 58, 134, 164, 216, 219, 308, 315, 320, 333
N-acetyl-tyrosine 314
N-aceytl-transferase 194
N-acetyl-cysteine, some substances rendered less toxic by 165
Nail fungus 259
Naloxone 88
Narcissism, age of 443
Narcolepsy 26
Narcolepsy-like syndrome 292
Nardil 87, 259, 267, 291, 313, 397
National drug abuse 34
Natural estrogens 183
Nausea 143, 202, 242, 279, 282, 330, 394
Necrosis 248
Necrotic debris 68
Neoplasms 272
Nephritis 202
Nephrotic syndrome 143
Neptazane 58, 334
Nerves 184
Nerves, numbness or pain in 336
Nervous excitability 202
Nervousness 29, 90, 339
Neuro-psych test 55
Neurobiochemical imbalance 195
Neuroendocrine substances 285
Neurologic disorder (seizures or psychosis) 259
Neurological and psychometric techniques 55
Neurological disease 289
Neurological obesity 290
Neurological/somatization disorders, diary for 378
Neuromuscular disorders 390
Neuromuscular reeducation 438
Neuropathies of the feet in diabetes 395
Neuropeptide Y 246
Neuropeptides 285
Neuropsychiatric testing 13
Neuropsycho-Spiritual Development 385
Neuropsychological evaluation 54, 56, 282
Neuropsychological examination, the 372
Neuropsychological screening 55
Neuropsychological test 56
Neuropsychological testing 443
Neurotransmission in the brain 112
Neurotransmitters 50-52, 111, 168, 171, 182, 201, 285, 290
Neurotransmitters 301, 302, 311, 312, 313, 314, 316, 342, 414
Neurotransmitters, amino acids as precursors of 302
New age movement 439
Newborns, high elevation of tyrosine in blood 240
Nickel 3
Nicolar 331
Nicorette 90, 202
Nicotine 182, 296, 338, 397
Nicotine patches 202
Nicotinic acid 244
Night sweats 342
Nightshade family (potatoes, tomatoes, eggplants and peppers)393, 394
Nipples, sore 356
Nitrates 308
Nitrogen sparing 306
Noracymethadol 3
Norepinephrine 3, 171, 172, 246, 314, 316, 317, 366
Norethisterone 347
Norfloxacin 3
Norgesic 173

Norgesterol 347
Norival 321
Norpramin 84, 366
Numbness 226, 292, 369, 394
Numbness in the hands and toes 438
Nutrasweet 90, 221, 311
Nutri-Fast 120
Nutrient beatitudes 297
Nutrient diuretics 146
Nutrient formula contents 322
Nutrients, essential 298
Nutrients, essential -- conditionally essential nutrients 298
Nutrition/Malnutrition, marginal, basic causes 298
Nutritional facts and fancies 99
Nutritional, hormonal, and metabolic disorders 44
Nutritional ten commandments 428
Nutritional testing for vitamins, benefits of 332
Nuts 78, 129
Nuts and seeds 113
Oat bran 82
Obesity 84, 87, 91, 93, 112, 134, 144
Obesity 187, 193, 339, 350, 389, 390
Obesity, DHEA, treatment for obesity 189
Obesity, diet pills for 338
Obesity, gross 390
Obesity, neurological 290
Obesity, risk of 338
Obsessive adherence to rules 433
Obsessive compulsive disorder 287, 306, 320, 442
Obsessive compulsive rituals 25
Obsessive thoughts 173
Obstetrics 339
Obstructive pulmonary disease 389
Occlusive arterial disease 236
Occupational asthma 389
Octacosanol 319
Oedipus conflict 443
Oil, borage 11, 75, 76, 182, 291, 320, 349, 393, 340
Oil, canola 99
Oil, cod liver 318
Oil, corn 99
Oil, evening primrose 393
Oil, fish 75, 76, 87, 114, 120, 173, 182
Oil, fish 237, 238, 242, 246, 247, 259, 264
Oil, fish (EPA) 3, 60, 73, 77, 79, 218, 221, 311, 320, 340
Oil, fish, and sudden death 246
Oil, fish, anticoagulates the blood 247
Oil, fish, can repeat 331
Oil, fish, uses of 318
Oil, linseed 75, 321
Oil, olive 84, 99, 142, 212, 243, 280, 340
Oil, omega 3 393
Oil, peanut 76
Oil, polyunsaturated 75, 247, 318
Oil, primrose 11, 60, 73, 76, 134, 146, 218, 239, 240, 320, 393
Oil, safflower 75, 79, 99, 143, 291, 321
Oil, safflower or sunflower 247
Oil, soy bean 99
Oil, sunflower 75, 99, 143, 243
Oils and fats 113
Oils, cooking, that contain silicone additive 243
Oils, hydrogenated 247
Oils, polyunsaturated oils (safflower, sunflower) 114
Oleic acid 143
Olivopontocerebellar atrophy 319
Omexins 75
Onion 134, 237, 238, 239, 240
Onion extracts 3
Opiates 311
Opioids 12
Opium 164
Oplopanax horridum 79
Optifast 111, 120
Oral contraceptives 313, 329

Oranges 99
Orap 290
Organ transplantation 270
Organics 15, 164
Ornithine 62, 305, 315, 401, 418
Orthomolecular approach 114
Osteoarthritis 161, 270, 311, 319, 320
Osteoarthritis, nutrition and 393
Osteogenesis imperfecta 362
Osteoporosis 64, 87, 143, 144, 187, 193 241
Osteoporosis 319, 332, 326, 328, 339, 342, 361
Osteoporosis and diet 363
Osteoporosis and nutrients 362
Osteoporosis, causes of 362
Osteoporosis in menopausal women 341
Otitis 315
Otitis media 315
Otitis media ear infections 144
Out-of-body experiences 368
Ovarian activity 199
Ovarian cysts 120
Ovaries 184, 186, 187, 188
Ovary goes to sleep 187
Overeating, ... 439
Oxalate 277, 363
Oxiracetam 43
Oxy-Cholesterol in food 101
Oxygen 365
Oxygen 402
Oxylated glycine 296
Oyster shells 361
Oysters 147
Ozone 205
P300 diagnosis and testing 26, 27
P300 wave (see also BEAM) 13, 26, 33, 48, 84, 183, 320, 321
Pacemakers 168
Pain 36, 226, 336, 353
Pain and nutritional supplements 311
Pain, chronic 310, 311
Pain in the neck 283
Pain relief 302, 311
Pain tolerance, increase 417
Pain upon inhalation 390
Painkiller 311
Palms, increased lines on the 75
Palpitations 3, 336, 365, 369, 438, 439, 441
Pamelor 173
Pancreas 183, 187, 188, 219, 289, 329
Pancreatic diseases 219
Pancreatic enzymes 215
Pancreatin 57
Pancreatitis 280, 301
Pancreopause 187
Panic 295
Panic anxiety attacks 365
Panic attacks 90
Panic disorders 369
Pap smear 67, 340, 342
Pap Smears, understanding 358
PAP (prostate acid phosphatase) 398
Paralysis in one or both diaphragms 390
Paranoia 32, 36, 124, 173, 327, 425
Parasites 270, 271, 272
Parathyroid glands 292, 312
Parathyroid hormone, calcitonin 339
Parathyroid hormones 253, 261
Parenteral Nutrition 406
Parkinson's disease 13, 15, 22, 25-27, 43, 45, 48
Parkinson's disease 144, 185, 188, 292, 311-315, 319
Parkinson's disease is a result of dopamine def... 337
Parlodel 34, 259, 267, 271, 280, 291, 292
PATH Medical weight loss program 88
Pavlov's dogs 285
Paxil 84

PCP (phencyclidine) 14
Peace, some signs of inner 433
Peace through love of God and neighbor 429
Peanut butter 76
Pears 99
Pectin fruits (apples, bananas) 247
Pellagra 92, 144, 313
Pelvic irradiation 271
Pelvic pain 350
Pelvis stress fractures 241
Penicillamine 305
Peptic ulcer disease 93, 336
Peptic ulcers 223, 437
Peracitin 309
Pergamol 397
Pergolide 292
Periactin 173
Perimenopause 342
Periodontal disease 71, 320
Perioperative malnutrition 401
Perioperative nutrition 406
Peripheral neuropathy 336
Peritoneal adhesions 403
Peritonitis 404
Pernicious anemia 45, 77
Persantine 239
Personality 184
Personality, a new science of 372
Personality, antisocial disorder 381
Personality, avoidant disorder 383
Personality, borderline disorder 382
Personality, clues to basic 372
Personality, dependent disorder 383
Personality, disorders 22, 380
Personality, disorders, references regarding 384
Personality, histrionic disorder 382
Personality, multiple, disorder 384
Personality, narcissistic disorder 383
Personality, new tests 372
Personality, obsessive compulsive disorder 384
Personality, paranoid disorder 380
Personality, schizotypal disorder 380
Personality testing 55
Personality type 55
Pesticides 15, 185, 308
PET, Positron Emission Tomography, scanning 68, 225, 247, 279, 359
PET scanning at PATH 247
PET scanning, pre-PET scan instructions 248
PET scanning, whole body 68, 248
Peyronie disease 397
PH changes 253
Phagocytosis 261
Pharmaceutical purchases 200
Pharmacist, your, and this office 335
Phencyclidine 14
Phenelzine 259
Phenobarbital 28, 281, 367
Phenol 73
Phenolic acids 61
Phenothiazines 7, 8
Phenylalanine 3, 14, 43, 48, 13, 195, 199, 202, 255, 271
Phenylalanine 280, 292, 301, 305, 314, 316, 319, 366, 397
Phenylalanine, fatigue and pain relief 311
Phenylalanine is an antidepressant 311
Phenylketonurics 311
Phenytoin 28
Phlebitis 226, 239, 240, 339
Phoschol 337
Phosphate 407
Phosphatidyl choline 337
Phosphetamin 259
Phospholine 310
Phosphorous 401
Phosphoserine 27

Photosensitivity 146, 259, 312
Phytates 124, 363
Pick's disease 45
Picolinic acid 313
Pigmentary glaucoma 334
Pilocarpine 58, 334
Pilonidal cysts 403
Pineal gland 48, 194
Piperidines 8
Pituitary gland 184
Placebo mechanism 285
Placentas 75
Plant sterols 62
Plants 48, 195, 208
Plaque forming LDL's 339
Plaquenil 292
Plasma albumin 402
Plastics 308
Platelet aggregation 239, 240
Platelet clotting factor 313
Platelet elements of blood 59
Platelets 239, 240
Plethysmography 229
Pleural effusions 389, 390
Pleural fibrosis or tumor 390
Pleurisy 390
Pleurisy, rib fractures or incisions 390
PMS 48, 195, 287, 319, 328, 320, 336, 349, 350, 441
PMS and BEAM 349
PMS, current research into 349
PMS, hot flashes 342
PMS-like symptoms 340
PMS, perimenstrual tension 349
PMS, progesterone, natural, using for 350, 351
PMS, syndrome 311, 394
PMS, tension 328
PMS, what can be done about it? 351
PMS, what causes it? 351
PMS, what it is not 351
Pneumococcal bacteremia 258
Pneumococcal disease 258
Pneumococcal meningitis 258
Pneumococcal pneumonia 258
Pneumococcal polysaccharide vaccine 258
Pneumoconiosis 390
Pneumonectomy or lobectomy 390
Pneumonia 3, 202, 389, 390
Pneumonia shots 254
Pneumothorax 390
Poliomyelitis 390
Pollen counts 2
Pollen, ragweed 2
Pollens 2, 7
Pollutants, indoor, sources 205
Polyamines 62
Polycythemia 60
Polycythemia vera 393
Polynuclear leukocytes 403
Polyp 146
Pondimin 48, 92, 290
Porphyria 44
Porphyrins 335
Post-endarterectomy follow-up 226
Post-exercise test 232
Post-traumatic stress disorder 287
Postmenopausal 143
Postmyocardial infarction 312
Postnatal blues 344
Postnatal psychosis 344
Postoperative morbidity 404
Postoperative recovery 161
Postphlebitic ulcers 226
Postsurgical patient 403
Postsurgical tracheal stenosis 390

Potassium 79, 114, 144, 242, 259, 312, 319
Potassium citrate 277, 278
Potassium deficiency can cause muscle spasm 242
Potassium, importance of 417
Potassium iodide 57, 203
Poultry 212
Poverty 299
Prayer 3, 285, 437
Prealbumin 404
Prednisone 59, 183, 198, 339, 394
Pregnancy 59, 301, 305, 310, 311, 319, 328, 353, 390
Pregnancy/cholesterol 245
Pregnancy, difficult 328
Pregnancy, ectopic 340
Pregnancy, hypertension of 328
Pregnancy, nausea of 218
Pregnancy, nutrition and 355
Pregnancy, substance abuse and 355, 356
Pregnancy, utilization by pregnancy trimester markers 354
Pregnant women 226
Premarin 197
Premature infants 312
Premenopausal women 199
Premenstrual tension 146
Preventricular arrhythmias 312
Primrose 243
Prison population 26
Probenecid 393
Procardia 336
Products for Achieving Total Health (PATH) 319
Progesterone 27, 34, 78, 146, 148, 184
Progesterone 187, 189, 191, 199, 340, 349
Progesterone administration 345
Progesterone and miscarriages, update on 348
Progesterone and PMS 350
Progesterone, conception on 348
Progesterone course, timing of 346
Progesterone differs from progestogens 347
Progesterone dosage 346
Progesterone, drug interactions with 346
Progesterone effects 348
Progesterone enhances lactation 344
Progesterone/estradiol/testosterone 191
Progesterone for postpartum (postnatal) depression 344
Progesterone, natural and synthetic 343
Progesterone, natural, new ideas 345
Progesterone, natural, side effects? 343
Progesterone, natural, using for premenstrual syndrome 351
Progesterone needs to be taken along with estrogen 339
Progesterone, oral, most asked questions about 343
Progesterone, oral, why? 345
Progesterone, overdose of 347
Progesterone, prophylactic, for postnatal depression 345
Progesterone, side effects of therapy 347
Progesterone therapy, principles of 344
Progesterones, natural 183
Progestogens, synthetic 347
Prolactin 271
Proline 302, 315, 401
Prolixin 7, 34
Prolonged immobilization 437
Promethazine 7
Proscar 398
Prostaglandin E2 239
Prostaglandin inhibitors 350
Prostaglandins 1 and 3 239
Prostate 147, 289
Prostate, benign prostatic hypotrophy 398
Prostate, enlarged 329, 339
Prostate problems 186, 341, 398
Prostate, PSA (prostatic specific antigen) 270, 398
Prostigmin 337
Protein 298, 363
Protein and amino acid balance 401

Protein powders, commercially available 300
Protein, skeletal 404
Protozoal infections 44
Proventil 3
Provera 340
Proverbs and healthy emotions 425
Prozac 4, 34, 80, 84, 85, 87, 92, 173, 202
Prozac 267, 271, 336, 349, 350, 366, 394
Pruritus 128, 147
Pseudodementia 196
Pseudogout 147
Psoriasis 62, 76, 77, 78, 148, 150, 187, 308
Psychiatric Diagnostic Lab of America 198
Psychiatric disorders 337
Psychiatric disorders, five symptoms of 376
Psychiatric problems 198
Psychiatry and the doctor-patient relationship 46
Psychodiagnostic examination, the 373
Psychological and spiritual factors 90
Psychological disorders 12, 36, 53
Psychological stress 394
Psychological tests, computerized 376
Psychological therapy 365
Psychology, and death 426
Psychology, stages of dying 426
Psychometric testing 372
Psychometrics 443
Psychoneuroimmunology 285
Psychosexual disorder 369
Psychosis 90, 201, 285, 288, 296, 308, 309, 328, 349
Psychosis, and antipsychotic drugs 25, 321, 336
Psychosis, organic etiology of symptoms 369
Psychotherapy 85, 202, 285, 372
Psychotic patients 301
Puberty 339
Pulmonary disease 197
Pulmonary disorders 389
Pulmonary embolism, high risk for 226
Purines 393
Putrescine 62, 253, 261
Pyroluric 125
Qualudes 90
Quercetin 2, 143, 203, 320, 337
Quinine 242, 296
Quinine toxicity 296
Radiated foods makes certain toxic amino acids 213
Radiation 203, 308
Radiation exposure 77
Radiation-induced fibrosis 390
Radioactive barium 203
Radioactive cesium 203
Radioactive iodides 203
Radioactive strontium 203
Radiotherapy 402
Radon 205
Ragweed pollen 2
Raisins 84
Rare arrhythmia such as torsade de points 328
Rare deficiency syndromes 409
Rare diseases information 260
Rash 203, 220, 307
Rash, generalized urticarial 347
Rashes 189
Ratios of T-helper to T-suppressor ratios in various diseases . . . 271
Rauh Ha Kodesh 445
Raynaud's syndrome 226, 331
Raynaud's syndrome 437, 441
Reactive hyperemia test 232
Recipe, Beef Stroganoff 157
Recipe, Better Butter 152
Recipe, Better Butter Spreads 114
Recipe, Brand New High Protein Breakfast 159
Recipe, Chinese Steamed Fish With Cashews 153
Recipe, Fresh-Start Tomato Juice 114, 151

Recipe, Frozen Fruit Juice 89
Recipe, Have-it-your-way Fillet Souffle 154
Recipe, Healthy Heart Spread 156
Recipe, Hypertension Shake 156
Recipe, Jicama-chili Pepper Relish 155
Recipe, Oatbars 158
Recipe, Pizza 158
Recipe, Pumpkin Cake 159
Recipe, Tangy Cucumber Dressing 152
Recipe, Tuna Kabobs 153
Recipe, Two-step, Two-herb Pesto 154
Recipe, Two-way Total Health Salad 156
Rectal bleeding 350
Rectal fissure 128, 147
Rectal pain 350
Red meat 243
Red pepper extract 85
Reduce anxiety 439
Reglan 173
Regrets 173
Relationships Between Biofeedback and Religious Terminology . 435
Relaxation techniques 285
Religion, materialistic 426
Religious Addiction 433
Religious views of death 426
REM (Rapid Eye Movement) 34
Renal and hepatic disorders 43
Renal dialysis 279
Renal failure patients 277, 280
Respiratory failure 3, 147
Respiratory infections 198
Retardation, mental 307, 313
Retardation, mental and physical 309
Retin-A 66, 73, 75, 76, 78
Retinal detachment 329
Retinitis pigmentitis 312
Retinitis pigmentosa 58, 312, 333
Retinoic acid 402
Retinoids 62
Retinol binding protein 404
Retinylacetate 402
Reverse transcriptase 403
Reye's syndrome 309, 329
Rheumatoid and osteoarthritis 270
Rheumatoid arthritic patients 339
Rheumatoid arthritis 255, 271, 309, 336, 358, 394
Rheumatological disorders 393
Rhinitis 220
Rhinitis, atopic 75
Rhinitis, seasonal allergic 2
Rib fractures 390
Ringworm 431
Riopan 221
Risk for injury 98
Ritalin 38, 69, 87, 254, 283
Rosacea 200
Rubidium 320
Runner's high 241
S-adenosylmethionine 310, 311, 320
Safe sex and family planning 399
Salad dressings 80
Salad dressings, dietary information for 97
Salad vegetables 113
Salads 247
Salicylates 87
Sallow skin 215
Salt 114, 280, 296
Sarcoidosis 59, 390
Sasparilla 148
Saturated fats 90, 126
Saw palmetto herb 398
Schizo-affective disorder 287
Schizophrenia, see also Psychosis
Schizophrenia 12, 13, 15, 22, 26, 28, 32, 37, 52

Schizophrenia 90, 92, 147, 170, 183, 255, 281, 287, 301
Schizophrenia 309, 310, 313, 321, 329, 368, 380, 393, 400
Scleroderma 59
Sclerosis 308
Sclerotic hardening 234
Scopolamine 218
Scripture, key chapters of 425
Scriptures on Abortion 434
Scurvy 92, 305, 403
Scurvy, subclinical 403
Seasonal Affective Disorder (SAD) 370
Sedentary people 241
Seeds 124
Seizures 14, 25, 40, 308, 328, 329, 336, 339, 349
Seizures, children's 282
Seizures, estrogen may increase 14
Seizures, kinds of 295
Seizures, nutritional control 295
Seldane 259
Selenium 3, 11, 60, 76, 77, 79, 134, 164, 202
Selenium 215, 237, 240, 243, 247, 255, 264, 270, 308
Selenium 319, 325, 326, 330, 331, 349, 401, 403, 408
Selenium sulfite 78
Self-esteem 414
Self-esteem, inflated 366
Self-esteem, poor 36
Senile dementia 15
Senility 62, 234
Sense of smell 184
Sensitivity, overly 375
Sensory oriented 372
Sepsis 307, 401, 415
Sergelide 292
Serine 301, 315
Serositis (pleuritis, pericarditis) 259
Serotonin 12, 50, 84, 100, 194, 201, 253, 261, 302
Serotonin 308, 313, 316, 317, 350, 365, 366, 367, 394, 417
Sex 12, 147, 355, 397
Sex, aphrodisiac. 314
Sex, as a mood healer 355
Sex, barometer of brain health and brain 397
Sex, condoms do not insure safe sex 399
Sex drive 147, 241, 314, 397
Sex drive, basic rules of 398
Sex drive, in women 339
Sex drive, increasing 339, 397
Sex drive, low 314
Sex drive, sexual brain health and increasing the 397
Sex hormone levels 245
Sex hormones 339
Sex hormones and cholesterol 245
Sex, infertility and impotence 397
Sex, libido, decreased 342
Sex life, improved 183
Sex, male's sex life is usually absent after eighty 339
Sex, painful intercourse 350
Sex, safe 399
Sex steroids 199
Sex, stimulating 147
Sexual difficulties 36, 173
Sexual dysfunction 233
Sexual function, decreased 187
Sexual hormone functioning 187
Sexual libido 339, 340
Shaking 365
Shampoos 338
Shark cartilage 64
Shell fish 3, 78
Shopping list, healthy choice 160
Short bowel syndrome. 404
Shoulder, frozen 437
Shoulder pain 350
Sickle cell disease 329
Seizure, antiseizure drugs 336

Sight 184
Sigmoidoscopy 328
Silicon 364
Silver 308
Sinus Histiocytosis X 271
Sinusitis 3
Sishium Jampos 84
Sjogren's syndrome 148
Skin 184
Skin color, change of 226
Skin diseases 301, 329
Skin, disorders 441
Skin problems 73, 76
Skin sensitivities 394
Sleep 11, 148, 320, 328
Sleep apnea syndrome 34, 390
Sleep disorders 3, 98, 195, 308, 312, 320, 441
Sleep EEG 394
Sleep hormone 194
Sleep, need more than usual 370
Sleep, trouble falling asleep 334
Sleepiness 282
Sleeping better 296
Sleeping rhythms 320
Sleepwalking 368
Slim-Fast 120
Smell and taste, loss of 329
Smoker's hack, preventing 308
Smokers 337
Smoking 3, 216, 221, 296, 333, 356, 439
Smoking, techniques for stopping 202
Sneezing 205
Social difficulties 36
Sodium 221, 312, 364
Sodium citrate 234
Sodium fluoride 296
Sodium, role of 417
Sodium selenite 330
Sodium valproate 291
Soft drinks 349
Solitude, preference for 29
Somatic conditions 36, 283
Sorbet 100
Soy milk 196
SPECT scan 225
Speech disorders 202
Sperm 310
Sperm function 397
Spermidine 62
Spermidine (a cancer maker) 310
Spermine 62, 253, 261
Spices 130
Spicy foods 221
Spinal deformity/kyphosis/scoliosis 390
Spinal muscle atrophy 307
Spiritual awareness 145
Spiritual Behavior Inventory, Abridged 423
Spiritual distress diagnosis 425
Spirituality 423
Spirometry, benefits of 389
Spirometry or PFT 389
Splenectomy 59
Sponge 399
Sporonox, for nail fungus 259
Sports and Exercise 413
Spotting in the premenstrum 347
Spring and mineral waters 113, 131
Sprouted grains 124
Starvation 307
Stature, short 7
Stelazine 87
Steroid, anabolic 403, 415
Steroid therapy 78
Steroid therapy, natural 184

Steroid treatment 291
Steroids   14, 66, 75, 183, 187, 198, 199, 254, 259, 285, 330, 333, 393
Stomach, "butterflies" in 283
Stomach flu 330
Stomach trouble 173
Stomach, upset 1, 282
Stomatitis 270
Stone formation 143
Stones, oxalate 278
Stool abnormalities 221
Strep faecium 216
Streptococcus pneumoniae 258
Stress 1, 84, 145, 171, 216, 221, 305, 314, 338, 393, 436
Stress, and neurotransmitters 317
Stress hormone cortisol 184
Stress intolerance 38
Stress regulation 264
Stress related withdrawal syndrome 167
Stress states 307
Stress thallium testing 247
Stroke 80, 200, 225, 226, 237, 240, 247, 292, 359
Stroke, prevention 238, 240
Stroke, small 237
Stroke, symptoms of 237
Stroke, T.I.A.'s (small reversible strokes), geriatric patients 226
Stroke, victims of 226
Strontium 71, 203, 319
Strychnine 431
Stuffy nose 203
Subclavian steal syndrome 226
Sudden death 246
Sugar 78, 92, 92, 127, 131, 241, 243, 338, 365, 367
Sugar, addiction 90
Sugar, content in certain manufactured foods 83
Sugar, cravings 100, 148
Sugar, glycemic index of foods 80
Sugar metabolism 329
Sugarholism 148
Suicidal patients 313
Suicide 202
Sulfites 3
Sulfonamide 259
Sulfur 326, 330
Sulfur amino acids 305
Sunflower seeds 212
Superego 444
Superior limbic keratoconjunctivitis 58, 333
Supernatural experiences 368
Superoxide dismutase 403
Support groups, listing 379
Surgery 305, 307, 328, 401, 415
Surgery, colorectal 404
Surgery, correlating nutritional status with outcome 404
Surgery, recovery from 305
Surgical patients 403
Swallowing, difficult 328
Swallowing, trouble 291, 292
Sweating 220, 365
Sweating, feeling faint, trembling or 365
Sweaty hands or cold hands 438
Sweet bay 83
Swimming 241
Swimming, in chlorine 204
Symmetrel 291, 292
Synapse 171
Synarel 357
Syzygium Jambos 79
T-cell functions, abnormal 285
T-cell or immune system ratios and health 267
T-cell ratios 267
T-cell Ratios: Modulation by Nutrition: Case Report 273
T-cell tests 254
T-cells 254, 270
T-helper cell function 274

T-helper cell counts 271
T-helper cells 264, 267
T-helper immune system 255
T-helper/T-suppressor ratio 264, 270, 272, 291
T-suppressor cells 264, 267, 271
T.I.A.'s (small reversible strokes), geriatric patients 226
Tachycardia 404
Tagamet 216, 221, 254, 270
Talkative 366
Tamoxifen 62
Tamoxifen and megace: hormonal manipulation 64
Tardive dyskinesia 319, 337
Tardive dyslexia 307
Tartrazine 259
Tasks, inability to complete 38
Taste and smell, loss of 329
Taste and smell, bad sense of 353
Taurine 11, 48, 58, 77, 114, 195, 215, 295, 301, 302, 319, 340
Taurine, anticonvulsant and antianxiety 312
Taurine for high blood pressure, seizures and depression 312
Taxol 62, 64
TB vaccinations 254
Tea 87, 216, 221, 243, 296, 349
Tegretol ... 11, 28, 34, 173, 242, 281, 282, 288, 296, 336, 366, 367
Tegretol protocol 288
Tegretol protocol, revised 288
Telangiectasia 262
Temper, explosive 38
Temper, tantrums 36
Temporal lobe abnormalities 22, 40, 281, 288
Temporal lobe disorder 194, 336
Temporal lobe epilepsy 441
Temporal-Mandibular Joint Dysfunction (TMJ) 71, 178, 394
Tenderness 350
Tenderness around the kidneys 350
TENS 311
TENS unit (Transcutaneous Electric Nerve Stimulation 161, 168
                                                  178, 182
Tenuate 48, 92, 290
Terfenadine 259
Testicles 187, 188
Testosterone 59, 184, 186, 187, 191, 199, 398
Testosterone, coronary artery disease, correlation of low 186
Testosterone, estrogens and progesterones, natural 364
Testosterone excess 339
Testosterone levels 14
Testosterone, natural 184
Tetracycline 73, 74, 394
Tetracycline-like effect 320
Thalamus 33
Thalidomide 431
THC (tetrahydrocannabinol) 14
Theobromine 32
Theophylline 3, 308
Theta activity 49
Theta wave 437
Thiazides 393
Thinking difficulties 36
Thoracic outlet syndrome 226
Thoracoplasty 390
Thorax 277
Thorazine 173
Thoughts and emotions 284
Thoughts, bad 285
Three Paths to Healing Model 430
Threonine 124, 301, 302, 304, 305, 309, 315
Throbbing 394
Thrombocytopenia 259
Thromboembolic disease 339
Thromboembophlebitis 407
Thrombophlebitis 226, 342
Thrombosis 149, 236, 247
Thymidine 267
Thymus 184

Thymus cells 267
Thymus extracts 254
Thymus function 253
Thymus gland 185
Thymus hormone and T-cell life 267
Thymus injections 270
Thymus pause 267
Thyroid 187, 188, 196, 254, 314, 349
Thyroid, and estrogen deficiency 77
Thyroid, Armour 184
Thyroid, cabbage and beans, antithyroid 124
Thyroid, conditions 198
Thyroid, deficiency 69
Thyroid disease 431
Thyroid, disease. 85, 333
Thyroid, function 197
Thyroid, hormone, low 187
Thyroid, hormones 253, 261
Thyroid, hormones and iodine 197
Thyroid, hypothyroidism 394
Thyroid, masses obstructing the trachea 390
Thyroid, problems 2, 31
Thyroid, stimulation test 196
Thyroid, stress test or TRH screen 197
Thyroid, T3 and T4 187
Thyroid, therapies, natural 183
Thyroiditis 59
Tibial fractures 241
Tic douloureux 149
Tics 290
Timoptic 58, 334
Tin 308
Tingling hands and feet 365
Tingling sensation 394, 283
Tinnitus 242, 296
Tinnitus 441
Tobacco (also a nightshade) 394
Tofranil 38, 365
Tofranil protocol 185
Tolerogens 261
Tonsillectomy 253
Tooth decay 148
Tourette's syndrome 149, 290, 337
TOVA tests 55
Toxemia 319
Toxic chemicals 319
Toxic epidermal necrolysis 271
Toxic exposures 13
Toxic heavy metals 325, 326
Toxic metal accumulation 320, 325
Toxic metals 164, 201, 235
Toxicity, N-acetyl-cysteine, some substances rendered less toxic by 165
Toxins (e.g., lead, cadmium, aluminum) 196
Toxoplasma virus 270
TPN solution 238
Trace element study, your 330
Trace elements 280, 325
Trace metals 349
Trace metals and clotting 239
Trancelike states 368
Tranquilizers 296
Transference 442
Transferrin 404
Transient ischemic attacks (T.I.A.'s) 226
Trauma 307, 328, 401, 406, 415, 418
Trauma, emotional, damages the immune system 37
Traumatic experiences 53
Trembling 283, 365
Tremor 173, 309, 328
Tremor, factors increasing physiological 35
Tremor, movement 292
Tremors, classification of common 35
Trexan 182
Triavil 173

Trichloracetic acid	73
Trichomonas	279
Trigeminal	149
Triglyceride levels	239
Triglycerides	114, 148, 149, 241, 320, 321, 359
Triglycerides, high, and high cholesterol	243
Slim-Fast	120
Trimeprazine tartrate	7
Trophic nails	228
Tryglicerides, lowered triglycerides	196
Trypsin	124
Tryptophan	11, 14, 32, 43, 48, 69, 80, 85, 87
Tryptophan	90, 100, 124, 147, 148, 194, 195, 199
Tryptophan	254, 271, 280, 292, 296, 301, 302, 304
Tryptophan	306, 308, 313, 316, 331, 365, 394, 418
Tryptophan foods	111
Tryptophan, sleep and antiaggression nutrient	313
Tuberculosis	3, 271, 390
Tugor, poor turgor (normal rigidity)	215
Tumors	45, 248
Tumors, noncancerous	120
Tums	216, 221
Twelve-step program	90
Twenty-four hour blood pressure monitor	251, 252
Tylenol	87
Tylenol (may affect the hemoglobin of baby)	353
Type A (overachiever) personalities	221, 247
Tyramine	116
Tyrosine	3, 14, 27, 34, 43, 48, 69, 70, 79, 84, 133, 195
Tyrosine	197, 199, 202, 240, 246, 271, 292, 301, 305, 306
Tyrosine	311, 314, 316, 319, 320, 321, 331, 365, 366, 397
Tyrosine, antifatigue adrenalin builder	314
Tyrosine foods	111
Tyrosine, newborns, high elevation of tyrosine in blood	240
Ulcer, benign chronic peptic	404
Ulcerative colitis	218
Ulcers	198, 221, 439
Ulcers, conventional treatment	221
Ulcers, healing	273
Ulcers, ischemic	226
Ulcers, non-healing	226
Ulcers, topical zinc heals ulcers	240
Ultra Fuel	321
Ultrabright light systems	335
Unconscious, involuntary processes	438
Unconscious mind	369
Unhappiness	90
Unreality	15, 25
Unstable hypertension	342
Uric acid	278
Uric acid crystals	393
Uric acid, elevated, and gout	393
Uric Acid, elevated	393
Urinary difficulty	292
Urinary methylmalonic acid, to detect B-12	333
Urinary tract infections	320
Urinate, urge to, when the bladder is not full	279
Urination, difficulty in	279
Urination, frequent	438
Urination, increased	291
Urination, urgency to urinate	350
Urine, blood in	279, 350
Urine, burning	350
Urine, maple syrup urine disease	307
Urine sample, some guidelines for selecting a specimen	327
Urticaria vasculitis	7
Uterus	199
Vaccination, TB	254
Vaccinations	254, 255, 258
Vaccines	268, 353
Vaccine, hepatitis and measles vaccine	268
Vaccine, influenza	331
Vaccine, pneumococcal polysaccharide	258
Vaccine, polio	268
Vaccine, who should receive pneumococcal polysaccharide vaccine	258
Vaccines, medicines and religion	432
Vaccines, pertussis and rubella	268
Vagina, dry	342
Vaginal deodorants, avoid	279
Vaginal dryness	342
Vaginal foam	399
Vaginal infections	150
Valine	301, 302, 307
Valium	11, 12, 87, 171, 173, 199, 255, 280, 321
Valproate	282, 282
Valproic acid	296
Valvular incompetency	226
Vanadium	71, 320, 366
Vanilla extract	212
Varicose veins	93, 225
Varicosities	226
Vascular and venous blood testing	228
Vascular patient history	228
Vascular testing, indications for non-invasive	227
Vasculogenic impotence	226
Vasodilan	242
Vasotec	84
Vegetables	78
Vegetarian amenorrheic women	199
Vegetarianism, Dr. Fuhrman's Strict Vegetarian Diet	126
Vegetarianism, hair loss due to vegetarianism	77
Vegetarianism, lacto-ovo-	124
Vegetarianism, problem of	124, 125
Vegetarianism, vitamin B-6 and zinc deficiency and	124
Vein thrombosis	226
Veins, distended	340
Venous insufficiency	226
Venous phlebitis	225
Venous reflux test	230
Ventricular fibrillation	246, 314
Verapamil	25, 48, 247
Verses of Peace and Healing	429
Vertigo	228, 291, 292
Violent behavior	287
Viral	254
Viral illness, intermittent	273
Viral illnesses	254
Virus infection	271
Vision, impaired	234
Vistaril	173
Visual Evoked Responses	22
Visual loss	292
Visual-spatial disorder	291
Vitamin	318, 338, 363
Vitamin A	60, 73, 75, 77, 87, 246, 259, 274, 312, 318, 319, 331, 402
Vitamin A and D	78
Vitamin A Complex - the Antiviral Formula	319
Vitamin A drops	58
Vitamin B-1	92, 235
Vitamin B-12 deficiencies can imitate MS	291
Vitamin B-12 shots	149, 292, 255
Vitamin B-12	43, 62, 124, 134, 235, 253, 331
Vitamin B-12 deficiency	333
Vitamin B-6	3, 11, 28, 60, 69, 70, 79, 85, 114, 125, 134, 143, 146
Vitamin B-6	182, 218, 234, 235, 241, 247, 277, 278, 280, 281, 295
Vitamin B-6	296, 310, 311, 312, 313, 319, 328, 331, 349, 394, 416
Vitamin B-6 and magnesium deficiencies	278
Vitamin B-6 and zinc deficiency and vegetarianism	124
Vitamin B-6 deficiency	77
Vitamin B-complex	28, 34, 238, 264, 281, 338
Vitamin B-complex, benefits	416
Vitamin B-vitamins	311
Vitamin B-vitamins	11, 84, 100, 296, 311
Vitamin biotin	307
Vitamin C	2, 3, 4, 7, 57, 60, 62, 71, 76, 85, 92, 134, 143
Vitamin C	203, 216, 235, 237, 238, 240, 241, 243, 246, 247, 255
Vitamin C	279, 291, 296, 311, 314, 315, 319, 337, 366, 393, 394
Vitamin C Complex - the Allergy (Antihistamine) Formula	320

Vitamin C deficiency, ... 301, 333
Vitamin C promotes the absorption of all iron in both food 357
Vitamin C and wounds 403
Vitamin D 278, 280, 328, 361, 363
Vitamin D-3 270
Vitamin D and C 75
Vitamin D-deficiency rickets 124
Vitamin D deficiency 301
Vitamin D supplements. 339
Vitamin E 4, 58, 60, 62, 76, 85, 87, 111, 134, 202, 221
Vitamin E 237-240, 242, 243, 255, 259, 264, 270, 280
Vitamin E 319, 320, 339, 340, 397, 403
Vitamin E, anticlotting ability 239
Vitamin E, dry 76
Vitamin E, inhibits platelet aggregation 239
Vitamin E therapy 397
Vitamin Ester-C 337
Vitamin folate 331
Vitamin, folic acid deficiency 60
Vitamin, folic acid 60, 62, 134, 142, 219, 240
Vitamin, folic acid 246, 310, 314, 353, 362, 366
Vitamin, folic acid (protects against birth defects) 353
Vitamin, inositol 11, 28, 79, 100
Vitamin K, deficiency 240
Vitamin multivitamin, Path Save is a 320
Vitamin niacin 11, 69, 73, 79, 92, 147, 242, 243, 247, 288
Vitamin niacin . . . 296, 311, 313, 321, 331, 340, 365, 393, 394, 397
Vitamin niacin, lowering triglycerides (type 4) 243
Vitamin niacin, reduces cholesterol 247
Vitamin niacin therapy 331
Vitamin niacin, wonders of 332
Vitamin niacinamide 34, 69, 79, 84, 296, 319, 331, 393, 394
Vitamin nicotinic acid 84
Vitamin pantetheine 243, 320
Vitamin pantothenic acid 243, 296, 312, 394
Vitamin riboflavin 60, 134, 241, 253, 261, 331
Vitamin Stress Formula. 319
Vitamin testing 332
Vitamin thiamin, riboflavin , ... 331
Vitamin thiamine 27, 79, 135, 331, 366
Vitamin thiamine deficiency 403
Vitamin topical vitamin A 403
Vitamins 60, 87, 124, 135
Vitamins, boost the immune system 331
Vitamins, minerals and wound healing 402
Vitamins, taking your 331
Vivactil 34
VLDL's 101
Vomiting 279, 282, 291, 307, 330, 350
Von Gierke's disease 393
Walking, gait difficulty 292
Walking, how much? 242
Walking is an exceptionally good form of exercise 241
Water 402
Water, chlorinated 204
Water, hard 247
Water, soft water 247
Water supply 203
Weakness 292
Weight control, brain, area of battle for 87
Weight, excessive, or fluid retention 349
Weight gain 340
Weight lifters 307
Weight loss 312, 336
Weight loss, PATH Medical program 88
Weight loss, some new ideas 100
Weight loss, The Fast Path to Weight Loss 88
Weight, overweight patients 226
Wellbutrin. 4, 34, 69, 80, 87, 92, 173, 259
Wellbutrin 267, 280, 291, 349, 365, 366, 394, 397
Wheezing 3, 205
Whiplash 22, 438
Whiplash and head trauma 37
White flour 92

White potatoes 99
Whole body PET scan 248
Wilson's disease (high copper) 301, 329
Wilson's disease, hepatolenticular degeneration 44
Withdrawal symptoms 1
Withdrawal syndromes 44
Woman, large-breasted 339
Women and heart disease 359
Women, immature nulliparous 347
Women who smoke 400
Women's health 339
Wood stoves and fireplaces 205
Worry 365
Wound contraction 403
Wound healing 328
Wound healing, nutrients which may affect 401
Wound healing, poor 328
Wound healing, retarded 329
Wound healing, vitamins, minerals and 402
Wound infections 404
Wrinkles 76
X-ray treatments 431
Xanax 11, 12, 173, 202, 296
Yeast 88, 150, 211, 217
Yeast infection 89
Yocon (yohimbine chloride), Yohimex 397
Yogurt 3
Zantac 216, 221
Zinc 11, 60, 62, 70, 75, 76, 77, 78, 79, 82, 87, 92, 100
Zinc 114, 124, 125, 134, 135, 164, 201, 202, 215 219, 221
Zinc 239, 241, 243, 247, 253-255, 264, 267, 270, 280, 296
Zinc 308, 311-313, 319, 320, 325, 326, 329, 330, 331, 338
Zinc . . 349, 340, 353, 357, 366, 393, 394, 397, 398, 400, 403, 408
Zinc and selenium deficiencies 84
Zinc Complex - the Trace Metal Formula 320
Zinc deficiency 77, 305
Zinc in combination with erythromycin 76
Zinc lozenges 255
Zinc oxide 78
Zinc, topical zinc heals ulcers 240
Zoloft 394
Zostrix 395
Zyderm 73